Pharmaceutical Particulate Matter

Analysis and Control

Interpharm Press Editorial Advisory Board

Chairman: Michael J. Groves
Institute for Tuberculosis Research, USA

Michael Akers
Eli Lilly & Company, USA

Andrew Balo
Baxter Healthcare, USA

Per O. Bremer
Institutt for Energiteknikk, Norway

Samuella Emrich
Northgate Research, USA

Roland Jeppsson
KabiVitrum, Sweden

Jean Lanet
Technique d'Aide Aux Affairs, France

Frank Leo
Automated Liquid Packaging, USA

Theodore H. Meltzer
Capitola Consulting, USA

Wayne Olson
Armour, USA

Rodney Pearlman
Genentech, USA

Michael Rubenstein
The Liverpool Polytechnic, UK

Dean Snyder
DeanCo Ltd., USA

Pharmaceutical Particulate Matter

Analysis and Control

Thomas A. Barber
Baxter Healthcare

Illustrations by John G. Williams
Photomicrography Section by Damian S. Neuberger

Interpharm Press
Buffalo Grove, IL

NEW BOOK CONCEPTS

Interpharm Press specializes in publishing books related to applied technology and regulatory affairs impacting the biotechnology, chemical, cosmetic, device, diagnostic or drug manufacturing industries. If you have a manuscript in progress, or are planning to write a book that will be applicable to development, medical, regulatory, manufacturing, quality or engineering professionals, please contact our editorial director.

SOCIAL RESPONSIBILITY PROGRAMS

Interpharm Resources Replenishment Program

Interpharm Press is significantly concerned with the worldwide loss of trees, and the impact of such loss on the environment and the availability of new drug sources. Losses to tropical rain forests are particularly remarkable in that only 3% of all possible endangered plant species have been evaluated for their active drug potential.

Interpharm Press commits to replant trees sufficient to replace those destroyed in meeting the paper needs for Interpharm's publications and advertising. Interpharm is actively supporting reforestation programs in Bangladesh, Israel, Kenya and the United States.

Pharmakos-2000

To foster the teaching of pharmaceutical technology, Interpharm Press has initiated its Pharmakos-2000 program. Under this program, one copy of this book is being sent, at no charge, to every College and School of Pharmacy worldwide. The program covers all 504 establishments listed by the Commonwealth Pharmaceutical Association (CPA) and the Federation Internationale Pharmaceutique (FIP).

It is hoped that this book will be a suitable reference resource to faculty and students advancing the theory and practice of pharmaceutical technology.

10 9 8 7 6 5 4 3 2 1

ISBN: 0-935184-29-5
Copyright © 1993 by Interpharm Press, Inc. All rights reserved.

All rights reserved. This book is protected by copyright. No part of it may be reproduced, stored in a retrieval system, or transmitted in any form or by any means, electronic, mechanical, photocopying, recording, or otherwise, without written permission from the publisher. Interpharm Press actively prosecutes infringers of its copyrights in the courts, and pays a reward for information and evidence regarding cases where a breach of copyright occurs. Additional measures to discourage copyright infringement (such as, but not limited to, the casting of souls into eternal damnation) are also taken where appropriate. Printed in the United States of America.

Where a product trademark, registration mark or other protected mark is made in the text, ownership of the mark remains with the lawful owner of the mark. No claim, intentional or otherwise, is made by reference to any such marks in this book.

While every effort has been made by Interpharm Press, Inc. to ensure the accuracy of the information contained in this book, this organization accepts no responsibility for errors or omissions.

Interpharm Press, Inc.
1358 Busch Parkway
Buffalo Grove, IL 60089, USA

Phone: + 1 + 708 + 459-8480
Fax: + 1 + 708 + 459-6644

We respectfully dedicate this book
to health care professionals and their patients.

Contents

Preface	*xv*
Acknowledgements	*xvii*

I. Introduction   1

GMP Principles   *1*
Compendial Requirements   *4*
    Particle Distribution   5
    Particulate Matter Control   6
    Standards   8
Summary   *19*
References   *19*

II. Visual Inspection   22

Visual Inspection   *23*
    Manual Inspection   24
    Reproducibility of Visual Inspection   33
Automated (Machine) Inspection   *34*
    Application of Automated Systems   44
Compendial Requirements   *44*
Summary   *46*
References   *47*

III. Instrumental Particle Counting   50

The Coulter Principle   *51*
Light Extinction Counting   *54*
    Laser Versus White Light Extinction Sensors   59
    Error Sources   70
    Recent Developments   73
Spectrex (Phototron) System   *75*
Particle Size Standards   *77*
    Emulsion Polymerization   78

Suspension Polymerization 79
Swollen Emulsion Process 80
Storage and Handling of Standard Particles 81
Use of Commercial Standards 82
USP Particle Count Reference Standard 84
Alternative Count Standards 85

Automated Light Extinction Counting — 87

Validation of the Robotic Assay — 89
Operational Validation 92
Validation of Data Collected 93

Summary — 96

References — 96

IV. *Microscopy* — *100*

Structure of the Compound Microscope — 102
Lens Aberrations 103
Objective Lenses 107
Working Distance of Objectives 109
Resolving Power 110
Oculars (Eyepieces) 111
Condenser Lens 111

Reflected Illumination — 112

Dark-Field Microscopy — 112

Refractive Index — 114

Polarized Light Microscopy — 115
Interference 116
Birefringence and Extinction 118
Refractive Index Determinations 121
Dispersion Staining 122

Isolation and Handling of Particles — 123

Hot Stage Methods — 125

Microscope Calibration — 126

Measurement of Particle Size — 127

Techniques for Microscopic Particle Counting — 129

Enumeration of Particles in Parenteral Products — 134

Summary — 139

References — 139

V. Instrumental Analysis for Particle Identification — 143

Particle Identification—Electron Microscopy — 145
   Transmission Electron Microscopy — 146
   Electromagnetic Lenses — 149
   Scanning Electron Microscopy — 152

Application of X-Ray Spectroscopy — 160
   Elemental Composition Analysis — 162

Infrared Microspectrophotometry — 165
   Mass Spectrometry — 169
   LAMMA — 169
   Secondary Ion Mass Spectrometry — 172

X-Ray Diffraction Crystallography — 177

Summary — 183

References — 183

VI. Environmental Particulate Matter Monitoring and Control — 187

Applicable Standards — 189

Principles of HEPA Filtration — 192
   HEPA Filter Particle Retention Characteristics — 197
   In-Use Testing of HEPA Filters — 197

Environmental Particle Monitoring — 201
   Laser Versus White Light Counters — 203
   Remote Particle Monitoring — 208

Application of Federal Standard 209-D — 212

Federal Standard 209-E — 215
   Isokinetic Sampling — 219
   Sampling of Compressed Gases — 223
   Tubing Transport of Particulate Matter Samples — 226

Large Particle Monitoring — 229

Personnel Monitoring — 231

Summary — 232

References — 233

VII. Process- and Product-Related Particles — 237

Packaging Materials — 240
   Solution and Formulation Components   *243*
   Dry Powder Drug Materials   *246*
   Product-Container Interactions   *248*
   Process Point-Generated Particulates   *249*

Particulate Matter Problem Solving — 253
   Philosophical Considerations   *255*
   Sampling for Large Particles   *259*

Summary — 260

References — 261

VIII. Particle Population Analysis — 266

Particle Size — 268

Particle Shape — 271

Particle Size Distributions (Particle Number) — 281
   Distribution of Extraneous Particle Counts   *294*
   Average Diameters   *294*

Instrumentation and Methods — 298
   Nephelometry   *303*
   Laser Diffraction   *306*
   Photon Correlation Spectroscopy   *309*
   Microscopy and Image Analysis   *312*
   Sieving   *318*
   Light Extinction Counting   *323*
   Sedimentation   *328*
   Adsorption and Porosimetry   *330*
   Porosimetry   *334*
   Application of Adsorption and Porosimetry   *337*

Aerosol Population Analysis — 338

Summary — 344

References — 345

IX. Collection and Isolation of Particulate Matter   **350**

Filter Structure and Application   *352*

Retention Ratings, Pore Size, and Porosity   *359*
- Mechanism of Liquid Filtration   *361*
- Determination of Retention Ratings   *364*
- Wettability and Refractive Index   *365*

Filtration Apparatus   *366*

Collection of Particles for Analysis   *367*
- Isolation of Particles for Identification   *368*
- Powder Sampling   *371*
- Collection of Particles from Environmental Air   *376*
- Microscopic Analysis of Airborne Particles   *379*
- Monitoring of Components and Parts   *385*
- Sampling of Clean Room Garments   *386*
- Testing of Clean Room or Surgical Gloves   *389*

Summary   *390*

References   *390*

X. Process Control of Particulate Matter   **393**

Process Design   *394*

Process Control   *398*
- Statistical Process Control   *399*
- Process Stability and Capability   *403*
- Control Charting   *407*
- Batch Sampling   *420*

Summary   *428*

References   *429*

XI. Medical Devices   **431**

Parenteral-Type Devices   *433*
- Sources and Control of Particulate Matter in Devices   *434*
- Process Design   *437*
- Patient Concerns   *440*

Analysis of Particulate Matter in Devices *442*	
Autologous Transfusion Devices *448*	
Blood Filters *449*	
Choice of Particle Counting Methods	*449*
GMP Control of Device Particulates	*450*
Current Regulatory Issues *453*	
Device-Related 483s *459*	
Device Specific Particulate Matter Issues *460*	
Consideration Regarding Particulate Matter Requirements *461*	
Safe Medical Devices Act of 1990	*463*
Summary	*465*
References	*466*

XII. Patient Issues Related to Particulate Matter   **470**

Circulatory Transport	*471*
Human Injury by Particles	*473*
Animal Studies	*474*
Liposome Research	*476*
Infusion of Blood-Related Materials	*478*
Phlebitis and Particles	*479*
Conclusions Regarding Patient Risk	*480*
Summary	*480*
References	*482*

Appendices   **487**

1. *Photomicrography of Particulate Matter*	*487*
Sample Preparation *488*	
Instrumentation *489*	
Film *493*	
Light Balancing Filters *495*	
Color Compensating Filters *496*	
Polarized Light Techniques *497*	
Illustrations *498*	

xiii

    2. *Vendor and Equipment Information*   *504*
        Particle Counters (Airborne and Solution)   *504*
        Light Extinction Counter Sensors   *505*
        Counter Calibration Software   *505*
        Calibration Materials   *505*
        Visual Inspection Systems   *506*
        Image Analysis   *506*
        Electrical Zone Sensing Counters   *507*
        Laser Diffraction Particle Analyzers   *507*
        Lamma Instrumentation   *507*
        Light Microscopes   *507*
        X-Ray Spectrometers   *508*
        Electron Microscopes   *508*
        Photon Correlation Spectrophotometers   *509*
        Laser Light Scattering Liquid Counters   *509*
        Micro (Submicron) Particle Samplers   *509*
        Microfiltration Supplies   *509*
        Clean Room Supplies   *509*
        Particle Analysis Equipment (General)   *510*
        Powder Analysis Equipment   *510*
        Secondary Ion Mass Spectrometers   *511*
        Laboratory Robots   *511*
        Additional Sources of Supplemental Information and Standards   *511*
        Software for Data Reduction   *513*

    3. *Trademarks*   *514*

Index   **519**

    Name   *519*
    Subject   *524*

The color photomicrographs found near the middle of this text are described on pages 498 to 503 in Appendix I.

Preface

I originally set out to write this book in the belief that a need existed for a text that would provide basic information regarding the analysis of particulate matter in the pharmaceutical industry. Although many books deal with the principles and theoretical aspects of particle identification and enumeration, no single text is dedicated to the applications of particle analysis in the pharmaceutical industry. Thus, a considerable body of practical information has not been readily available. This book represents my effort to share some of this information with other particle analysts in this specialized field.

The goal of pharmaceutical manufacturers is to serve the patients and health care professionals who depend upon their products. The best interest of the health care consumer is served by the cooperative activity between manufacturers, regulatory agencies, and compendial groups that is essential to the development and production of high quality pharmaceutical and medical products. Therefore, I also have included a discussion of patient issues involving particulate matter and standards-setting activities.

The great majority of the pharmaceutical products manufactured in the world today are produced in total compliance with compendial requirements and contain extremely low levels of particulate matter. The high level of concern that pharmaceutical manufacturers have for the quality and efficacy of their products has resulted in significant decreases in product particle burden over the past decade. Furthermore, because of the competitive environment in which pharmaceutical products are developed, manufactured, and marketed today, only the manufacturer with a conscientious commitment to customer satisfaction can be successful. The maintenance of extremely low levels of particulate matter in products adds to the customer's perception of product quality and safety.

A further incentive to writing this book arose from my recollections of having entered this field from another discipline more than 15 years ago. Looking back on my process of learning has suggested that sharing insights might make the way easier for others. Understandably, the contents of this book come in some part from my own experience and hence reflect my interests and views. I have made a concerted effort to discuss all of my topics objectively.

Parts of the text have been rewritten several times in response to changing technology or discussions with colleagues. The analysis of particulate matter of all kinds is a constantly evolving field, particularly with regard to pharmaceutical and medical products. I have tried to provide the most current information, but readers are forewarned: Once a technology is within their grasp, vigilance is required to stay abreast of changes, many of which afford ways of collecting better data or decreasing time requirements.

This text deals with the aspects of particle analysis that should be most useful to a laboratory manager or technician. Some theoretical material has been included where necessary for intelligent application of the techniques described. References are provided for those readers who desire to pursue the subject matter in greater detail. It is the thesis of this book that almost anyone with undergraduate training in the basic scientific disciplines and laboratory techniques can gain a useful knowledge of the subject matter in a relatively short time. An application-oriented technology rather than a pure science, particle analysis combines knowledge from a number of areas with a logical approach to problem solving rather than comprehensive knowledge in a single field such as chemistry or physics. In pharmaceutical particle analysis, the people who become most adept are generalists rather than specialists.

An important word is appropriate here regarding selection of instruments. My description of forms of analysis or specific instrument function is in no way intended to indicate a preference for one specific instrument over another. I am, however, guilty of saying more about instruments with which I am familiar or for which a greater amount of descriptive literature is available. Because the technology for single particle counters for either airborne or solution-borne particles is still evolving, the market environment is intensely competitive. I advise the reader to investigate instruments available and seriously evaluate their performance criteria prior to any purchase.

When I began to write this book, it was my intent to deal only with technical subjects related to the analysis and control of particulate matter in pharmaceutical and medical products. It became obvious early on that this approach would not be appropriate because of the extent that GMP, compendial requirements, and regulatory issues impact the interpretation of some types of particulate matter data. Therefore, I have included a minimal amount of discussion on these nontechnical subjects. With regard to these discussions, I must emphasize that any and all subjective judgments, opinions, and viewpoints expressed in this book are my own and not necessarily those of Baxter Healthcare Corporation or any organization representing manufacturers of medical devices or injectable products.

I wish my readers well and hope that the information they find in this book will help them gain expertise in a most interesting and challenging area of endeavor.

Acknowledgements

I am deeply grateful to those numerous individuals who provided me with assistance and encouragement in the preparation of this manuscript. At the professional level, I have been fortunate to have the invaluable assistance of other particle analysts, quality and production managers, statisticians, and analytical chemists who made it possible for me to extend my knowledge into new areas of technology.

Specifically, I would like to acknowledge the patient technical assistance of the following: Mr. Alvin Lieberman (Particle Measuring Systems), Dr. Chuck Montague (Pacific Scientific), Mr. Jules Knapp (R&D Associates), Dr. Benjamin Liu (University of Minnesota), Dr. Holger Somer (Met-One), Mr. Terry Munson and Mr. Robert Sorenson (FDA), Mr. Joseph Belson (USP), Dr. David Fairhurst (Brookhaven Instruments), and Dr. David Nicoli (Particle Sizing Systems). My thanks also go to vendors (Millipore Corporation, Seradyn Inc., Hiac/Royco, and the Eisai Company) who allowed material to be included in the text.

I also owe a great debt of gratitude to those at Baxter Healthcare Corporation with whom I work, who made it possible for me to complete the task of writing this book. I extend my thanks to understanding and supportive supervisors, Dr. Barrett Rabinow and Dr. Theodore Roseman; to the secretaries who dealt with my numerous revisions and changes to drafts and offered editorial assistance, Ms. Myrna Storm and Ms. Marsha McKinney; and to my fellow professionals at Baxter, Dr. Damian Neuberger, Ms. Christine Pavek-Hicks, Mr. Matt Lannis, and Mr. William Lu.

As will be obvious to the reader, Mr. John Williams is an artist and technical illustrator of rare skill. It would have been impossible to write this book without John's dedicated collaboration and the patience and attention to detail that his drawings display. I would like to express my deepest gratitude to John for his efforts. Likewise, I also must thank Dr. Damian Neuberger for his superb photomicrographs and the written material he contributed.

The particle analyst is literally blind in the consideration of the numbers that are collected without the light shed by statisticians and statistical treatment of data. Those skilled in the art who have contributed to this effort include Dr. Harold Sargent, Dr. Howard Seipman (deceased), Dr. Kewei Pu, Dr. Wayne Taylor, and Mr. Jim Mellon. Because of their skill in application of statistical principles, they have helped me over the years in a wide range of projects as diverse as regulatory issues and high school science projects.

During my career I have grown to hold critical comment on work that I do (and those who offer it) in high esteem. A constructive critic is a true friend. In this regard, I must offer my sincere thanks to Dr. Michael Groves of the Department of Pharmaceutics at the University of Illinois. Mike's unfailing ability to criticize the material that I write has been as valuable as his persistent friendship and willing assistance whenever needed.

Finally, I must express my appreciation to my employer, Baxter Healthcare Corporation, whose commitment to product quality, customer satisfaction, and advancing technology made it possible for me to complete this book.

Tom Barber

I

Introduction

The analysis and control of particulate matter in pharmaceutical products is a complex subject (Benjamin 1990; Kalm 1987). In addition to the particulate matter contained in large volume parenteral solutions administered to patients, particles generated by or contained in small volume injectables (especially reconstituted powders), administration sets, syringes, needles and ampoules, and those resulting from the procedure of intravenous therapy itself are a concern. DeLuca et al. (1988) and Ho (1967) will serve as excellent sources of reference regarding a wide range of subjects of interest to the particle analyst. The 1986 paper by Borchert et al. is also very useful both in regard to sources of particulate matter and applicable analytical methods.

GMP Principles

In any consideration of particles in injectable products, our definition of extraneous particles becomes extremely important. This definition must be made based on a consideration of GMP principles, applicable means of analysis, and patient well-being. Particulate matter in injectable products may be defined as randomly sourced extraneous material of heterogeneous chemical composition that is not amenable to analysis by chemical means due to the extremely low levels present and its diverse composition. There are three important concepts embodied in this definition. (1) Particulate matter currently exists at extremely low levels in injectable products and there is no demonstrable evidence of adverse patient effects. (2) The material cannot be monotypic, but rather results from a variety of sources inherent in a GMP-controlled production process. (3) The material is not amenable to chemical analysis due to the small mass that it represents and its heterogeneous composition. Thus, the appropriate analytical methods for enumeration of this material must be sensitive physical tests that detect size and quantitate the material based on its optical properties.

Of extreme importance to this definition is the concept of GMP control of particulate matter in pharmaceutical products. If a particulate material from a single source becomes dominant in a product, control of the production process is lacking. Monotypic particulate matter is not random in occurrence and frequently may be analyzed at high levels of sensitivity. Specifically, materials such as silicone oil microdroplets from an elastomeric closure or syringe piston do not fall within this definition; such container-related materials are inherent in the product and can be quantitated at high sensitivity by chemical means.

The ultimate goal of our consideration of particulate matter in pharmaceutical products is its control at levels far below those at which there is any issue of patient well-being. Although the manufacturers of injectable products, compendial bodies and regulatory agencies share this goal, there is a distinct divergence in philosophy regarding how this control is to be attained. The charters of the world's various compendia address the assurance of product safety and efficacy, that is, patient well-being. In this regard, it is reasonable that pharmacopeia include tests and limits for extraneous particulate matter. The critical consideration so often overlooked in discussions of particulate matter is the extremely low level of particulate matter present in products produced under current GMP conditions. The products currently produced in Japan, the United Kingdom, Europe, and the United States have an extraneous particle burden so low as to make any issue of adverse patient effects nonexistent.

Regulatory agencies and the compendia have historically placed their reliance on limiting allowable number of particles as a means of achieving control. This approach is useful, and particulate matter limits worldwide have had some effect on increasing product quality with regard to particle content. The unfortunate aspect of the limits approach is that it does not represent the ultimate measure of control. Dependent on the degree to which a manufacturer incorporates uniformity as a feature of their process, units tested for compliance with limits may or may not accurately represent untested units of a batch. An example of the shortcomings of this approach is provided by the current USP <788> assay for particles in small volume injections (SVI). The assay result for this test is an estimate of the average per-container particle count based on light extinction counting of a 10-unit pool. No measure of between-unit variability of these counts is obtained. Thus, individual units with particle counts in excess of limits might conceivably get into the field. Lower limits would have little or no effect on this situation since variability is not assessed.

Although more requirements or tighter limits may be attractive from a regulatory standpoint, the desired result with regard to an assurance of patient protection cannot be achieved by this means. The only sensible, practical, and totally effective control of particles in product is achieved by GMP (Akers 1985). Good manufacturing practices, as specified by a large number of compendial and regulatory documents worldwide involve: (1) the definition and operation of a manufacturing process that does not generate nonrandom particle populations and is thoroughly validated in that regard, and (2) monitoring of the crucial parameters of that process to ensure that it continually operates within the established operating range. Tightly controlled, well-validated processes allow a high degree of control over particles in product.

This philosophy of GMP control of particulate matter has significant implications regarding enforcement activities. Grounds for enforcement activity are provided by GMP regulations presently in force (Munson and Sorenson 1991). If a process is validated to produce units with low levels of particles and is strictly controlled and adequately monitored, the product generated will, by definition, have a well-controlled particle burden. It is interesting to consider what value particulate matter limits really have. While limits may have the beneficial effect of restricting the activities of a few manufacturers operating poorly controlled processes, regulatory activities against such vendors will almost invariably be based on the failure to follow GMP rather than the actual particle burden of product. There is an unfortunate tendency on the part of some compendial groups to view tighter particulate matter limits as an assurance of higher product quality. Even more unfortunate is the tendency of some to view higher numbers of requirements and more restrictive limits as a measure of compendial stature. These views in no way promote patient well-being. In the contemporary pharmaceutical manufacturing environment, the manufacturer and the GMP process protects the patient rather than compendial requirements and regulatory activity.

With regard to the simplest case, large volume injection (LVI) solutions, the United States Pharmacopeia (USP), the British Pharmacopoeia (BP), and the Pharmacopoeia of Japan (JP) each specify allowable levels of extraneous particles that may be present on a per mL or per unit basis. This allowance is made in recognition of the fact that it is impossible to manufacture injectable products totally free of particles (Groves 1973). Products manufactured under the strict conditions of GMP control in the United States, Europe, and Japan will invariably contain some amount of extraneous particles. Implicit in the compendial requirements is the philosophy that particles in excess of those levels resulting from conscientious application of GMP are not allowable. Thus, although the compendial limits may differ significantly between countries, the concept of control is quite similar.

Compendial Requirements

Of all the compendial requirements placed on injectable products, particulate matter has historically been an area that receives a significant amount of attention and a single product characteristic that is most likely to involve subjective judgments. Correctly or incorrectly, the particulate matter burden of a product has been taken by some health care practitioners, academic investigators, and regulatory personnel as an indicator of overall product quality. This is unfortunate, since particulate matter is, realistically, only a single parameter by which product suitability or conformity to requirements may be judged. One reason particulate matter receives so much attention is that it may constitute an obvious defect in product. The pharmacist, physician, nurse, or patient cannot reasonably be expected to detect a departure from product requirements with regard to pH, potency, drug concentration, or osmolarity. Particles, however, may be detected by simple visual inspection, or in the case of subvisible particles, quantitated by fairly simple tests. Thus, there is a reasonable (if subjective) inclination to emphasize and be acutely aware of the occurrence of particulate matter.

Several rationales have been presented to justify guidelines, limits and concerns regarding particulate matter (Groves and DeMalka 1976). Some argue that realistic particle standards should be consistent with the capabilities of existing technology and in this sense are a measure of good manufacturing practices. Others believe that particle limits are necessary to control the cumulative particulate matter "insult" the patient receives. In the United States, the USP LVI and SVI requirements have been rationalized on both accounts. Numerous articles have been published concerning the size and numbers of particles in LVI and SVI (see DeLuca et al. 1986). These studies have utilized a variety of methods for counting particles, including the microscope and light extinction, light scattering, and electrical zone-sensing instrumental particle counting techniques.

Particle Distribution

Particle size distributions have been reported for particles in parenteral products. It has been observed that sometimes there is a log-log relationship of particle size and number, and some workers have been able to summarize their data using the following equation (Groves and Muhlen 1987; Muhlen 1986).

$$\ln N = \ln N_{1.0} - M \ln D$$

where N is the cumulative number of particles at the threshold of diameter (D), $N_{1.0}$ is the value of N, $D = 1.0$ μm, and M is the slope of the log-log plot. Based on the result of these size distributions, a variety of limits have been suggested for both LVP and SVP solutions. While the premise of a log-log distribution of particles in parenterals has received some support, it is unclear whether or not the extraneous particle population in injectables actually conforms to any single distribution. The data obtained with any method of particle enumeration will be inextricably linked to the method used. Thus, a given unit of injectable product will contain one distribution of particles by light extinction, another by Coulter counter, and yet a third by microscopy. Thus, to make any general statements regarding particle distribution in an unqualified fashion is at best tenuous.

Further, light extinction particle counters do not see all types of particles equally well, and the size assigned a particle will depend critically upon shape and refractive index. Thus, the distribution of particles detected will depend on the particle type being counted. In fact, the historical data on which a log-log distribution is based shows a considerable variability of distribution and could as well be shown to fit Poisson, negative binomial, or other distributions. This data has sometimes been compared without regard to the precision or accuracy of individual data points or the types of counters used (Barber 1987). In some cases light extinction counter data has been considered with Coulter data. In short, it would appear that in some cases data has been interpreted in favor of theory in disregard of technical and scientific principles.

Unfortunately, most published material purporting to summarize the occurrence of particles in parenteral solutions represents too few data points to be widely indicative of marketed product. Some of the instruments used, especially light extinction counters, show less than 50% sensitivity at the particle sizes counted in early (pre-1970) studies. Also, historical sampling techniques for instrumental counting (small aliquots and inadequate particle suspension) have been shown to alter particle distributions (Knapp and Abramson 1990). Counting of parenteral solutions with the multichannel light extinction instruments currently available shows that significant discontinuities can exist between the wide-set thresholds used in previous studies. Given the widely known tendency of light extinction counters to undersize large particles, it would be particularly unfortunate to base limits on a hypothetical log-log distribution since these particles typically are not correctly represented in the data base. Based on all of these considerations, limits precluding numbers above a certain value at a specific size appear to be a better choice for the present than any requirement based on an assumed distribution.

Particulate Matter Control

Despite the conscientious efforts of a manufacturer to totally eliminate particulate matter, some low number of particles will occur in injectable products and medical devices; the number of particles occurring is invariably below any level that might raise issues of patient well being. The user of a parenteral product—a pharmacist, doctor, or nurse—may also inadvertently put particulate matter into the product during intravenous therapy administration. Particulate matter found in parenteral products arises from a number of sources and has been generally classed as being either intrinsic or extrinsic in origin (Groves 1973). Intrinsic particulate matter consists of material originally in a solution that is not removed by filtration prior to filling or particles that occur due to precipitation reactions in the solutions. Extrinsic particles are those that enter the product or its container during the filling operation—rubber, metal, or plastic coming from container product contact surfaces.

From the manufacturer's viewpoint, there are generally four components of particulate matter control that pertain irrespective of the product type and manufacturer. These are:

- Process design,
- Process and environmental particulate matter monitoring,
- Enumeration of particles in product, and
- Particulate matter identification.

The first item (process design) is of overwhelming importance. Design of a process to eliminate particles results in more positive control than any removal of particles after the process is in place. Currently, the industry's emphasis in all four of these areas has turned from particle control to particulate matter source elimination. During manufacture, it is necessary to protect the product from particles related to the process by which it is made, for example, fillers, mixers, cappers, and the product container itself. Frequently, in troubleshooting, it becomes necessary to measure particulate matter added to the product at each step in the process.

With regard to environmental particulate matter, current standards for nonviable particles in the pharmaceutical industry are less stringent than those observed in the microelectronics or aerospace industries. For product that will be sterilized after filling (terminally sterilized), microbes are not an issue; particulate matter present at the current low levels constitutes no patient risk whatsoever, and has a minor implication with regard to product quality. For aseptically-filled product that will not be terminally sterilized, the particulate matter burden may be indicative of microbial content and particle burden, and is a more serious concern. For the latter type of product, exposure to particulate matter is more strictly controlled. For aseptic fill operations, the equivalent of Class 100 conditions per Federal Standard 209-D are mandated. For terminally sterilized product, higher environmental particle levels that result in product with an acceptably low particle burden are acceptable.

The enumeration of particles in product and the assessment of product particle burden in comparison to the applicable limits has been a subject of great interest to manufacturers, regulatory agencies, and compendial groups. Historically, many of those concerned with particulate matter in pharmaceutical products have believed that the particle burden of LVI solutions is the principle source of particles to which patients are exposed. This belief is likely erroneous, but a series of compendial particulate matter standards for LVI product have been proposed and implemented in different countries. Some have been adopted and are currently enforced

(United States Pharmacopeia, British Pharmacopoeia, Japanese Pharmacopoeia). These are summarized in Table I.

Table I. Various LVI Solution Particulate Matter Limits

Counting	Method	Limits Counts (per mL)					
		≥2 µm	≥3.5 µm	≥5 µm	≥10 µm	≥20 µm	≥25 µm
U.S. (USP XII)	Microscopic	—	—	—	50	—	5
Australia	Coulter	1000	250	100	—	5	—
	LE*	1000	250	100	—	—	—
Great Britain	Coulter	1000	—	100	—	—	—
	LE*	500	—	80	—	—	—
Japan (JP XI)	Microscopic	—	—	—	20	—	2
European Pharmacopoeia	Coulter	—	—	100	50	5	—
	LE*	—	—	100	50	5	—

*Light Extinction Particle Counting

Standards

The history of development of the present USP requirement for particulate matter is interesting.

> **1942—USP XII: Appearance of Solutions or suspensions:** Injections that are solutions of soluble medicaments must be clear and free of any turbidity or undissolved material that can be detected readily without magnification when the solution is examined against black and white backgrounds with a bright light reflected from a 100-watt Mazda lamp or its equivalent.

> **1947—USP XIII: Clarity of Solutions:** Injections that are solutions of soluble medicaments must be clear and substantially free of any turbidity or undissolved material that can be detected readily without magnification when the solution is examined against black and white backgrounds

with a bright light reflected from a 100-watt Mazda lamp or its equivalent.

1955—USP XV: "Injections" <1>: Every care should be exercised in the preparation of all products intended for injection, to prevent contamination with microorganisms and foreign material. Good pharmaceutical practice requires also that each final container of injection be subjected individually to a physical inspection, whenever the nature of the container permits, and that every container whose contents show evidence of contamination with visible foreign material be rejected.

1975—USP XIX: Present Microscopic Test (<788>) Limits: The large-volume injection for single-dose infusion meets the requirements of the test if it contains not more than 50 particles per mL that are equal to or larger than 10 µm, and not more than 5 particles per mL that are equal to or larger than 25 µm in effective linear dimension.

1980—Supplement No. 3 USP XX: 5-HMF Disclaimer— Note: For dextrose-containing solutions, do not enumerate morphologically indistinct material showing little or no surface relief and presenting a gelatinous or film-like appearance. Since in solution this material consists of units of the order of 1 µm or less and is liable to be counted only after aggregation and/or deformation on the membrane, interpretation of enumeration may be aided by testing a specimen of the solution with a suitable electronic particle counter.

1985—USP XXI: Small Volume Injection Requirement added to <788> for Light Extinction Counting—Interpretation: The small-volume Injection meets the requirements of the test if it contains not more than 10,000 particles per container that are equal to or greater than 10 µm in effective spherical diameter, and/or 1000 particles per container equal to or greater than 25 µm in effective spherical diameter.

The first subvisible product particulate matter requirement implemented in the United States was for LVI solutions. These products are defined as solution products for injection that have a volume greater than 100 mL. The current USP standard for LVI solutions is no more than 50 particles ≥10 µm per mL and no more than 5 particles ≥25 µm per mL in longest linear dimension as determined microscopically. Small volume injections are products for injection with a volume of 100 mL or less. Establishing standards for small volume parenterals is complicated by the wide variety of unit sizes and product types. Nevertheless, the USP standard applies to all SVIs irrespective of product type and size. This inclusion of all product types in a single requirement appears particularly unfortunate, since dry powder dosage forms have particle burdens that differ significantly from those of terminally filtered SVI product. These limits, which had an effective date of January 1, 1986, were 10,000 particles ≥10 µm and 1000 particles ≥25 µm per container.

The identification of particulate matter is often pivotal to the decrease of numbers of particle present in product or the resolution of issues related to particulate matter, that is, "particle problems." Most major pharmaceutical companies have impressive capabilities in this regard, having learned that costs and turnaround times of outside specialty laboratories may not be consistent with uninterrupted production. The most powerful analytical techniques available to the chemist who works with bulk materials are now available to the pharmaceutical particle analyst. In particular, the techniques that are applied include light microscopy, atomic spectroscopic methods (SEM/EDXS, electron microprobe, ESCA, Auger electron spectroscopy), and molecular spectroscopic techniques (infrared spectroscopy, Raman spectroscopy, and mass spectrometry) (Borchert et al. 1986). With regard to actual identification of particles, the pharmaceutical manufacturer's capability typically exceeds those of other industries; this is an inevitable consequence of the often time-critical need to identify and eliminate particle sources.

A consideration of the available literature indicates that the particle burden to which a patient is exposed is related not simply to injectables but rather to the whole process of intravenous therapy. The proportional contribution to the total particle burden from various component sources cannot be assessed with any great degree of certainty. Information available from industry data and various published reports (Borchert et al. 1986; Endicott et al. 1966; Pflag 1966; Johnson et al. 1970; Illum et al. 1978a, 1978b; Illum 1980; Williams and Barnett 1973; Taylor 1982; Akers 1985; and Groves 1973) suggest the relationship of Figure 1 to be a useful approximation. It is interesting that a significant number of

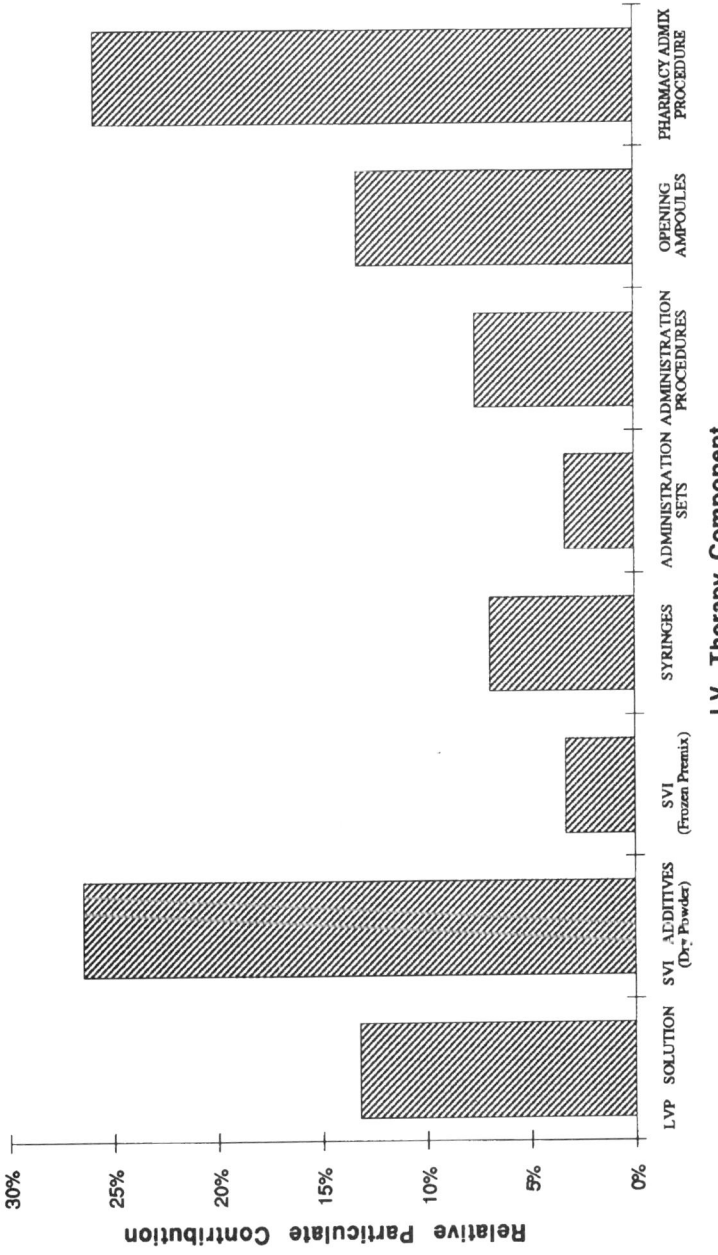

Figure 1. Sources of particulate matter in parenteral solutions.

particles in the solutions administered to patients result from sources beyond the control of the manufacturer.

The desirability of controlling product particle burden by means of process control rather than compendial limits is also true with regard to medical devices. During the past decade, there have been several discussions between industry and the various regulatory and enforcement authorities regarding whether or not particulate matter requirements for devices are necessary or desirable. In this case, as in others, assurance that a clinical need has been identified should be confirmed prior to determining whether or not a standard should be developed. Any proposals for particulate matter limits must be tempered with the knowledge that there is no significant evidence regarding adverse clinical effect of particles from devices. If a need were to be identified for a specific product, controls should logically be established for that product.

Comparing the particulate matter level in the medical devices evaluated by manufacturers and independent investigators to the particulate matter levels indicated as acceptable per the USP monograph for large volume injections for single-dose infusion, it appears that devices in general do not significantly contribute to particulate matter levels being infused into a patient (see chapter on medical devices). Additionally, it appears that products produced under controlled conditions meet customer expectations as evidenced by the absence of customer complaints regarding subvisible particulate matter and the very low number of complaints related to large, visible particles that have been received, based on the millions of devices used annually. The USP monograph for large volume injections for single-dose infusion states that the solution passes the test "if it contains not more than 50 particles per mL that are equal to or larger than 10 µm and not more than 5 particles per mL that are equal to or larger than 25 µm in effective linear dimension." These ranges are significantly above the level of particulate matter in commonly used medical devices.

Differences in devices and their use further complicate establishment of a standard, and it is evident that a single standard could not possibly address the entire range of devices and problems. A Dacron® vascular graft and a winged cannula cannot be expected to shed comparable numbers of particles since the Dacron® vascular graft has a much greater surface area and has the potential to continually release some small number of particles throughout its life span. Other medical devices, such as syringes and blood oxygenators, have material such as silicone or surfactants purposely applied to aid in the product's function.

Eliminating these additives to control particulate matter could adversely effect the function of the product. Failure to allow for the particulate matter generated as a result of the additives within some allowable limits range could also result in an unwarranted rejection of the product.

In summary, the main points that underscore the general lack of need for a device particulate matter requirement are as follows:

- The absence of any clinical evidence indicating that particulate matter requirements on medical devices would benefit patients;
- The impracticality of requirements for devices due to the many different types of devices and the lack of any uniformly applicable test method;
- The fact that only GMP will control device particulate matter burden (testing to demonstrate compliance with requirements may represent cost without benefits); and
- Present availability of detailed GMP requirements for device manufacture that have proven capable of controlling device particulate matter burden.

With regard to any proposal for particle limits, an evaluation of the cost-benefits ratio should also be made to ascertain if the costs encountered to comply with a standard are equal to the expected benefit. In a worst-case scenario, small companies might be unable to continue operating due to inordinate cost increases. Increased manufacturing costs as a result of implementation of an additional standard of unsubstantiated benefit will inevitably result in increased cost to the consumer that would appear to be particularly undesirable at a time when the medical community around the world is attempting to control costs. Process controls and effective implementation of the applicable GMPs have continued to be the medical device industry's methods of choice for reduction of particulate matter levels.

Disposable Syringes

A recent USP proposal (*Pharmaceutical Forum* Nov.–Dec. 1990) of a requirement for disposable syringes and the response received provides an interesting study in the difficulty of generating requirements for devices:

> **Particulate matter**—Proceed as directed for Procedure under Large-volume Injections for Single-dose Infusions in the

chapter Particulate Matter in Injections <788>. Unless a needle is an integral part of the unit, attach a needle that has been flushed thoroughly with membrane-filtered water. For sample preparation, select 10 syringes or cartridges having a capacity of less than 50-mL, or 3 syringes or cartridges having a capacity of 50-mL or greater. Fill each previously unfilled syringe to its rated capacity with membrane-filtered water, then expel the contents into a suitable, cleaned volumetric flask. Repeat this procedure two more times collecting the expelled contents in the same flask. Use the same flask to collect the contents from all the syringes or cartridges. Examine the sample visually for foreign matter. Using the same sample, proceed as directed for Large-volume Injections for Single-dose Infusions in Particulate Matter in Injections <788> except that the whole sample shall be passed through the filter. Count and size the total number of particles collected on the upper surface of the filter. Calculate the average number of particles per syringe or cartridge.

Interpretation—The syringe or cartridge meets the requirements of this test if it is essentially free of visible particles or foreign matter and the sample contains not more than 10 particles equal to or greater than 10 µm in effective linear dimension and not more than 1 particle equal to or greater than 25 µm in effective linear dimension per 1 mL nominal volume of the tested syringe or cartridge. If the sample does not conform at this stage, retest using pooled material from a second sample of twice the number of specimens (20 or 6) from the same batch. The requirements are met if the results conform to the criteria stated above.

The manufacturers of this type of product offered a number of critical comments on the proposal. Regarding the method of testing, it is difficult to understand why "single use" syringes would be flushed three times to collect effluent for the test. This part of the test seems inconsistent with the use of the syringes. The proposed requirement as written means that a 1-mL syringe, a difficult-to-inspect mechanical device, which must be actuated three times using the test, may contain only 10 particles ≥10 µm and 1 particle ≥25 µm. A 1-mL ampoule, a clear, nonshedding container with no moving parts may contain 10,000 particles ≥10 µm and 1000 ≥25 µm. In this case, the proposed syringe particulate matter standard is 1/1000 of that allowable for an SVI. A comparison of particles allowed from these different product groups is shown in Table II for purposes of comparison.

Table II. Comparison of LVI and SVI Limits and Proposed Limits for Syringes

USP Product	# of Particles ≥ 10 μm	# of Particles ≥ 25 μm
LVI (1000 mL)	50,000	5,000
SVI (per container)	10,000	1,000
Empty Syringe—1 mL (proposed)	10	1
Empty Syringe—20 mL (proposed)	200	20

Data from syringe manufacturers indicate that a number of syringes produced by domestic and foreign manufacturers will not meet the proposed limits. Based on the author's experience, most of the failures would occur in the 1- to 3-mL size range. Some of our testing suggests that there are more than twice as many particles per syringe in the 1-mL to 3-mL volume range as in the 5-mL to 10-mL range. This again indicates the unsuitability of a single limit. Some glass syringes incorporate a ground glass plunger bearing on a ground glass barrel surface. Here the number of actuations becomes very critical, since more actuations simply generate more glass fragments.

In the case of syringes, a consideration of the purpose of the proposed limits and the trends shown in the testing of syringes by manufacturers are given rational consideration; development of a more suitable, realistic limits proposal will result. A better alternative for the requirement would be to modify the test method to incorporate a single flush of each syringe tested. This has the benefit of not generating artifactually elevated numbers of particles from the syringes tested so that the test articles appear to have a higher particulate matter burden than they actually contain.

Visual Inspection

Limits on the occurrence of visible-size particles in medical products and injectables is another particularly pertinent example of the benefits of process control of particulates and the difficulty of establishing requirements. It is, in effect, impossible to perform a uniform critical visual inspection of injectable solutions using human inspection. This is due to the fact that visual inspection by a human analyst is dependent on variables, including

- Morphology of the particle;
- Type and intensity of illumination;
- Vision of the inspector;
- Inspector training;
- Container transparency and size; and
- Time of inspection.

Any human inspection thus incorporates a very high level of variability.

In recognition of the physical limitation of the visual inspection process, the major pharmacopeia have described acceptable product as "essentially free" (USP), "practically free" (BP) or "free of particles" visible under specific conditions (JP). These descriptions are generally imprecise and only apply to certain types of product. A recently suggested improvement to the USP requirement would substitute "no evidence of" (visible particles) for "essentially free." This constitutes no improvement or clarification, and, worse yet, implies an absolute standard. The only control for visible-sized particles in product is obviously a process that eliminates larger particles through process design and control.

Automated inspection has been suggested as a means of eliminating particles of visible size. A 100% inspection process as a means of eliminating units containing particles ≥100 μm in size is most practical for ampoule product, for which a very critical automated visual inspection can be applied. Although SVI vial units can also be inspected automatically, vial product may have particles adherent to the closure that are released during transport, so visible particles undetected by the inspection at manufacture may be detected by the user. Dry powder vials cannot be inspected at manufacture because visual inspection is a destructive analysis. Ampoules are the product type most readily 100% inspected, and are also the product type that most often contains the highest levels of particles (glass fragments) when used. It is also impossible for the manufacturer to inspect LVI product critically enough so that assurance of no visible particles can be obtained. This is due to the fact that particles not present in the solution when inspected may be released during transport or storage, and to the inadequacy of both automated and manual inspection of LVI product. Translucent plastic containers cannot be inspected critically by either automated or manual means. The consideration of visible particulate matter effectively leads to the conclusion that the control of particulates by inspection is not practical for the majority of injectable products. Particulate must be controlled by a carefully validated and monitored process operated strictly under the principles of GMP.

Parenteral Emulsions

The combined input of regulatory agencies, compendial groups and the manufacturers is most important if reasonable, technically sound standards are to be developed. An example is provided by the USP's recent efforts to develop a requirement for the emulsion "globule" size distribution in parenteral emulsions that appeared in the July–August (1991) issue of *Pharmacopeial Forum.*

> Parenteral emulsions used in total parenteral nutrition (TPN) are most frequently aqueous suspensions of soybean oil, safflower oil, or a mixture of the two combined with an emulsifying agent. The size distribution of the emulsified oil droplets is critical to the properties of the product, since there is some evidence that larger size globules can be retained in the capillaries of the lungs due to capillary filtration. The pertinent characteristics of a fat emulsion for parenteral use thus include the mean size of the microdroplet particle distribution and the distribution of the globule sizes as expressed by the standard deviation of the distribution. These values allow control of the percentage of particles outside a specific distribution. Importantly, it may also be desirable to know the volume percent of total oil represented by particles of greater than a specific size, such as 5 µm.

The originally proposed requirement, prepared with negligible input from industry, incorporated two analytical methods: (1) electrical zone sensing (Coulter principle) and (2) photon correlation spectroscopy (PCS). As discussed in later chapters of this book, these two instruments differ greatly in principles of operation; one (the electrical zone sensing model) is a single particle counter while the other (PCS) measures collective light scattering properties of the emulsion. This dual approach is basically flawed, in that some form of equivalence is implied between the two types of analyses. In fact, no equivalence exists, and the difference in principles of operation of the two instruments raises serious technical doubts regarding the validity of the proposed method. Another negative feature of the proposal is that vendor-specific identification of the PCS instrument to be used is included. Compendial methods must be sufficiently rugged so that assays become principle-specific, rather than instrument-specific, if they are to be successfully applied in routine fashion.

A further inherent disadvantage in both of the proposed methods is the extensive dilution of the emulsion material required (typically 1:1000 or greater). Diluted samples of any material for population analyses result in a bias in favor of the large numbers of small particles that are not affected to any significant extent by the dilution procedure. In a parenteral emulsion, the geometric mean particle size may be in the range of 0.3–0.4 µm. The particle size distribution is heavily skewed toward the small (submicron sizes) with millions of submicron particles present for each 1000 particles of 5 µm or larger. Thousand-fold dilution results in a concentration of submicron particles that is effectively unchanged while the concentration of large particles is seriously decremented. The PCS devices can only accurately assess particle size distributions below about 3 µm due to the fact that this measurement is based on particle Brownian motion. Particles of 0.1–0.5 µm size are emphasized in this analysis. Instruments operating on the Coulter principle become an effective measuring tool only at particle sizes of <0.4 µm. The possible great disparity of analytical results is obvious.

As a result of industry comments on this proposal, the USP has agreed to withdraw the Coulter-type counter from the requirements proposal. This is a decided improvement, but leaves us with the PCS-type instrument that does not provide an analytical result for particles larger than 3 µm when the larger particles of concern are those over 5 µm in size. A better approach would involve the use of two instruments to span the entire range of emulsion distributions, namely the PCS-type instrument to determine mean particle size and a laser diode light extinction instrument or microscope to count particles greater than 5 µm.

The inadequate requirements proposals discussed above that have involved publication of inadequate methods in the *Pharmacopeial Forum* followed by withdrawal of the proposal upon industry comment are indicative of a procedural defect in the standards development process. Happily, the procedure for establishing compendial requirements, which resulted in the unsatisfactory requirements proposals discussed earlier, has been the subject of significant changes. More recently, the approach of obtaining in advance of the publication of the requirements proposals the technical input from manufacturers of the products involved and instrument vendors has been taken. The result is requirements proposals that are technically sound and appropriate to the product to which they apply. It has proven particularly critical to obtain the consensus of manufacturers, since the producers of pharmaceutical products invariably have a thorough understanding of the principles of analyses related to their products. Recent cooperative activities between industry and the USP, such as those involved in development of an improved microscopic test for subvisible particles in solutions, suggest that this course will become the standard operating procedure in the future.

Summary

The occurrence of low numbers of heterogeneously sourced particles is inevitable in the manufacture of injectable products and medical devices. The numbers of particles that occur in product manufactured under conscientiously applied GMP are extremely low. There is no practical issue of adverse patient effects due to the particle burden of current product. This low level of particulate matter has been reached through the efforts of manufacturers toward product improvement rather than being due to regulatory activity. Based on a rational consideration of particulate matter occurrence, the numbers of particles in product cannot be further reduced by either additional requirements or tighter limits, since these have no effect on the manufacturing process. The manufacturing process itself is our sole available control on particulate matter. Ample GMP regulations are currently in place to provide for enforcement activities against noncompliant manufacturers. Good manufacturing practice, rather than monitoring or regulatory or compendial requirements, controls particles. It is the manufacturer's commitment to product quality that has resulted in the current high quality levels, cost effectiveness, and efficacy of parenteral solutions.

References

Akers, M. J. 1985. *Parenteral quality control: Sterility, pyrogen, particulate, and package integrity testing.* New York: Marcel Dekker, Inc., 143–197.

Barber, T. A. 1987. Limitations of light blockage particle counting. Paper presented at the meeting on *Liquid Borne Particle Inspection and Metrology,* May 11–13, Washington, D.C.

Benjamin, F. 1990. Particulate matter: A historical review. In *Proc. PDA Int. Conf. on Particle Detection, Metrology and Control,* 28–65. Arlington, VA.

Borchert, S. J., A. Abe, S. D. Aldrich, L. E. Fox, J. E. Freeman, and R. D. White. 1986. Particulate matter in parenteral products: A review. *J. Parenteral Sci. and Technol.* 40:212–239.

British Pharmacopoeia. 1988. Vol. II:756. London: Her Majesty's Stationery Office.

DeLuca, P. P., S. Bodapatti, D. Haack, and H. Schroeder. 1986. An approach to setting particulate matter standards for small volume parenterals. *J. Parenter. Sci. Technol.* 40:2–13.

DeLuca, P. P., B. Conti, and J. Z. Knapp. 1988. Particulate matter II. A selected annotated bibliography. *J. Parent. Sci. and Technol.* 42 Supplement.

Endicott, C. J., R. Giles, and R. Pecina. 1966. Particulate matter: Its significance, source, measurement and elimination. In *Proc. Symp. on Safety of Large Volume Parenteral Solutions,* 62–75. Washington, D.C.: FDA.

Groves, M. J. 1969. The size distribution of particles contaminating parenteral solutions. *Analyst* 94:992–999.

Groves, M. J. 1973. *Parenteral products.* Hinemann Medical Books, Ltd., p. 316.

Groves, M. J. 1992. An improved method for calculating data from particulate matter limit tests of small volume injection solutions. *Pharmacopeial Forum* 16:4100–4101. United States Pharmacopeial Convention, Silver Spring, MD.

Groves, M. J., and S. R. DeMalka. 1976. The relevance of pharmacopeial particulate matter limit tests. *Drug Dec. Commun.* 2 (3):285–324.

Groves, M. J., and E. Muhlen. 1987. The parenterals numbers game—Newer ways of looking at particulate contamination. *J. Parent. Sci. Technol.* 41 (4):116–120.

Ho, N. F. H. 1967. Particulate matter in parenteral solutions. I. A review of the literature. *Drug Intel.* 1 (1):7–11.

Illum, L. 1980. Characterization of particulate contamination released by application of parenteral solutions. 3. Particulate matter from syringes. *Arch. Pharm. Chem. Sci. Ed.* 8:109–115.

Illum. L., V. G. Jensen, and N. Moller. 1978a. Characterization of particulate contamination released by application of parenteral solutions. 1. Particulate matter from administration sets. *Arch. Pharm. Chem. Sci. Ed. 6:93–102.*

Illum, L., V. G. Jensen, and N. Moller. 1978b. Characterization of particulate contamination released by application of parenteral solutions. 2. Particulate matter from cannulas. *Arch. Pharm. Chem. Sci. Ed.* 6:169–174.

Johnson, K. T., C. D. Helper, and J. P. B. Gallardo. 1970. Particulate contamination in vials of sterile dry solids. *Am. J. Hosp. Pharm* 27 (December):968–976.

Kalm, M. 1987. Historical review of particulates. In *Proc. PDA Conf. on Liquid Borne Particle Inspection and Metrology*, 70–74. Washington, D.C.

Knapp, J. Z., and L. R. Abramson. 1990. A systems analysis of light extinction particle detection systems. In *Proc. Int'l. Conf. on Particle Detection, Metrology and Control*, 283. Arlington, VA.

Muhlen, E. 1986. An index for the particulate contamination in parenterals—Its fundamentals and its application to quantitative determination by photometric control and fully automated image analysis. Paper for presentation at the Congress of the F.I.P., September 9–13, Helsinki.

Munson, T., and R. Sorenson. 1991. *Sterile pharmaceutical manufacturing: Applications for the 1990s,* ed. M. J. Groves, W. P. Olson, and M. H. Anisfeld, 163–184. Buffalo Grove, IL: Interpharm Press.

Pflag, S. C. 1966. Large volume parenteral solutions procured by the military. In *Proc. Sym. Safety of Large Volume Parenteral Solutions,* 10–14. Washington, D.C.: FDA.

Taylor, S. A. 1982. Particulate contamination of sterile syringes and needles. *J. Pharm. Pharmacol.* 34:493–495.

The Pharmacopoeia of Japan. 1986. 11th Ed.:20–21. Tokyo: Yakuji Nippo, Ltd.

The United States Pharmacopeia. 1990. 22nd Ed.:1596. Easton, PA: Mack Printing Company.

Williams, A., and M. I. Barnett. 1973. Particulate contamination in intravenous fluids, administration sets and cannulae. *Pharm J.* 211:190–198.

II

Visual Inspection

There are many technical publications associated with visual inspection methodology. Some of the most useful references are listed at the end of this chapter. The papers by Knapp and Kushner (1980a, 1980b, 1982) and Knapp et al. (1983) are the most comprehensive references on this subject and deal with manual and automated (machine) inspection and the relationship of these two methods. Historically, there has been a significant level of interest in particulate matter of visible size in injectable products (Archambault and Dodds 1966; Kramer 1970; Sandell and Ashlund 1974). The level of visible particles in product is believed by many to provide an indication of process control, and a significant increase in visible particles has been suggested to be an indicator of a poorly controlled manufacturing process. The commonly used term *visual inspection* is in itself something of a misnomer. Although the analysis referred to is performed to detect particles within or approaching the visible size range, it is not always performed using human vision. Of all the types of particulate matter analysis that may be applied to parenteral products, visual inspection has the potential for the most highly variable result (Archambault and Dodds 1966). Conduct of the test will differ greatly based on whether the inspection is performed by manual or automatic means and whether the product evaluated is a large volume (i.e., greater than 100 mL) solution unit, a dry powder vial, or an ampoule of a liquid dosage form.

Visual Inspection

It is not uncommon to hear 50 μm quoted as the minimum particle size detectable in the visual inspection of injectable products. Particles far too small to be visually detected singly can be visually detected if they are present in high numbers due to their collective light scattering effect (e.g., immiscible liquids), and will be visible to the human eye. For example, silicone oils employed to lubricate containers and/or closures may be seen visually or by light extinction techniques. Semisolids such as partially solubilized lyophilized cake or silicone-cake agglomerates in dry powder drugs are also in this category. Air bubbles are especially prone to cause false failures in visual inspection. Subvisible 5–10 μm crystals of precipitated insolubles may be seen when present in numbers of 1000–2000. Haziness or "tornado" swirls in parenteral fluids are examples of such groups of small particles. The 50 μm figure may be challenged, since the minimum size particle detectable in a visual inspection by a human analyst is critically dependent on a number of factors, including:

- Nature of the particle (color, shape, opacity, reflectance);
- Type and intensity of lighting;
- Visual acuity of the inspector;
- Inspector training;
- Container clarity;
- Container volume;
- Interval of inspection; and
- Analyst fatigue/psychological factors.

The technical principles and critical parameters for automated and manual inspections differ significantly. Thus, the following discussion of visual inspection methodology is separated according to whether the test is performed using human analysts or machines.

Manual Inspection

Manual (human) inspection of parenteral solutions for particles of visible size is most commonly performed on large volume injection (LVI) solutions. For reasons that will be discussed in a following section, containers of 100 mL and greater size are not ideal subjects for a machine inspection and the adequacy of the automated inspection of large volume units of injectable solutions generally decreases as the solution volume increases.

A generalized inspection procedure for product of 50 mL and greater volume in glass containers may be conducted as follows:

1. The solution container must be free of attached labels and thoroughly cleaned. Use a dampened nonlinting cloth or sponge to remove external particles.

2. Hold the container by its top and carefully swirl the contents by rotating the wrist to start contents of the container moving in a circular motion. Vigorous swirling will create air bubbles, which should be avoided. Air bubbles will rise to the surface of the liquid; this helps to differentiate them from particulate matter.

3. Hold the container horizontally (about 4 inches below the light source) against a white and black background. Direct light should be shielded from the eyes of the inspector and the solution volume viewed on an axis normal to that of the incident light, so that particles are detected on the basis of scattered light.

4. If no particles are seen at this stage, invert the container slowly and inspect for any heavy particles that may not have been suspended by swirling.

5. Reject any container evidencing visible particles at any time during the inspection process.

Representative times of inspections for product between 50 mL and 100 mL are 10 to 20 seconds; 30 seconds to 1 minute usually suffices for units between 250 mL and 1 L.

Smaller volume containers are currently not commonly inspected by manual means. When manual inspection of ampoules was common practice, "clips" that held 10 units were often used, and an inspection time of 30 seconds to 1 minute was commonly employed for a group of 10. Despite efforts by manufacturers to standardize visual inspection methodologies. a large number of manual techniques have been used. Typically, these have in common the use of separate black and white backgrounds, illumination on an axis normal (at 90°) to the viewing axis so that particles are visualized based on the light that they scatter, and some means of pacing (timing) so that each unit is inspected for the same interval. Most companies using manual inspection have documented criteria for inspector training and some have requirements for inspector visual acuity. Figure 1 shows an inspector using one type of "light box" in current use. Historically, many different types of devices have been designed and used (Figures 2a and 2b) for visual inspection in pharmacies.

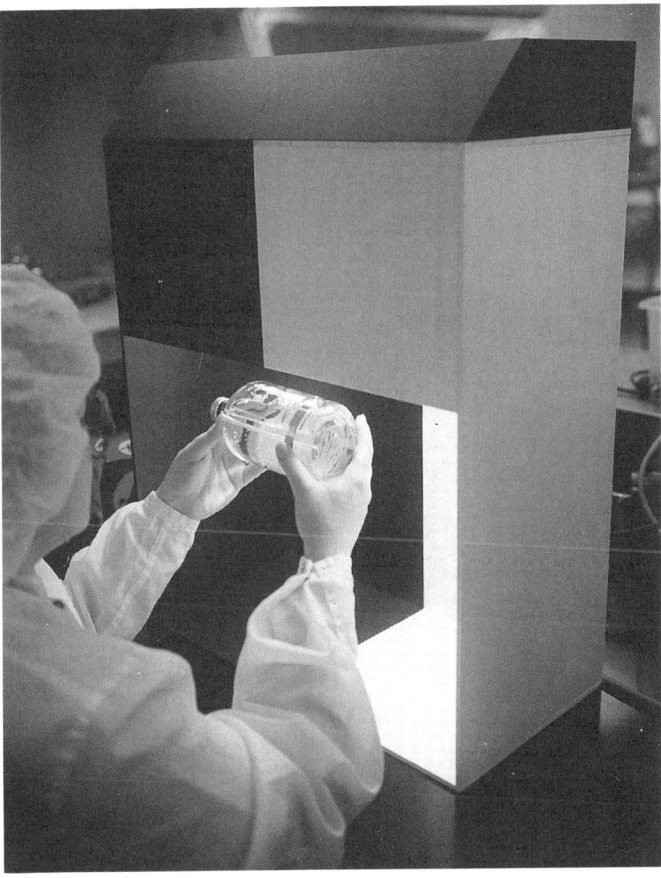

Figure 1. Manual visual inspection using a black and white background light box.

26 *Pharmaceutical Particulate Matter*

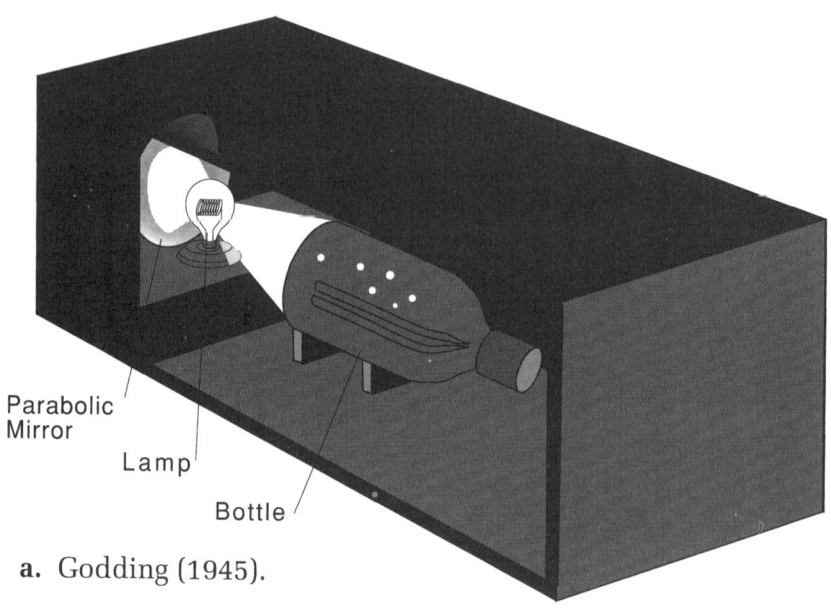

a. Godding (1945).

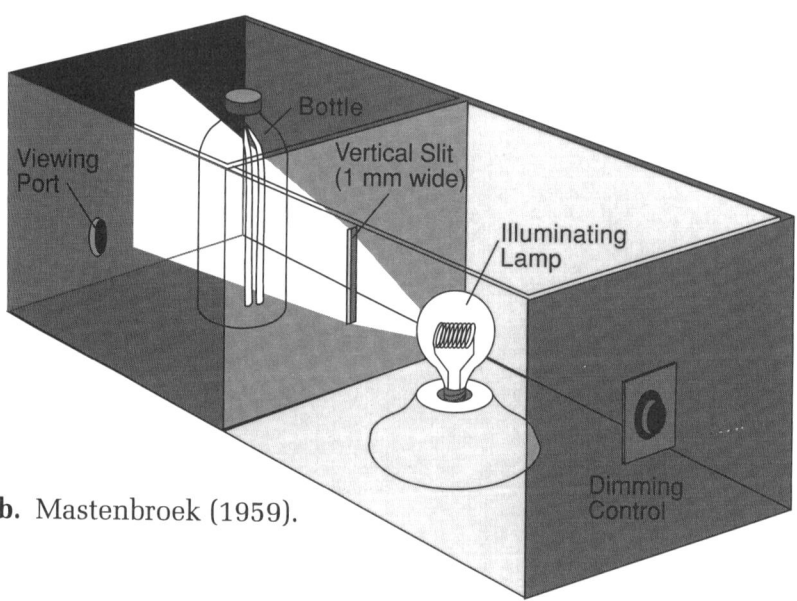

b. Mastenbroek (1959).

Figure 2. LVI inspection devices.

The devices shown in Figures 2a and 2b are primarily of historical interest; although they provide for critical inspection, they do not allow easy manipulation of the unit being inspected and do not enable the analyst to work quickly enough to inspect large numbers of units. The latter is almost invariably a key consideration in manual inspection.

One other type of device for manual inspection should also be mentioned here. It is manufactured by the P. W. Allen Co. of London, England. The ampoule viewer (Figure 3) allows inspection of single ampoules in polarized light at a magnification of 2×. The incorporation of magnification provides enhanced detection. Single manual inspection of ampoules is, of course, impractical for inspection of large numbers of units. Figure 4 shows the Allen liquid viewer. This device also allows the analyst to view the unit inspected between two (crossed) polarizer sheets and provides enhanced detection of some types of particles (such as paper fibers) in glass LVI units. One potential disadvantage of this unit is that it may not enhance detection of isotropic particles above that attained in indirect unpolarized light. In fact, it may give lower detection sensitivity for this type of particle than conventional inspection. Further, it is of somewhat limited use for plastic LVI containers since the extruded plastic sheeting or tubing of which these containers are made may be anisotropic and produce extinction

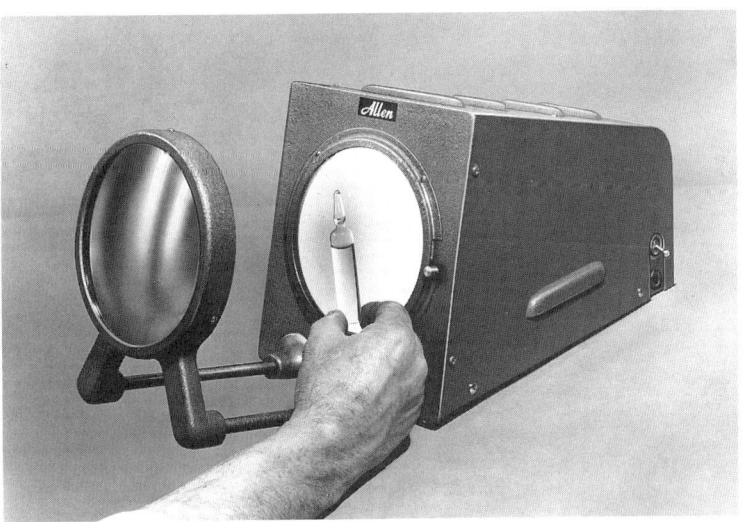

Figure 3. Ampoule viewer (Allen, Ltd.).

28 *Pharmaceutical Particulate Matter*

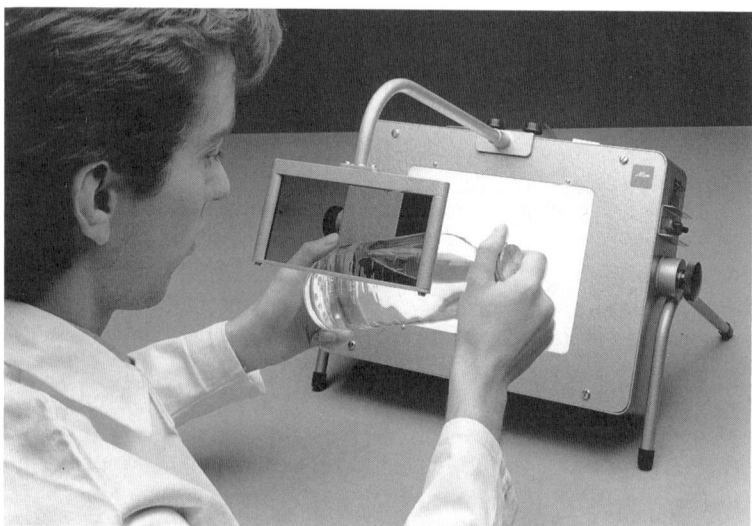

Figure 4. Allen liquid viewer (Allen, Ltd.).

---

patterns in polarized light that confuse the analysis. These devices receive fairly wide use in the United Kingdom; their application in lieu of a conventional inspection using indirect white light will obviously require validation by anyone contemplating changing their visual inspection method.

Besides manual inspection systems, numerous semiautomatic machines have been developed that use people for the detection of particles, but present the units for inspection automatically (Knapp 1987). These systems have a significantly higher throughput than manual processes because they perform most of the mechanical manipulations normally done by human analysts. These include such operations as swirling containers, inverting samples, stopping containers, and removing defects. Some authors claim that these machines reduce eye strain for the operators and provide improved inspection quality by providing more critical imaging than is possible with manual systems.

Reproducibility of Manual Inspection

There have been a number of attempts to assess the objectivity of the visual methods used for inspection of ampoules. Early evidence of the lack of objectivity was presented by Sandell (1953), who used six inspectors to assess a group of one hundred 5-mL ampoules. Each ampoule was marked and examined repeatedly by each of the inspectors, for a total of 20 inspections. The rejection rates varied between 2% and 23% (mean value 11.6%), illustrating the uncertainty of the method. Of the 100 ampoules, 51 were rejected on at least one occasion, but the worst ampoule was only rejected on 14 times out of the 20 checks, a probability of rejection of $^{14}/_{20}$ or 70%.

The results of this test are shown in Table I and clearly indicate that the manual inspection yielded unreliable results. In addition, the author suggested that if the real probability of rejection for units of a batch fell below 50%, a single inspection would be ineffectual so that final inspection for particulate matter could be neglected. This suggestion has some merit, but it seems reasonable that visual inspection would be necessary to remove those individual units with a higher than 50% probability of rejection.

Table I. Rejection Rates for 100 Ampoules Inspected 20 Times by Six Inspectors (Sandell 1953)

Number of Ampoules	Number of Times Rejected
1	14
1	12
2	11
4	10
2	9
1	8
2	7
4	6
3	5
6	4
4	3
7	2
14	1

These data illustrate a basic principle of visual inspection. It is extremely important that those conducting visual inspections understand that the process is probabilistic and not deterministic in nature. With a deterministic process, multiple inspection of the same set of containers would result in the same containers always being rejected. The rejection probability is one of two values, 0 for good units and 1 for defective units. In contrast, with a probabilistic process, each container will have some associated variable rejection probability that may be any value between 0 and 1.

Knapp and Kushner (1980b) carried out the first carefully designed experiments to determine whether human inspection was deterministic or probabilistic. In these studies, 1000 vials were examined by five inspectors 10 times each, for a total of 50 inspections, and rejection records were maintained for each vial. The summary of these results, Table II, demonstrates the range of rejection probabilities. Only 2 vials were rejected on 100% of the inspections; approximately 10% of the containers were rejected 10% of the time.

Table II. Results of Knapp and Kushner (1980b) Experiments

Rejection Probability	Number of Vials
0.0	805
0.1	98
0.2	33
0.3	17
0.4	11
0.5	10
0.6	8
0.7	6
0.8	5
0.9	5
1.0	2

Knapp et al. (1983) also defined a relationship between rejection probability and particle size. Vials with the smallest particles fell into the lowest rejection probability groups and those with the largest particles had the highest rejection probability. In summary, larger particles result in a higher detection probability. The probabilistic nature of particle detection must be considered in any compendial test.

The findings of Knapp and his co-workers are consistent with the function of the human visual process (Blackwell 1946, 1959). Accordingly, any description of visual inspection methods must include a consideration of the capability of the inspector, the size of the particle, the background illumination level, and the contrast of the particle against its background.

The existence of rejection probability zones was also introduced by Knapp and his group (Knapp and Kushner 1980b), and this key principle is commonly used for assessing the effectiveness of visual inspection systems. The range of the rejection probability, ρ, is divided into three regions:

$$0.0 \leq \rho < 0.3 \text{ Accept Zone}$$
$$0.3 \leq \rho < 0.7 \text{ Gray Zone}$$
$$0.7 \leq \rho \leq 1.0 \text{ Reject Zone}$$

The region of low rejection probability, into which the great majority of units from a controlled manufacturing process will fall, is the "Accept Zone." Higher rejection probability, the "Gray Zone," is affected by changes in the inspection process and includes a wide range of rejection probabilities. The region of most certain rejection probability was termed the "Reject Zone." This group of samples will invariably be rejected by an effective visual inspection process.

The importance of the assessment that a visual inspection (manual or machine) as a probabilistic process cannot be overemphasized. The most critical implication of this finding is that standards requiring "no visible particles" cannot be implemented or enforced. Total freedom of a product from any defect can only be achieved if the defect is an attribute, that is, it is by the means of inspection employed either present or absent with absolute certainty. A deterministic inspection procedure is essential to either the total elimination of a defect or the allowance of a specific level. A probabilistic process cannot achieve either of these ends. Another key consideration (particularly with manual inspection) is the occurrence of false rejection, or the rejection of good product.

Detection Limits of Manual Inspection

There has been considerable discussion regarding the lower size limit of particles that are visible to the unaided human eye. Saylor (1966) concluded that clear solutions in glass vials effect some magnification and, under specific conditions, it was possible for some inspectors to detect particles as small as 50 µm in size. Using a 100-watt lamp and examining against a black and white background, Brewer and Dunning (1947) were surprised to find that inspectors were rejecting ampoules that contained multiple particles of glass

1–2 mm in size. These authors had previously come to the conclusion from a literature survey and by consultation with ophthalmologists that a person with 20/20 vision under the inspection conditions should be able to detect particles of about 50 µm. That inspectors could detect very small glass particles is understandable based on the highly reflective nature of these particles and the high numbers that are occasionally found.

Later work of Knapp and Kushner (1982) and Knapp et al. (1983) provided useful information concerning detection limits for human visual inspection. The ampoules that were inspected in this study were characterized beforehand with regard to particle content using a holographic technique. A 10-second paced inspection of two ampoules at a time with a 3× magnifying lens, a diffuse light source, and a white/black background was used in performing multiple inspection of the ampoules. The light intensity on the samples was approximately 225 foot-candles and validated inspectors were used. In these studies, an approximate 70% rejection probability was obtained for a spherical particle with a diameter of 65 µm. Equivalent rejection probability using the same inspection conditions with the unaided eye would theoretically result in a 70% detection probability for a 100-µm spherical particle.

The visual inspection process for vials and ampoules has also been extensively studied by manufacturers. In results discussed by Borchert et al. (1986, 1987) at Upjohn, a set of one thousand 10-mL ampoules containing particles as shown in Table III was used. The particles were fluorescent-dyed polystyrene divinylbenzene spheres. All inspectors examined the entire group without magnification in an inspection booth with standard lighting and background conditions. Paced inspection was used with a "clip" of 10 ampoules being examined every 38 sec. The analysts chosen for the studies included both quality assurance and production inspectors. The results of one such study with 14 inspectors is shown in Table IV. Based on these data, the 70% rejection probability would occur for a spherical particle with a diameter between 100 and 165 µm. Despite the differences in inspection rates, magnification, and other conditions, these results were believed to be generally comparable with the earlier findings of Knapp. These experiments and those of Knapp et al. (1981a, 1981b, 1983) suggest that 100 µm rather than 50 µm is a reasonable lower size limit for reproducible detection in a manual inspection.

Table III. Ampoule Particulate Matter Test Set (Borchert et al. 1986)

Number of Ampoules	Number of Particles/Ampoule	Size of Particles (µm)
50	1	165
75	1	100
875	—	—

Table IV. Average Results for Inspection of 10 mL Ampoule Material from Table III (Borchert et al. 1987)

Category	Mean Rejection Probability (%)
Good	1.1
One 100-µm particle	59.0
One 165-µm particle	82.0

Reproducibility of Visual Inspection

A second, most important, characteristic of a visual inspection system is its reproducibility (Boucher 1965). If the same set of samples is examined multiple times under identical inspection conditions, one can define the rejection rate for an individual inspector or a group of inspectors. This information is critical to definition of the inspection process. In general, the performance of a manual inspection is not highly reproducible. This was clearly illustrated when a 1949 FDA court action against a U.S. manufacturer was dismissed because the FDA expert, while on the witness stand, could not distinguish his rejects in a group that included randomly selected material. There is variability in the capability of individual inspectors and the performance of each inspector can change significantly with time. For the ampoules described in Table III the rejection probability varied from 19% to 84% for 100-mm particles and from

64% to 96% for 165-μm particles. Knapp and Kushner (1982) found that for 23 inspectors testing the same group of vials, the reject rate varied from 13.7% to 49.3%.

Human inspection systems also invariably have a detectable false reject rate. The false reject containers are classified with samples having a very low rejection probability. Several factors can lead to the rejection of units that do not contain any detectable particles. Inspectors occasionally mistake an air bubble for a particle. If several samples are examined at the same time, human error may result in the removal of a good sample instead of a defective one (Hayashi 1980). In some drug formulations, immiscible components of the formulation will confuse the visual inspection. It is possible that as many as 1% of the total units rejected from a given group inspected may be false rejects. A critical issue in the inspection of reconstituted dry powder vials regards the differential solubility (different dissolution rate) of large and small particles of drug; large particles that dissolve more slowly may be perceived as extraneous particles.

Automated (Machine) Inspection

The foregoing discussion shows that the manual inspection process is a complex procedure due to the many variables involved. Automated inspection is no less difficult to deal with. Although this process appears generally to be more reproducible than human inspection, detection efficiency and sensitivity (both of which are functions of machine design) remain critical issues that must be addressed (Klein and Reuter 1978; Martyn 1970). A number of machines using different detection methods are commercially available. Although these machines are based on different electronic principles, there are common mechanical features. The paper by Knapp (1987) provides a description of available automatic and semiautomatic inspection machines. The units inspected are generally spun at a high rate of speed and the movement of the container is stopped immediately before the sample is examined. This has the effect of causing particles to rise from the bottom of the container to the top of the solution, then spiral downward after the container rotation has stopped. This spin-stop procedure results in particles being sensed as moving objects and significantly enhances detection. On most systems the spin speed can be varied. The interval between the deceleration of the container and the observation time is typically short in duration. This is necessary in order to detect heavy particles, such as glass fragments, that will settle quickly.

Visual Inspection   35

Conversely, if the interval between braking and detection is too short, bubbles will not have sufficient time to escape the solution and will not be distinguished from particulate matter contamination, thus resulting in false rejects.

The Eisai AIM series of inspection machines are widely used both in the U.S. and other countries (vendor communication 1991). The functional layout of an Eisai machine is shown in Figure 5. Figure 6 illustrates how the static division (SD) particle detection head functions. Immediately before reaching the light beam, each container is spun at high speed and stopped with proper timing so

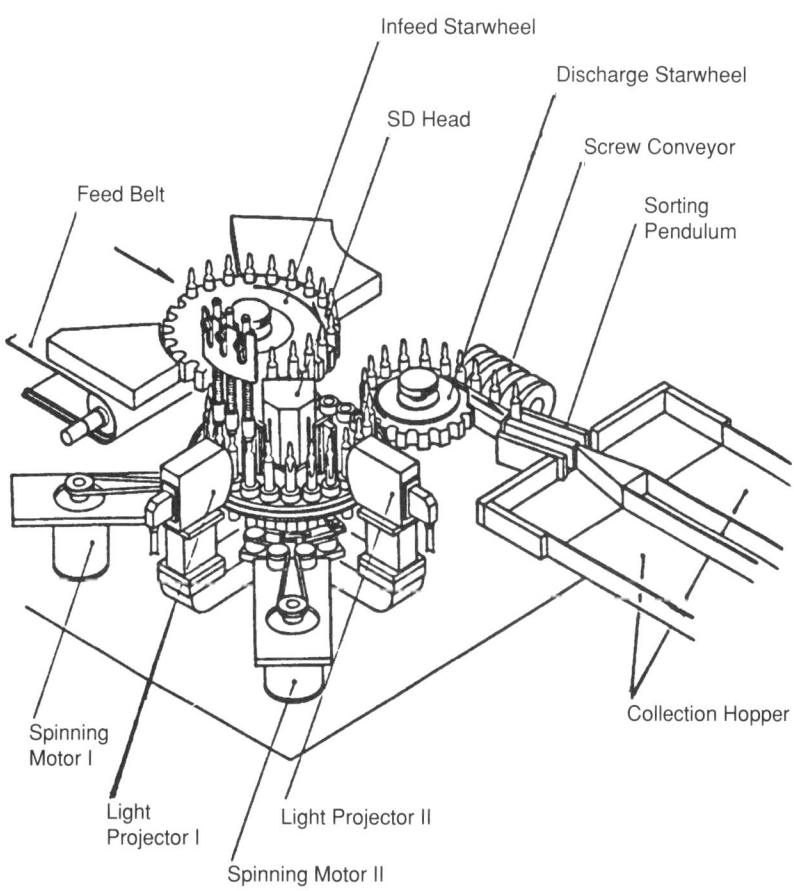

Figure 5. Functional layout of Eisai automatic inspection system for ampoules (Eisai, Ltd.).

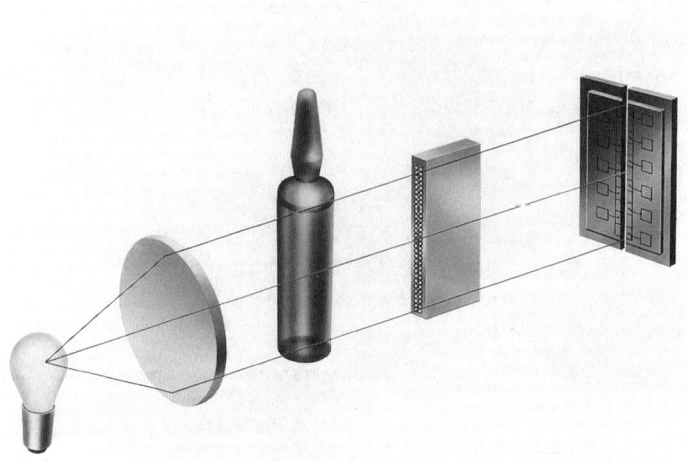

Figure 6. Detection system of Eisai automatic inspection machine (Eisai, Ltd.).

---

that only the liquid in the ampoule or vial enters the light path. If there is any particulate matter rotating with the liquid, the light transmitted through the liquid is blocked and a shadow is cast by the moving particulate matter. All Eisai machines employ a double check system that inspects each vial twice to ensure a maximum detection rate. Performance of the test is not affected by the presence of flaws or stains on the surface of the container, or the color of the particulate matter. According to the vendor, colored particulate matter is detected as accurately as noncolored particulate matter. The machine provides solution level detection simultaneously with particulate matter inspection so that empty, overfilled, or underfilled units may be rejected.

The sensor consists of a photodiode array that converts the shadow to an electrical signal. The photodiode array senses this moving shadow and evaluates its size in accordance with a preset detection sensitivity that may be based on particle size or on a manual inspection result. Only those ampoules/vials containing particulate matter outside of predetermined sensitivity levels are rejected. The photodiode array design results in an increased sensitivity over designs using a single photodiode; the shadow cast by a particle most frequently falls on only one diode of the array so that the signal-to-noise ratio is significantly increased over that which would result if a single large photodiode were used. In addition to high throughput (5K to 10K units/hour), two other operational factors typically enter into a manufacturer's decision to purchase an inspection machine. First, the potential sensitivity of some machines is greater than that of a human analyst. In experiments conducted by Eisai (Table V), a machine set for maximum sensitivity proved capable of near 100% detection of particles of sizes that were not detected with good efficiency by trained inspectors. Although the size of the insoluble foreign material detected was not specified by the vendor, the relative detection efficiency of multiple manual inspections and a single machine inspection was notably in favor of the machine. This high level of detection by the machine was based on two inspections; under some circumstances, double inspection by two human inspectors will significantly increase the level of detection in manual inspections. Secondly, when percent detection for particles of a given size is plotted against particle size threshold, machines (dependent on the model in question) typically show a very steep detection rate curve (Figure 7). It is interesting that even with these highly efficient machines, the detection process remains probabilistic.

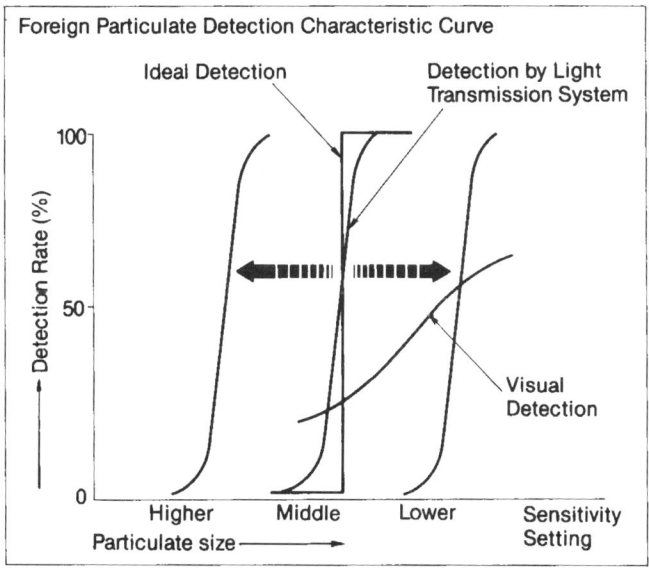

Figure 7. Particulate matter detection curve for AIM machine inspection (Eisai, Ltd.).

Table V. Detection Ratio of Foreign Matter in 2 mL Ampoule (Eisai, Ltd.)

Insoluble Foreign Matter*	Inspection by the Naked Eye	Automatic Inspection Machine
Small size glass	46%	98.8%
Middle size glass	54	100.0
Large size glass	65	100.0
Small size dust**	42	99.1
Middle size dust	60	100.0
Large size dust	89	100.0

*Small = 20 µm to 40 µm; middle size = 40 µm to 60 µm; and large size = >60 µm.
**Nonglass particulate matter.

Significant differences between automatic systems are found in the manner in which particles are detected. In the case of the Eisai machine, as discussed above, a light beam passes through the container and illuminates a linear array of photodiodes. A particle will cast a shadow on one or more of the detectors, resulting in a signal that is compared to a threshold voltage. If the signal is greater than the threshold voltage, the sample is rejected. Thus, with the Eisai machine, the threshold voltage is the sensitivity parameter. Besides this method of detection, image analysis technology and light scattering have also been utilized.

A second general operational category of automated visual inspection machines consists of those based on video imaging. The Takeda AK series machines represent the state-of-the-art of this type. With the Takeda machine (Figure 8), a video image of the solution unit, illuminated from below, is recorded with a TV camera. This image, which is projected onto a master frame, is digitized in memory. The master is then compared to successive frames of digitized video data from the unit inspected. Two inspections and 24 frames/inspection are used. If any of the digitized images are not identical to the master, an error signal results. Rejection sensitivity is determined by defining the number of error signals that correspond to a defect. Video detection systems have the advantage of allowing particles to be visualized and, in some cases, identified on line as a basis for troubleshooting.

Visual Inspection 39

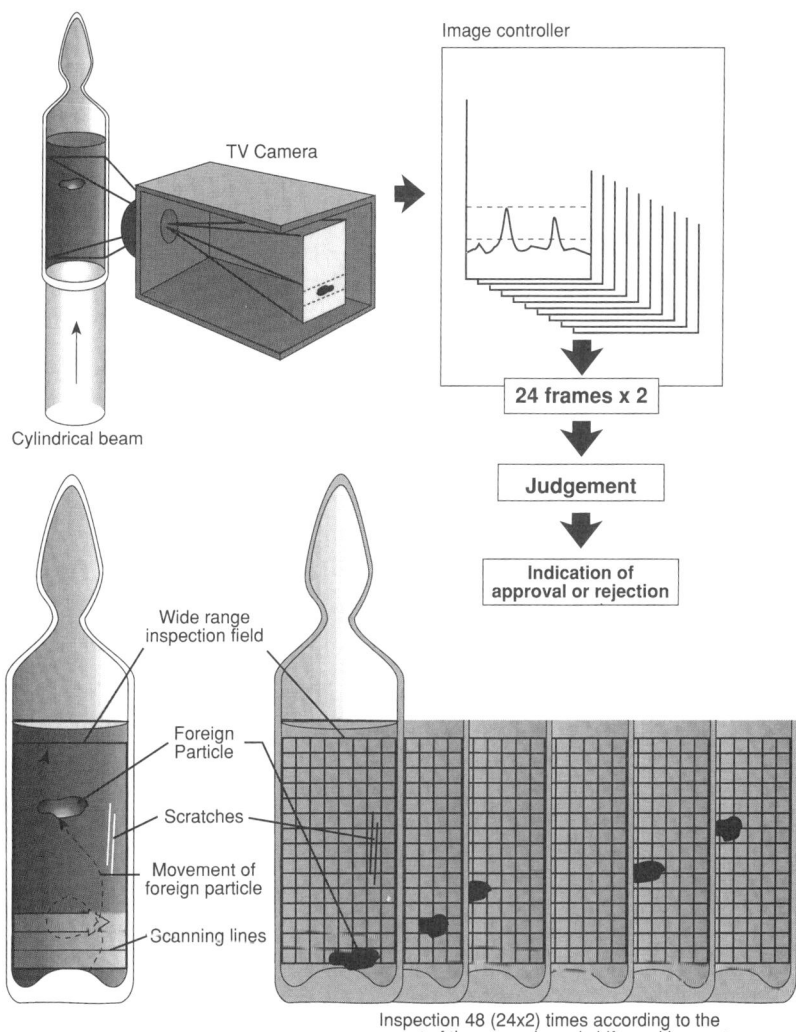

Figure 8. Operation of Takeda AK Series inspection machine (MTC Corporation).

The Takeda machines operate on the basis of light reflection off of particulates, as detected by two stationary solid state CCD TV cameras, whose highlighted image signals are recorded by computer. Judgments by the computer are made at rapid speed, comparing the original image against those appearing on subsequent frames. A total of 24 frames appear on each camera. Consequently, each vial/ampoule receives double inspection.

The method of inspection includes an electronic shift masking system. A direct image of the ampoule/vial appears on the TV monitor. The electronic mask size can be adjusted vertically and horizontally to include a wide range or specific areas of body and bottom of ampoules/vials. The highlighted signals appear in the monitor and only those in the mask are used to compare against the master image frame. At this point, computer judgment is made regarding good, recheck, or reject. This procedure occurs on each camera for each container. Foreign particles, minute and large, are discernible by their movement as they appear on the TV as grid lines. Scratches on the container are also detected by their stationary position on the grid. Sensitivity adjustments are easily made at the control panel to establish predetermined levels of rejection. A sensor detects empty containers that are automatically rejected. A key element of the system is a high-intensity halogen lamp (650 watts). This lamp generates a cylindrical high-beam with uniform intensity through the bottom of the ampoules/vials.

The data processing unit provides comprehensive information for analysis and production quality control. The data is recorded and printout is available on the total number of ampoules/vials inspected, and the number of good, rejected, and rechecked on each production run. In addition, a detection analysis mode (test mode) establishes specific sample standards for good and reject product. This mode is used for periodic validation testing to assure machine reliability.

Data collection and printout capability are available for production and detection modes as follows:

- Total number of vials inspected,
- Number of good vials,
- Number of rejected vials,
- Day of week,
- Date,
- Time (start and end),
- Clip sensitivity settings (body/bottom),
- Name of product,
- Lot number,

- Size of ampoule/vial,
- Parameter settings,
- Surface defect value,
- Ratio,
- Comment (operators' notes), and
- Rotation speed.

The data is retrievable and can be used for future production requirements.

As with human inspection, machines must be evaluated in terms of their critical key characteristics, including size detection limit, reproducibility of particle detection, and false reject rate. In general, the detection limit of machines is as low or lower than the human process. For any particular automated system the detection limit depends primarily upon the setting of the sensitivity parameter. If the response of a human inspection is well characterized, a machine inspection may be adjusted to the same sensitivity based on the use of spherical polystyrene latex particles of appropriate size. For example, if a 100 μm particle is the smallest particle that falls in the reject zone of the normal manual inspection, the machine sensitivity may simply be adjusted to give an equivalent reject rate for particles of this size.

It is interesting to note that manufacturers of visual inspection machines discuss precision and sensitivity of inspection primarily with regard to ampoule or small volume vial product. Both the human eye and automated detection systems are limited by the size of the three-dimensional solution volume that they can critically inspect within a given time and considerations of geometric optics. Ampoule inspection is, in effect, a relatively easy procedure, since swirling of the ampoule will tend to ensure motion of a particle within the focal volume of the instrument or of the human eye. The thin column of solution in an ampoule requires a shallow depth of field for inspection and the small solution volume results in minimal scattering of both the illuminating and imaging radiation (light). The fact that many of the particles found in ampoules are dark also tends to enhance levels of detection.

Eisai has overcome some of the difficulties associated with inspection of large volume units through extensive modification of their standard machine that is used for small volume product (Figure 9). The large volume container machine uses paired detectors for each detection station in place of the single detectors of the

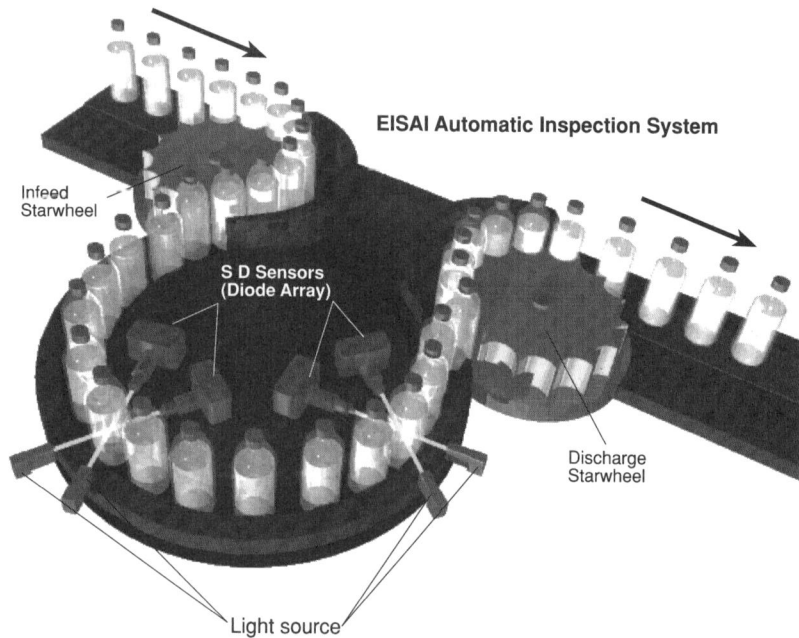

Figure 9. Eisai large volume container inspection machine.

ampoule inspection device. This design has the effect of significantly increasing the critical view volume of the machine and reportedly results in a high detection efficiency for particles of ≥40 μm in size in the critical lower half of the volume of the large containers.

Similarities exist between machine and human particle detection based on the limitation imposed by the critical inspection volume. Simply stated, there will be some limited volume within which the means of detection used may focus critically enough for particle detection. The number of critical inspection volumes in a given unit will depend both on the height and thickness of the solution volume. As larger container volumes are considered, a number of critical inspection volumes must be inspected, and there is no assurance that a moving particle in a container will be within a volume inspected at the time of inspection. With manual inspection, this is compensated for to some extent by the tendency of the human eye to "home in" on or be attracted by the motion of a particle. In the case of a machine that projects a shadow of the particle on a detector, the maker must ensure either: (1) that a particle intersecting any portion of the path of illuminating radiation produces a sufficiently well-focused shadow on the detector; or (2) that sufficient time of inspection must be allowed for a particle traveling in a helical path to move into a critical inspection volume. Similarly, with video systems, at least one comparison frame must contain a digitized image of the particle. The resulting more difficult requirements for larger volumes tend to make inspection of large volume solution units more difficult. Increasing the duration of the inspection has historically been used as a means of increasing detection capability in the inspection of LVI units.

In summary, advantages accruing to the use of automatic inspection machines that are cited by vendors and users of these machines include:

- The number of people engaged in the inspection process is significantly decreased;
- Health problems related to visual inspection, such as stiff shoulder, eyestrain, tendonitis, and so forth, are avoided;
- Consistency of particle detection is enhanced and is free from subjective human errors;
- Extensive training of personnel to perform visual inspection;
- Inspections can be conducted in an ordinary workroom without special lighting;
- Statistical evaluation of inspection results is facilitated; and,
- As a result of the more reproducible detection of smaller particles by the machine, better quality control methods may be introduced in the process from solution preparation up to filling.

Importantly, the comprehensive probabilistic theory and statistics regarding confidence of detection developed for ampoules are not directly applicable to LVI. Further, no manufacturer has as yet developed a viable inspection machine for the flexible plastic LVI containers in which much LVI product is packaged. Thus, the only referee test for the presence of particles of visible size in LVI remains a carefully performed microscopic assay performed on the total volume of solution from the unit tested. Instrumental counting methods will generally not detect particles of visible size reproducibly because of the small sample aliquots used and the low numbers of these particles that are encountered.

Application of Automated Systems

The purchase of any of the automated inspection systems presently marketed requires a large capital outlay. Their validation against an existing manual inspection process is also a nontrivial issue (Borchert et al. 1985; Digaetano 1975). The only standard for validation available in most cases is a manual process with a large amount of associated historical data (Brownley 1967). The selection of a machine must be the subject of careful consideration. The level of vendor support in terms of both validation and maintenance must be investigated, and users of the machine in question should be consulted in order to obtain information regarding the extent of satisfaction with the machine and its durability in use. While the vendors of automatic inspection machines typically claim a sensitivity and reproducibility of results exceeding those of a manual inspection, these capabilities must be tested. One method of performing this testing is to require the vendors to perform an inspection of some significant number of vials (e.g., 1000) that have been repeatedly inspected using the manual process to be duplicated. Sufficient information is provided in the referenced literature so that an objective evaluation before purchase and one site validation can be performed using the standard measurement of reject zone efficiency.

Compendial Requirements

The three most widely used compendia are the United States Pharmacopeia (USP) (1990), British Pharmacopoeia (BP) (1980) and the Japanese Pharmacopoeia (JP) (1986). None of these deal with visual inspection and the detection of visible-sized particles in any suitably definitive fashion, although the JP does attempt to specify an inspection method.

> **USP:** Good pharmaceutical practice requires that each final container of injection be subjected individually to a physical inspection, whenever the nature of the container permits, and that every container whose contents show evidence of contamination with visible foreign matter be rejected; (reconstituted dry powder dosages are essentially free of particulate matter).

BP: Injectable preparations that are solutions, when examined under suitable conditions of visibility, are clear and practically free of particles.

JP: When the outer surface of the container is cleaned, injectable solutions or solvents for drugs to be dissolved before use must be clear and free from foreign insoluble matter that is readily noticeable when inspected with unaided eyes at a luminous intensity of about 1000 luxes (93 foot-candles), directly under an incandescent electric bulb. As for injections contained in plastic containers, the inspection is performed with unaided eyes at a luminous intensity of 8000 to 10,000 luxes (740 to 930 foot-candles) with an incandescent electric bulb placed at appropriate distances above and below the container.

As discussed above, the inspection rate, the amount of magnification, the visual acuity of the inspectors, the type of illumination and background that are used, and other factors, can have a significant effect on the detection of particulate matter. It is impossible to specify an absolute compendial requirement (i.e., absence of any visible particulate matter) due to the highly variable (probabilistic) nature of the inspection process for particles of visible size. This is a basic problem that the USP, BP, and JP have wrestled with for many years. While it is not possible to specify that product will have no visible particulate matter, the GMPs and the attention of manufacturers in the various countries subject to these compendia to the issue of large (visible-sized) particles in product has resulted in product that has an extremely low particle burden for particles of visible size.

Application of a 100% inspection process as a means of eliminating units containing particles ≥100 µm in size is unquestionably practical for ampoule product, for which a very critical visual inspection can be applied. Although small volume injections can also be inspected automatically, vial product may have particles adherent to the closure that are released during transport. Thus, visible particles undetected by the 100% inspection at manufacture may be seen by the user. Dry powder vials cannot be inspected at manufacture because visual inspection is a destructive analysis for this product type. Ironically, ampoules are not only the product type most readily 100% inspected, but are also the product type that most often contains the highest levels of large particles (glass fragments) when used (Uhlir 1973, 1974). It is impossible for the manufacturer to inspect LVI product critically enough so that assurance of no visible particles can be obtained. This is due not only to the fact that particles not present in the solution during the manufacturer's inspection may be released during transport or storage, but to the critical parameters of both automated and manual inspection and the general unsuitability of many plastic container types for inspection. Translucent plastic containers cannot be inspected as critically by either automated or manual means.

This effectively brings us to the same consideration that has been reached regarding the occurrence of subvisible particles in parenterals. The control of particulates by inspection is not practical for the majority of injectable products. Particulates must be controlled by a carefully validated and monitored process operated strictly under the principles of GMP. The manufacture of LVI product in Japan is illustrative of this principle. Much of LVI product in Japan is marketed in translucent polyethylene containers that cannot be critically inspected by either human or automated methodology. Nonetheless, the levels of particles of visible size in these containers are very low (such particles are almost nonexistent). This low level of particulate matter is achieved through manufacturing steps that are designed and validated to generate product with an extremely low level of visible-sized particles. These include a high level of attention to container component cleanliness, and laminar airflow protection of the container with HEPA-filtered air at all process points. Thus, a suggestion for compendial groups who struggle with requirements for visible particulate matter is to require control by careful process validation and monitoring rather than to rely on compendial requirements that include such phrases as "essentially free," "practically free," or "bear no evidence of." These requirements are of limited usefulness and are, therefore, unenforceable.

Summary

Visual inspection of parenteral products is a complex undertaking. Both manual and automatic analyses involve significant error sources. For manual procedures, validation of inspectors and inspection methodology are necessary if a reproducible result is to be obtained. The primary consideration must be the definition of the reject probability for particles of a given size with the system used. Objective evaluation of automated systems can only be performed on the basis of a thoroughly understood manual process. Automatic systems are highly effective for the inspection of small volume liquid vials and ampoules, but far less useful for containers of greater than 100 mL volume.

References

Archambault, G. F., and A. W. Dodds. 1966. Macroscopic light-testing procedure for large volume parenterals. *Safety of Large Volume Parenteral Solutions,* 15–17. Washington, D.C.: FDA.

Blackwell, H. R. 1946. Contrast thresholds of the human eye. *Journal Opt. Soc. Am.* 36:624–643.

Blackwell, H. R. 1959. Development and use of a quantitative method for specification of interior illumination levels on the basis of performance data. *Illum. Eng.* LVI:317–353.

Borchert, S. J., A. Childers, L. Fox, D. Myer, and A. Reynhout. 1987. Preparation of standards and metrology. In *Proc. PDA Conference on Liquid Borne Particle Inspection and Metrology,* 122–166. Washington, D.C.

Borchert, S. J., R. Gaines, and J. R. Kraska. 1985. Validation of the Eisai visual inspection system. In *Proc. Europe Conf. on Visible and Subvisible Particles in Parenteral Products,* (October):224–260. European Org. Q.C.

Borchert, S. J., R. J. Maxwell, R. L. Davison, and D. S. Aldrich. 1986. Standard particulate sets for visual inspection systems: Their preparation, evaluation, and applications. *Journal of Parenteral Science and Technology* 40:6–18.

Boucher, C. L., and H. A. Sloot. 1965. An improved method for visual inspection of injections. *Pharm. Weekblad Ned.* 100:253–262.

Brewor, J. H., and J. H. F. Dunning. 1947. An i*n vitro* and *in vivo* study of glass particles in ampoules. *Journal of the American Pharmaceutical Association* 36:289–299.

British Pharmacopoeia. 1980. Vol. II. London: Her Majesty's Stationery Office.

Brownley, C. A. 1967. Statistical analysis of parenteral product rejects. *Bulletin Paren. Drug Assoc.* 21:77–97.

Digaetano, T. N. 1975. Optimizing the Einhart autoskan inspection system using the EVOP method. *Bull. Paren. Drug Assoc.* 29:183–197.

Eisai Ltd. 1991. Personal communication.

Godding, E. W. 1945. Foreign matter in solutions of injection. *Pharm. Jour.* 154:124–132.

Hayashi, T. 1980. Studies on the particulate matter in parenteral solutions: Part I. Occurrence and size distribution of particulate matter in parenteral solutions. *Yakuzaigaku* 40:62–67.

Klein, H. J., and E. W. Reuter. 1978. Automatic electronic inspection device for the detection of particles in ampoules. *Pharm. Ind.* 40:1357–1366.

Knapp, J. 1987. Process control by non-destructive testing. In *Proc. PDA Conf. on Liquid Borne Particle Inspection and Metrology*, 521–562. Washington, D.C.

Knapp, J. Z., and H. K. Kushner. 1980a. Implementation and automation of a particulate detection system for parenteral products. *J. Paren. Drug. Assoc.* 34:369–393.

Knapp, J. Z., and H. K. Kushner. 1980b. Generalized methodology for evaluation of parenteral inspection procedures. *J. Parent. Drug Assoc.* 34:14–61.

Knapp, J. Z., and H. K. Kushner. 1982. Particulate inspection of parenteral products: From biophysics to automation. *J. Paren. Sci. Tech.* 36:121–127.

Knapp, J. Z., H. K. Kushner, and L. R. Abramson. 1981a. Particulate inspection of parenteral products: An assessment. *J. Paren. Sci. Tech.* 35:176–185.

Knapp, J. Z., H. K. Kushner, and L. R. Abramson. 1981b. Automated particulate detection for ampoules using the probabilities particulate detection model. *J. Paren. Sci. Tech.* 35:21–35.

Knapp, J. Z., J. C. Zeiss, B. J. Thompson, J. S. Crane, and P. Dunn. 1983. Inventory and measurement of particulates in sealed sterile containers. *J. Paren. Sci. Tech.* 37:170–179.

Kramer, W. 1970. Inspection for particulate matter essential to I.V. additive program. *Drug Intel. & Clin. Pharm.* 4 (Nov):311–313.

Mastenbroek, G. G. A. 1959. The problem of particles in infusion solutions. Ph.D. diss., University of Amsterdam.

Martyn, G. W. 1970. Utilization of RONDO unscrambler and strunck units in ampoule inspection. *Bull. Paren. Drug Assoc.* 24:231–244.

Sandell, E. 1953. Inspection control during ampoule filling. *Farmacevtisk Revy* 52:859–870.

Sandell, E., and B. Ashlund. 1974. Visual inspection of ampoules. *Acta Pharm. Sued.* 11:504–508.

Saylor, H. M. 1966. Particulate matter, II—Visual inspection. *Bull. of Paren. Drug Assoc.* 20:31–44.

The Pharmacopoeia of Japan. 1986. 11th Ed. Tokyo: Takeji Nippo, Ltd., 20–21.

The United States Pharmacopeia. 1990. 22nd Ed. Easton, PA: Mack Printing Company, <788>:1596.

Uhlir, A. 1973. Testing of ampules for undissolved impurities. Part I: Evaluation method. *Pharm. Ind.* 35:356–371.

Uhlir, A. 1974. Testing of ampules for undissolved impurities. Part 2: Evaluation method. *Pharm. Ind.* 36:582–597.

III

Instrumental Particle Counting

Specifics regarding counting and sizing of particles using light extinction counters and electrical zone sensing (the Coulter principle) are contained in the references cited for this chapter. The general discussion provided here is intended to provide the reader with a basic familiarity with this instrumentation. The primary advantages of electronic particle counters are their automated characteristics and the rapidity with which they allow performance of particulate matter analysis. There also are disadvantages to their use. Electronic particle counters cannot discriminate between various types of particles; data collected are subject to artifact and require review by a well-trained analyst. The instruments are relatively complex in operation, and they require a time-consuming calibration at regular intervals. Comparisons of the count data obtained by instrumental and microscopic methods of counting particles in parenteral products are discussed in the references (DeLuca 1977; DeLuca et al. 1988; Schroeder and DeLuca 1980; Montanari et al. 1986; Hopkins and Young 1974). As I stated in the preface, any purchase of instruments of this type should be based on a thorough understanding of the instrument's operating principle and capabilities; the counters presently made by a number of vendors are very competitive in terms of performance and purchase price.

The Coulter Principle

The Coulter technique allows determination of the size and number of particles suspended in an electrolyte solution based on their passage through a small orifice in a glass tube that separates two electrodes of opposite potential. The principle is illustrated in Figure 1. The changes in resistance as particles pass through the orifice generate voltage pulses of amplitudes proportional to the volumes of the particles. The pulses are amplified, sorted, and counted, and from the resulting data the number and size distribution of the particulate matter may be determined (Lines 1967a,

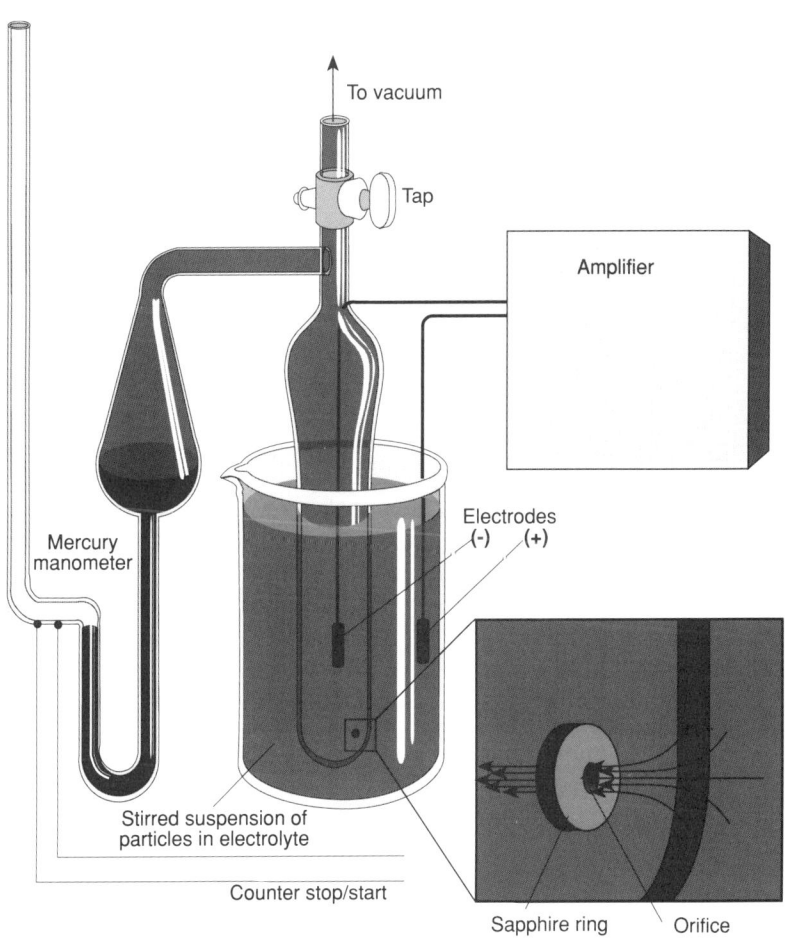

Figure 1. Operational principles of the Coulter counter.

1967b, 1981). Coulter instruments were the first automatic instruments to be widely applied for counting particles in parenterals (Kinsman 1969; Amaker and Boymund 1967).

The amplified voltage pulses produced by particles are passed to a pulse collection circuit having multiple adjustable threshold levels. On some models the threshold levels and pulse amplitudes may be visualized on an oscilloscope on the instrument as the analysis is conducted. In the total mode of pulse collection, all pulses above a given threshold level are counted, and this count represents the number of particles larger than some volume proportional to the appropriate size threshold setting. The Coulter instruments currently marketed, such as the Multi-sizer, allow counts to be separated into a large number of channels so that a relative frequency distribution or population analysis may be performed. This is accomplished by simply collecting a series of counts between each of a number of sequentially increasing threshold settings. Aperture tubes are available for direct insertion into solution units (Lines 1967b).

Coulter counters employ an aperture tube with an aperture of known size that is immersed in a volume of the parenteral solution to be tested. The ratio of particle diameter to orifice diameter should be 2% to 60% for the optimum proportionality of resistance change and particle volume. A 30 µm or 50 µm aperture tube is thus generally acceptable for counting particles in the ≥2 µm size range; a 100 µm aperture is appropriate for counting at the USP size ranges of ≥10 µm and ≥25 µm. Apertures suitable for counting over a range of 0.4 µm to 1200 µm are also available. As noted, the Coulter principle is based on the fact that change in resistance between the instrument electrode is directly proportional to the volume of the particle. The Coulter counter thus sizes a particle as a three-dimensional object, in contrast to light extinction counters that see a particle in two dimensions and size particles based on area of light extinction. The Coulter principle of measurement is thus less sensitive to particle shape.

One significant disadvantage of the Coulter method is the requirement for an ionic (conducting) diluent if the solution to be tested is not itself ionic in nature. Sterile sodium chloride for injection (0.9% concentration) is commonly used as a diluent. The diluent solution itself (or the dilution process) may also add a significant number of particles to the sample, and thorough filtration of the diluent solution is desirable. Blank controls must also be utilized, and the particulate matter contribution caused by the added electrolytic solution may be subtracted if desired. A more acceptable procedure is to filter the diluent at the 0.45 µm size using a recirculating filtration device offered by the vendor. For apertures of <30 µm in size, a 4–5% sodium chloride concentration is satisfactory, but for larger apertures 1% electrolyte concentration should be used.

The Coulter instruments employ a mercury-filled manometer to sample from 500 µL to 2 mL of the I.V. solution tested. Counts of extraneous particles in LVI collected in this small volume may be too low for appropriate statistical strength, necessitating repetitive counting or counting for longer intervals. Due to the positioning of the aperture and the low flow rate of solution through it, large particles may be drawn into the orifice in disproportionately low numbers, resulting in undercounting (Harfield and Wood 1972; Blanchard et al. 1977). As with any instrumental analysis, air bubbles adversely affect accurate counting. Air bubbles are eliminated by either minimized agitation during sampling, or application of a vacuum before measurement or sonication. Electrical background noise, vibration, and electrical fields also contribute to some error in counting. The Coulter analysis is also more time-consuming than other types of instrumental analysis. Despite these drawbacks, particulate matter in the subvisible size range present in intravenous solutions can be accurately counted using Coulter counters, if the user takes the time necessary to understand and master the technology before beginning to count for record (Barnett 1987; DiGrado 1970).

The Coulter principle for particle counting was discovered in the late 1940s. The available instruments have been updated successively since that time, and the current microprocessor-based instruments provide for a high level of versatility in use. The Multisizer II model allows data collected to be displayed on the instrument monitor in a wide range of formats. Optimum resolution for the sample tested may be obtained by selecting the number of size classes (channels) into which the size distributions can be subdivided. The instrument contains a multi-channel analyzer board, and from 16 to 256 channels of data can be obtained over a 30:1 dynamic size range on the full range analysis. Use of Narrow and Window modes allows the equivalent of 25,600 channel size resolutions to be obtained.

The British Pharmacopoeia (BP) recognizes the Coulter counter as one of the two official methods for performing compendial particle assays (the other is light extinction). In the United States, the instrument is not often applied for compendial counting, but remains very popular for particle population analyses where dilution factors and small sample volumes are not necessarily detrimental to the accuracy of the resulting data. One advantage of the Coulter counter in the analysis of flake-like or acicular (needle-like) particles is the precision of the count result. These particles are sized based on the conversion of their volume to an equivalent spherical volume. This is a decided improvement over the light extinction counter that "sees" flakes or aciculars as being different sizes depending on the aspect presented to the sensor.

Light Extinction Counting

The key reference for this means of counting was presented in the paper by Carver (1969). The method is currently widely used in the pharmaceutical industry in the U.S. and abroad (Montanari et al. 1986). The data obtained from light extinction counters result from complex interactions between a small particle moving at high velocity, and an intense light beam in the narrow confines of the particle counter sensor (Figure 2). In the sensor, the sample fluid travels through a narrow rectangular passage 0.025 mm^2–0.5 mm^2 in cross section in front of an illuminated window. The light from an incandescent lamp or laser is formed into a collimated beam at the window, and directed through the liquid sample stream and onto a photodiode. As long as the number of particles in suspension does not exceed a specified concentration, the particles will pass through the sensor view volume individually. Whenever a particle traverses the light beam, the intensity of light reaching the photodiode is reduced and an amplified voltage pulse is produced by the sensor. In theory, the amplitude of the pulse is proportional to the projected area of the particle in a plane normal to the light beam, and the particle size is registered as the diameter of the circle having an equivalent projected area. The sample solution maybe passed through the sensor cell by applying either pressure or vacuum; pressure sampling has obvious advantages for viscous liquids such as concentrated dextrose solutions.

The analog signal from the sensor is sent to a counter unit, and converted into a digital form that can be read and stored in memory by a dedicated microprocessor. As with the Coulter counter, pulses are sorted and counted within channels determined by preset voltage amplitude thresholds in order to measure particle size distributions. In the differential mode of counting, the pulse produced by the particle is recorded as a count only in that channel with a range in mV that includes the pulse produced by the particle; in the total or cumulative mode, the pulse from the particle triggers a count in

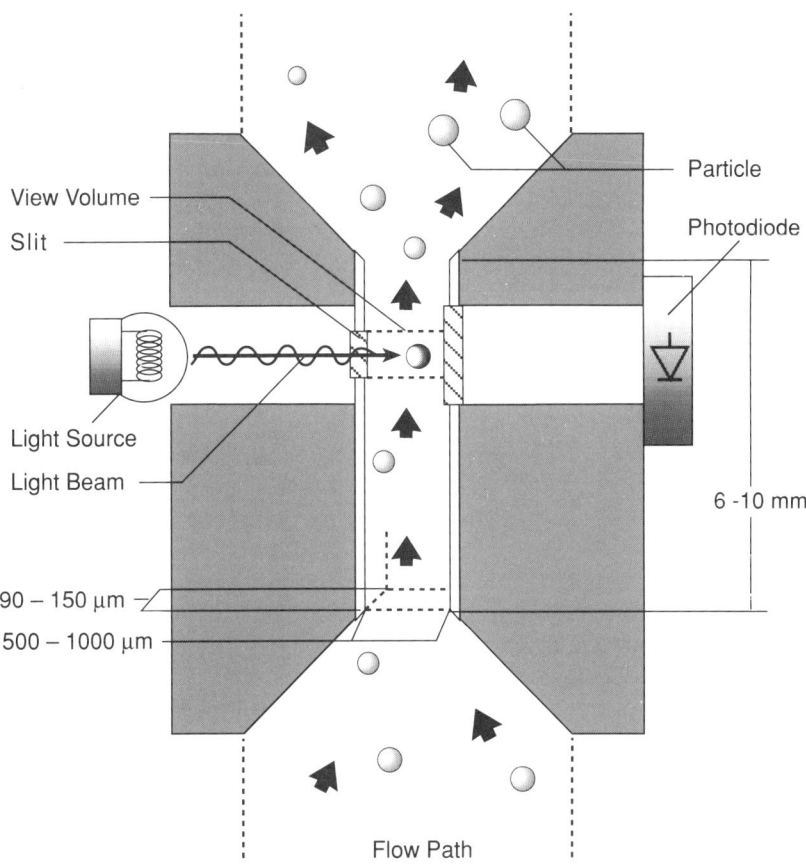

Figure 2. Light extinction particle sensor.

all channels with a threshold setting in mV below that of the pulse produced by the particle. Contemporary light extinction sensors can count up to 40,000 particles/mL at a flow rate of 5 mL/minute; sensor characteristics (flow rate, sensitivity, and concentration limit) vary extensively dependent upon design and intended use.

The stated theoretical relationship between the size of the particle and the amplitude of the voltage pulse in light extinction counting produced is given as:

$$E_o = \frac{\lambda}{A} E_b$$

where E_o = pulse amplitude from photo-detector
 λ = maximum projected area of the particle
 A = area of the window
 E_b = 10 V, the base voltage from the photo detector

The interaction of a particle with light in the view volume of a light extinction sensor is not as simple as this relationship suggests (Figure 3). This equation is generally appropriate, but it does not take into consideration refractive index, light absorption, and light scattering effects; all of which can impact the result obtained in light extinction counting.

Resolution is a key factor in the performance of light extinction sensors. This term describes the range of pulse voltages that will be produced by the sensor for particles of a single size. Poor resolution (i.e., broadening of the pulse response distribution) will result in decreased accuracy and precision of count data. Nonuniform illumination in the sensor is the primary cause of variances in sensor response for particles of the same size. This variance is typically several percent of the mean diameter of particles in the 5 µm to 20 µm range. Under normal sampling conditions, however, the particles are randomly distributed throughout the cell, and a statistical averaging process applies to the pulses generated.

Most currently used light extinction counters have white light sensors with size measurement ratios of 1:60. Vendors commonly

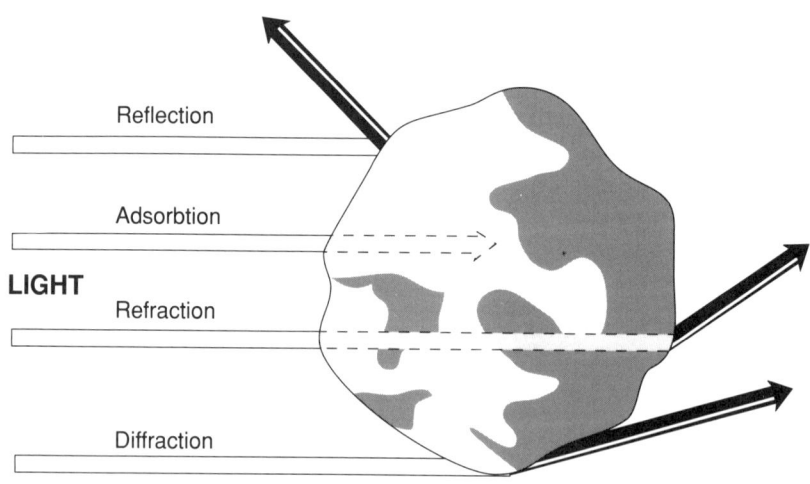

Figure 3. Interaction of particle with incident light.

specify dynamic measurement range in the sensor technical description or model designation. A 1-60 sensor can measure particles from 1 µm to 60 µm, while a 2.5-150 sensor can measure particles ranging from 2.5 µm to 150 µm. Over the past several years, light extinction counter systems have progressed significantly with regard to technology, user friendliness, and automation. Hiac/Royco, Climet, Particle Measuring Systems, Rion, and Met-One all currently offer systems operating on this principle.

The light extinction particle counting method is the USP compendial test for particulate matter in small volume injections (SVI) (United States Pharmacopeia 1990). The test is summarized in Figure 4. The current test provides for pooling 10 units and performing counts on the pooled volume. This is generally adequate for ampoule product or vial product of <20 mL volume, but SVI units of 25 mL and greater are more appropriately tested on a single unit basis.

The user should also be aware of the potential pitfalls of using this method. Results of the instrumental assay cannot be expected to agree in any predictable fashion with those of a microscopic test (Rebagay et al. 1977a, 1977b; DeLuca 1977; DeLuca et al. 1987; Schroeder and DeLuca 1980). Product types analyzed should be well-understood with regard to inherent sources of artifact, including production of gas bubbles, refractive index effects, and droplets of dispersed immiscible liquids. The various potential sources of error are outlined in detail in referenced publications (Barber 1987; Barber and Williams 1990). The user should also be aware that although light extinction sensors with a similar dynamic range have a generally similar response to particles found in parenterals, there may be specific sensitivity differences related to particle refractive index, or type of sensor illumination used (white light, diode laser, gas laser) that should be investigated before an instrument is purchased or applied to a broad range of product types.

Before proceeding, I must briefly reemphasize the current wide availability of light extinction counting systems suitable for use in counting particulate matter in pharmaceuticals and medical products. I have based the following discussion of laser and white light sensors on Hiac/Royco instrumentation, but principles of operation of sensors manufactured by other vendors are sufficiently similar so that the same considerations apply. Other vendors of counters with light and/or laser sensors include Climet, Malvern, and Met-One. Particle Measuring Systems has both laser diode and gas laser sensors, and their units feature an extremely high level of automation and user-friendliness. Rion instruments are made in Japan and,

58 Pharmaceutical Particulate Matter

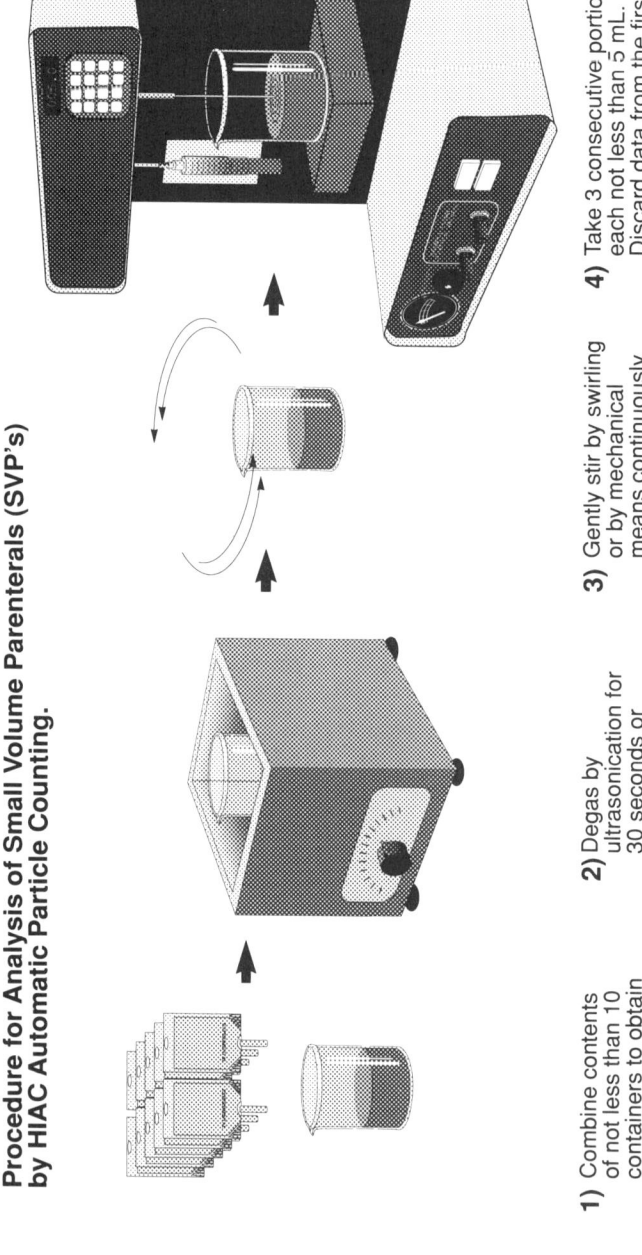

Figure 4. USP <788> light extinction test for SVI.

based on limited the reports I have received, they are also appropriate for pharmaceutical applications.

Laser Versus White Light Extinction Sensors

The function of these two types of light extinction sensors is well-discussed in the papers by Holger Sommer (1990a, 1990b, 1991). Much of the following information is drawn from these references. Some amount of pressure is being placed on pharmaceutical users of light extinction instruments to convert from the older model white light sensors to the newer laser diode models by the instrument manufacturers. Prior to replacing white light sensors with the newer laser diode type, the user should become familiar with the functional difference between the two. The laser diode sensors embody a number of advantages. Since monochromatic light is produced by laser diodes, all optical elements can be optimized for the laser diode wavelength. This theoretically results in better resolution, since the measuring volume is more accurately defined as to height, and is more uniformly illuminated; particles of the same size passing through different parts of the view volume would be expected to give pulses of similar magnitude. In all current generation light extinction sensors, the height of the view volume or sensing zone is defined by the thickness of the ribbon of illuminating radiation in the solution path, rather than by an aperture. The dimension of the radiating area of the laser diode (laser cavity) is orders of magnitude smaller than the tungsten filament of an incandescent light bulb, resulting in a smaller measuring volume height. This improves both the concentration limit and the dynamic range of the sensors.

Long source lifetime is probably the most desirable feature of the laser diode. White light extinction sensors generally suffer from short bulb life (approximately 500 hours maximum, in the author's experience). Heat has a detrimental effect on bulb life because the bulb is enclosed and typically not well-cooled. The sensitivity of the filament to mechanical vibrations affects the performance of white light extinction sensors and limits their applications in environments with mechanical vibration. The laser diode is insensitive to vibrations within reasonable limits. Despite the considerable advantages of the laser diode sensors, the user should be aware that these sensors may potentially detect and count some types of particles differently than white light sensors, and that their calibration differs significantly from that of white light models. The operational principles of the two types of sensors are discussed below along with some practical considerations related to their use.

White Light Sensors

Early white light extinction sensors were of very simple design (Carver 1969). In these models, a tungsten bulb with an integral lens illuminated the window of a microcell, and the light beam thus formed illuminated the flow passage of the sensor. Because of generally poor definition of the light beam, poor collimation, and intensity variations across the beam, these sensors featured rather poor resolution. Figure 5 shows an assembly drawing of an early Hiac/Royco CMH-type sensor. Despite its disadvantages, this type of sensor was compact, rugged, and was widely used.

The resolution and the concentration limit of the extinction sensor was improved when imaging optics were applied in forming the sensor light beam. The Hiac/Royco HR-type sensor, introduced in the early 1970s, used a nonadjustable lens system to project an image of a 100 µm slit aperture (illuminated by the filament of a low voltage incandescent bulb) into the flow passage of the sensor, thus defining the view volume of the sensor more precisely. Figure 6 shows this sensor type. The optical dimension (height) of the measuring volume in this design depends on the quality of the imaging optics. A more uniform illumination of the view volume improved the resolution with this design. In addition, the reduced size of the view volume permitted higher concentrations of particles to be counted than with the earlier Hiac/Royco models.

In the HA series of HR white light sensors (Figure 7) particle size resolution can be optimized by adjusting sensor alignment with a pulse-height analyzer. The more sophisticated optical

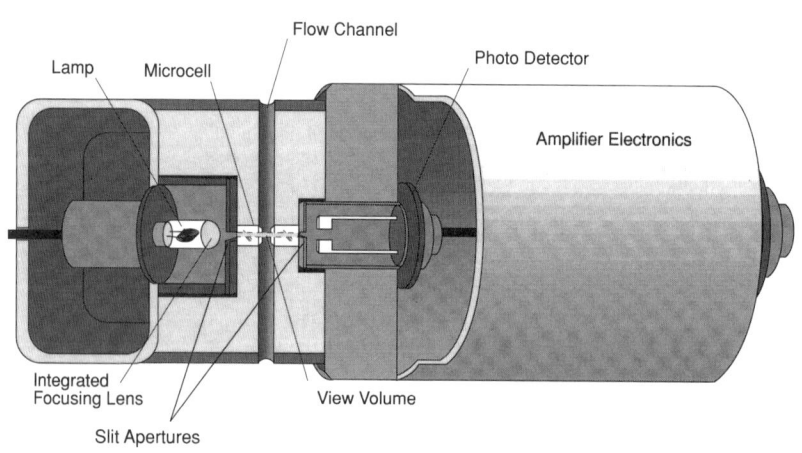

Figure 5. Hiac/Royco CMH-type light extinction sensor.

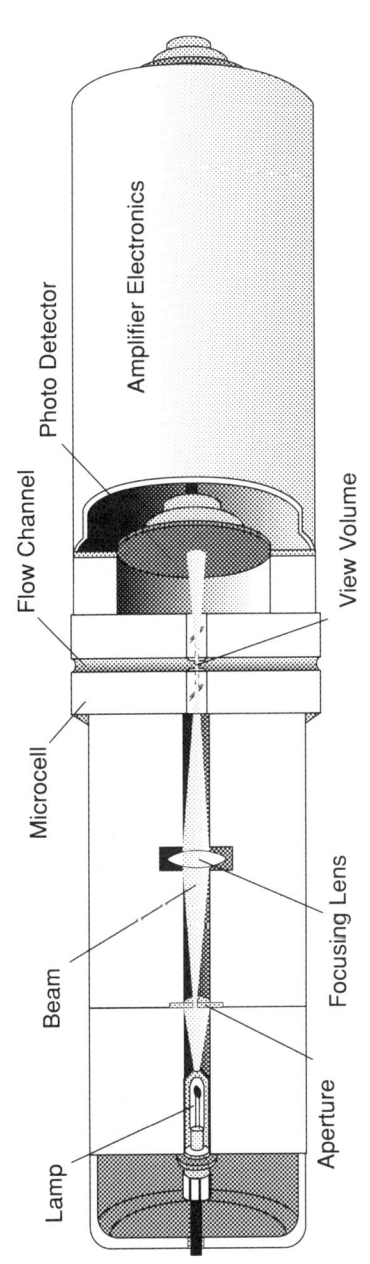

Figure 6. Hiac/Royco HR-type white light extinction sensor.

system consists of four moveable components that can be aligned to optimize resolution. Vibration sensitivity of the HA series sensors is shared between the light source and optical components. Sensor performance in the HA series is not dependent on tolerances of machined parts and optical components, but can be improved by compensating parts imperfections with alignment procedures. Through this design, almost identical responses to calibration materials by different sensors can be achieved.

Importantly, the particle size response of a white light sensor is typically characterized by a simple power law relationship between particle diameter and pulse height. This results in a straight line response curve for log size versus log voltage within the dynamic range (Figure 8).

Laser Diode Sensors

Figure 9 shows the optical arrangement of a typical laser diode sensor. The laser diode is mounted on a rigid, thermally conductive metal support to keep it near ambient temperature, thus prolonging its lifetime. The typical laser diode source life at 25°C is

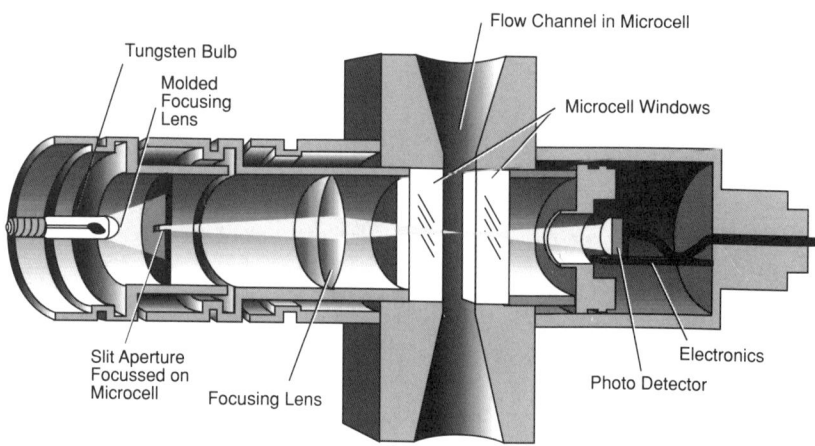

Figure 7. HR HA-type white light extinction sensor.

---

optimistically estimated by the vendor to be one million hours or longer at the nominal 3 mV output of the laser. While this figure may not be achieved, the source life is far greater than that of an incandescent bulb. The laser is a gallium aluminum arsenide type, with an active laser cavity of about 20 µm × 10 µm in cross section. The illumination from the laser diode is uncollimated. It emerges in a flattened cone with half angles in the range of 10 degrees by 40 degrees. This point light source is imaged by high numerical aperture optics (a collimating and focusing lens) and focused into the center of the microcell. To provide uniform illumination of the entire depth of the microcell, a negative cylindrical lens is placed between the cell and the collimation optics. This optical arrangement provides a very uniform ribbon of light in the flow passage, providing the potential for excellent particle size resolution.

One major difference between these two types of sensors is view volume size. With laser light, optics can be optimized for a single wavelength and a view volume height of 20 µm to 50 µm can be achieved. This results in a higher illumination power density and a lower particle size sensitivity limit. With the white light sensor, this view volume height is more likely to be 100 µm to 150 µm.

The intensity of the light passing through the cell is monitored by a high-speed photodetector that is mounted directly to the sensor circuit board. The change of intensity on the detector due to the presence of a particle in the measuring volume is registered as an

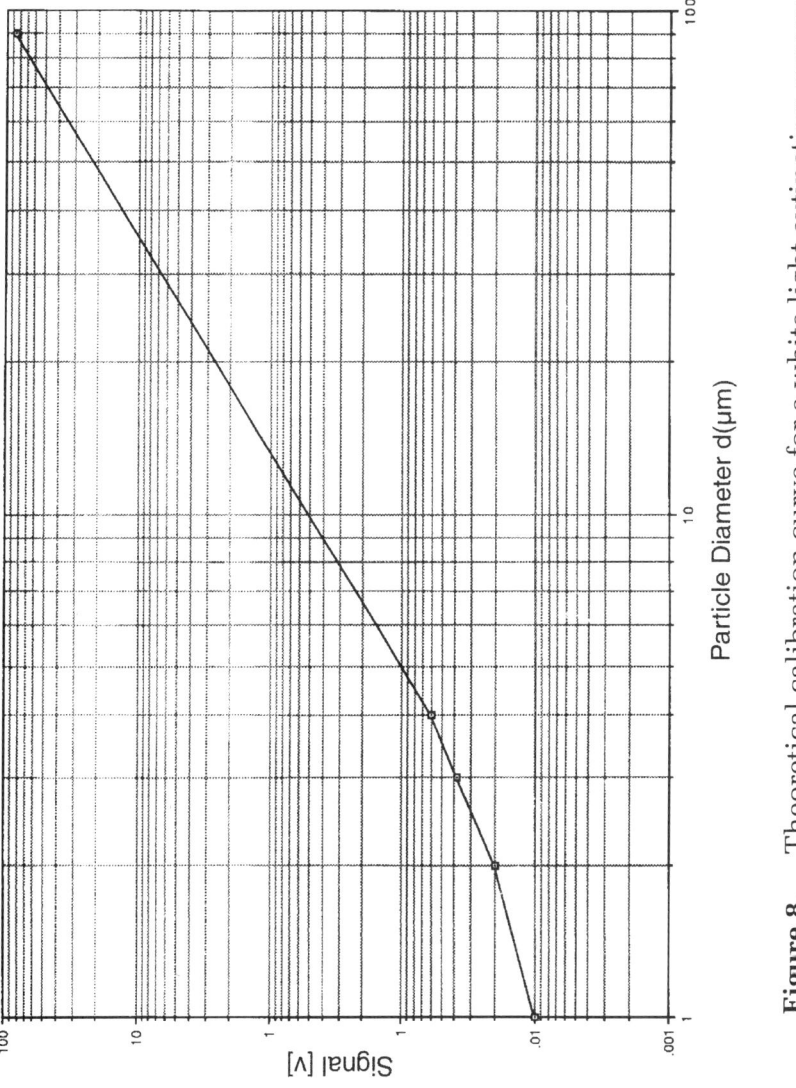

Figure 8. Theoretical calibration curve for a white light extinction sensor.

inverted pulse. The signals are converted to pulses acceptable by standard electronic counting and sizing circuitry, which determines the particle sizes from the height of the signal pulses. The laser power is adjusted automatically so that the power reaching the detector is constant. This maintains the accuracy of the calibration curve independent of the absorbance of the carrier fluid.

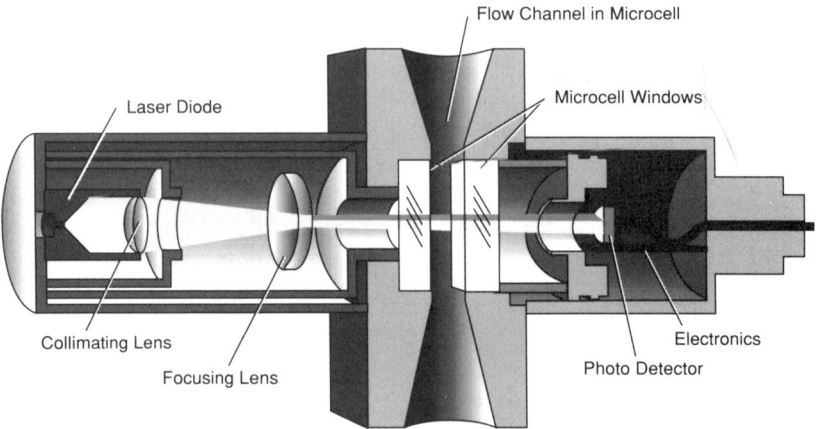

Figure 9. Hiac/Royco HR LD-type sensor.

A theoretical calibration curve for a Hiac/Royco HR–LD laser diode sensor is presented in Figure 10. This complex curve is obviously different from that of the HR–HA series white light extinction sensor (Figure 8), which is characterized by a simple power law dependency between the electrical signal (pulse height) and particle diameter. The complex laser diode calibration curve shows a low end sensitivity extending to about 1 μm. In the range from 1 μm to 2 μm, the slope of the calibration curve effectively varies from 3 to 6. In the range of 2 μm to 5 μm, the slope of the curve changes, showing a lower rate of increase for pulse height versus particle diameter. The response from particles with diameters between 5 μm and 20 μm follows a square power law. Particles larger than 20 μm (the view volume height) elicit a linear response. Between 20 μm and 50 μm, a slope of 1 is observed, indicating that the measuring volume height is defining the maximum particle dimension that can be measured. The complexity of the curve may be further increased if different rates of gain (electronic signal amplification) are applied for particles of different sizes. According to one design, a higher rate of gain is applied for pulses from particles of 2 μm to about 13 μm, and a second gain rate with lower slope is applied for larger particles.

A fundamental explanation of the laser diode sensor calibration curve may be found in the principles of light scattering and extinction phenomena. Simplified, extinction is the loss of light intensity, due to scattering of a portion of the light of the illuminating beam

Instrumental Particle Counting 65

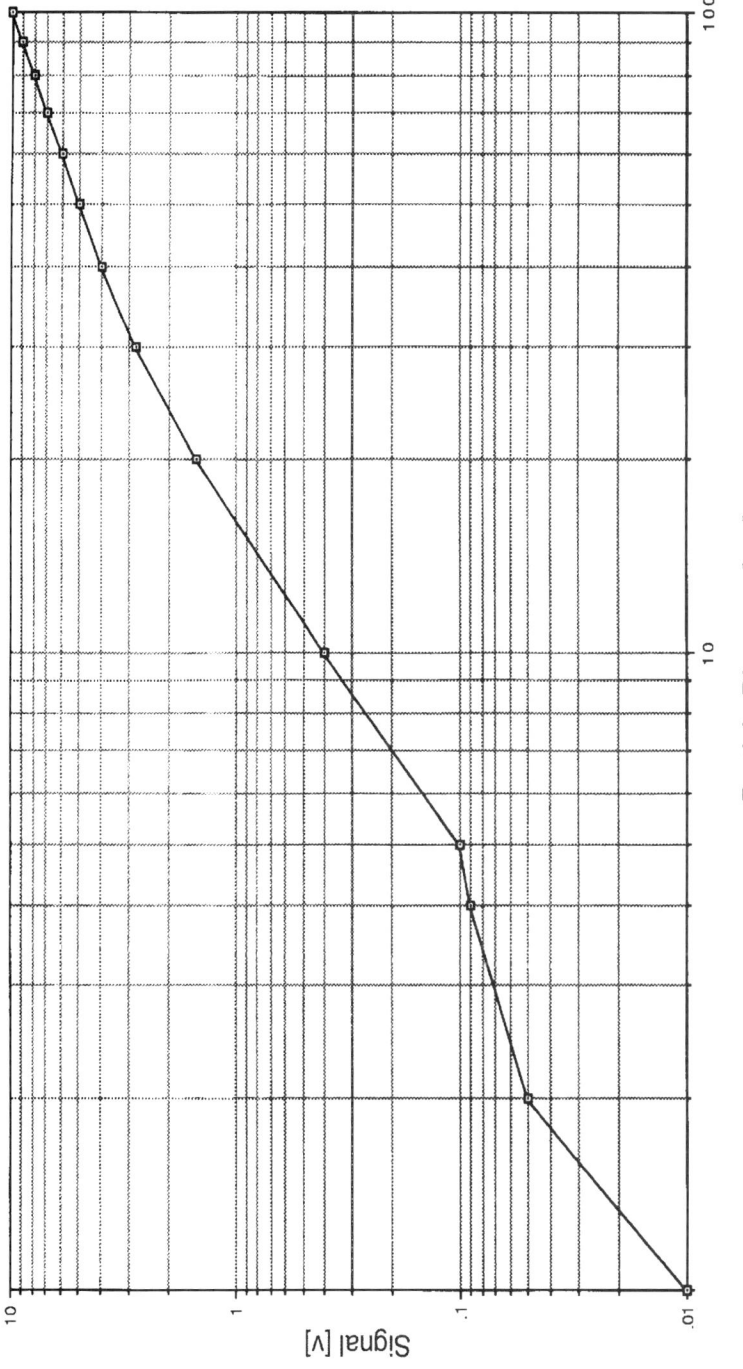

Figure 10. Typical calibration curve of Hiac/Royco laser diode extinction sensor Model HR–LD 160.

in the sensor, falling on a particle. It is a complex combination of physical phenomena (absorption, refraction, reflection) as discussed earlier. In the size range between 1 μm and 2 μm, the slope of the curve is approximately 6. This indicates that the extinction signal is predominated by Rayleigh scattering effects. Generally, for particles in this size range, the uniform increase of scattering removal of light from the sensor beam results in a uniform increase of pulse height with increase in particle size.

For particles greater than about 2 μm in size, the effect of scattering in removing light from the beam becomes less uniform. Particles in this size range tend to scatter light in a forward direction, toward the detector; so much of the scattered light is not removed from the beam. Furthermore, at the 2 μm to 5 μm range, particles begin to interact with light according to the principles of geometric optics, and combined scattering and diffraction effects produce lobed or irregular scattering patterns in front of the particle. These diffraction patterns may result in particles of larger sizes removing less light from the beam than smaller particles, so that oscillations in the calibration curve result. Thus, within the 2 μm to 5 μm range, smaller particles may generate higher scatter signals than particles of larger size, and thus also generate higher extinction signals (due to a removal of light from the beam that is disproportionate to their size). This effect is not noted with white light sensors, due to the compensating effect of the various wavelengths of height in the illuminating beam. For extinction sensors, the calibration curve, both measured and theoretical, is nearly monotonic. With these sensors, the mixture of wavelengths of light in the beam from the source tends to block out the nonlinear regions of the curve seen with the laser sensor in the 1 μm to 5 μm region of the curve.

Application of White Light and Laser Diode Sensors

The practical considerations in switching to a laser diode sensor from a white light sensor may be summarized as follows:

- Difficulty of user maintenance;
- Differing calibration principles;
- Increased small particle sensitivity;
- Count differences due to nonlinear response curve;
- Morphology-dependent sizing of particles;
- Resolution differences;

- Use of USP count standard; and
- Implications with regard to the manufacturer's historical particle count database.

The first consideration is probably not an issue for the majority of labs that test pharmaceutical products. Most labs using white light sensors of Hiac/Royco manufacture rely on the manufacturer's service personnel to change bulbs on HA-type sensors and optimize bulb alignment. The relatively small number of labs that perform their own bulb changes to minimize costs and down time will not be able to perform this maintenance with the laser sensors. Specialized equipment is required, and the diodes themselves are extremely fragile and liable to damage by static electrical charge during installation. Hopefully, the long life of the laser diode will offset this problem almost entirely.

Depending on the application, the selection of calibration procedures for the laser diode sensor may be extremely important. The foregoing discussion explained that the calibration response of the laser sensors was significantly more complex than that of the earlier white light models. As is obvious from inspection of the curve in Figure 10, a larger number of size standards will be required to characterize the responses of the laser sensor if particles below 5 μm are to be counted. However, vendors of laser diode sensors are in agreement that an adequate calibration for counting at the 10 μm and 25 μm thresholds may be achieved using the USP <788> method, with only three standard sizes; if the USP Particle Count Reference Standard (PCRS) is to be used, a 15 μm calibrant particle should also be used.

The greater "low end" sensitivity of the laser sensors is also problematical. Where the white light Hiac/Royco HA-type sensors were limited to 2 μm as a low-end sensitivity limit, some laser sensors (by virtue of a stronger signal-to-noise relationship at lower particle size) can be calibrated to provide valid counts at the 1 μm size. Realistically, the laser diode sensors must be assumed to have the potential for acquiring higher counts at lower sizes. It will be up to the individual user to determine whether or not this occurs. This may be a significant issue if counts must be collected at ≥2 mm per the BP.

Because of the nonlinear response curve of the laser sensors, it is not possible to derive a simple best-fit calibration line, even if only the 10 μm and 25 μm sizes will be counted. A curve can be fit using a segmented line constructed by simply drawing straight line segments between supporting calibration points. A better fit can be obtained using the software routines introduced as part of the automation package in Hiac/Royco Model 8000 counters, or by use of a cubic spine equation. The latter is simply a mathematical means of fitting a curve to points not on a straight line. The greatest problem with either method of calibration is that between any two calibration points the curve only provides an approximation of the true response. If a laser sensor is to be used to size particles in multiple channels below 20 µm (i.e., for population analysis) the use of more standards should be considered. Precise sizing can only be insured by using standard particles close to the individual threshold settings. This latter peculiarity of the laser sensor can be a significant consideration if the user intends to use the USP 15 µm PCRS. It may prove impossible to split the 15 µm peak if a 15 µm calibration point is not generated with standard spheres and included in the calibration curve.

Although the potential resolution of laser sensors is better than that of white light sensors, this higher level of performance cannot be taken for granted. The factors that detrimentally affect resolution in white light sensors also affect the laser diode type. These include:

1. Dark areas at the edges of the microcell walls (shadows);
2. Divergence of the beam in the view volume;
3. Nonuniform intensity across the measuring volume; and
4. Nonuniform response of the photo detector surface.

Factors 1–3 result in uneven illumination in the sensor viewvolume. This nonuniform optical performance causes particles traveling at identical velocities through different portions of the measuring cell to generate different signal pulse heights. Because of the more precise collimating of the laser beam in the view volume, the beam intensity may be non-gaussian and contain satellite intensity peaks due to diffraction of the beam itself. Poorer resolution may theoretically result than with the white light sensor (i.e., ≥6%), unless the sensor elements are critically aligned to take advantage of the unit's higher performance potential. Unlike the situation with white light sensors, resolution for laser diode sensors may vary significantly over the dynamic range. Best resolution is typically found if the portion of the curve used follows a square law relationship (5 µm to 20 µm in Figure 10). Calculated resolution of the laser diode sensors with a segmented line calibration curve may vary from that determined if a spline fit is used.

Based on the different optical characteristics of laser diode and white light sensors, it is reasonable to conclude that particles of different color, transparency, and refractive index will be detected with differing sensitivity by the two types of units. Before using laser sensors in our laboratory, we performed a significant amount of testing using instruments equipped with sensors of the two types. The testing involved Hiac/Royco 4100 and 8000 units, a Particle Measuring System Micro LPS unit, and a Climet CI-1000. In the great majority of cases, counts collected with laser diode or laser-based (Micro-LPS) systems fell within the range of data generated by the Hiac/Royco HR-120 HA white light sensors. Test suspensions used included NIST glass spheres, AC fine test dust, and carbon particles. Parenteral materials evaluated ranged from sterile water to reconstituted dry powder antibiotics.

This results suggest that laser-based sensors are readily applicable to counting extraneous particles in parenterals or in other medical products. In the usual situation (where small numbers of randomly-sourced particles with heterogeneous optical properties are present) it would seem reasonable that any over-counting or over-sizing of one particle type would be compensated for by the undercounting of some type with different optical properties (i.e., any differences should "average out").

In our own experience, transparent, flake-like particles and amorphous particles were the only types of particles for which laser diode sensors gave counts differing from white light sensors. These monotypic materials of high transparency may be expected to be counted differently by the laser sensors based on the specific wavelength of light involved. The amorphous particles are globular protein or drug agglomerates that consist largely of water. These materials would be expected to have an "average" refractive index very close to that of an aqueous suspending medium. This effect may prove to be an issue with the present <788> requirement's use of light extinction counters to resolve the microscopic count problems arising with dextrose solutions that contains similar amorphous materials.

The potential issues arising from monotypic materials with laser sensors are not deemed serious by the author. Such materials fall outside the randomly-sourced particles of heterogeneous composition present in parenteral solutions and are rarely encountered; for any use of light extinction counters, it will continue to be the burden of the user to understand the response of the sensor to different types of particulate matter and/or different solution types. The best general statement to be made is that a user should thoroughly evaluate any type of sensor being considered for purchase and understand its performance characteristics with regard to materials that will be analyzed.

Despite this favorable result in our testing, a number of questions remain unanswered regarding the comparison of data from laser and white light sensors. Our experience in the use of the laser sensors indicates that some models of these sensors can be used to count particles between 1 µm and 2 µm in size with acceptable accuracy. As mentioned earlier, this implies a greater sensitivity at the 2 µm size, which is a concern for those performing BP counts. The comparison of the two sensors at small particle sizes is not simplistic, however, since sensor resolution also enters into the equation. The laser sensors theoretically incorporate higher resolution at the 2 µm size than do their white light-based counterparts. Lower resolution at the 2-µm size with a white light sensor may result in higher counts at 2 µm, due to the log normal or Poisson particle distribution in many materials and the much higher numbers of particles present at small sizes. This would occur, because in addition to wide pulse distributions for mono-size standards, low resolution implies that particles below a specific size threshold may be counted as being above the threshold (Figure 11).

Error Sources

Due to the current wide application of light extinction counting for enumeration of particles in pharmaceutical products, potential count error sources are of increased interest. Limitations of the method are addressed in the papers by Barber 1987, Chrai et al. 1987, Blanchard et al. 1976 and 1978, Ernerot et al 1970, and Grundelman and Goldsmith 1987. Significant error sources may be summarized as follows.

Particle Size and Shape Bias

With respect to any type of particle other than a sphere, as discussed in the preceding section, light extinction instruments assign sizes that are lower than those obtained by a microscopic assay. Spheres are the only particles that are counted and sized in a generally predictable fashion by light blockage counters. Spherical particles occur infrequently in parenteral solutions. Further, since randomly determined cross sections of irregular particles are viewed by a light blockage counter as they pass through the sensor view volume, a polydisperse size distribution of counts will be

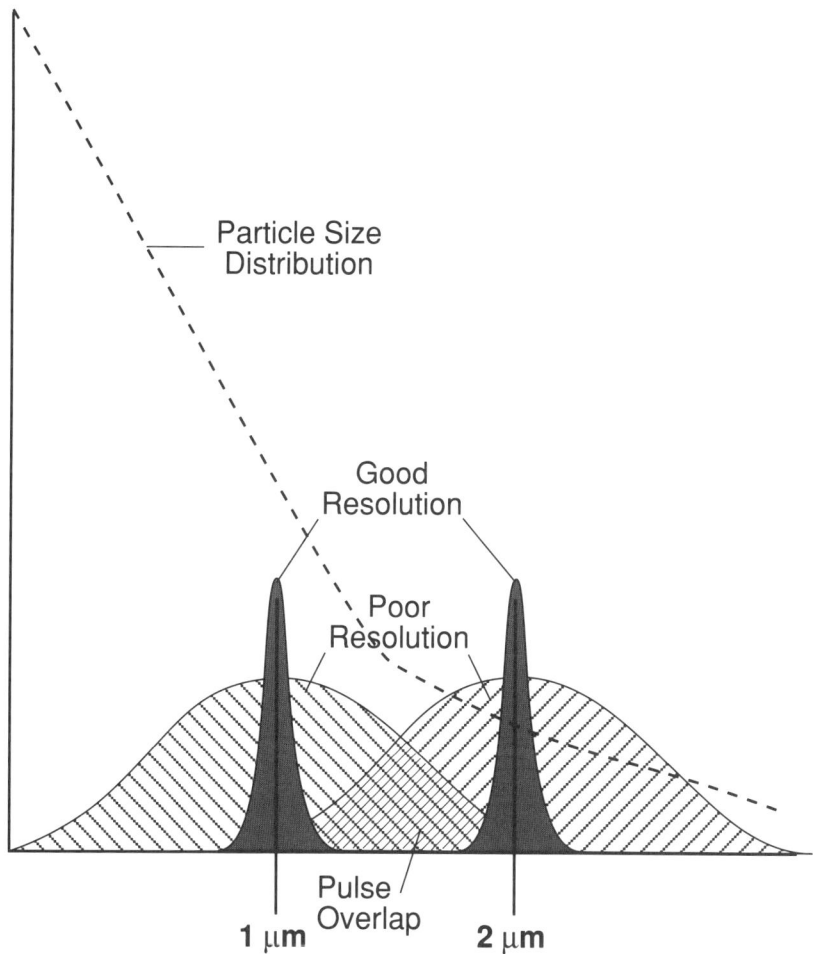

Figure 11. Resolution effects on count accuracy.

---

recorded for a population of nonspherical particles of the same size and shape. This error is most serious with fibers.

Sampling Effects

In particle counting of parenteral products, as in any endeavor involving statistical inference, larger samples more accurately represent the population from which they are taken. Hence, sampling small aliquots of a solution volume gives a more variable result and a less accurate estimate of the particle population in a solution unit than will be gathered with a larger sample. The sampling mechanism of light extinction counters compounds this problem, in that the sample aliquot is taken from a small region of the solution volume. Large particles are not as easily entrained in the solution entering the sample probe as are small ones. Unless continuous agitation is used, the settling of particles >20 µm in size may remove them from the area of the sample probe (Blanchard et al. 1977). Generally speaking, particles ≥20 µm (including fibers) are underrepresented in light extinction counts.

Coincidence Counting

The simultaneous presence of two or more particles in the sensor view volume of a light blockage particle counter results in coincidence counting. The outcome is decreased counts at the size threshold of the particles involved, and increased counts at higher thresholds where multiple small particles register as one large one. Severe coincidence effect is denoted by closely similar counts in adjacent channels.

Interferences from Immiscible Fluids

Immiscible liquids in drug formulations, emulsified materials, or silicone fluids from elastomeric closures can all cause artifact. Agitation of solutions in containers with silicone-coated closures can result in a transient, unstable dispersion of immiscible in the solution. Drug products in suspensions or solutions containing dispersed organics, such as ethanol and propylene glycol, products containing benzyl alcohol, or surfactants, are difficult to assay by light extinction counting. The presence of extremely low chemical concentrations of silicone oil dispersed as microdroplets can result in significant count artifact.

Between-Instrument Variability

Variation in counts between two instruments of identical make and model, calibrated by the same procedure, may exceed ±20% for a given sample of pharmaceutical product.

Refractive Index and Light Scattering Effects

The interaction of a solution-borne particle with white light in the sensor of a light blockage counter is characterized by a complex interaction of diffraction, refraction, absorption, and reflection effects (Knollenberg and Gallant 1990). The total extinction effect or attenuation of incident light results from a combination of these four light-particle interactions. The interaction of light with the particle is further modulated by the nature of the fluid in which the particle is suspended. Extinction efficiency for absorbing particles (carbon) is the sum of the scattering and absorption efficiencies. The variation of light scattering with particle transparency, refractive index, and size has serious implications for the sizing accuracy of light extinction counting when particles of different transparency, size, color, and surface textures are present in a sample. Dark colored or opaque particles may be sized significantly above their actual physical dimensions.

Air Bubbles

The analyst must be constantly aware that gas bubbles generated by the negative pressure in a sensor, or present due to agitation of a sample, will be counted as particles. While large bubbles (≥20 μm in size) are removed effectively by letting solutions sit before analysis, bubbles of smaller size (i.e., 5 μm to 10 μm) are less effectively removed even by ultrasound, and may impact the analysis as an error source. Some solutions, notably those containing bicarbonate, evolve gas in a sensor to give erroneous counts if vacuum sampling is used.

Recent Developments

Over the past five years, technical advances in light extinction particle counting and an increased user knowledge base related to these instruments, has made possible great strides in the application of this mode of particle counting in pharmaceutical labs.

Improvements in instruments systems include:

- Compact, user-friendly system design;
- Integrated sensor design (counter and sensor in one unit);
- PC-based data processing;
- Automated calibration procedures;
- Storage of calibration data for interim checks of instrument calibration;
- Interactive software function (WINDOWS®);

- Real time multichannel data presentation; and
- Reporting and data presentation options.

Benefits that accrue to the use of these newer instruments include not only simple, relatively trouble-free operation, but the ability to perform the USP <788> calibration and resolution determination in minutes instead of the hours originally required (Barber et al. 1990).

An instrument that embodies all of these improvements is Particle Measuring Systems' Automatic Particle Sampling System (APSS 200) with Liquilaz sensor (Figure 12). The bench top area required for this instrument is approximately one square foot. The system has three components. The first of these is a syringe-operated liquid particle sampler (LS-200), the mechanism whereby a sample is delivered though the sensor and then to a waste container. The second component of the system is the laser diode sensor. The new solid-state Liquilaz extinction sensor is a "smart" sensor in that all of the electronics are contained in the sensor, and the signals that represent particle data are transmitted directly to a personal computer. This system utilizes a solid-state 780 nm laser diode light source. In addition, it has several new features for adjustment and calibration of various lenses and detectors that are usually transparent to the user, but appreciated by those who maintain the sensor. Resolution is stated to be less than 7% at 2 µm.

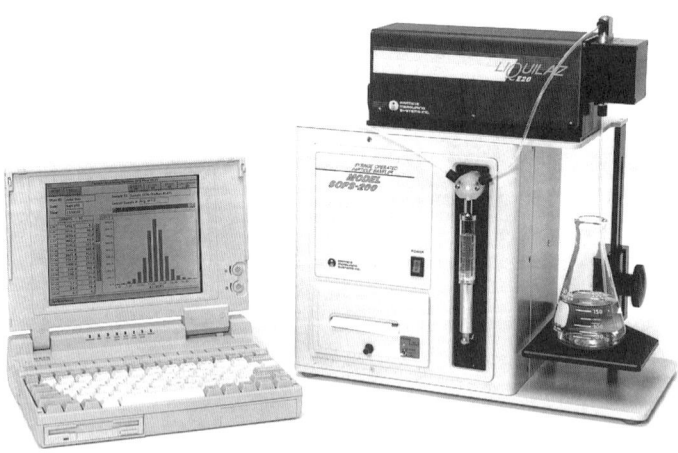

Figure 12. Particle Sampling System APSS 200 with Liquilaz sensor (Particle Measuring Systems).

The most significant refinement in the system is the data handling. The data system is a PC (IBM compatible 386 or faster microcomputer). User screens are manipulated using the WINDOWS® operating system. The system incorporates software-settable thresholds for particle size. For calibration, the user provides calibration suspensions with particles of the proper size and known variance, and the calibration curve for operation of the instrument is automatically determined. The instrument uses six calibration particles: of 2 µm, 5 µm, 10 µm, 15 µm, 20 µm, and 30 µm nominal diameters. It assesses the relative standard deviation, coefficient variation, or percent resolution of each monodispersed distribution, and (if within the desired specification) allows the instrument to proceed with the calibration. If percent resolution is not within the desired specification, the instrument will not proceed with the calibration. After the calibration curve is established utilizing those calibration particles, the data are recorded by the computer and stored in its memory. An operator can recall this data to check the history over a period of time, but can utilize only the most recent calibration performed. Any sample volume desired can be used for calibrating the instrument. If a sample volume larger than the syringe currently installed on the LS-200 is selected, multiple strokes are taken until the required sample volume is taken. Complete calibration can be performed in less than 30 minutes.

An additional consideration regarding this and other microprocessor-based counters is the validation of software governing the calibration and counting function of the instruments. For APSS 200, the manufacturer will supply the purchaser with validation documentation generated during development of the instrument, as well as the source code for software. This material should significantly decrease the extent of validation activities the user will need to perform in-house.

Spectrex (Prototron) System

This instrument (Figure 13) constitutes a unique methodology for counting particles in parenteral solutions. The instrument uses a focused He-Ne laser beam that moves in a circular (revolving) scan pattern to detect particles suspended in a liquid in a transparent (glass) container. As the beam strikes a particle, the forward-scattered light is sensed. A photodetector records the light pulses that are counted and measured. The design of the optical system ensures that only particles inside the vial are counted. Neither the glass walls nor particles in the air affect the count, as they are "out of focus."

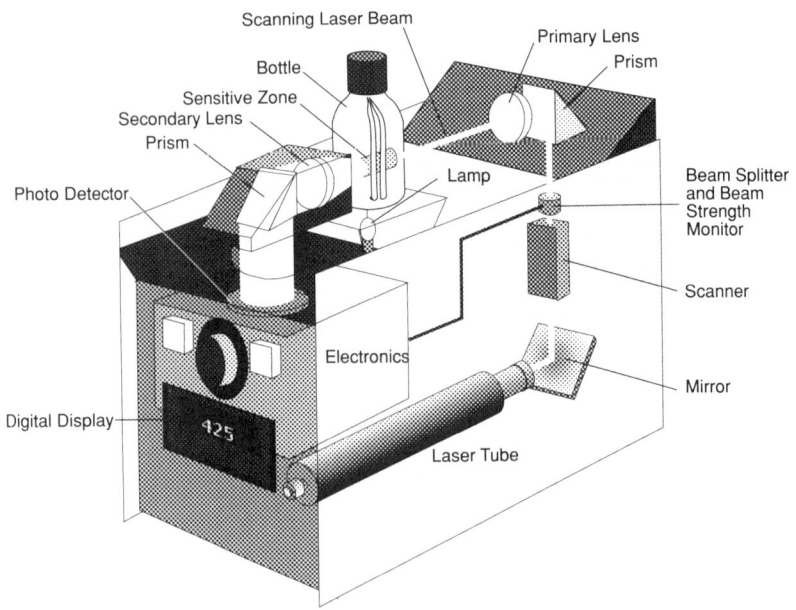

Figure 13. Spectrex Prototron particle counter.

According to the vendor's information, the laser beam focuses inside the bottle in a 2-cm long "sensitive zone." The secondary lens picks up scattered light (in the annulus around the target) from all particles in the path of the scanning laser beam. However, the photon detection electronics registers only those particles in the "sensitive zone" that are larger than the size specified by the threshold setting. Optical discontinuities in the glass of the container must be avoided. Once the count button is pushed, the revolving laser beam scans a total volume of 10 mL in 15 seconds, and the digital readout displays the average number of particles with sizes above the threshold limit in 1 mL of liquid. By taking sequential measurements, qualitative size distribution data can be developed, or the threshold selector can be locked to provide statistical quality control data at one particle size setting. The instrument also incorporates a lamp below the container being inspected that may be used for manual detection of large particles. Interfacing the counter unit to a microcomputer allows population (multiple threshold) analyses to be performed in automated fashion with the vendor's software.

This instrument has been investigated for the enumeration of pharmaceutical contaminant particles (Groves 1974; Blanchard et al. 1976). Although the low numbers of randomly-distributed extraneous particles in a parenteral solution do not present an ideal analyte for this means of analysis, counts comparable to microscopic or light extinction data may be obtained if conditions of analysis are carefully chosen.

Aside from measurement of extraneous particles, a promising application of the instrument would appear to be in dissolution rate measurements for solids (Henley and Portnoff 1990). In this application, the powder-solute system of interest is mixed in a transparent container, and the instrument is used with a computer data station to provide counts for particles greater than a given threshold as dissolution proceeds. The total time required for a single dissolution run on many powders using the device is less than 10 minutes. During this time, the instrument can perform 100+ scans of the drug-in-water test system and trace the progressive shift in particle size distribution as dissolution occurs. The time required for a similar assay by chemical methods to determine release of the drug is at least 1 hour.

Particle Size Standards

Particle size standards made of polymeric materials play an important role in the particle testing of parenteral products. They have a number of uses, including:

- Calibration of electronic counters and sizing equipment;

- Testing of filters and microfiltration equipment;

- Measuring the efficiency of mixing systems; and

- Model particles for visual inspection, container cleaning, and other quality control procedures.

Polymer materials used in the production of standard particles include polystyrene, carboxylate modified latex and polyvinyltoluene. Particles <5 μm in size are usually prepared by emulsion polymerization. The result of this process is a series of particles with extremely uniform size distributions. This uniformity is measured by the standard deviation or coefficient of variation

(CV). The CVs are are typically around 1%. Large polymer particles >5 μm in size are most easily produced by suspension polymerization. The CVs for particles made by this process are typically larger than for particles made by the emulsion process. The newest particles available are large uniform polymer particles produced by a hybrid type process that might be called "swollen emulsion polymerization." They can be made in diameters from 2 μm to 20 μm with CVs of 3% or less.

Standard particles have been produced on space shuttle flights. Emulsion polymerization carried out in the weightlessness of space can produce uniform particles of up to 15 μm in diameter, with size distributions as narrow as submicron particles produced under more conventional conditions on earth. This process is expensive and production volume is also limited. The CVs for space particles are only marginally better than those currently made by the emulsion polymerization process on terra firma.

Particle standards suitable for calibration purposes in pharmaceutical particle analysis are available from several vendors, including Duke Scientific (Palo Alto, CA), Coulter Electronics (Hialeah, FL), and Seradyn Inc. (Indianapolis, IN). A discussion of the use of standard reference materials for counter calibration procedures is provided by Barber et al. (1990). A great deal of information regarding the manufacture, handling, and use of polymer particle-size standards is available from vendors. Stan Duke will send the user (on request) reprints of publications regarding the sizing and use of sphere standards. This vendor provides the majority of standard spheres used for calibration by pharmaceutical manufacturers (Duke 1988; Duke and Layendecker 1989; Duke et al. 1989). An excellent illustrated booklet thoroughly covering the various aspects of production, storage, and handling (Bangs 1988) is available from Seradyn Inc. The information provided in this booklet serves as the basis for the following discussion.

Emulsion Polymerization

When surface-active agents or "surfactants" are dissolved in water in concentrations above a critical level (CMC), they associate with one another to form micelles. In these micelles the surfactant molecules are arranged with their hydrocarbon (oleophilic or hydrophobic) ends together and their polar (or hydrophilic) ends facing outward into the water. Emulsion polymerization starts with an aqueous solution of a surfactant such as sodium dodecyl sulfate, or any of a variety of other anionic or nonionic surfactants. If a hydrocarbon monomer, such as styrene, is mixed into such a surfactant solution, it will become emulsified or uniformly dispersed, due to the fact that the styrene is compatible with the hydrophobic centers of the micelles. Some of the styrene will be dissolved in the water as single molecules, but most of the material will enter and swell the micelles already present in the surfactant solution.

Next, a water soluble polymerization initiator, such as potassium persulfate ($K_2S_2O_8$), is added to the system. Upon heating, the persulfate ion decomposes into two sulfate free-radical ions: $S_2O_8 \rightarrow 2SO_4$. Each free-radical ion reacts with a styrene molecule to form a new sulfate ion/styrene free-radical, which in turn reacts with another styrene molecule. This process forms oligomers and short polymer chains of styrene with a sulfate ion on one end. Each sulfate free-radical ion will initiate a polystyrene chain, and each chain will continue to scavenge unreacted styrene until all the styrene is consumed or until the free-radical reacts with another free-radical to terminate polymerization. When polymerization is complete, each polymer chain will have a sulfate ion on both ends, and the chains will occupy the space formerly occupied by the monomer in the swollen micelles (Figure 14). The resulting polystyrene balls are "uniform latex particles." The term *latex* is used because the process evolved from synthetic rubber production, and it has an appearance similar to a latex emulsion. This one-step polymerization can be used for particles as large as 2 µm–3 µm in diameter.

Suspension Polymerization

Originally designed for producing ion-exchange beads, this process has been extended downward to produce particles in the size range of 4 µm to 90 µm. It is most commonly used with styrene copolymerized with 4 or 5% divinylbenzene (S/DVB). This process differs from the emulsion process in two important ways. Suspension polymerization uses a colloidal suspending agent such as colloidal silica in place of the surfactant. The monomer or comonomer mixture is vigorously agitated in water in the presence of the colloidal agent(s). The negatively charged colloidal particles coat the oil (monomer) droplets that result, and also surface stabilize the droplets during and after polymerization to prevent coalescence. More violent agitation results in smaller particles, and the increased exposed oil/water interface area requires more suspending agent to stabilize the smaller particles. If insufficient colloid is available, the particles coalesce until a stable system is obtained, so that the exposed oil/water interface matches the available colloid. The process is sometimes called "limited coalescence polymerization" for

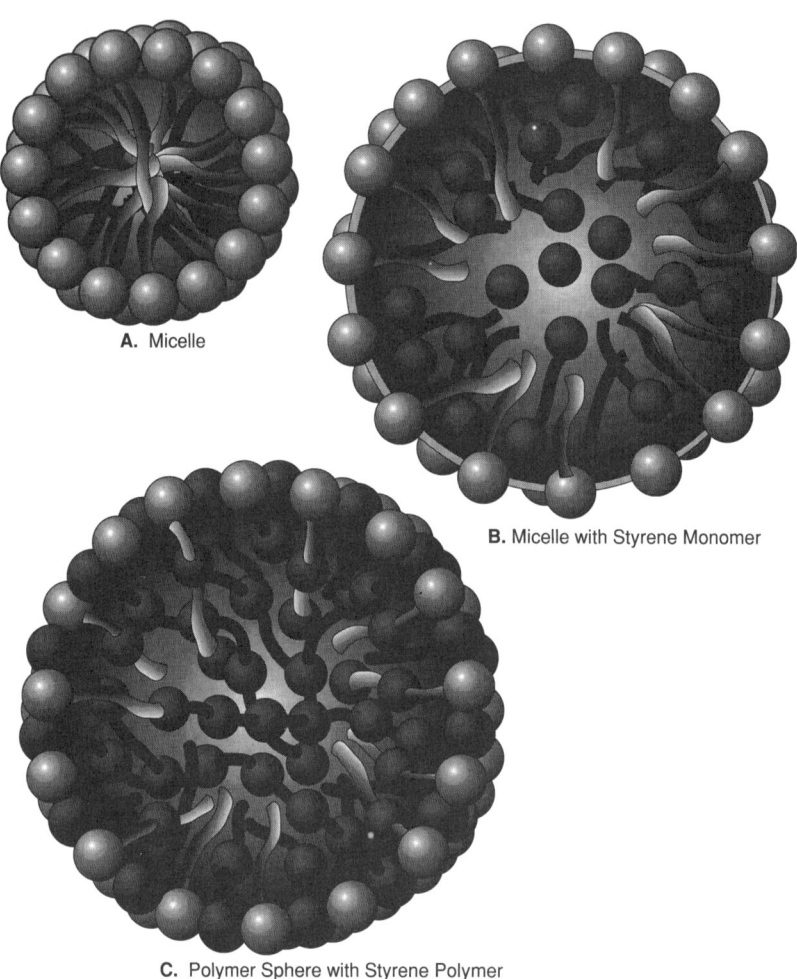

A. Micelle

B. Micelle with Styrene Monomer

C. Polymer Sphere with Styrene Polymer Terminated by Free Radical Molecules.

Figure 14. Polystyrene latex sphere chemical structure.

---

this reason. An oil-soluble polymerization initiator or catalyst (such as benzoyl peroxide) is used to catalyze polymer formation. All polymerization takes place inside the oil-phase. This process is of limited value in the production of standard spheres because of the size variability of the resulting particles.

Swollen Emulsion Process

A process for making standard particles of 5 μm to 20 μm in size with an extremely low size variation was discovered by a

Norwegian researcher (Ugelstad et al. 1982). This process entails use of a special group of chemicals that permit the two-step polymerization of uniform particles as large as 25 µm. This process allows preparation of uniform spheres in large sizes (2 µm to 20 µm). These particles are almost as uniform as the smaller particles prepared by emulsion polymerization, and the process requires significantly fewer steps than conventional emulsion polymerization. After the initial emulsion polymerization step, a swelling agent, dodecyl chloride, is added that permits swelling of the submicron polymer particles by large volumes of monomer. The resulting 2 µm to 20 µm monomer-swollen particles are then polymerized. Most of the particles produced to date by this process have been polystyrene or S/DVB, but other monomers and comonomers can be used. These particles are stabilized with sodium dodecyl sulfate (SDS) and carry a negative surface charge.

Storage and Handling of Standard Particles

Standard polymer particles are typically furnished by vendors as aqueous suspensions, stabilized by surface-active agents. The material is generally pasteurized (70°C, 24 hours) after packaging, and no antimicrobials are added. Room temperature storage is recommended. Refrigerated storage is also acceptable if one guards against freezing. Freezing can cause irreversible flocculation (aggregation) of the particles. Latex standard spheres that have been frozen have the texture of cottage cheese. The bottles should be tightly capped to prevent water loss and a consequent change in the percent of solids, or drying of particles. Dried particles will be irreversibly agglomerated. Dilutions of particles should be made with deionized water; electrolytes can also cause agglomeration of particles (Wilkison et al. 1986, 1987).

Standard latex particles larger than approximately 0.5 to 0.625 µm settle upon standing. Larger diameter particles settle more quickly. Agitation using a table shaker, wrist-action shaker, rollers, or other devices will resuspend them. Depending on particle diameter and settling time, it may take several hours of agitation to fully redisperse settled, agglomerated particles. Mild ultrasonic agitation may also be used, but ultrasonic energy should be used carefully. If too intense, it can overheat and irreversibly flocculate the particles. The dispersion of particles can be checked by examining them under a light microscope. When properly dispersed and diluted to about 10 ppm (parts per million), single particles should be present, with only an occasional doublets. If clumps of particles are visible, the suspension should be agitated longer. The proper surfactant can be used to assist redispersion.

Dilution of a sphere suspension before use is often necessary; it is essential to avoid extraneous contaminant materials being added to the system by the diluent or by the procedure used to make the dilution. This can often be done simply by adding deionized water and thoroughly redispersing. The act of dilution can destabilize a polymer dispersion if the stabilizing surfactant is diluted out too far. This problem can be overcome by the simple expedient of diluting the suspension with a solution containing the surfactant in order to maintain a minimum packing area of surfactant on the surface of the latex. Anionic surfactants, especially alkyl sulfonates or sulfates such as sodium dodecyl sulfate, typically work well, as do nonionics like Triton® X-100 or Tween® 20. Suggested detergent concentrations are <0.1%; higher concentrations can result in foaming.

The analyst should ensure any dilution made is stable by counting at appropriate intervals of time following dilution. If the count is found to decrease or increase, this is a good indication that the state of dispersion is changing, and the system is not stable. In order to avoid adding extraneous materials that can interfere with the procedure, dilutions should be made in a clean environment, such as a laminar flow hood using glassware with surfaces repeatedly rinsed with filtered water to give a low blank count.

When electrolytes must be used as a diluent, special attention should be paid to particle stability. Surfactants of the nonionic type may be appropriate in this case. The nonionic surfactants stabilize the particles by a steric-hindrance mechanism rather than by mutually repulsive negative charges. Latex particles can also be suspended in nonaqueous liquids that will not dissolve or swell them. Polar liquids (like methanol) that mix with water can be added directly to dry the particles. This is as simple as centrifuging and decanting a few times to extract the water. The same surfactants that stabilized the particles in water should work in other polar systems. Dispersion in nonpolar liquids, such as a linear hydrocarbon that is not miscible with water, may involve more steps. It may be possible to change phases from water to methanol, for example, and then to change from the intermediate medium to the final or intended dispersing medium. Another way to change liquids is to dialyze from one phase to another. This is a much more gradual process and less likely to cause the particles to flocculate.

Use of Commercial Standards

Commercial standards are available in certified sizes (ranging from 0.02 μm to 1000 μm in diameter) from the vendors mentioned in the beginning of this section. Aerosol particle counters are routinely calibrated with standard sphere sizes from 0.02 µm to 3.0 µm. Liquid filtration systems may be challenged with a wide range of sphere sizes in the form of either monodisperse or polydisperse suspensions. Particles from 2 mm to 100 µm in diameter are most commonly used to calibrate liquid-borne optical particle counters.

For particle counters used to determine the levels of particulate matter in parenteral products according to the compendial requirements, service engineers or users generally adjust the responses of the instruments using certified monodisperse polystyrene latex dispersions with diameters approximating 10 µm, 20 µm, and 30 µm (for USP counting) or 2 µm and 5 µm (BP). Newer instruments allow the user to perform the calibration procedures based on internal software. Unfortunately, some users are still reluctant to actually carry out the calibration procedures themselves, despite the relative simplicity of the procedure and the need to check any particle counting instrument at frequent intervals.

The use of polymeric microspheres for calibration of automatic particle counters will always be questionable, in that these materials represent ideal particles unrelated in shape and refractive index to contaminant particles that will be counted or recorded. These standard particles, nonetheless, represent the only uniform approach that is widely available to users, and they have distinct advantages over other reference materials such as the AC fine test dust. The user must constantly be aware of the aspects of use of the polymeric microspheres that may result in erroneous calibration data. The two most serious issues are the tendency of the spheres to form agglomerates (doublets, triplets, or larger clumps) under some conditions, and to adhere tenaciously to parts of the test system, including the sensor probe, and windows.

With regard to particles suitable for calibration of counters, those available from the Japanese Synthetic Rubber Company (JSR) are worthy of mention here. Two types of particles are marketed by JSR. These are the Stadex line, intended for use as size standards, and Clintex, which are made up in controlled number suspensions. At this writing, however, the Clintex numerical standard particles are not available in sizes larger than 5.5 mm, so their usefulness as a particle count standard for counters applied in USP testing is questionable. The Stadex monosize particles are available over a size range of 0.042 µm to 1.041 µm, so their usefulness for liquid borne counters in the pharmaceutical industry is not great. Both types of JSR standards find application in the calibration of airborne particle counters and the liquid borne particle counters used in the electronics industry.

In this discussion, I have deliberately omitted any reference to the use of AC fine test dust as a standard material, as well as any discussions of the NIST non-latex standard materials (such as the 1003 polydisperse glass sphere standard), the BCR materials that have fairly wide use in the U.K. and Europe, and the quartz test dusts available from Particle Technology Inc. These materials are all useful for a wide range of applications of electronic counters in other industries, such as in the testing of hydraulic fluids, but are not generally applicable to the aqueous systems in which the pharmaceutical analyst is interested. The suitable refractive index of latex materials, their ready availability and high quality, and ease of use make them the method of choice in applications covered by this book.

USP Particle Count Reference Standard

In 1991 the USP began marketing a particle count reference standard (PCRS) intended to allow a count accuracy check for light extinction particle counters without resorting to the difficult comparison of the microscopic test. The results of testing this standard are specified in <788> (*Pharmaceutical Forum,* May–June 1990). The experience with this standard to date provides an interesting commentary on the previously described variability of the light extinction particle count assay between laboratories.

Because the <788> counter calibration method is a half-count procedure, the USP Subcommittee of revision determined that the PCRS should be composed of 15 µm particles. This size is sufficiently above the 10 µm threshold so that, in theory, all of the particles will be counted at the 10 µm threshold, and half of the particles counted at the 15 µm threshold. The PCRS consists of a vial that contains 25 mL of a dilute suspension of mono-dispersed polystyrene spheres with a mean diameter of 15 ±0.18 µm. The diluent is particle-free water with added dispersants and preservatives. A sample blank is provided in an identical container, and consists of the diluent without particles. The approximate shelf-life of the PCRS was expected to be 3 years; stability studies on the standard are being run concurrently with issuance of the PCRS.

A collaborative study was conducted by USP to determine the count per mL of the candidate reference standard. This procedure is somewhat questionable, akin to voting to determine the most popular value for a reference material. The study was conducted in two phases. Phase I was a 13-laboratory pilot run to uncover any problems with (a) the instructions for the standard procedure; and (b) the capability of the laboratories to run the test. Each participant received a copy of instructions, the test method, report forms, and two sets of the standard. Comments from the participants and analysis of the data allowed refining of the instructions. Some of the participants uncovered procedural problems in Phase I that were solved before proceeding to Phase II.

In Phase II, each of the 13 participants received the revised instructions, report forms, and ten sets of the PCRS. Each participant reported the counts obtained at the ≥10 µm and ≥15 µm threshold. The results of the round-robin test were not promising. The appropriate mean count determined with the 10 µm threshold was determined to be 3750; the ratio of ≥10 µm counts to ≥15 µm counts chosen, based on the study, was 1.5 to 3.5 (2 would be ideal). The range for ≥10 µm counts selected was 3250 to 4250. The range chosen seems wide on initial consideration, but even so, 40% of the data collected were outside of the chosen limits, and only three of the 13 participating labs were in limits on all of the 10 vials they tested. Wider limits (≥10 µm 2680–4460), ≥10 µm to ≥15 µm ratio of 1.5–4.2 would be necessary to bring 90% of data collected into compliance. This standard would appear to be a step in the right direction with regarded to facilitating the <788> test, but some improvement is definitely necessary. It is difficult to accept a standard with this range of variability as being suitable for compendial test.

In fairness to the makers of this standard and to the USP, I must add one further comment. It is not likely that the standard itself is the source of any significant component of the variability noted. The majority of the imprecision of the test data obtained with the standard must be considered to result from the unsuitability of monodisperse material as a count standard, and/or the variation of technique and calibration procedures between laboratories.

Alternative Count Standards

One inherent difficulty in the USP approach to the PCRS would seem to be that monosize standard spheres with a narrow distribution make poor count standards. The threshold setting for a specific particle size that is determined from a calibration "curve" can be expected to differ from the threshold that will split the pulse distribution of a monosize standard of the same size. Thus, with the PCRS, a fairly slight deviation in the slope of an instrument calibration curve with regard to the actual thresholds may be expected to result in a failure to meet the count ratio criteria. Further, minor instrumental "drift" that has no practical effect regarding the result of a compendial test, may also result in failure to split a monosize standard pulse distribution at a specific size.

A more appropriate control for particle sizing and counting for light extinction counters would seem to be a polydisperse material with a continuous distribution of sizes over the size range of interest, for example, 2 μm to 50 μm. Such a material with a distribution approximating log normality would be insensitive to minor instrument drift during day-to-day operations, but would indicate significant changes in the particle size response curve. Such a product would meet the need for a sample to check the calibration and precision of parenteral product particle counters on a daily or weekly basis. When the observed cumulative count or the count per channel varies excessively from the expected count using such a standard, the instrument will require a more exhaustive check using monosized standards, or technical assistance from the vendor. Duke Scientific is presently testing a standard of this type; current plans are to make the standard available in late 1992.

Another alternative to use of the PCRS is to prepare standards in one's own laboratory. This operation has historically been avoided by counter users, but can be used to obtain a standard of good precision and stability. One vendor of standard spheres (Duke Scientific) provides certified specifications for numbers of spheres in each bottle of standard with a ±5% SD. Given that the number of spheres in a bottle of standard is known, and the material evenly suspended, careful dilution procedures will allow a standard with a precision exceeding that of the USP standard to be prepared in the laboratory for in-use validation and calibration of light extinction counters.

The materials needed are:

1. Ultraclean sample cuvettes (e.g., sample cuvettes from Coulter Electronics);
2. 0.1 μm filtered water from a cartridge filter or pressure vessel;
3. 0.1 μm filtered alcohol;
4. Analytical balance with 1 mg or better accuracy;
5. Low intensity sonic bath;
6. HEPA hood or bench;
7. Clean wipes;

8. Fixed volume micro pipettes for 100 µL delivery; and

9. Appropriate standard materials of known concentration.

All containers used should be cleaned thoroughly with the filtered alcohol and water and let dry. Sphere suspensions are mixed by a combination of gentle rolling on a flat surface, slow inversion 20–30 times, and 20–30 second sonication at low energy (≈500 Watts). Once the standard is mixed, 100 µL of standard suspension is pipetted from the bottle (after the top is removed) and added to the tared sample container. Inversion of the stock suspension must be continued until the moment the standard is pipetted, since spheres of 5 µm size or greater will settle very rapidly. The sample tubes plus standard are weighed and 25 mL of diluent is added, followed by a final weighting. After sonication, the number of particles in the diluted standard may then be determined based on the dilution factor applied to the original suspension. The precision of this method in practice is typically very good, with multiple diluted samples from a single vial of standard giving better then ±5% reproducibility.

A final alternative to a control standard for daily use is found in the polydisperse sphere suspensions made available by the vendors of standard particles. These are available in various size ranges from 2 µm to 100 µm. If evenly dispersed, and counted on a counter calibrated by a validated procedure (such as USP <788> method), such polydisperse suspensions constitute a control material that can be applied on a daily or less frequent basis to evaluate instrument performance between calibrations.

Automated Light Extinction Counting

The role of cost-efficient operations in today's laboratory environment is critical. To expedite new product development, laboratories must be able to rapidly produce accurate and precise test results. In the current regulatory and compendial environment, pharmaceutical laboratories are often required to perform more tests than were previously required to develop new products. As competitive pressures and customer requirements drive the demand for higher product quality, product specifications become tighter and designing least-cost schemes of laboratory analysis becomes increasing difficult. Time economies in particle counting assays are as important as with other types of tests.

Manually performed light extinction particle counting has two components: (1) preparation of the sample units for testing by laboratory technicians and (2) data collection and recording. The technician's role is primarily to identify the sample units, open them, and present them to the counter. This task consists of six discrete steps:

1. The analyst selects the unit to be tested, verifying the identification through use of a data system display or the appropriate sample request form. (Use of bar code identification is an obvious enhancement here.)

2. This unit is inverted 10–20 times to effect removal of particulate matter from its inner surfaces and disperse particles prior to counting.

3. The port of a plastic unit is cut off with scissors to allow the counter sample probe to enter the solution; for glass units, the neck of the bottle is washed and the closure ring and stopper are removed.

4. The analyst then inserts the counter sample probe into the solution volume and initiates counting by pushing the "start" button on the counter. Three 5 mL (or larger) volume sample aliquots are routinely tested.

5. As counts are collected, the analyst scrutinizes the data to determine whether air bubbles are being counted, or if other artifacts are responsible for high counts or count variation. If these conditions are present, additional sample volumes are counted.

6. Data collected from the aliquots sampled from a unit are inspected by the analyst before being sent to an intermediate database or recorded for supervisor review.

The simple manual procedures listed above are characteristic of a process to which automation can be successfully applied; many similar manually intensive tasks are currently performed by laboratory robots. In a large laboratory, it is not uncommon to expend 4000–5000 man-hours annually in nonautomated light extinction testing at a significant cost. A robot system in this application can perform the work of two technicians manually performing particle counting using an instrumental counter. As in other applications, the use of robotics allows the manufacturer to get out of the loop of hiring more technicians to perform more work.

We purchased a Zymark ZP100-3 system for our laboratory and used it to effect automation of the compendial particulate matter assay currently performed manually with Hiac/Royco particle counters. A total purchase price of 81.6K reflected the capital costs necessary to send accurate data to a control database from the RS232 interface of the robot controller. The hours spent in interfacing the robot to the database were minimal, since data is presented in exactly the same format as with the manual analysis previously interfaced.

The performance criteria for our system included: (1) unattended operation, (2) fail-safe measures preventing incorrect unit identification; and (3) of extreme importance, logic that allows scrutiny of counts collected for artifact before data is sent to a database. By transferring this work to a Zymate® system, the technicians responsible for a given set of tests now spend only the time necessary to set the system up and load units to be tested. Additional benefits include improved precision of data and the ability to test outside of normal working hours.

The system purchased was based on the standard Zymate® format, with workstations arranged in a circle about a central mechanism that effects movement of a "hand" that transports the bags analyzed between stations. The sampling of solution bags by a Hiac/Royco 4100 system interfaced to the robot and movement of the robot is controlled by a standard Zymark controller unit. A microcomputer (PC) interfaced to the controller is used for programming the controller and data inspection during operation of the unit. A benefit of this configuration is that the PC also serves as an intermediate database. Figures 15 and 16 show general design details of the robot workstations, bag holders and the robot hand.

Validation of the Robotic Assay

For any analytical system used to collect data related to pharmaceutical products, system validation is an extremely important concern (Lieberman 1987). The validation performed must conform to the principles accepted by the Food and Drug Administration (FDA). A thorough validation, described in summary below, was performed prior to the implementation of the Zymark System for light extinction particulate matter assays. There were two major components to the validation of this automated assay: (1) verification that the robot performed all programmed functions; and (2) verification that the analytical result obtained was consistent with the manual assay. The latter is extremely important, due to the fact that data collected must be screened for artifacts of various

90 *Pharmaceutical Particulate Matter*

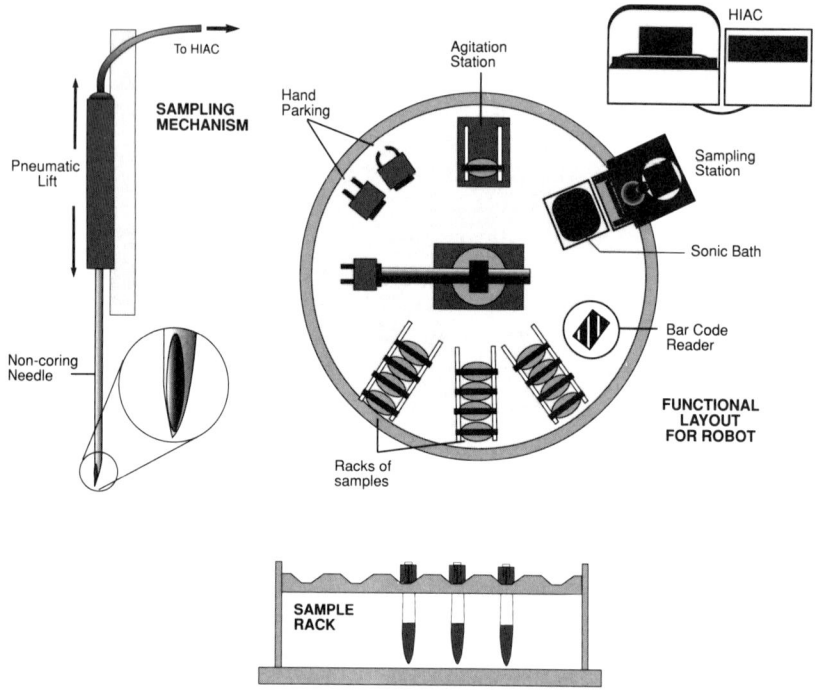

Figure 15. Functional layout of Zymark robot and sampling mechanism.

---

types. In the manual assay, this screening is performed by a trained analyst whose expertise and attention to the data collected provide the final check on the accuracy of counts obtained.

Validation of a robotic system consists of obtaining functional assurance of the entire system. For an analytical system, data must be at least as precise and accurate as that of a manual assay. The validation of computer-based robotic systems has become more demanding as the complexity of such systems and the available power of micro-computers has expanded. Fortunately or unfortunately, as the usefulness of laboratory robotics has increased, so has extent of validation required. This is particularly true in the pharmaceutical industry, since it is regulated by the FDA.

Per the FDA policy in this respect, a formalized validation of any hardware/software system must include (at a minimum) the following components:

Instrumental Particle Counting **91**

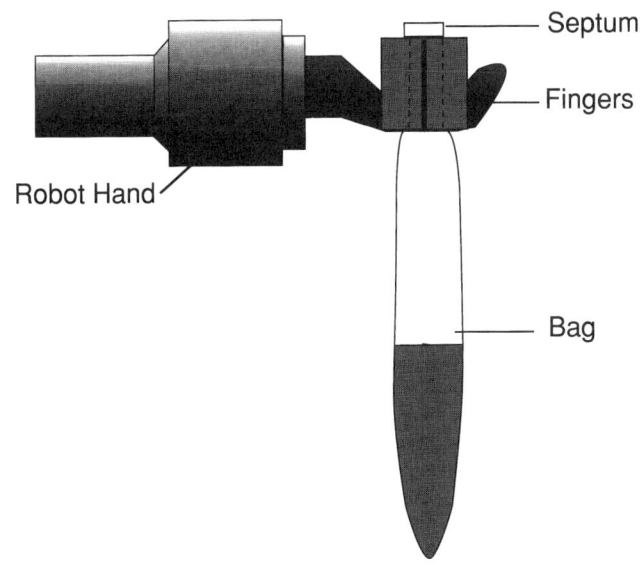

Figure 16. Robot "hand" and bag holder assembly.

1. A written test plan based on the relevant aspects (i.e., features and function to be used) of the requirements definition for all critical system modules, telecommunication, data storage, etc.);
2. Expected results for each test are documented prior to executing the actual test;
3. Actual results for each test are documented;
4. For discrepancies between expected and actual test results, incidences must be logged and resolved before the validation process can be completed;
5. Test steps must include boundary level testing for all inputs (terminal, digital, analog, etc.); and
6. Test conditions should be used that prove both that the system performs as intended, and that it does not perform as is not intended.

Of course, all validation documentation is collected per GLP and treated as original data (i.e., signatures, dating, review, etc.). Despite the regulatory pressures involved, the pharmaceutical manufacturer must develop objective, conscientious validation protocols that are technically valid and defensible, rather than to attempt to address all possible points that might be raised by an auditor. Unfortunately, there are no specific regulatory guidelines for robotics systems that clearly define acceptable validation. In this situation, unfamiliarity of field inspectors with robotic systems could conceivably lead to technically minor points being given undue emphasis. Past experience shows that auditors are not likely to question robotic systems if the FDA's principles of validation for computerized systems are observed.

Validation of our system was conducted in two stages. First, an operational validation was conducted to ensure that the system operated as intended (up to and including the review of data obtained from the test). Once we obtained assurance that the system operated properly, we compared data obtained in the robotic assay to that of the manual test.

Operational Validation

Critical operational steps validated in this stage were the following:

1. Tracking of unit identification and rack position;
2. Verification that counts collected as shown on the instrument were accurately sent to remote monitor and database;

3. Selection of samples from proper rack position;
4. Adjustment of test parameters for container size when samples of different volume are mixed;
5. System flags for counter errors (e.g., overconcentration);
6. Control of number of aliquots taken with regard to unit volume (MAXIMUM SIPS); and
7. Ensuring that the robot took appropriate action if artifacts were present in data—excessive variability of counts between sequential aliquots, unusual relationships of counts between channels, etc. (CHECK RESULTS).

The first five items proved relatively easy to validate, either operating according to test criteria on the first attempt, or being brought on line with slight modifications of the original programming. One unforeseen physical failure mode encountered was the occasional piercing of the side of a bag by the cannula, due to the bags having a slight "bend" from being folded over in their packing cartons. When this occurred, the drawing of air by the sampling needle resulted in a baseline fail message and an aborted cycle.

The most problematical step proved to be item 7. The collection of data free of artifacts, as mentioned earlier, is the most important job of the trained human analysts who operate these counters in pharmaceutical labs. The most frequent source of artifactual counts is air bubbles, which may be large (≥ 25 µm in size) and reflect only in higher channel count, or may be smaller (particularly if the solution being counted has some degree of surfactant activity) so that smaller bubbles are emulsified and prevented from fusing to form larger bubbles. Instrumental artifacts are also frequently encountered whereby one of a series of three counts from a sample will "spike" in one or more channels due to the influence of external electrical fields or vibration on an instrument. The final version of the CHECK RESULTS 1 and 2 programs, although simple in execution, resulted in the collection of data as free of artifacts as manually collected data.

Validation of Data Collected

Any validation procedure must begin with a consideration of the technical aspects of the manual assay and its robotized counterpart. This is particularly important with regard to the compendial light extinction particle count assay. This test is not a chemical assay, such as a titration, for which standards of accuracy and precision are established and readily available. The instrumental particle test is simply intended to indicate whether or not a number of particles in a tested unit are within limits. Specific human factors, such as differences in the way the analysts agitate or enter a solution nit, have an effect on the outcome. Typically, when two identical Hiac/Royco 4100 instruments (same sensor and counting electronics) calibrated by the same method are used to count an ideal standard suspension of mixed latex spheres, a variation of ±10% or greater will be noted between counts from the two instruments. In counting non-ideal particles, (i.e., extraneous particles in parenteral solutions), this between-instrument variability increases to in excess of 20%. With regard to the variability of test articles, between-unit variability of particle counts also increases as unit size decreases, so that a considerable variability component from this source is introduced into the assay result. Although a great deal of effort has been put forth in individual laboratories to minimize the effect of these variables, their impact on the test is still significant in the manual test.

For validation of our Zymark System, a simplistic approach was used based on the characteristics of the assay involved. The light extinction particle counting assay described in chapter <788> of USP XXII is a limits test, or pass-fail assay. The desired result is a simple prediction of whether a batch or other sample group tested exceeds or meets the established compendial limits. Given the variability of the light extinction test, it is impractical to test a sufficient number of units to determine actual numbers of particles present in a unit with any reasonable degree of confidence. Therefore, the primary goal of validation was to ensure that the robotic assay resulted in a determination of batch suitability that was in agreement with the manual assay result, (i.e., that the probability of failure of a tested batch was the same for both assays).

In consideration of all these factors, we chose to analyze data obtained in four specific areas:

1. Numerical agreement between assay results for two sample groups from the same batch of product, one tested manually, the other robotically;

2. Occurrence of the same count distribution in manually and robotically tested samples;

3. An agreement for mean results of testing across a specific product type, for example, SVI drug units, LVI flexible containers, etc; and

4. Assessment of equivalence of the two assays with regard to prediction of probability of a batch exceeding or meeting compendial limits.

Again, item 4 was considered to be the most meaningful test. The procedure involved in testing involved fitting a distribution to the data for five particle sizes counted, as a first step. This distribution is typically found to be a Poisson log normal or negative binomial distribution. With the data distribution, mean assay result, and sample size known, it became possible to predict what fraction of all possible sample groups of a specific size from a given population (e.g., batch) would give a failing result. This probability was invariably extremely low (10^{-6} or greater) and was generally the same for the manual and robotic assay.

Based on the data comparison, the counts obtained from the robotic test were equivalent to those obtained by the manual assay. In fact, the count-to-count comparison (Step 1) only infrequently showed significant variation between particle counts at given sizes between the manual and robotic assay. These differences were nonuniform with regard to particle size, and typically involved robotic counts that were slightly higher than manual counts. It should be observed in this regard that a difference at the ≥ 25 mm size observed frequently resulted from a comparison of a mean of 0 counts in one assay, and a fraction of 1 count by the other. The differences in counts observed were technically nonsignificant in view of the between-analyst and between-instrument variability that is observed with the manual assay. Data grouped by product types showed no significant variation between robot and manual assay. A comparison of data distributions in the two tests by product code showed robot and human data to have identical distributions.

Regarding validation of both robotic and manual light extinction counting procedures, I must make one additional exceedingly important comment. In regard to the application of in-use validation standards, the more frequently a validation of the counting procedure is performed, the less likely the generation of erroneous data. In some chemical analyses (e.g., gas chromatography) a standard may be run with each sample. This approach is not feasible with particle counting, but a generally similar practice can provide enhanced confidence in data. Particle standards generated in the laboratory can be applied for this purpose. It is relatively simple to generate count standards using the techniques described above, and use them on a daily basis for manual counting. Such standards may be monitored for count stability using a counter designated as a standard instrument, on which key electronic and physical parameters are closely monitored. If an analyst applies standards of this type before and after each day's counting, appropriate functioning of an instrument during a day's work is increased. Similarly, standards may be placed among the units of a group to be run robotically.

Summary

Light extinction and electrical zone-sensing counters provide a time-effective means of counting extraneous particles in parenteral solutions. The light extinction assay is used worldwide in the enumeration of particles in parenteral solutions. Advantages for using light extinction particle counters generally outweigh the disadvantages. The assay is easy to perform, and when applied in a controlled environment to a product that is well characterized with regard to the expected particle burden, it is an effective screening tool. The method is the official USP test for particulate matter in small volume injections (product of 100 mL or less volume). It has proven generally suitable in this role. When used by appropriately skilled personnel so that accuracy of data is maximized, the speed of the light extinction test becomes a significant advantage. The light extinction particle counting assay may be automated with a consequent decrease in time required for the test and increased precision of data.

References

Amaker, P., and P. Boymund. 1967. The control of the presence of foreign particles in an injectable solution with the aid of the Coulter counter. *Pharm. Act. Helv.* 42:357–340.

Bangs, L. D. 1988. Uniform latex particles. *Seradyn, Inc.* (Particle Technology Division), Indianapolis, IN.

Barber, T. A. 1987. Limitations of light blockage particle counting in the analysis of parenteral solutions. In *Proc. PDA Conf. on Liquid Borne Particle Inspection and Metrology,* 317–375. Washington, D.C.

Barber, T. A., and J. Williams. 1990. Analysis of dry powder antibiotics by light obscuration counting. In *Proc. PDA Int. Conf. Particle Detection, Metrology and Control,* 502–537. Arlington, VA.

Barber, T. A., M. D. Lannis, J. Williams, and J. Ryan. 1990. Application of improved standardization methods and instrumentation in the USP particulate test for SVI. *J. Parent. Sci. Technol.* 44:185–203.

Barnett, M. I. 1987. Resistance modulation particulate measurement. In *Proc. PDA Conf. on Liquid Borne Particle Inspection and Metrology,* 222–233. Washington, D.C.

Blanchard, J., J. A. Schwartz, and D. M. Byrne. 1977. Effects of agitation on size distribution of particulate matter in large volume parenterals. *J. Pharm. Sci.* 66:935–938.

Blanchard, J., J. A. Schwartz, D. M. Byrne, and D. B. Marx. 1978. Comparison of two methods for obtaining size distribution characteristics of particulate matter in large volume parenterals. *J. Pharm. Sci.* 67:340–344.

Blanchard, J., C. Thompson, and J. Schwartz. 1976. Comparison of methods for detection of particulate matter in large volume parenteral products. *Am. J. Hosp. Pharm.* 33:144–150.

Carver, L. D. 1969. Light blockage of particles as a measurement tool. *Ann. NY Acad. Sci.* 158 (3):710–721.

Chrai, S., R. Clayton, L. Mestrandrea, T. Myers, R. Raskin, M. Sokol, and C. Willis. 1987. Limitations in the use of Hiac/Royco for product particle counting. *J. Parent. Sci. Technol.* 41 (6):209–214.

DeLuca, P. P. 1977. Need for improved microscopic methods and understanding of correlations between microscopic and automatic mothods. *Bull. Parenteral Drug Assoc.* 31:173–178.

DeLuca, P. P., B. Conti, and J. Z. Knapp. 1987. An overview of technical issues in particle detection. In *Proc. PDA Conf. on Liquid Borne Particle Inspection and Metrology,* 376–380. Washington, D.C.

DeLuca, P. P., B. Conti, and K. Z. Knapp. 1988. Particulate matter II. A selected annotated bibliography. *J. Parent. Sci. and Technol.* 42, Supplement.

DiGrado, C. J. 1970. Liquid borne particle counting in the pharmaceutical industry. III. Method evaluation. *Bull. Parenteral Drug Assoc.* 24:62–67.

Duke, S. D. 1988. Particle retention testing of 0.05 to 0.5 micrometer membrane filters. In *Proceedings of the International Tech-*

nical Conference on Filtration and Separation, (March):525–532.

Duke, S. D., R. E. Brown, and E. Layendecker. 1989. Calibration of spherical particles by light scattering using photon correlation spectroscopy. *Particulate Science and Technology* 7:223.

Duke, S. D., and E. B. Layendecker. 1989. Improved array method for size calibration of monodisperse spherical particles by optical microscope. *Particulate Science and Technology* 7:209.

Ernerot, L., I. Helmstein, and E. Sandell. 1970. Some factors influencing the measured content of particulate matter in infusion fluids. *Acta Pharm. Suecia* 7:501–508.

Groves, M. J. 1974. The nuclepore prototron counter for the detection of particles in I.V. solutions. *Pharm. J.* 213:581–582.

Grundelman, G. P., and S. H. Goldsmith. 1987. User experience with liquid borne particle counters. In *Proc. PDA Conf. on Liquid Borne Particle Inspection and Metrology*, 495–506. Washington, D.C.

Harfield, J. G., and W. M. Wood. 1972. Standard calibration materials in the Coulter counter. Excerpt from *Particle Size Measurement* (edited by M. J. Groves and J. Wyatt-Sargent 1990). *Soc. Analyt. Chem.* 293–298. London, England.

Henley, M. W., and J. B. Portnoff. 1990. Development of an electronic technique for determining rate of solution of solid products. *Pharm. Tech.* (September):26–29.

Hopkins, G. H., and R. W. Young. 1974. Correlation of microscopic with instrumental particle counts. *Bull. Parenteral Drug Assoc.* 28:15–25.

Kinsman, S. 1969. Electrical resistance method for automated counting of particles. A*nn. NY Acid. Sci.* 158 (3):703–709.

Knollenberg, R. G., and R. C. Gallant. 1990. Refractive index effects on particle size measurement by optical extinction. In *Proc. PDA Int. Conf. on Particle Detection, Metrology and Control*, 154–182.

Lieberman, A. 1987. Particle counter validation for measuring particulate matter in injections. In *Proc. PDA Conf. on Liquid Borne Particle Inspection and Metrology*, 301–316.

Lines, R. W. 1967a. Particle counting in small containers. *Bull. Parenteral Drug Assoc.* 21:118–123.

Lines, R. W. 1967b. An insertable orifice tube for i*n-situ* contamination counts of solutions in opened ampoules and vials using the Coulter counter. *J. Pharm. Pharmacol.* 19:701–705.

Lines, R. W. 1981. Particle counting by Coulter counter. *Anal. Proc.* 18:514–519.

Montanari, L., F. Pavanetto, B. Conti, R. Ponci, and M. Grassi. 1986. Evaluation of official instrumental methods for the determination of particulate matter contamination in large volume parenteral solutions. *J. Pharm. Pharmacol.* 38:785–790.

Rebagay, T., H. G. Schroeder, and P. P. DeLuca. 1977. Particulate matter monitoring II. Correlation of microscopic and automatic counting methods. *Bull. Parent. Drug Assoc.* 31:150–155.

Schroeder, H. G., and P. P. DeLuca. 1980. Theoretical aspects of particulate matter monitoring by microscopic and instrumental methods. *J. Parent. Drug Assoc.* 34:183–191.

Sommer, H. T. 1990a. Optical sizing of single particles (Hiac/Royco laser). In *Proc. 2nd Int. Congr. Optical Particle Sizing,* 612–618. Tempe, AZ.

Sommer, H. T. 1990b. Performance of monochromatic and white light extinction particle counters. In *Proc. PDA Int. Conf. on Particle Detection, Metrology and Control,* 269–282. Arlington, VA.

Sommer, H. T. 1991. Performance of optical particle counters: Comparison of theory and instrument. Paper presented at IES 36th Ann. Meeting, 6–10 May, San Diego, CA. (per Hiac/Royco, Silver Springs, MA.).

The United States Pharmacopeia. 1990. 22nd Ed. Easton, PA: Mack Printing Co., <788>:1596–1598.

Ugelstad, J., P. Mork, A. Berge, T. Ellengsten, and A. Khan. 1982. Swollen emulsion polymer particles. In *Emulsion polymerization,* ed. I. Pirma, 383–430. New York: Academic Press.

Wilkinson, M. C., J. Hearn, F. H. Karpowicz, and M. Charley. 1986. The storage and handling of polymer latices used as particle standards. *Part. Charact.* 3:56–62.

Wilkinson, M. C., J. Hearn, F. H. Karpowicz, and M. Charley. 1987. The stability of latex particulate in aqueous suspensions. *Partic. Sci. Technol.* 5:65–82.

IV

Microscopy

This chapter provides a summary discussion of the basic principles of identifying, characterizing, and enumerating particles using visible light microscopy (see also Appendix 1). For many years, prior to the invention and development of the various modern modes of microchemical analysis, the particle analyst was limited to the application of stereomicroscopes and compound light microscopes for the analysis of particulate matter. Methods for particle identification, sizing, and counting using light microscopy were highly developed during the first half of this century and the methods developed remain applicable today.

The key to the effective application of the light microscope in particle analysis is the availability of an experienced analyst. The mental database of the human analyst allows quick identification of particles seen previously, and an experienced analyst can size and count particles with a speed and precision approaching that of an automated microscopic image analysis system (Barber et al. 1989). The problem is that experienced microscopists with comprehensive skills applicable to particle analysis are not easily found. Without well-directed training, years of experience may be required to acquire competence in particle analysis with the light microscope. In the majority of pharmaceutical particle analysis labs today, reliance is typically placed on expensive, complex microanalytical instrumentation to provide analytical answers rather than human experience. This situation occurs primarily because of the limited numbers of skilled microscopists available.

There is a simple solution to the problem posed by the short supply of experienced microscopists. This involves training of laboratory technicians to utilize light microscopy in a relatively narrow range of analytical endeavors in which the instrument is most useful. In a laboratory that will be constrained with regard to capital for acquisition of expensive instruments, the lab manager is well advised to acquire a light microscope and develop structured training for individuals who will be responsible for its subsequent application. Although extensive training and years of experience may be required to acquire a broad-based expertise in light microscopy, the basic skills required for identification of a very high percentage of all particles that will be encountered in pharmaceutical products or pharmaceutical manufacturing environments may be acquired in a relatively short time. Similarly, the acquisition of near-automatic skills for rapidly and accurately sizing particles may be acquired quickly (McCrone 1978). The actual time required for training will vary dependent on how frequently the analyst is required to use the microscope. In the author's experience, analysts can become adept at particle enumeration in about two months with daily practice. Largely because the microscope is used to identify particles on a less frequent basis, acquisition of the ability to use the microscope in an analytical role will take longer (4–6 months).

Acquiring the skills to make effective use of light microscopes quickly is dependent on teaching the use and application of the instrument as a technology rather than a science. Simply stated, the best progress will be made by teaching an analyst only the basic skills needed to operate a light microscope and to identify particles by sight or by simple manipulations of polarized light. A basic feature of this approach is the use of comparison standards that allow the analyst to see what a particle looks like and file this information in his or her mental database. For accurate and precise sizing of particles, a methodology should be chosen that allows the analyst to size particles based on comparison to a circular rather than a linear scale, making a direct smaller-than-bigger-than comparison rather than an incremental judgment (Draftz 1990; Kirnbauer 1970).

The following sections of this chapter are intended to give the beginning analyst basic information on how the microscope works and how to apply it in the analysis of pharmaceutical particulate matter. A brief description of the simple applications of the polarizing light microscope and microscopic tests related to the identification of particles are provided. Some of the critical terminology that relates to the use of microscopes is also defined. More detailed information is readily available from the references at the end of this chapter (Rebagay et al. 1977a, 1977b; Schroeder and DeLuca 1980; McCrone and Delly 1973a, 1973b, 1973c, 1973d; McCrone and Stewart 1974; McCrone et al. 1979; McCrone and Martin 1964). Also see the reference by Delly (1988) for an elegant summary description of light microscope function. If the analyst is seeking the single most useful text regarding microscope use, including polarized light microscopy, the author can strongly recommend McCrone's book entitled *Polarized Light Microscopy* (1987).

Structure of the Compound Microscope

The compound microscope is based on the magnifying power of combinations of lenses that are arranged so that their magnification is multiplied or compounded (Figure 1).

The magnification, M, of an image produced by a simple lens is equal to

$$\frac{\text{image size}}{\text{object size}} \quad \text{or} \quad \frac{\text{image distance}}{\text{object distance}}$$

In a compound magnifying system, magnification takes place in two or more stages. A second lens system may be placed so that it produces a further magnified image of the primary image produced

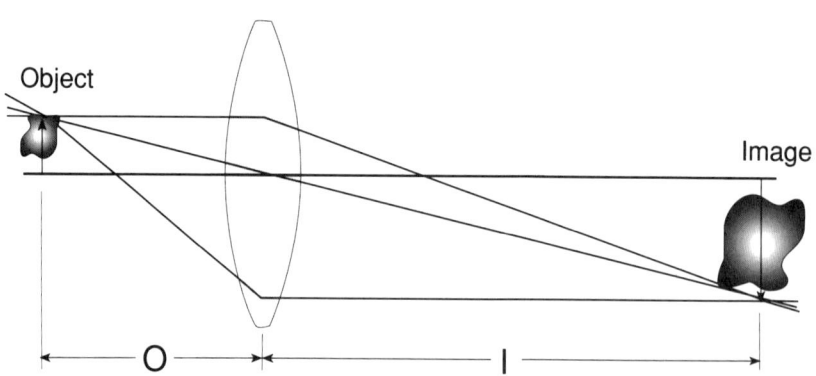

Figure 1. Formation of a projected image by a biconvex lens.

by the convex lens shown in Figure 1. The total magnification is the product of the magnification of the first lens and the second lens. This is the basic principle of a compound magnifying system. The analyst looks at the primary image with an ocular lens that produces an enlarged secondary image or virtual image. The brain sees this virtual image, rather than the real image formed on the retina; there is no real image at the point where the virtual image appears to be (Figure 2).

The first lens in a microscope is called the objective, since it is nearest the object being magnified. This lens projects a magnified image of the specimen at a fixed position called the primary or intermediate image plane in the ocular. The primary image is located about 1 cm from the top of the body tube of the microscope. The distance from the objective upper focal plane to the primary image is the optical tube length (Figure 3). Light rays emerging from the eyepiece (ocular) converge at a point called the eyepoint. In practical use the lens of the eye is placed exactly at this spot. The distance from the eyepoint to the virtual image, or final image, within the microscope system is about 250 mm (~10 inches), which is the generally standard close-viewing distance.

Lens Aberrations

A lens aberration is a failure of a lens to produce an exact point-to-point correspondence between an object point and an image. Spherical aberration is shown in Figure 4. Light in ray paths near the center of the lens is focused at different points on the optical axis compared to that in paths near the periphery. This can be reduced using only the central zones of the lens, placing aspherical surfaces in the lens system that compensate for the defect, or through the use of glasses with different refractive indices (e.g., crown glass and flint glass) and curvature in a doublet or triplet array.

Chromatic aberration (Figure 5) is caused by refractive index variation of the lens material with wavelength of light. A lens accepting white light from an object will form a blue image closest to the lens, a red one further away. Achromatic lenses that minimize this effect are combinations of two or more lens elements of materials having different refractive indices.

Objectives are divided into types according to how they are corrected for the various aberrations. There are achromats, semiapochromats, and apochromats. In achromatic lenses, chromatic aberrations are generally corrected for two colors, and spherical

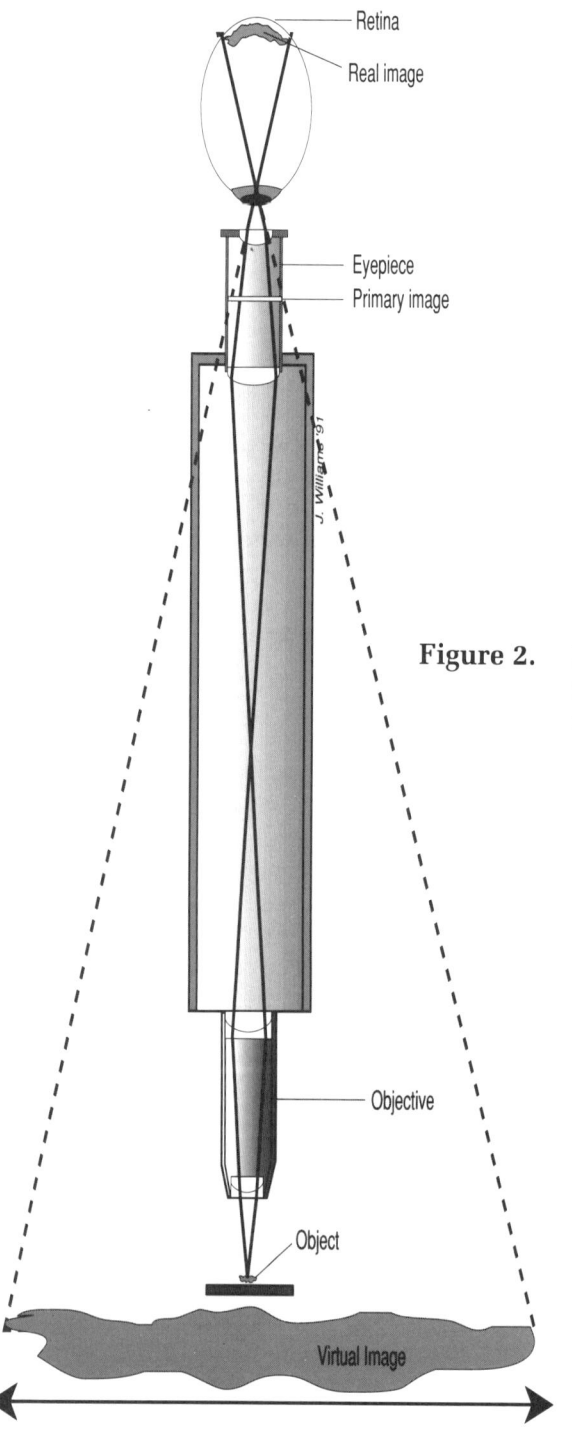

Figure 2. Image formation in the compound microscope.

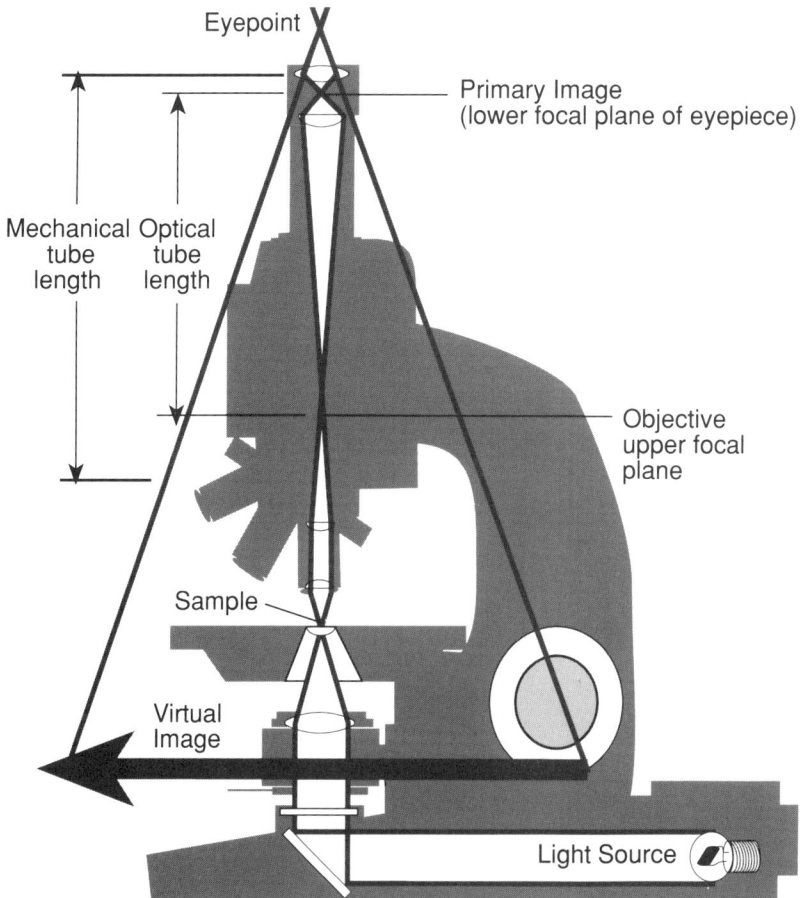

Figure 3. Optical parts and path of light through the compound microscope.

aberration is corrected for one color. Semiapochromatic lenses incorporate correction for both defects in two colors. Apochromats are corrected for chromatic aberrations in three colors and spherical aberration in two.

Images from objectives may also exhibit some curvature of field due to the different lens thickness through which the on-and-off axis image forming rays must pass (Figure 6). When the image is sharp in the center of the field, it may be less sharp at the periphery (plane of focus "C" in the figure); if the image is made sharp at the periphery, it may be blurred at the center of the field of view (plane

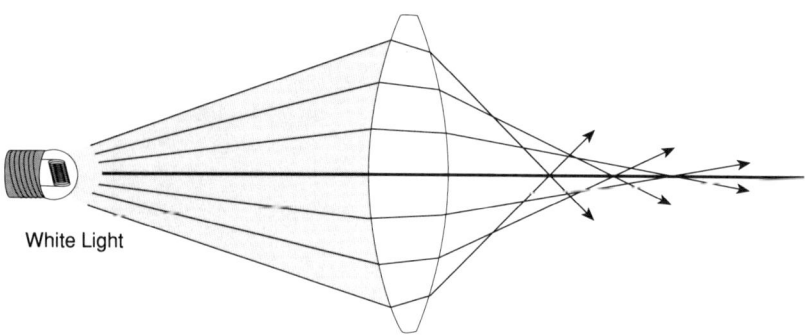

Figure 4. Spherical aberration by a convex lens.

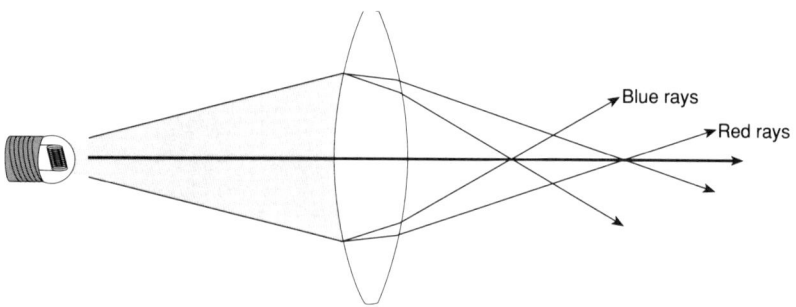

Figure 5. Chromatic aberration.

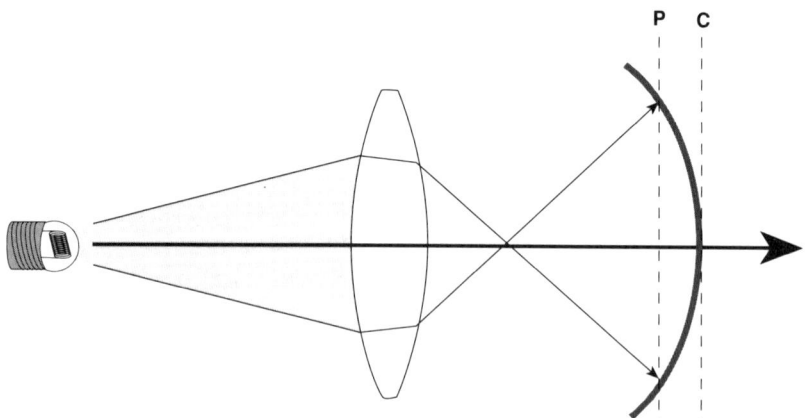

Figure 6. Curvature of field.

of focus "P" in the figure). Thus, besides the several types of objectives classified according to chromatic and spherical corrections, there are also plano or flatfield objectives. These flatten the image, correcting for field curvature through the use of additional lenses; these lenses are usually within the objective itself, but may also be in the body tube. Plano or flatfield objectives are important in photomicrography (see Appendix 1), where it is essential to have the image in focus across the entire field, and in particle counting.

Objective Lenses

Objectives are the most important optical element of the compound microscope. They form the primary (intermediate) image of the object that is then magnified by the ocular. The magnification of a single lens or lens system depends upon its focal length (Table I). Magnification is achieved through curvature of the lens—the higher the curvature, the shorter the focal length. Lenses of different focal length, therefore, have different angular acceptance of diffracted light waves from the specimen (Figure 7). Lenses of shorter focal length (higher magnification) have the greatest angular apertures; that is, the largest acceptance angle of image-forming rays.

The numerical aperture (NA) of a lens system is related to angular aperture (AA) by the relationship

$$NA = n \sin \frac{AA}{2}$$

where n is the refractive index of the space between the coverslip and the objective front lens and AA is the angular aperture of the lens, that is, the angle through which it accepts illuminating radiation. The highest numerical aperture for a non-oil immersion objective, with a refractive index for air of 1.00, is, on this basis, 1.00. In actual practice, a numerical aperture of about 0.95 is the highest achievable for a dry objective lens. The higher the NA, the greater the resolving power of an objective; so a high numerical aperture is desirable. Increasing the NA logically involves increasing the angular aperture and/or increasing the refractive index of the space between the specimen and the objective. Given a practical maximum focal length and angular aperture, the easiest way of increasing the numerical aperture is by increasing the refractive index of the medium in the space between the coverslip and the objective. Objectives intended for this use are termed oil immersion objectives. Oil immersion objectives have a practical maximum NA of about 1.4.

Table I. Representative Performance of Microscope Objective Lenses

Focal Length (mm)	Magnification	Angular Aperture (degrees)	Numerical Aperture	Working Distance (mm)	Depth of Field (µm)	Field of View (mm*)	Resolving Power (µm)
30	5	10	0.10	25	16	5	3.0
15	10	30	0.25	7	8	2	1.22
8	20	60	0.50	1.3	2	1	0.61
4	40	80	0.65	0.7	1	0.8	0.47
4	40	116	0.85	0.5	1	0.6	0.36
1.6	90	120	1.28	0.2	0.4	0.35	0.20

*Measured with a 10× eyepiece.

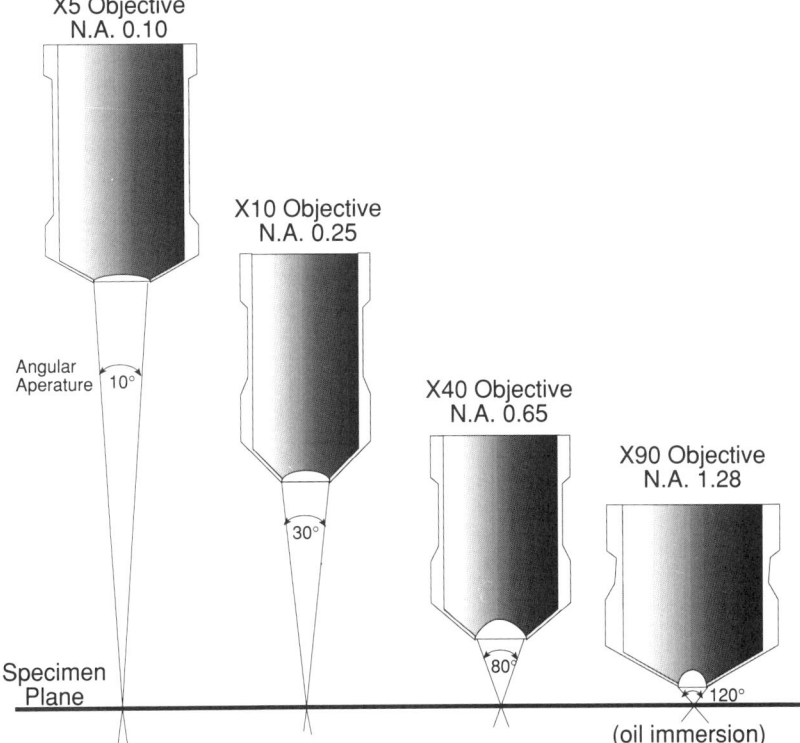

Figure 7. Angular and numerical aperture of objectives.

Working Distance of Objectives

The distance between the front lens or lens mount of an objective and the top surface of the cover glass on a specimen slide or surface of a membrane is the working distance for the objective. Working distance governs the allowable movement of the objective in obtaining critical focus of the specimen image. Generally speaking, working distance decreases as the focal length of the objective decreases and magnification increases (Table I). For oil-immersion objectives, the working distance is measured in fractions of a millimeter.

Resolving Power

In geometric optics, it is assumed that light travels in straight lines, but this assumption is not always valid. Bending of light rays is the basis of the diffraction effect that limits microscopic resolution. A beam passing through a pinhole aperture creates a bright spot larger than the pinhole with alternating bright and dark rings appearing on either side of the central bright spot. The intensity of successive rings decreases as a function of the distance from the central spot. For this reason, the image of a point of light produced by a lens is not a point but rather is a larger spot of light surrounded by dark and bright rings (Airy disc).

If:

λ = the wavelength of the light, and
θ = one-half the lens AA,

then the diameter, D, of the first dark ring may be defined as:

$$D = \frac{1.22\lambda}{\sin\theta}$$

For a minimal diffraction disc size to result with light of a given wavelength, the lens aperture must be as large as possible. Shorter wavelength light also produces a smaller diameter disc pattern and theoretically better resolution. The resolving power of various objectives is shown in Table I.

Diffraction effects determine image resolution. If two points are to be seen as separate in an image, their diffraction discs must not overlap more than one half their diameter. The ability to distinguish image points is called resolving power and is expressed as one half the diameter of the diffraction disc.

If:

λ = the wavelength of the light, and
NA = the numerical aperture of the objective,

then the limit of resolution for two discrete object points, a distance R apart, is defined as:

$$R = \frac{0.61\lambda}{NA}$$

Thus, with a wavelength of approximately 550 nm for white light and assuming a numerical aperture of 1.2, two points separated by about 270 nm (0.27 µm) can be resolved. Better resolving power can be achieved only with light of shorter wavelength. Short wavelength ultraviolet light (220 nm) lowers the resolution limit to about 0.1 µm. Diffraction is the single most critical factor limiting resolution, but the practical resolution of detail observed in a magnified image also depends on the illumination, specimen contrast, cleanliness of the optics, and acuity of the human eye.

Oculars (Eyepieces)

The ocular, or eyepiece, provides the second stage of compound magnification. It provides a magnified image of the primary image formed by the objective. The usual magnifications available in oculars ranges from 5× to 30×, with the most common oculars in the 10× to 20× range. A rule of thumb for oculars is that the maximum useful total magnification for a microscope is about 1000 times the numerical aperture (*NA*) of the objective. Magnification in excess of this value gives no additional resolving power and thus results in useless magnification. Only higher-power oculars will give full use of the resolving power of high *NA* objectives; a 10× or 15× ocular may provide too little magnification for the eye to see the detail resolved by high quality objectives.

Wide-field eyepieces allow large areas to be examined and are useful for examining membrane filters and particle counting. Long relief eyepieces are made for those who must keep their glasses on when viewing through the microscope. Viewing with glasses is necessary when the user has eye defects that cannot be corrected with the microscope, such as astigmatism. Generally, the near-sighted or far-sighted may use a microscope without glasses, since the necessary correction may be made with the microscope, but the convenience of leaving glasses on for data recording must also be considered.

Condenser Lenses

The third major optical component of a compound microscope is the condenser lens assembly, or substage condenser. The condenser lens provides a conical beam of light that illuminates the specimen. Light from the condenser converges on the specimen, and the light diverges in passing through the specimen to form an inverted cone, the included angle of which fills the objective lens. The angular size of the cone of illumination is controlled by a variable diaphragm located beneath or within the condenser. This diaphragm is called the aperture diaphragm or substage diaphragm. The correct focus of the condenser and the proper opening of the aperture diaphragm are of extreme importance in microscopic viewing of a sample with transmitted light.

One of the most important points to consider in choosing a condenser is the numerical aperture. The angular aperture of the illuminating cone of light from the condenser must be matched to the angular aperture of the objective for best image resolution. If a condenser is used dry with an oil immersion NA 1.40 objective, the NA realized will not be greater than 1.0. To obtain the benefits of objectives with NAs greater than 1.00, a condenser with an NA greater than 1.0 must be used and oil must be placed between the condenser and the bottom of the slide.

Reflected Illumination

Transmitted, nonpolarized light is of limited usefulness for the analysis or counting of particles. There are two general procedures for illuminating particles from above. One makes use of auxiliary illuminators; this is generally called lateral or reflected illumination. The second makes use of illumination from the objective lens of the microscope itself. This procedure is commonly called vertical, episcopic, or incident illumination. Bright field incident illumination is directed downward onto the specimen through the objective lens using a half-silvered mirror; the dark-field incident mode uses mirrors or lenses at the periphery of the objective lens to project light on the sample at angles of 20°–45° (Figure 8).

Particles on a membrane filter, can best be examined using vertical lighting. Auxiliary light sources may also be used. For particle analysis, external illuminators may be placed at the side of the instrument with the light directed downward onto the particles. The source must deliver sufficiently intense illumination and should be used at as high an angle with respect to the horizontal as possible to achieve this end. This is in conflict with the current USP <788> method for counting particles collected on filters that recommends low angle reflected illumination.

Dark-Field Microscopy

Dark-field transmitted light technique produces a black background image with particles that are brilliantly illuminated. This is accomplished by equipping the light microscope with a specific type of condenser that directs the light path from the source of

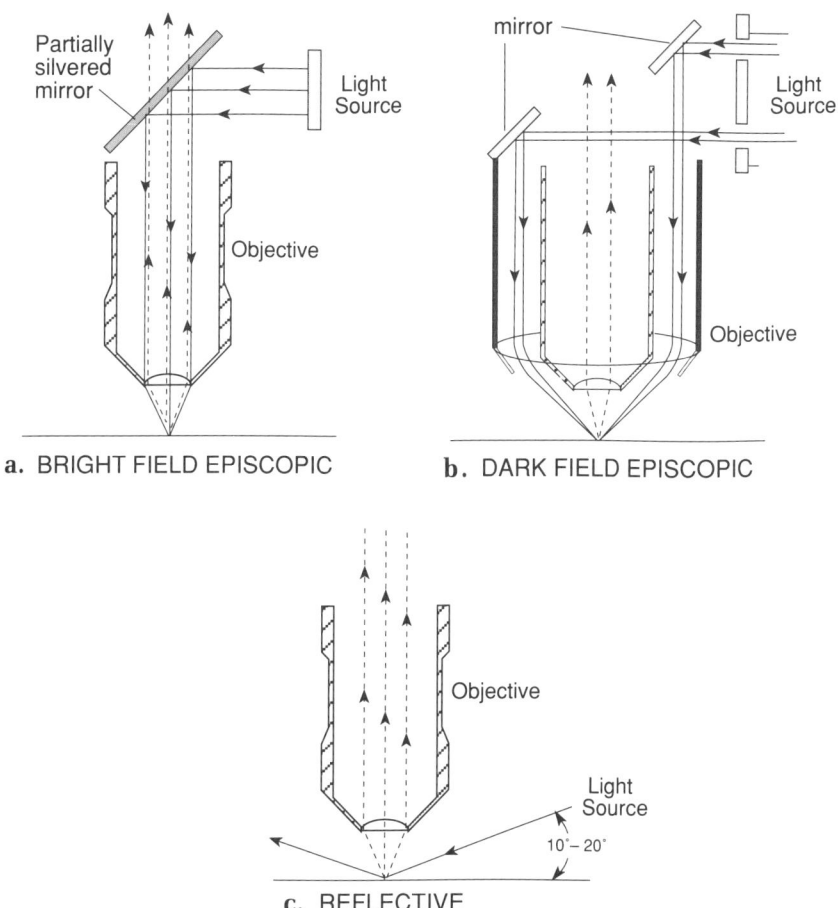

Figure 8. Vertical illuminators.

illumination through the specimen but outside the angle of acceptance of the objective (Figure 9). Thus, if the specimen is transparent and homogeneous, the light directed through the condenser does not enter the objective and the entire field of view is dark. If, however, the transparent medium contains objects that differ from it in refractive index, there will be a scattering of light by reflection and refraction. The scattered light will enter the objective, and thus the object will appear bright in the otherwise dark microscopic field. Dark-field microscopy may be useful for the examination of particles in a transparent film or on a slide.

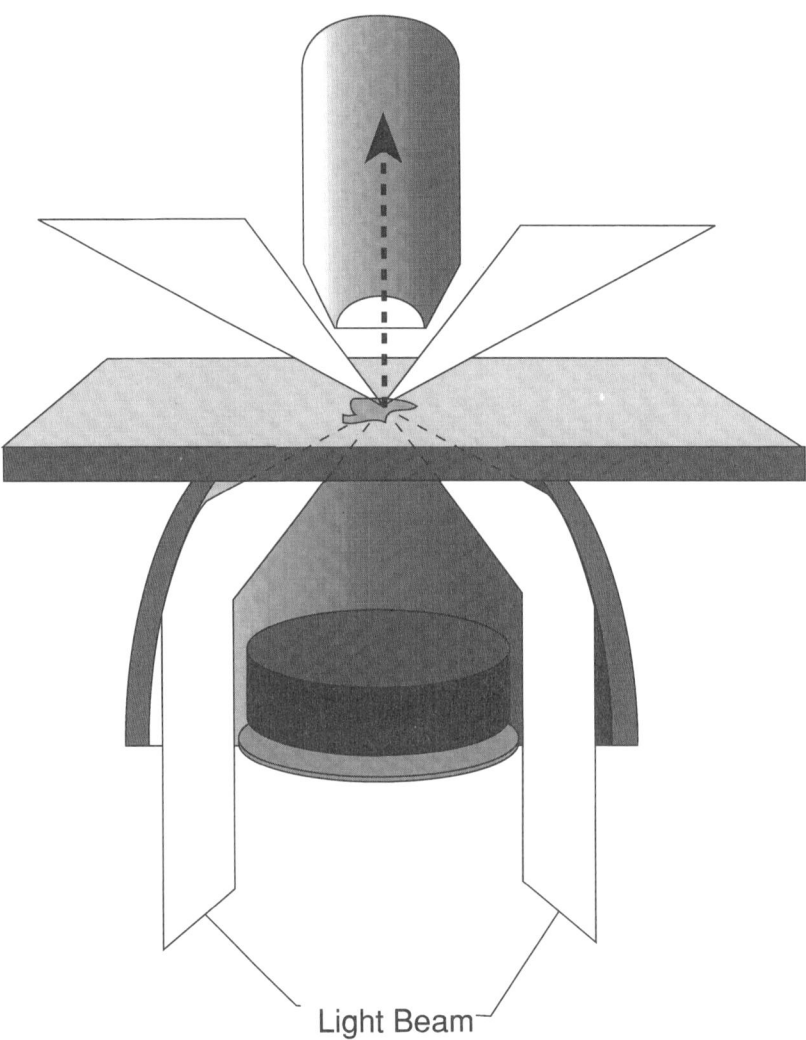

Figure 9. The path of light through a dark-field condenser.

Refractive Index

Light travels more rapidly in a vacuum or in air than in solid or liquid media. The ratio of the speed of light in a vacuum to its speed in a transparent solid or liquid medium is termed the refractive index (n). That is:

$$n = \frac{V_v}{V_m}$$

where V_v is the speed of light in a vacuum and V_m is the velocity in another medium. This relationship is responsible for the deviation of light rays by glass lenses; it is also responsible for a number of phenomena observed when light microscopes are used in particle identification. Glass, for example, with a refractive index of 1.52, allows light to travel at a velocity of about 66% of its speed in a vacuum.

Transparent, colorless particles will be visible in a given medium only if the n of the particle differs to some extent from that of the liquid. Glass fragments may be seen in water due to the relatively large difference in n between the two materials (1.5 vs 1.33). A series of refractive index liquids are available that have closely specified refractive indexes and may be used as suspending media to determine the n of unknown particles. Refractive index liquids are available for use in microscopy with a range of refractive indices from 1.3 to 2.10.

Polarized Light Microscopy

The polarized light microscope is an invaluable aid in identifying particles. The color plates in this book illustrate the morphology in polarized light of particles typically present in pharmaceutical products. Ordinary unpolarized light consists of a bundle of rays having a common propagation direction (linear axis) but different vibration directions. The rays of polarized light have a single vibration plane. Polarized light may be produced from ordinary light by reflection, by double refraction with a suitable crystal, or by absorption.

The completeness of polarization of reflected light depends on the optical properties of the reflecting surface and on the angle of incidence (and hence, angle of reflection). Some transparent substances at specific characteristic angles of incidence may be nearly perfect polarizers. For each transparent substance, the angle of reflection giving maximum polarization is called the Brewster angle. The angle for maximum polarization, i, is about 57° for most optical glasses with refractive indices of approximately 1.5.

Most crystalline materials show different properties of light absorption and transmission on different axes. Such crystals are called pleochroic. A pleochroic compound showing very strong absorption in one direction and very weak absorption perpendicular to that direction will transmit polarized white light with the plane of vibration corresponding to the weak absorption direction. Early polarizing filters were composed of such crystals. Such polarization of white light by absorption depends on all visible wavelengths being absorbed. Strong polarization of light in the visible range does not necessarily equate to polarization in the ultraviolet and infrared (invisible) ranges. The function of one type of polarizer (Nicol prism) in producing polarized light by reflection is shown in Figure 10.

Interference

Interference between light waves traveling in mutually parallel ray paths is a second key principle in the use of the polarizing microscope. Two light rays from a coherent source arriving at a point in phase will reinforce each other. This is known as constructive interference (Figure 11). If they are completely out of phase, they show destructive interference and cancel each other (Figure 12). Two light rays from a single source can interfere destructively by various mechanisms. One is reflection of a light ray by a thin, transparent film or by transparent layers of a crystalline material. One ray (A) is reflected from the top surface and one from the bottom surface of the film or crystal (B). The distance traveled by the second ray in excess of that traveled by the first is twice the thickness of the film or greater if the incidence is at an angle (Figure 13). With white light, the difference in distance traveled may

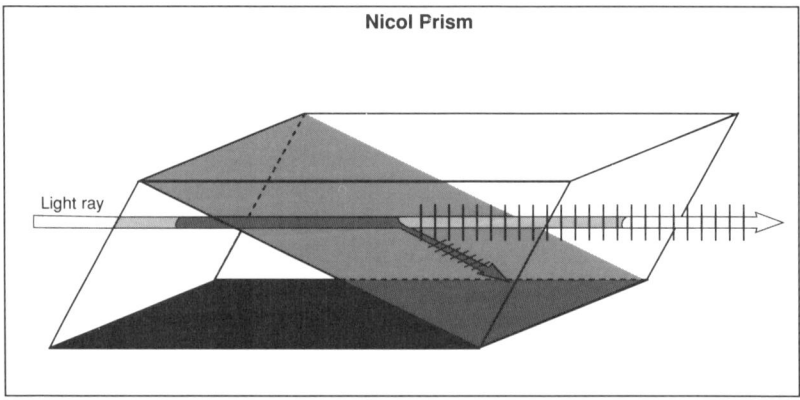

Figure 10. Polarization of light by a nicol prism.

Microscopy 117

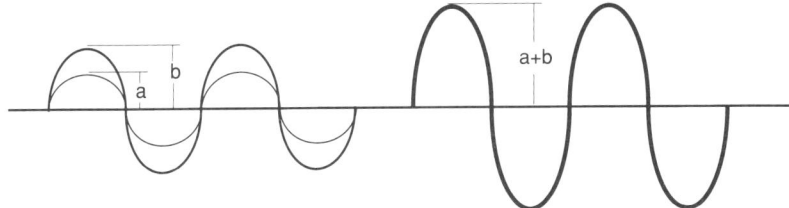

Figure 11. Constructive interference between two in-phase light beams.

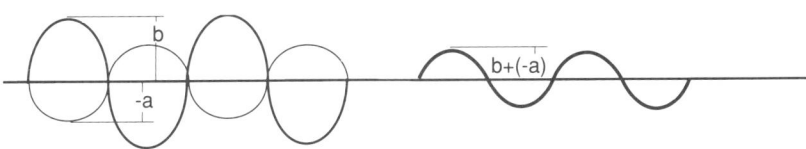

Figure 12. Destructive interference between two out-of-phase light beams.

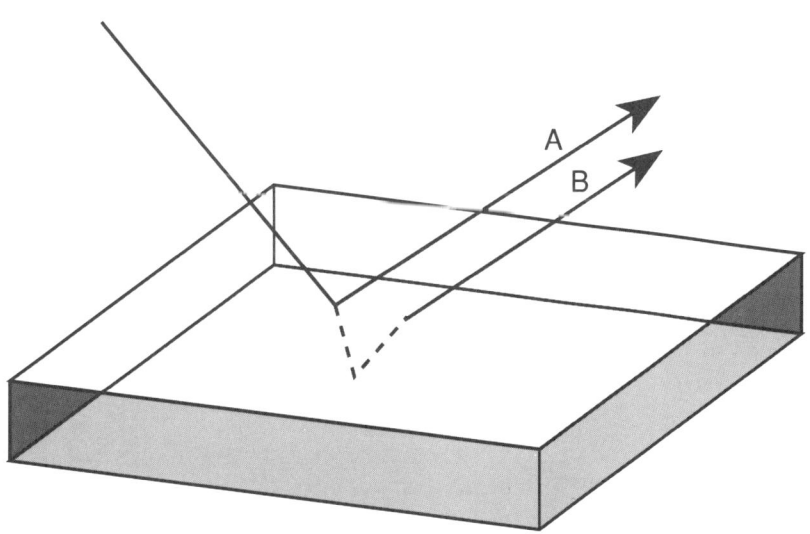

Figure 13. Thin film interference.

offset wave trains sufficiently to cause the light in the ray paths of different length to form colors when they recombine (interference colors).

Birefringence and Extinction

Knowing the principles of polarization of light and interference between light of various wavelengths in mutually parallel ray paths, it is relatively easy to understand the use of the polarizing microscope in particle identification. The simplified design of a polarizing microscope involves a polarizing crystal plate inserted between the sample and the light source (polarizer). This serves to polarize the incident light that passes through the specimen (Figure 14). A second polar (analyzer) is inserted above the specimen so that light that has passed through the specimen may also be polarized. Only light that has been polarized (i.e., vibrates in planes parallel to the axis of polarization of the analyzer) will pass into the ocular. If the vibration direction for the two polarizing plates is perpendicular (crossed polars), the field will appear dark.

If transparent particles are placed on a slide between crossed polars, some crystals will appear colored, others will appear bright, and some will be invisible against the black background. The crystals that appear bright, or colored are anisotropic and must have at least two principal refractive indices. Those that are invisible are isotropic and are either glasses, cubic crystals, or unoriented polymers. If the orientation of the crystals that appear bright or colored between crossed polars is changed by rotating the stage, they will be observed to disappear (become black) four times during complete rotation of the stage. These positions, 90° apart, are called extinction positions and may be used to determine the vibration axes of each crystal.

When polarized light enters an anisotropic crystal (a crystal with different indices of refraction on different axes), the light is resolved into components vibrating in two perpendicular planes. This splitting of plane polarized light into two components is called double refraction. Since the components follow two principal vibration directions having different refractive indices, they move through the crystal at different speeds; they emerge with one retarded by a definite amount that depends on the difference in the two refractive indices, $n_2 - n_1$ (birefringence), and the thickness. The actual offset of the wave fronts is called the retardation.

If the polars are crossed and the crystal is oriented so that one of its principal refractive indices (vector components) is parallel to

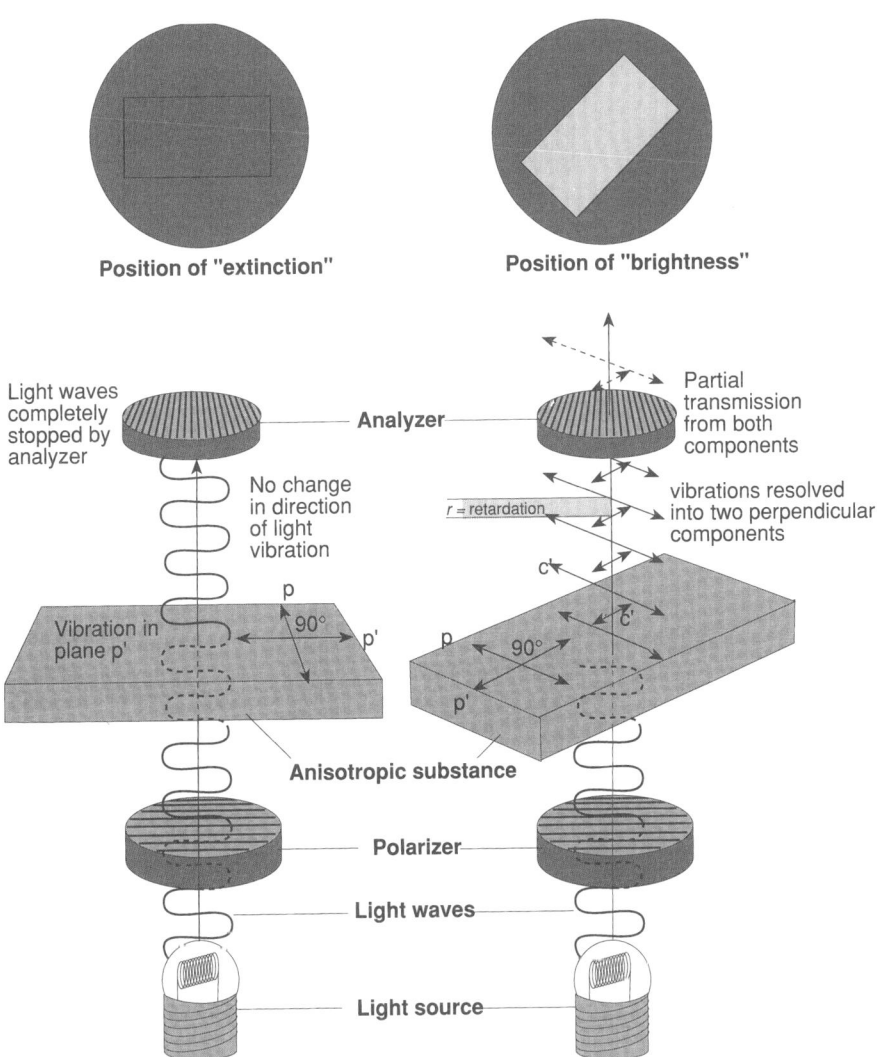

Figure 14. Polarizing light microscope.

the vibration direction of the polarizer, the second vector component becomes zero. All light emerging from the crystal has the same vibration direction as the polarizer and it will be absorbed by the analyzer if the analyzer plate has a vibration direction perpendicular to that of the polarizer (extinction). Both the crystal and the background will appear dark when the crystal is in an extinction position.

If a birefringent (anisotropic) crystal is oriented so that a principle axis of refraction is not parallel to the vibration direction of the polarizer, the emerging components of illumination will recombine in the vibration plane of the analyzer. Interference will destroy some wavelengths of light and reinforce others. Since one component is retarded, interference on recombination of the two components by the analyzer may cause the image to appear colored. The colors seen will depend upon the retardation, which depends upon both the thickness and the cross-axial differences in refractive indices (birefringence). If the crystal varies in thickness, several colors may be observed. The colors will be brightest when the crystal is between extinction positions.

Both interference colors and patterns of extinction are characteristics of different transparent materials. Calcium carbonate, calcium oxalate, skin cells, penicillin powder, starch, and other materials of interest to the particle analyst have their own interference colors and patterns. It is possible to use the polarizing microscope to perform detailed studies regarding the properties of crystalline materials. The methodology used for this purpose is covered in some detail in the references (Winchell 1964; McCormack et al. 1976; McCrone et al. 1973a, 1973b, 1973c, 1973d). The pharmaceutical particle analyst does not usually wish to perform studies on the crystalline properties of an unknown, but rather simply to identify it. For this purpose, a relatively unsophisticated use of the polarizing microscope is sufficient.

An example of this type of use is illustrated by McCrone's *Particle Atlas*. Some of the volumes of this series are profusely illustrated with color plates of many types of particles as seen under a polarizing microscope. These are invaluable to the analyst for "cognitive" identification of particles (i.e., identification by recognition). Almost without exception these micrographs were taken with "slightly uncrossed polars." The use of slightly uncrossed polars allows enough unpolarized light to pass through the specimen so that both anisotropic and isotropic particles are visible, and the extent of polarization present allows extinction patterns and interference colors also to be seen. Thus, an analyst can readily compare the morphology of the unknown with a picture. More importantly, the morphology of the unknown is easily compared with a particle of known identity.

The use of comparison standards and slightly uncrossed polars is a key principle in the identification of particles encountered in a pharmaceutical particle lab. Comparison standards to which an unknown may be compared are readily available, based on a little inductive reasoning. The situation is even further simplified by the fact that many pharmaceutical particulates are identifiable on sight (e.g., skin fragments, starch, talc, glass fragments, hair).

Because of the historical development of this form of analysis, a considerable reference base exists in the literature that can be used to gain a better understanding of the principle of polarized light microscopy in particle identification. With regard to cognitive identification (identification of particles by sight), the texts by McCrone are invaluable. Mason's (1983) *Handbook of Chemical Microscopy* provides information regarding a number of useful chemical methods. The 1980 paper published by DeLuca and Bodapatti as an FDA guideline is of historical and practical interest as are those of Godfray (1979), Oles (1978) and Trasen (1968a, 1968b). Many of the "spot tests" described by Fiegl and Anger (1972) and Chamot and Mason (1958) are useful for microscopic identification of particles.

Refractive Index Determinations

The polarizing microscope may also be used to determine particle refractive indices. This is performed using the polarizer and a range of refractive index oils that bracket the refractive index of the particle. The test performed is called the Becke line test. The Becke line is a bright ring of light (halo), at the periphery of a transparent particle, that moves with respect to the particle edge as the objective focal point is moved up and down through the particle (Figure 15). The ring will always move into the higher refractive index medium as the point of focus is raised and into the lower refractive index medium when the objective is lowered. The formation of the Becke line is due to optical effects that concentrate light at an interface between two materials of different refractive index. When the microscope is critically focused on a particle, no Becke line is visible. Raising the focal point shifts the image in focus to the region above the crystal, where the light becomes concentrated within the boundary of the higher index medium; the Becke line crosses the interface into the higher refractive index medium. Lowering the focus to a point below the best focus for the crystal causes the Becke line to cross the interface to the lower index medium. Using the Becke line test, the analyst can readily compare the refractive index of an unknown particle to that of a refractive index liquid. Refractive index media are available in a wide range of values that span the refractive index range of pharmaceutical contaminant particles.

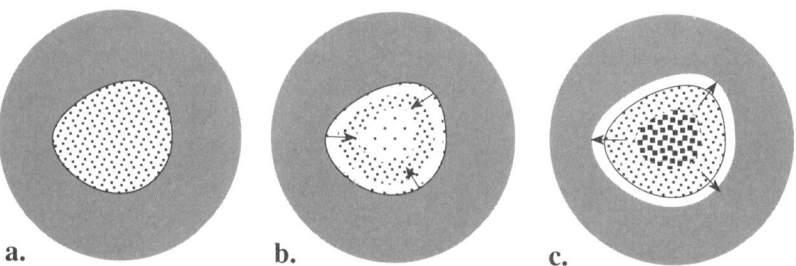

Figure 15. Becke line test:

    a. Particle in focus.

    b. Movement of line as focal plane raised (refractive index of particle higher than that of medium).

    c. Movement of line as focal plane raised (refractive index of medium higher).

Dispersion Staining

Transparent media (and particles) have different refractive indices for light of different wavelengths. This effect is termed refractive index dispersion. Dispersion staining is a simple particle identification technique based on the refractive index characteristics of a particle and of the liquid medium in which the particle is immersed. To produce dispersion staining colors, the particles and immersion liquids must have different dispersion curves that cross in the visible light region. At λ_b, the wavelength at which both the particle and the liquid have the same refractive index, the particle-liquid preparation becomes homogeneous with regard to refraction of light of that wavelength. Figure 16 illustrates the optical basis for the effects observed.

As discussed above with regard to the Becke line, refractive index effects will be noted at the particle liquid boundary if the two do not match in refractive index. If a particle and refractive index liquid match for yellow light, this color will be undeviated at the boundary and an annular aperture (stop) in the objective lens will portray the particles with a yellow boundary in a clear field. A central stop will allow only light that is deviated beyond a certain angle to pass (e.g., blue, so that the particles in question will appear

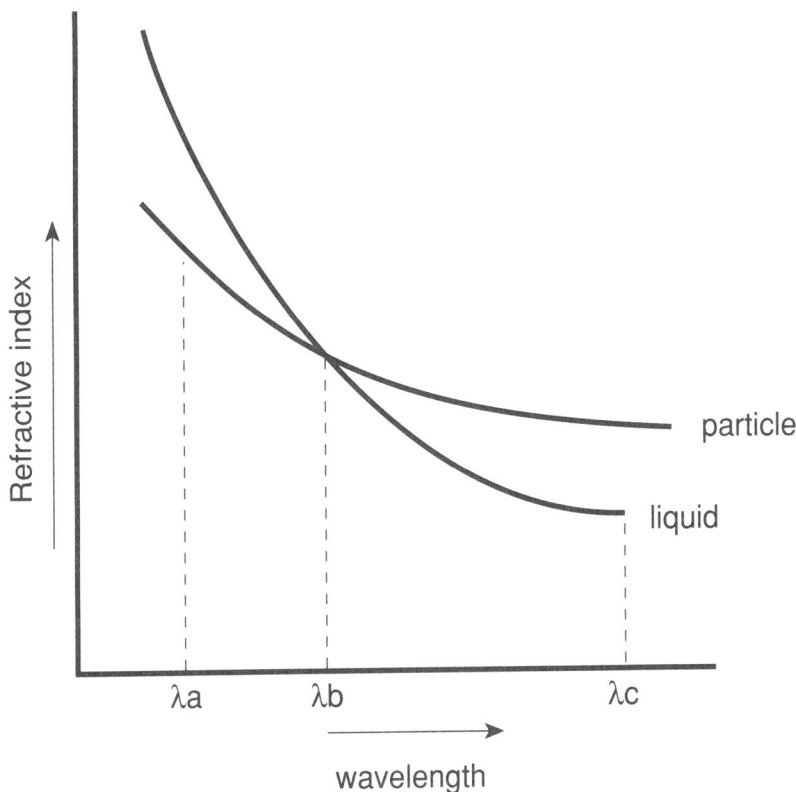

Figure 16. Dispersion curves for particle and liquid show refractive index match at λ_b.

blue). Obviously, the color dispersion characteristics for an anisotropic particle will be more complex than those of an isotropic material. This procedure is particularly valuable for identification of fibers, and is widely used in forensic microscopy (Fong 1982). Simplified for this purpose, the technique allows identification of a wide variety of fibers by means of the color observed in a single refractive index liquid. In this simplified application, a table is used to determine what color will be observed with a specific refractive index liquid-fiber combination.

Isolation and Handling of Particles

The paper by Teetsov (1977) provides an excellent discussion of how particles may be isolated for analytical procedures. The following brief information should also be useful (see also the chapter on particle collection and isolation). For bulk material such as a drug powder, a representative sample may be removed with a micro-spatula from different areas of the powder sample, or the material may be dispersed in a liquid in which it is insoluble and a drop of the resulting suspension transferred to a slide. When the particulate sample is dry, a drop of mounting medium is then placed over the particles which may be further dispersed by sliding a cover slip over the drop of mountant in a circular motion as necessary.

The most suitable mounting medium is a viscous liquid with a high refractive index. The Aroclor® series of chlorinated diphenyls or polyphenyls manufactured by Monsanto, have fallen out of favor due to environmental concerns. Other mountants that may be substituted are: Glycerol, Permount, Karo Syrup, Canada Balsam, or silicone oil. Aroclors may still be purchased, but their sale is controlled. Some very useful alternative PCB-free mountants are those of the Meltmount® series from Cargille. They are available in refractive indices ranging from 1.539–1.704. They have the beneficial properties of low cost and low melting point (65°C), and contain no volatile solvents.

Particles may be studied directly on the cellulose ester filters used to collect them from solution using reflected light or with transmitted light if a medium with a refractive index close to that of the filter material (about 1.54) is used to "clear" the filter. The particles may also be removed from the filter by scraping or picking, but this procedure will not generally give a complete or representative recovery. The most rapid procedure is simply to mount the filter in a Cargille liquid of approximately 1.5 refractive index or the manufacturer's recommended clearing index. The filter should completely disappear from view, leaving particles easily seen.

Particles can be removed from filters by dissolving the filter in solvent in a centrifuge tube (e.g., acetone), and centrifuging the particles to the bottom of the tube. The supernatant liquid is then pipetted off, the particles are washed with fresh solvent and a drop of the particle suspension is evaporated to dryness on a microscope slide. A drop of mounting medium and a cover slip are added to complete the preparation. Care must be taken in this procedure to avoid dissolving particles of interest or losing them when decanting the solvent. Particles can also be removed from filters by sonication in a liquid medium.

Transparent sticky tape is often used by forensic technicians to collect particles from a surface; the technique is also very useful for collecting particles in pharmaceutical manufacturing areas. A tape sample may be attached to a clean microscope slide while it is being transported to the laboratory for study. For quick examination a tape sample may be placed adhesive side down on a microscope slide and observed directly, or a small drop of a refractive index liquid may be placed between the slide and the tape in the area to be examined. This surrounds the particles with a uniform refractive index medium and improves the image. Refractive indices of particles relative to the medium may be estimated in this type of mount. As with particles collected on filters, the particles may be removed from the tape by solvent action. The adhesive surface of the tape is exposed and the tape sample is placed in a centrifuge tube with xylene. When the adhesive has completely dissolved, the particles are centrifuged to the bottom of the tube. The supernatant liquid is then pipetted or decanted off and the particles are washed in solvent before drying and mounting.

Hot Stage Methods

The polarized light methods described above work well for crystalline materials or for materials that have characteristic interference or extinction patterns, such as skin fragments. Although polymers other than fibers typically do not have these properties, they can be analyzed by polarized light microscopy. For most polymers, the melting point is a key parameter that may be sufficiently unique to provide for identification. In its simplest application, hot stage microscopy consists simply of determining the melting point of a particle in question and comparing it to a known comparison standard or to published data. This can be performed on a precise device such as the Mettlor hot stage or using less sophisticated methods devised in one's own laboratory. One (crude) method involves placing the unknown particle(s) and a comparison standard particle sandwiched between two glass slides that are heated with a soldering pencil. One begins with the soldering pencil in contact with the edge of the slides, then moves it slowly toward the particles so that an even rise in temperature results. Similar methods using a hot wire or an electrical cauterizing needle have also been used.

Totally satisfactory hot stage microscopy can be done without the purchase of a commercial hot stage, which is highly useful but also expensive. The analytical alternative here is the use of an electrically coated (EC) hot stage device. The use and calibration of this device is described in the article by McCrone (1981). The basis of the "device" is a 25 × 75 mm microscope slide that has a thin surface coating of chemically deposited SnO_2. The bond between the glass and the metallic oxide is persistent and electrically conducting; the passage of current through this thin layer generates heat that may be regulated with a variable transformer to give suitably precise control for melting point determination. Metal oxide coated slides are available from McCrone Research Institute (Chicago).

In use, the lead wires for a Variac are attached to the slide with conducting cement. A calibration is then effected using chemical melting point standards to generate a plot of voltage versus temperature. The device is then ready for use in melting point determination, using either published melting point tables or comparison standards to identify unknowns. A resistance thermometer may also be used to obtain direct temperature readouts.

Microscope Calibration

Light microscopes are easily calibrated using a stage micrometer scale (Bovey 1962). Such stage scales commonly have major divisions 100 µm (0.1 mm) apart, subdivided into 10 µm (0.01 mm) or finer divisions. These are used as a standard against which the divisions of the ocular scale (graticule) are calibrated. Each objective must be separately calibrated based on the correspondence between the stage scale and the ocular scale (Lanier et al. 1978). The ocular scale is first focused using the adjusting ocular of the microscope. Then, starting with the lowest power objective, the stage scale is focused and the two scales are superimposed in parallel alignment (Figure 17). At some point it will be possible to find a number of ocular divisions exactly equal to some whole number of divisions of the stage scale, expressed in micrometers (µm).

The calibration consists of calculating the number of micrometers (µm) on the stage scale per ocular scale division. To make the comparison as accurate as possible, a large part of the length of each scale must be used. For instance, in Figure 17, if four large divisions of the stage scale equal 80 ocular scale divisions, then

80 ocular scale division = 400 µm
1 ocular scale division = 400 µm/80 = 5 µm

Thus, when this ocular and scale are used with this specific objective and microscope tube length, each division of the ocular scale equals 5 µm and the scale can be used to measure an object on the microscope stage. A particle, for example, observed with the

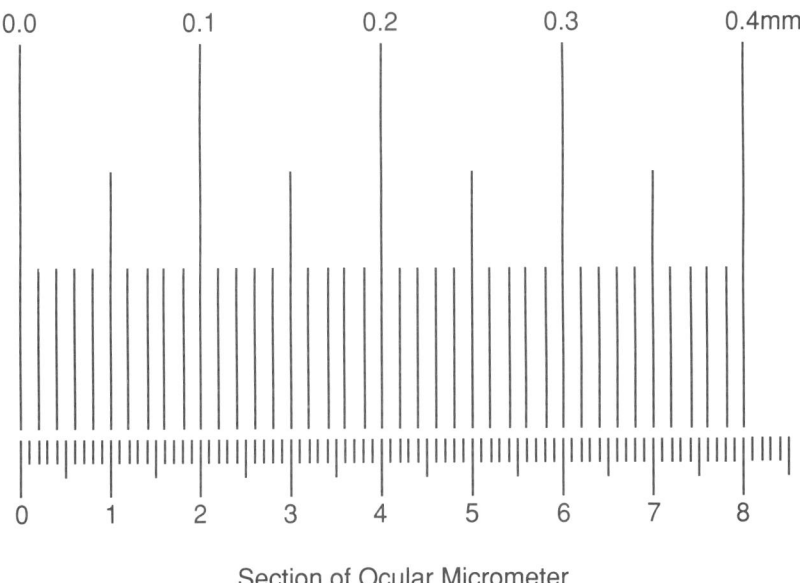

Figure 17. Comparison of stage scale with ocular scale.

---

calibrated objective measuring 10 divisions on the ocular scale, is 10 × 5 or 50 µm in diameter.

Measurement of Particle Size

The measurement of particle size varies in complexity depending on particle shape. The size of a sphere is defined by its diameter. The size of a cube may be expressed by the length of an edge or a diagonal, and the surface area, volume, and weight (if density is known). If the particles of interest are irregular in shape, the task becomes more complex. An irregularly shaped particle has a number of different dimensions that might be measured as "diameters." Figure 18 shows four statistical diameters commonly used in determining particle size. (See also the chapter on population analysis.)

Feret's diameter is the distance between parallel lines tangent to the particle profile and perpendicular to the ocular scale. The present USP measurement of particle size is in effect the maximum Feret's diameter with no regard given to the orientation of the

128 *Pharmaceutical Particulate Matter*

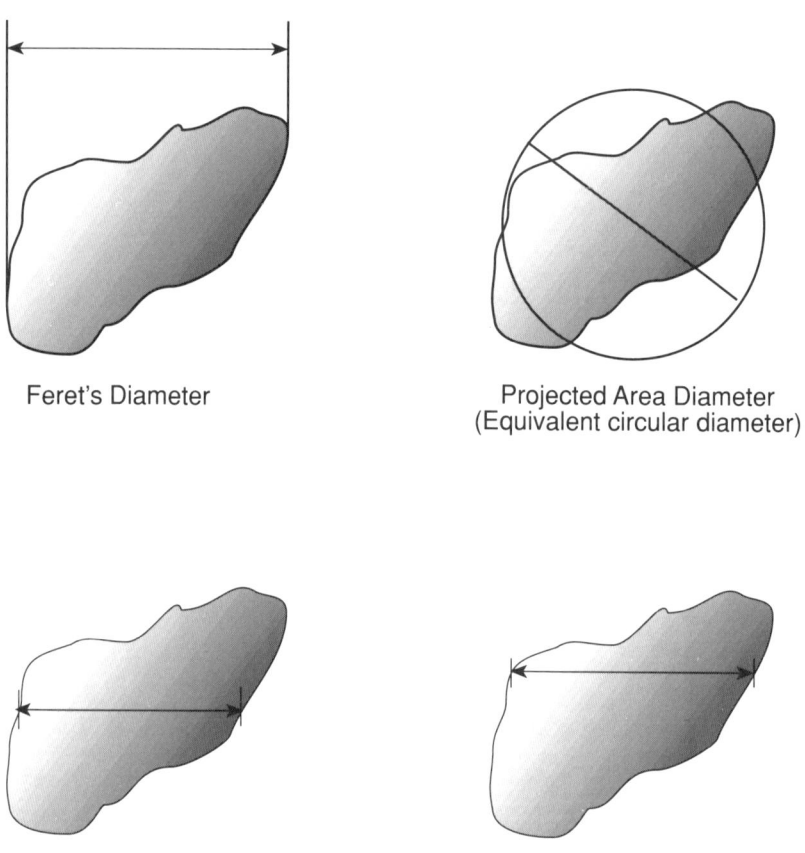

Feret's Diameter

Projected Area Diameter
(Equivalent circular diameter)

Martin's Diameter

Maximum Horizontal Intercept

Figure 18. Particle statistical diameters.

---

tangents. The maximum horizontal intercept is the longest horizontal diameter from edge to edge of the particle, parallel to the ocular reference line. Martin's diameter is one of the most frequently used for particle sizing. It is measured as the dimension (parallel to the ocular scale) that divides a randomly oriented particle into two equal projected areas. Projected area diameters are found by comparing the projected area of the particle with the areas of reference circles on an ocular graticule. In this analysis, two adjacent circles, one larger and one smaller in area than the particle, are used to define a size class into which the particle fits. The statistical diameter of the size class (and particle) is taken as the arithmetic or geometric mean between the diameters of the two circles.

Martin's diameter is a simple and widely used means of measuring and expressing the diameters of irregular particles, and is sufficiently accurate when averaged for a large number of particles. The more particles that are counted, the more accurate the average particle size will be. Platelike and needlelike particles must have a correction factor applied to account for the third dimension (thickness or width).

Techniques for Microscopic Particle Counting

The present USP <788> microscopic particulate matter test is shown in Figure 19. The general perception of the microscope as a simplistic means of particle enumeration is responsible for many of the shortcomings of this and other microscopic particle counting assays. There are a number of principles involving use of the microscope for the enumeration of particles in parenterals that must be observed if the results are to be reproducible. These are important enough to warrant their being summarized here. To begin with, the microscope must be uniformly adjusted for each analyst. There are four steps that should be followed each time an analyst sits down to perform counting.

1. Adjusting interpupillary distance,
2. Individually focusing oculars,
3. Adjusting auxiliary illuminator,
4. Balancing illuminator's light intensity, and
5. Squaring microscope stage.

The analyst first adjusts the interpupillary distance by decreasing or increasing the distance between the oculars like a pair of binoculars until a single image is obtained. The interpupillary distance as measured on the scale between the eyepieces is then recorded for future reference. The oculars must be individually focused for each user and for each eye. This is accomplished (with a specimen in place) by first defocusing the microscope so a bright field is obtained with no specimen detail visible, closing or covering the left eye, and rotating the right eyepiece diopter ring until the image of the graticule is in sharp focus. The left eyepiece is then focused to be parfocal with the right eyepiece. To do this, the microscope (not the eyepiece) is focused on some fine detail in the specimen, keeping the right eye open and the left eye closed. Then the right eye is closed or covered and the left eyepiece diopter ring is rotated until the specimen fine detail is in sharp focus. Then

130 *Pharmaceutical Particulate Matter*

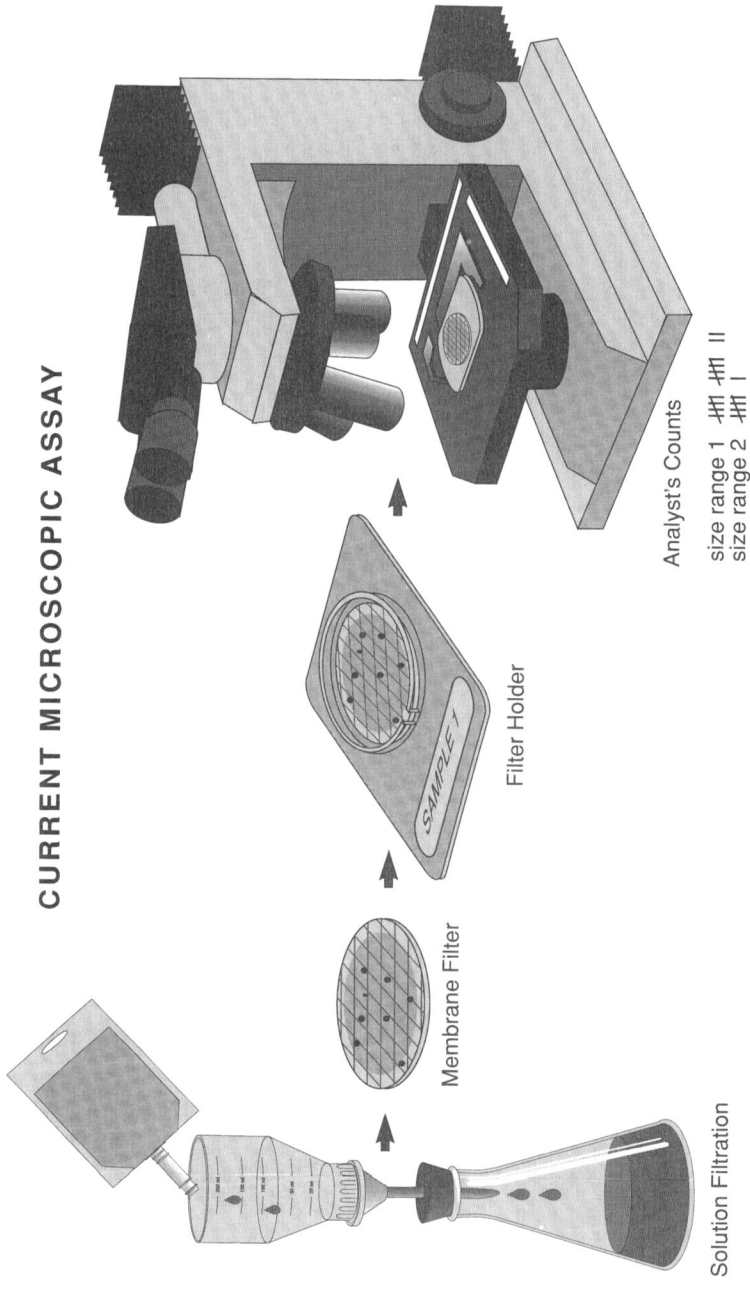

Figure 19. USP <788> Microscopic Particulate Matter Test

open both eyes. The specimen image should be in sharp focus in both eyepieces.

The lateral illumination is then adjusted by first increasing the lamp intensity by turning the transformer to the maximum setting in the black zone (typically 8 volts or 80% of full scale). The illuminator field diaphragm is fully opened, and the lamp filament is centered by tilting the illuminator horizontally and shining it on a nearby wall (or other perpendicular) flat surface 1–2 feet away. The lamp is focused to achieve a sharp image of the filament by rotating the focusing knobs on the side of the illuminator. The lamp filament is then centered by adjusting the centering screws. The analyst then rotates the lamp socket to verify the alignment; ideally, the filament image should rotate in one spot about its axis.

The illuminator must be placed in close proximity to the stage and in a specific angular orientation to the stage for optimal particle detection. First the illuminator is positioned on a diagonal (45°) with the microscope stage at the upper right corner of the stage. The front of the illuminator should be flush with the corner of the stage. Initially, the height of the illuminator should be adjusted to 3–5 centimeters above the microscope stage, then the tilt angle of the illuminator is adjusted so that the light beam is directed onto the portion of the specimen under the objective. The illuminator must be focused to give a bright spot of illumination, but the image of the filament should not be visible. While looking through the microscope eyepieces, the tilt and position of the illuminator are then aligned to achieve a bright, even illumination across the field of view. Particles on a membrane filter should have distinct dark shadows.

Finally, the microscope stage must be squared to be parallel with the eyepiece vertical and horizontal axes so that when a particle is moved across the field of view, it moves in a straight line rather than at an angle. The squaring procedure is accomplished in three steps: First the right eyepiece is rotated so that the graticule scale bar appears horizontal. Then a particle is placed at the center of the cross hair and moved by the microscope stage positioning control to the left and to the right the length of the horizontal cross hair. If the particle center stays on the horizontal scale bar, the stage is square to the eyepiece and no adjustment is required. If not, the stage is rotated until the particle traverses the field horizontally.

In addition to the adjustment of the microscope, the filtration process is a critical step in precise enumeration of particles and reproducibility of the assay. Cleaning of the filtration equipment may be conducted generally as described in the article by DeLuca and Bodapatti (1980). The general principle involved in cleaning is the exhaustive removal of adherent particles from any glassware or vessels or apparatus to be used in the test. This may be accomplished by soaking in a detergent solution, rinsing in distilled water, and a final rinse with a jet of filtered distilled (0.45 μm or lower retention rated filter) water (Figure 20). The final rinse should result in the water "sheeting" the entire rinse surface of the object being washed. A pressure vessel with filter on the dispenser nozzle may be substituted for the set up shown in the figure.

All of the steps in the filtration procedure are conducted wearing rinsed particle-free vinyl gloves in a Class 100 laminar airflow hood. For the whole volume filtration of a large volume injection (LVI), a 100 mL or more capacity filtration funnel should be used. The Gelman 25 mm polysulfone filtration setup with 200 mL twist lock coupling funnel (Gelman #4203) may be used. To assist in obtaining an even particle distribution, a metal diffuser screen (Millipore stainless support screen catalog #XX30 025 10) should also be used beneath the filter membrane. For filtration, the ultraclean filtration funnel is first assembled by placing the metal diffuser on top of the filtration base. A clean membrane filter is then centered on top of the diffuser using clean forceps to hold the filter edge, and then the filter funnel is attached to the base. The funnel is attached to a vacuum flask and the flask to the vacuum source. The neck of the unit to be sampled is rinsed, the unit is gently inverted 20 times, the stopper is removed and the desired sample volume is emptied into the funnel. To pool a number of small volume injection (SVI) vials, the vials are emptied into an ultracleaned beaker and then the beaker is poured into the filter funnel. Vacuum is applied to draw the solution through the filter. If the volume to be filtered is greater than the capacity of the filter funnel, additions of solution are made when the volume in the funnel is approximately $1/4$ to $1/3$ full.

Specific steps must be followed during filtration to ensure an even particle distribution on the analysis membrane. If care is not taken to ensure an even distribution, the concentration of particles in higher-then-countable numbers at the periphery of the membrane may occur, particularly if an entire LVI solution unit is filtered. As the final volume of solution is drawn out of the funnel, the analyst begins rinsing the funnel by directing a low pressure 10 psi stream of filtered distilled water in a circular pattern along the walls of the funnel, being careful not to direct the spray at the

Microscopy 133

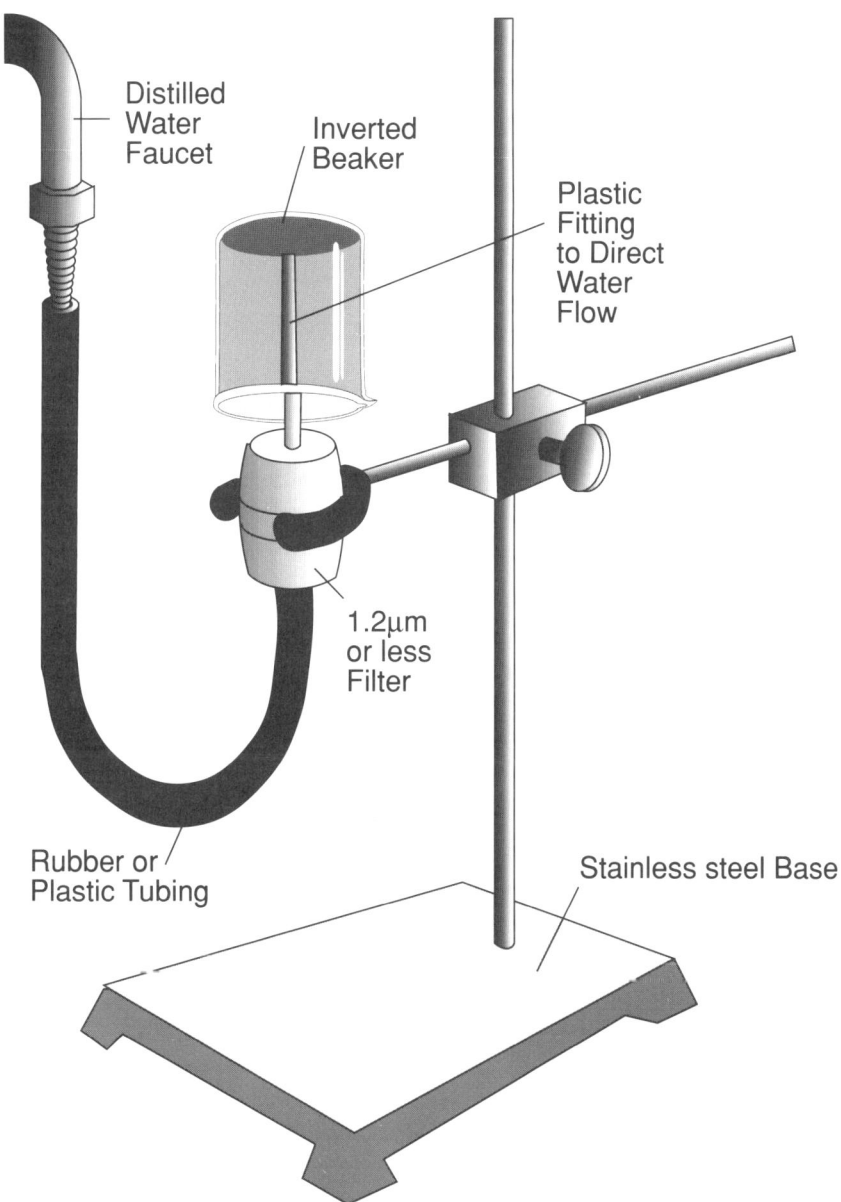

Figure 20. Final rinsing of glassware using filtered distilled water.

filter surface. Rinsing should stop before the volume in the funnel falls below 20 mL; the vacuum is maintained until all the liquid in the funnel is gone. Then the vacuum is turned off and the filtration funnel is removed from the filtration base. (Residual vacuum will hold the filter in place.) The vacuum in the filtration base is broken by disconnecting the vacuum hose from the side arm of the filtration flask or by opening a valve in the vacuum line. The filter is then removed with cleaned forceps to a labeled PetriSlide™ and secured in place with double sided tape. The membrane is allowed to air dry in a laminar flow hood with cover slightly ajar prior to viewing.

The following caution is of great importance: No laboratory should be engaged in the performance of microscopic particle counting without the inclusion of an ongoing process of analyst training and validation. This is typically conducted through the use of a set of "unknown" standard samples that are counted by each analyst on a regular basis. The scrutiny of counts from these membranes will allow the identification of analysts who need retraining due to their counts trending above or below the counts from the majority of the other analysts in the group. Additionally, an analyst should complete the count of any given membrane in a single sitting. Some laboratories require analysts to "warm up" by counting a standard membrane before beginning to count for each day. The goal of all of these procedures is to ensure that human analysts count so that precision and reproducibility are incorporated into the data collected.

Enumeration of Particles in Parenteral Products

There are potential major advantages that accrue in the use of microscopic test methods for the enumeration of contaminant particles in parenterals (Kirnbauer 1970). First, the microscopic test allows the particles counted to be visualized so that only "real" particles are counted; the method is not subject to interferences from gas bubbles and immiscibles, and refractive index effects that are encountered with light extinction counters are avoided. Further, there is uniform collection of particles of all sizes and the particle stratification (i.e., the overcounting of small particles) seen with both light extinction and electrical zone sensing instruments is avoided. Particles may often be identified in the preparation made for enumeration. Lastly, particles may be uniformly detected and sized based on their physical dimensions irrespective of their color, transparency, or refractive index.

The full potential for a compendial microscopic test method is not realized by the current USP <788> test method (United States Pharmacopeia XXII; Draftz 1990). Basically, this method requires the analyst to filter a 25 mL aliquot from the unit to be tested on a color contrast, gridded membrane filter and enumerate the particulate matter collected in two size categories (≥10 μm, ≥25 μm) based on the longest effective linear dimension of a particle. Low angle 10°–20° lateral illumination is used.

In the 25 years since the implementation of the USP <788> requirement, authors in the pharmaceutical industry, academia, and the regulatory agency have commented on method defects including: (1) possible count extrapolation errors resulting from the small aliquot sampled and the inability of the method to handle large numbers of particles; (2) the need for a more refined method with improved capabilities for particle detection; (3) the time consuming nature of the analysis and need for extensive analyst training; and, (4) the generally inadequate interpretation that can be made of the results (Porter 1977; Trasen 1968a; Rebagay et al. 1977a, 1977b; DeLuca et al. 1987; Delly 1980).

The Health Industry Manufacturer's Association (HIMA) in the U.S. has developed and proposed to the USP an improved microscopic assay (IMA) to be used as a replacement for the current USP <788> test for LVIs. The proposed new test differs from the USP assay in five fundamental elements. The new test involves the application of:

1. Particle sizing by circular area diameter (equivalent circular diameter),

2. Whole unit volume filtration,

3. Statistical (partial) counting of analysis membranes,

4. Episcopic as well as reflected illumination, and

5. Plain nongridded membrane filters.

The current USP procedure requires that a particle's maximum chord be used as a measurement of size. Particles are not actually measured for maximum dimension, but rather mentally compared to a linear graticule scale by the analyst. The linear measurement made in the present <788> method is responsible for a significant variability component in the test result (Beckett et al. 1976; Bovey 1962). In the absence of test data, the ≥10 μm size was apparently selected as a worst case dimension representing a particle of the size that might occlude capillary blood vessels. The basis of the ≥25 μm size range is uncertain. While there is still no data to support the importance of these sizes, parenteral manufacturers have been obtaining counts for particles of these sizes for years, resulting in a significant historical data base. The proposed IMA should provide better agreement between the particle sizes measured by the two different compendial methods, based on the equivalent circular area conversion produced both by light extinction counters and the IMA.

Much of the variability of data collected with the present USP microscopic test results from imprecision in sizing; the potential for error from this source in the present test is quite large (>±20%) (Heywood 1946). The linear scale is not only difficult to use for size comparison, but it is often located some distance from the particle being sized (British Standards 3625, 3406; Watson and Mulford 1952) Thus, mental transposition errors can be significant (Hamilton et al. 1952). Both of these errors will be eliminated in the new test. The USP IMA graticule has a circular field of view and sizing circles that correspond to 10 µm and 25 µm diameters (Figure 21) (similar to that described by Walton and Becket 1977). A

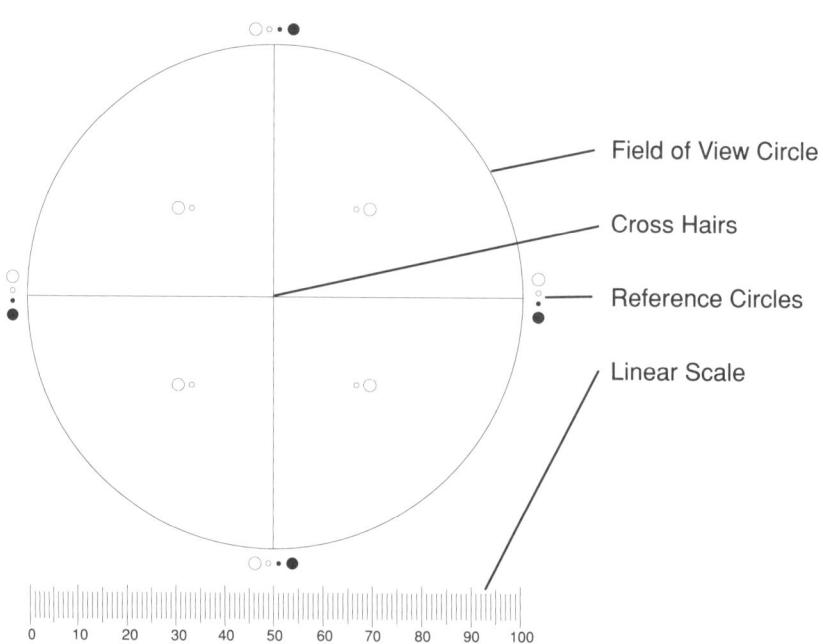

Figure 21. The proposed improved USP microscopic test graticule.

linear scale is included (outside the field of view) for use if measurement of particles by this method is necessary.

The USP <788> method defines the solution sample as the first 25 mL aliquot taken from an LVP solution. One of the problems commonly associated with this first 25 mL is that it may have a disproportionately high concentration of particles, especially particles larger than 25 µm in diameter. Some of these particles are low density materials that float and are decanted with the first 25 mL; others may be particles that were adhering to the neck, stopper, or port of the container before the closure was removed. These particles may detrimentally affect the accuracy of counts obtained from a 25 mL aliquot due to the sampling bias they cause. The simple solution to this problem is to sample the entire volume of an LVP unit for microscopical counting. Using the entire volume minimizes or eliminates bias in favor of large particles and should lead to improved assay precision. Sampling the entire volume also provides a better assessment of the average particle concentration delivered to a patient, and also eliminates the effect of blank contribution to the test result as a significant error effect (Trasen 1968a). Irrespective of sample size, it is imperative that the removal of the sample from the container be accomplished with as few steps and as simply as possible.

Poor particle detection in the present USP test, another critical issue, results from two factors: (1) the low angle of illumination prescribed (10°–20°), which results in some difficulty in obtaining a sufficient intensity of illumination; and (2) the fact that only reflected illumination is used. The latter results in an inability to detect flat, flake-like particles that reflect the incident illumination outside of the angle of acceptance of the microscope objective, and by virtue of their thinness, cast no shadow (Delly 1980). Particles of this morphology are often a dominant type in an SVI unit. This situation may be greatly improved through the use of a combination of oblique reflected illumination and episcopic illumination. The results of the HIMA testing show that a mixed cellulose ester filter viewed with oblique side lighting at a 10°–20° angle and episcopic fill-in illumination gives optimal particle detection.

With the improved assay, the user will be allowed the option of performing either a partial or total count of particles on an analysis membrane. With either procedure a confidence limit may be defined based on numbers of particles counted. Partial counting of sample membranes with larger numbers of particles will produce results comparable to those obtained with the current <788> procedure and yet reduce the time necessary for counting. A partial counting procedure simply specifies a predefined minimum number of particles and/or fields of view to be counted, based on a preselected confidence interval. If only a fraction of the membrane is counted, the elapsed time for counting particles from a total unit volume in this fashion will frequently be less than is required for a total count of particles from a 25 mL aliquot.

Knowledge of the statistical strength of the count data obtained from any analysis of a solution unit is of overwhelming importance. The new method will emphasize the use of statistical procedures to judge whether solution passes or fails the test. The current USP method does not employ a statistical decision making process or report an uncertainty (error range) in the numerical value obtained for each sample. This does not pose a problem for most LVP samples since they are usually very far below the current USP failure limit, but it becomes a serious issue if higher counts are obtained.

The distribution of particle sizes in a sample from an LVI or SVI unit approximates a Poisson distribution. With a Poisson distribution of particle sizes, the variability (standard deviation) of an assay result is to an approximation, simply equal to the square root of the number of particles counted, 1000 (±32), 100 (±10), 10 (±3.2). We can, therefore, preselect the desired precision for a test of whether a given sample is below or exceeds the limit by selecting the number of particles to be counted. With statistical counting, the higher the number of particles/field, the better the estimate one obtains of numbers of particles in the total unit volume. A statistical or partial count strategy is essential when the larger numbers of particles that may be present in an SVI unit are to be counted (Draftz 1990).

While it offers a number of significant advantages over the present microscopic and light extinction tests, it should be understood that the IMA is not being proposed as an ideal compendial particulate matter test (DeLuca et al. 1987). In fact, no single ideal test exists. What is gained in terms of better precision, improved particle detection, and the greater confidence in the pass-fail result in the test is offset, to some extent, by the significant amount of analyst training that will be required in method conversion and the time requirement inherent in performing any microscopic test. It is useful in this consideration to reflect on why a microscopic method is essential in particulate matter testing of parenteral products. First, microscopy constitutes the only means of making a direct measurement of particulate contaminant in parenterals. The light extinction test is an extremely time-effective ancillary method. When applied in a carefully controlled GMP environment to product for which the general particle burden has been well characterized, the instrumental method constitutes an adequate means of monitoring product particle burden. Since it is a secondary or indirect means of measurement, however, any result suspected of being in error will always have to be checked microscopically. It is most logical, therefore, to retain some form of microscopic methodology in the USP that will provide a compendial test that is unaffected by the interferences to which the light extinction test is subject.

Summary

Light microscopy constitutes the simplest and most cost-effective means for enumerating, characterizing, and identifying particles. The methods required can be applied by an analyst having only basic training in microscopy; the majority of the particulates encountered in parenterals may be identified on sight or through simple manipulations involving the polarizing light microscope. Microscopic methods of particle enumeration require more time than does the application of automatic particle counters, but microscopic methods are not subject to false counts due to air bubbles or artifact due to immiscible liquids. Improvements to the current USP <788> microscopic assay for particles in large volume injections have resulted in an improved test method that shows promise as a future compendial particulate matter referee test. In this era of high-tech analytical instrumentation, light microscopy remains a means by which a laboratory with limited funds and expertise can acquire the capability for analysis and counting of pharmaceutical particulate matter with a minimal outlay for equipment and personnel.

References

Barber, T. A., M. D. Lannis, and J. G. Williams. 1989. Method evaluation: Automated microscopy as a compendial test for particulates in parenteral solutions. *J. Parent. Sci. Technol.* 43 (1):27–41.

Beckett, R. K., R. K. Hey, R. Hirst, R. D. Hunt, J. L. Jarvis, and A. L. Richards. 1976. A comparison of airborne asbestos fiber counting with and without an eyepiece graticule. *Ann. Occup. Hyg.* 19:69–76.

Bovey, E. 1962. Graticules and fine scales: Their production and application in modern measuring systems. *J. Sci. Instrum.* 39:405–413.

Chamot, E. M., and C. W. Mason. 1958. *Handbook of chemical microscopy, Vol. I,* 3rd Ed. New York: John Wiley and Sons.

Delly, J. G. 1980. Problems of sizing particles using USP methodology. *Pharmacopeial Forum.* Rockville MD: United States Pharmacopeial Convention Inc. (July–August):357–376.

Delly, J. G. 1988. *Photography through the micropscope.* Publication P-2, 9th Ed. Rochester, NY: Eastman Kodak Co.

DeLuca, P. P., and S. Bodapatti. 1980. Guidelines for the identification of particles in parenterals. *FDA Guidelines,* no. 3 (July).

DeLuca, P. P., B. Conti, and J. Z. Knapp. 1987. An overview of technical issues in particle detection. In *Proc. PDA Conf. on Liquid Borne Particle Inspection and Metrology,* 376–380. Washington, D.C.

Draftz, R. G. 1990. Microscopical counting, sizing and statistical strategies for LVP contaminants. In *Proc. PDA Int. Conf. on Particle Detection, Metrology and Control,* 458–466. Arlington, VA.

Feigl, F., and V. Anger. 1972. *Spot tests in inorganic analysis.* 6th Ed. New York: Elsevier.

Fong, W. 1982. Rapid microscopic identification of synthetic fibers in a single liquid mount. *Journal of Forensic Sciences* 27 (2, April):257–263.

Godfray, M. F. 1979. Microscopy of contaminants of pharmaceuticals and their characterization. *Proc. Analyst. Div. Chem. Soc.* 16:160–161.

Hamilton, R. J., M. A. Holdsworth, and W. H. Walton. 1952. Factors in the design of a microscopic eyepiece graticule for routine dust counts. *Brit. J. Appl. Phys. Suppl.* 3:S101–S105.

Heywood, H. A. 1946. Comparison of methods of measuring microscopical particles. *Bull. Inst. Min. Metall.* 477:1–14.

Kirnbauer, E. 1970. Liquid borne particle counting in the pharmaceutical industry, I. Microscopic counting. *Bull. Parent. Drug Assoc.* 24:53–58.

Lanier, J. M., G. S. Oxborrow, and L. T. Kononen. 1978. Calibration of microscopes for measuring particles found in parenteral solutions. *J. Parenteral Drug Assoc.* 32:145–148.

Mason, C. W. 1983. *Handbook of chemical microscopy, Vol. I.* New York: Wiley Interscience Publishers.

McCormack, J., J. E. C. Harris, and H. J. Sullivan. 1976. Single particle characterization by optical microscopy and associated techniques. *Proc. Analst. Div. Chem. Soc.* 13:344–348.

McCrone, W. C. 1978. Identification of parenteral particulate contaminants. *Pharm. Technol.* 2 (May):57–59.

McCrone, W. C. 1981. Calibration of the E.C. slide hotstage. *The Microscope* 39:43–61.

McCrone, W. C. 1987. *Polarized light microscopy.* Ann Arbor, MI: Ann Arbor Science Publishers.

McCrone, W. C., and J. G. Delly. 1973a. *Principles and techniques.* Vol. 1, *The particle atlas,* 2nd Ed. Ann Arbor, MI: Ann Arbor Science Publishers.

McCrone, W. C., and J. G. Delly. 1973b. *The light microscopy atlas.* Vol. 2, *The particle atlas,* 2nd Ed. Ann Arbor, MI: Ann Arbor Science Publishers.

McCrone, W. C., and J. G. Delly. 1973c. *The electron microscopy atlas.* Vol. 3, *The particle atlas,* 2nd Ed. Ann Arbor, MI: Ann Arbor Science Publishers.

McCrone, W. C., and J. G. Delly. 1973d. *The particle analyst's handbook.* Vol. 4, *The particle atlas,* 2nd Ed. Ann Arbor MI: Ann Arbor Science Publishers.

McCrone, W. C., J. G. Delly, and S. J. Palenik. 1979. *Light microscopy atlas and techniques.* Vol. 5, *The particle atlas,* 2nd Ed. Ann Arbor, MI: Ann Arbor Science Publishers.

McCrone, W. C., and J. S. Martin. 1964. Identifying colorless transparent particles by microscopy. *Research/Development* (November):28–31.

McCrone, W. C., and I. M. Stewart. 1974. Microscopy. *Amer. Lab.* 6:13–17.

Methods for determination of particle size distribution. *Optical Microscope Method* 4:3406 (1963—Confirmed 1985). Available from British Standards Institution, British Standards House, 2 Park Street, London, UK.

Oles, P. J. 1978. Particle analysis and identification in the pharmaceutical industry. *Microscope* 26:41–48.

Porter, M. C. 1977. Detection of small particulates on membrane filters. *Bull. Parent. Drug Assoc.* 31:170–172.

Rebagay, T., H. G. Schroeder, S. Im, and P. P. DeLuca. 1977a. Particulate matter monitoring I. Evaluation of some membrane filters and microscopic techniques. *Bull. Parenteral Drug Assoc.* 31:57–69.

Rebagay, T., H. G. Schroeder, S. Im, and P. P. DeLuca. 1977b. Particulate matter monitoring II. Correlation of microscopic and automatic counting methods. *Bull. Parenteral Drug Assoc.* 31:150–155.

Schroeder, H. G., and P. P. DeLuca. 1980. Theoretical aspects of particulate matter monitoring by microscopic and instrumental methods. *J. Parenteral Drug. Assoc.* 34:185–191.

Specification for eyepiece and screen graticule. 1963. Standard 3625. Available from British Standards Institution, British Standards House, 2 Park Street, London, UK.

Teetsov, A. S. 1977. Techniques of small particle manipulation. *Microscope* 25:103–113.

The United States Pharmacopeia. 1990. 22nd Ed. Easton, PA: Mack Printing Co., <788>:1596–1598.

Trasen, B. 1968a. Detection and reduction of particulate matter in pharmaceuticals. *Chem. Eng. Progress* 64 (2):64–68.

Trasen, B. 1968b. Reduction of particulate matter in pharmaceuticals. *Drug and Cosm. Ind.* 102 (6):40–162.

Walton, W. H., and S. T. Beckett. 1977. A microscope eyepiece graticule for the evaluation of fibrous dusts. *Ann. Occup. Hyg.* 20:19–23.

Watson, H. H., and D. F. Mulford. 1952. A particle profile test strip for assessing the accuracy of sizing irregularly shaped particles with a microscope. *Brit J. Appl. Phys. Suppl.* 3:S105–S108.

Winchell, A. N., and H. Winchell. 1964. *The microscopical characters of artificial inorganic solid substances: Optical properties,* 3rd Ed. London: Academic Press.

V

Instrumental Analysis for Particle Identification

Light microscopic methods, as discussed in the previous chapter, often provide the simplest and most cost-effective way to perform particle counting and identification. However, light microscopic analysis of particulate matter has several limitations. With regard to enumeration of particulate matter, manual light microscopy becomes tedious and time consuming if large numbers of particles are to be counted. Thus, while light microscopy may be suitable for compendial testing of parenteral products when relatively small numbers of particles are to be counted, it is not practical for the enumeration of larger numbers of particles necessary for particle size distribution analyses. The use of light extinction counters provides an alternative, but this methodology also has serious limitations in that it provides no information on particle shape or other morphologic characteristics and is subject to artifact from microdroplets of immiscible liquids, air bubbles, or other sources.

Polarized light microscopy also is limited in its role. The foremost limitation is that particles must be of a unique morphology or be transparent in order to be identified by this method. Another serious practical limitation is that the power of the method is totally dependent upon the skill of the microscopist. Analysts skilled in the identification of particles using polarized light microscopy are relatively few in number, and have become increasingly harder to find over the years. Magnification is limited to approximately 1000× for both polarized light microscopy and nonpolarized transmitted light microscopy.

Thus, contemporary methods of particle identification and counting have come to be increasingly dependent upon instrumental methods of analysis and automated microscopy. General principles of the most widely applicable methods of these types are discussed in this section and in the appropriate references. The reference by Borchert et al. (1986) provides an excellent overview. With regard to particle identification, the particle analyst has adopted the three most basic chemical analytical techniques for his use. As the analytical chemist depends heavily upon x-ray spectroscopy, infrared spectroscopy, and mass spectrometry, those of us interested in the identification of particles frequently apply x-ray analysis (in combination with electron microscopy), microinfrared techniques, and micro methods of mass spectrometry. Transmission electron microscopy (TEM) and scanning electron microscopy (SEM) provide powerful means of examining particles at high magnification. Automated microscopy (image analysis) provides a rapid and precise means of sizing and counting large numbers of particles. Light scattering analyses (nephelometry, laser diffraction, photon correlation spectroscopy) provide us with ways of performing particle population analyses in short periods of time.

The method chosen for the instrumental analysis of particles is determined by the objectives of a specific study and the type of data required to meet those objectives (Aldrich 1990). For example, if the elemental composition of individual particles is required, then the most suitable means of analysis will be electron microscopy with x-ray microanalysis. The selection of an analytical approach has significant impact on sampling and particle collection. General considerations important in the selection of a mode of analysis involve whether or not it is labor-intensive, whether there are interferences in the analysis and corrections that must be applied, how contamination of samples will be avoided, and (importantly) the cost of the total analytical procedure.

Particle isolates differ from the traditional trace analytical sample by virtue of their dispersal: they are most often heterogeneously dispersed in a limited matrix and require isolation or localization prior to analysis. Light microscopy is most often an excellent first choice for any endeavor directed at particle identification. The typical path of analysis that is most successful in particle identification represents a step-wise progression from simple to complex techniques, and low to high magnification. Specific techniques used for particle identification include the following:

Visual Inspection

Low magnification examination (stereomicroscopy)

Compound light microscopic examination

Polarized light microscopy

- physical properties
- chemical composition
- crystallinity
- thermal analysis

Electron microscopy

- surface morphology

X-Ray spectroscopy

- elemental composition

Infrared microspectrophotometry

- molecular information

Mass spectrometry (LAMMA, SIMS)

- mass-specific molecular data

X-ray crystallography

- crystal structure-specific molecular data

Implicit in this scheme of identification is, of course, the fact that some isolates will be identified early on as the analysis is pursued and others may require the entire range of analytical processes. These latter cases are relatively few. Light microscopic techniques were discussed in the preceding chapter; the remainder of the section deals with electron microscopy and nonmicroscopic techniques.

Particle Identification—Electron Microscopy

Electron microscopic analyses are most often performed by analysts who specialize in this important and somewhat complex technology. This section is intended only to be an introduction to the method; the beginning particle analyst is directed to the references for a more detailed consideration. The little book by Wischnitzer (1981) is an excellent and widely-used introductory text, and the reference by McCrone et al. (1980) provides a wealth of specific information related to particle analysis. Electron microscopy can be used for the observation of particle size, shape, and morphology for counting particles or for determination of the chemical composition (x-ray spectroscopy). Electron microscopy may be applied in either transmission (TEM) or scanning (SEM) modes.

In TEM the sample is analyzed by detection of the transmitted electron beam and the 50–100 kilo electron volt (keV) electrons used must pass through the sample in order to obtain information about it. In SEM the electron beam is scanned across the sample in mutually perpendicular axes and the variation in the detected signal provides contrast information that is used in image formation. The resulting image reveals the surface features of the sample, giving a pseudo three-dimensional image. A scanning microscope typically employs a lower energy electron beam (1–30 keV) than a transmission instrument. A variety of detectors can be incorporated into an electron microscope system to be used for chemical analysis. These include energy dispersive x-ray (EDXS), wavelength dispersive x-ray spectroscopy (WDXS), electron energy loss spectroscopy (EELS), Auger electron spectroscopy, and selected area electron diffraction (SAED) for use with TEM systems.

The electron microscope does not eliminate the need for optical microscopy, but it provides an additional method that can be used in particle identification and analysis that offers its own special advantages. Although it is a powerful technique, electron microscopy should not be considered the ultimate method of analysis, but rather a complementary tool that can provide needed information about a specific particle sample. Optical microscopy, especially low magnification stereomicroscopy, should be used as a first step in all analyses by SEM or TEM. Preliminary particle identification, counting, sizing, and individual particle isolation and mounting for electron microscopy must be accomplished with the optical microscope.

Transmission Electron Microscopy

The function and application of electron microscopes is introduced in the basic text by Wischnitzer (1981); this book is an excellent investment for beginners who are looking for an introduction to this means of analysis. Figure 1 is a simplified schematic comparison of transmission light and transmission electron microscopes. The similarity between the two instruments is evident. Both microscopes contain a condenser lens to focus illuminating radiation upon the object being observed. In the light microscope this lens

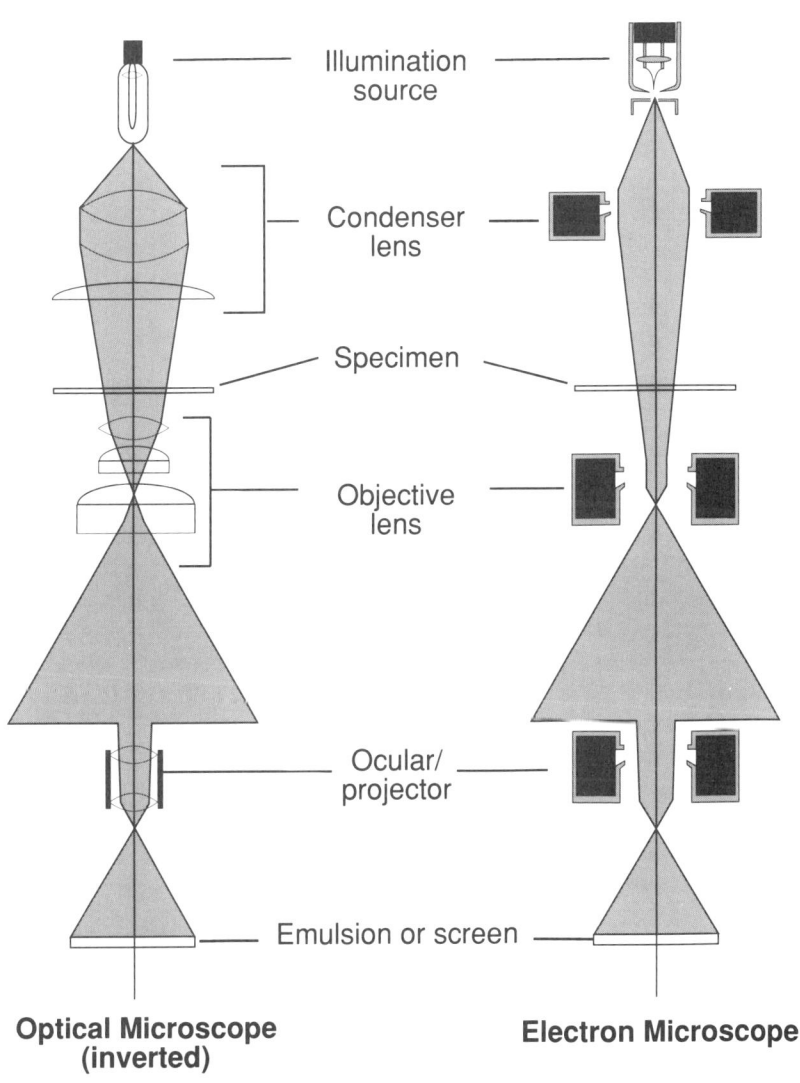

Figure 1. Transmission light and electron microscopes.

and other lenses are made of glass or a similar material. Glass is opaque to electrons, and in the electron microscope the lenses are cylindrical electromagnets formed by passing a current through a coil of wire precisely wound on an iron cylinder, the vertical axis of which is coincident with the optical axis of the microscope. The focal length of a glass lens is fixed and focusing with the light microscope is accomplished by moving the lens to an appropriate distance from the object. In the electron microscope, the focal length of the lenses is adjusted by varying the amount of current passed through the lens coil. As a result, the lenses of the electron microscope need not be moved in relation to the object; rather, the lens current is changed to achieve focus. The image of the electron microscope is viewed by allowing imaging electrons to fall upon a zinc or cadmium sulfide screen in which atomic electrons excited by the beam electrons emit a green-yellow light visible to the human eye as they return to their ground state. Image enhancement video systems are also applied for the purpose of imaging.

As discussed in the section on light microscopy, if we say that point-to-point resolution of a light microscope is 0.5 µm, we mean that two specimen points that are closer together than 0.5 µm will appear as a single object. When two points are separated by a distance greater than 0.5 µm, we will detect them as separate entities. The four principal factors that determine the resolution attainable with the light microscope—diffraction effects, chromatic aberration, spherical aberration, and astigmatism—also limit the resolution of the transmission electron microscope (TEM). In the case of the former instrument, resolution is ultimately limited by diffraction effects, whereas, in present day electron microscopy, resolution is limited by spherical aberrations in the objective lens. The great resolving power of the transmission electron microscope, which results from the short wavelength of electron illumination, is responsible for the high magnifications attainable with this instrument. In transmission microscopy advantage is taken of the fact that greatly increased resolution can be achieved by use of short wavelength electron illumination. In 1920, De Broglie postulated that any moving particle could be assigned a wavelength according to:

$$\lambda = \frac{h}{(mv)}$$

where h = Planck's constant
        m = mass of the particle
        v = velocity of the particle

For an electron, accelerated across a voltage potential difference v, this becomes:

$$\lambda = \frac{12.3}{\sqrt{v}}$$

For 100 keV electrons the wavelength is about 4.0×10^{-3} nanometers (nm) or about 10^{-5} times the wavelength of ultraviolet light. Using Abbe's equation it can be calculated that the resolution achievable with this wavelength illumination is approximately 0.25 nm. This is an approximate 10^3 increase in resolution over that achievable with light microscope.

In both transmission light and electron microscopes there would be no image if the object did not in some way interact with the illuminating radiation. In the light microscope, contrast results largely from the differential absorption of light structures in the object. In addition, as light passes the edges of objects in the specimen, diffraction patterns result from the interference of diffracted and undiffracted light and these diffraction patterns are reconstituted by the lens system into the final image. In the TEM, contrast is provided by electron scattering due to charge effects as the electrons pass through the object. Scattered electrons are removed from the beam and not focused on the screen; as a result, regions of the object that contain heavy metals, for example, are represented on the screen as dark areas.

Electromagnetic Lenses

Simple electromagnetic solenoids may be constructed by coiling a conductor around a hollow nonferrous core. Such a helix or solenoid unites the magnetic field of each coil of the conductor, has a north and south pole, and has an internal magnetic field as well as an external one. This sort of simple solenoid forms a simple, weak electromagnetic lens. Around and within any such cylindrical electromagnet, the field exists as concentric cylinders of magnetic flux lines. The central field in a solenoid is composed of flux lines of a density proportional, within limits, to the coil current. The field is uniform in the center of the solenoid, but at its ends the lines of force curve and diverge and form closed loops along the outer surface. The flux density is thus greater in the center of the loop than at any other point. The lines of force are parallel in the center of the solenoid and a permanent magnet placed in the center of the coil will orient itself perpendicular to the turns of wire.

With an electromagnetic lens (in reality a powerful solenoid), the path of an electron entering the central lens opening at some angle to the axis of symmetry is defined by resolution of a vector that acts perpendicular to the lens field flux lines and one that acts parallel to the field. The path will then be a straight line if the solenoid is not energized; if current is applied to the windings, the path becomes a summation of the linear and accurate vectors; that is, a spiral helical one. This principle results in the focusing action of electromagnetic lenses (Figure 2) in a transmission microscope. Regardless of their angle of entry, electrons entering the field at a given point complete the same number of turns as they pass from one end of the solenoid field to the other and are brought to focus at a single point behind the lens. As a result, the point at which an electron strikes an image plane will be precisely comparable to its relative position in the specimen plane before the lens. The path of an electron after leaving the lens field (behind the lens) and passing into an area where the lens influence is removed will again be a straight line at some angle to the optical axis determined by the original angle (θ) at which it entered the lens field. Electrons thus deflected and focused can form a diffuse magnified image on some behind-the-lens image plane. The end result is a lens system for electrons that mimics the focusing action of biconvex glass lenses for light.

The condenser lenses of an electron microscope allow a demagnified spot of illumination to be focused on the specimen. As in the light microscope, the role of these lenses is to allow optimum illumination by focusing the electron beam on the specimen. They are weak electromagnetic lenses with focal lengths measured in mm rather than the µm focal length of the objective. Instead of focusing a substage condenser, as with the light microscope, one simply changes beam focal conditions by varying lens current. The changeable focal length of the condenser lens in the electron microscope makes possible the simultaneous control of both α (the aperture angle of illumination) and beam intensity (electrons/unit area/time). Additionally, it makes the beam far more coherent than that obtained from the electron source (gun).

The imaging lens system of transmission electron microscopes consists of an objective lens and two or three projector lenses. Most commonly the final lens that projects an image onto the fluorescent screen is called a projector lens and those between it and the objective are called intermediate lenses. The objective lens forms the initial magnified image of the specimen. In so doing, it takes as its object field some portion of the specimen and projects a magnified image of that specimen in the front focal plane or object space of the lens beneath it. The final image projected on the fluorescent screen of the instrument will result from compound magnification

Instrumental Analysis for Particle Identification 151

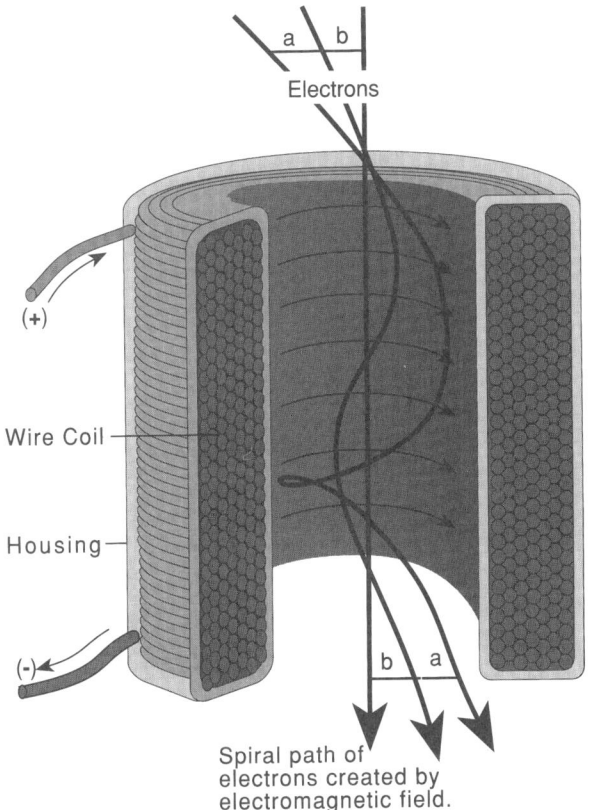

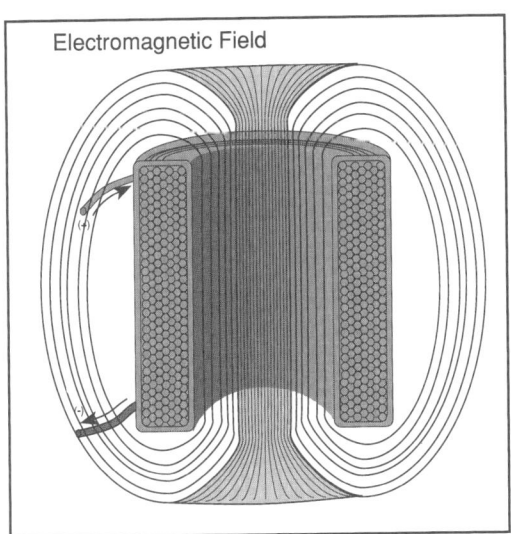

Figure 2. Electromagnetic lens construction and function.

of the objective and projector lenses and will consist of a complex contrast pattern resulting from the differential electron scattering properties of the specimen. An objective aperture placed beneath the specimen serves to remove or subtract electrons that are scattered from the beam at an angle greater than the acceptance angle for the lens below the objective.

As with the light microscope, the objective magnetic lens is the most critical component of the transmission microscope. In order to obtain a high magnification at the given image distance, which is fixed by the length of the column connecting the objective lens with the projector lens, the specimen must be situated close to the focal plane of the objective. The initial magnification provided by the objective lens is approximately 100× in most instruments. The quality of the objective lens determines the resolving power of the instrument. Usually the magnetic field of the objective lens is located eccentrically in relation to the axial extension of the lens coil in such a way that the field is close to the end of the coil at which the specimen is introduced.

Because of the weak penetration of electrons, TEM is only effective in revealing the internal structure of particles that are less than 50–100 nm thick. Thicker particles are revealed only in silhouette unless higher accelerating voltages are used. Three-dimensional information for thick particles can sometimes be obtained by shadowing the particles with evaporated metal (gold, platinum, palladium) atoms at a low angle with respect to the sample support surface.

Scanning Electron Microscopy

The image produced on the screen of a transmission microscope is generated by a continuous flow of electric current that varies in density over the screen area in response to specimen electron-scattering qualities. The TEM image is produced with a static beam spot that remains in one position on the specimen. In a scanning electron microscope the specimen remains in place and the beam is scanned in a rigidly controlled pattern of lines (raster) on the specimen surface. As the raster is scanned on the specimen surface, the beam spot dwells for a certain time interval at each of a large number of points on the specimen surface and excites from each spot a secondary electron signal. The image is formed by the variation in intensity of emitted secondary electrons at different sample points (Figure 3). The pattern of secondary emission and numbers of secondaries generated will depend both on surface contour and

Instrumental Analysis for Particle Identification   153

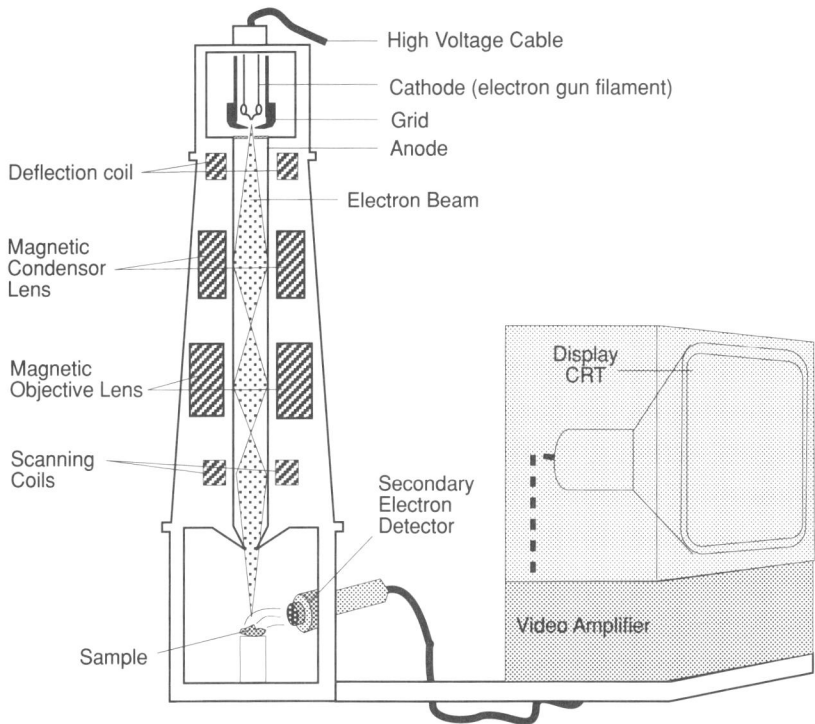

Figure 3.   Scanning electron microscope.

emissivity. A conductive, dry electron emissive, specimen surface is a necessity for conventional (high voltage) SEM.

Image formation in SEM results from collection of secondary electrons generated by the interaction of primary beam electrons with the specimen surface. Signal collection is effected by use of a phosphor- or aluminum-coated collector that converts the electron signal to photons that then impinge on a photomultiplier tube (PMT). The amplified signal from the PMT is used to intensity modulate the beam of a visual cathode ray tube (CRT) and form a television-type image to be interpreted by the eye of the viewer. The scanning microscope is somewhat similar in operation to a stereo dissecting microscope that forms an image using light reflected from the specimen surface; it may more properly be likened to a closed-circuit TV system that provides for high magnification of the imaged field (Figure 4).

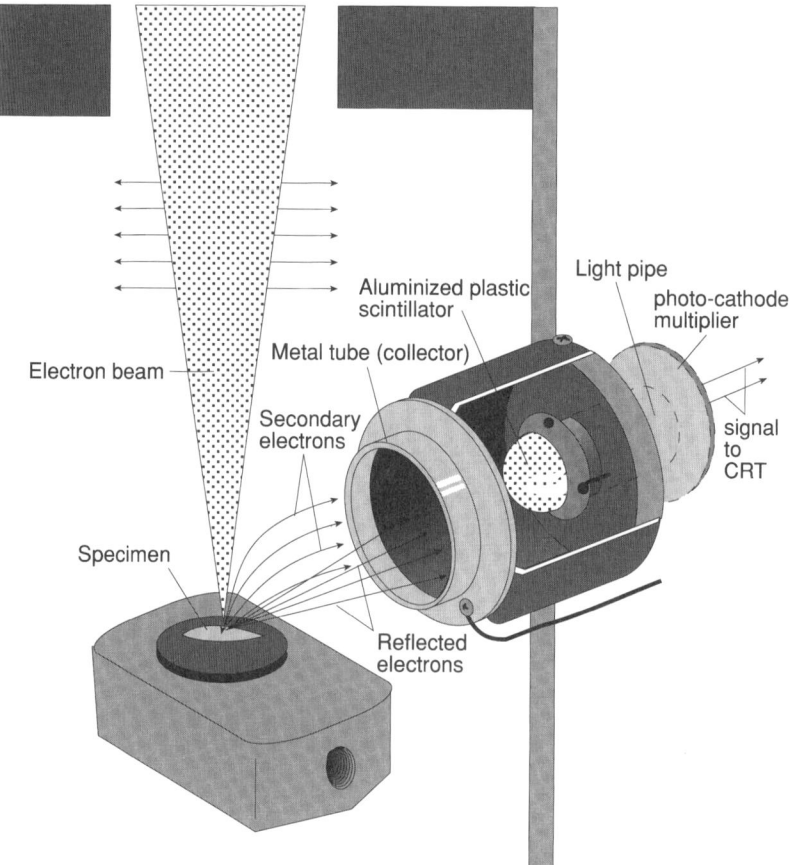

Figure 4. Electron collection in scanning microscope.

The specimen surface is located at the back focal point of the objective (second condenser) lens and is scanned by a small, intense, symmetrical beam spot that is generally 5 to 20 nm in diameter. A secondary electron signal is generated at the point of beam impact as the 5–20 keV electrons (primaries) excite or eject secondary electrons of 2–5 eV potential from the specimen surface. The secondaries emitted "see" the 50–100 V positive potential on the screen anode of the collector and are attracted to it as shown in Figure 4. Once secondaries are in close proximity to the screen anode, they are attracted by the much higher positive potential on the scintillator disc itself (usually 10,000–12,000 V negative) and accelerated across the space between the screen anode and the scintillator. They then strike the scintillator, a disc-like or hemispherical structure of clear plastic coated with either aluminum metal evaporated *in vacuo* or with a fine phosphor. As electrons impact onto the surface of the scintillator, photons are ejected from the opposite side of the phosphor or aluminized coat into a photomultiplier that generates the current used to modulate the imaging beam on the CRT monitor.

The resulting scanning electron microscope image is composed of a series of spot images (picture points) obtained by scanning the beam spot over the specimen surface and the CRT synchronously. Both are scanned in a precisely controlled raster pattern so that a series of imaging picture points is formed representing a series of secondary electron emitting specimen points. The degree of synchronization is such that the beam position on the CRT corresponds exactly to the position of the primary beam spot in the raster on the specimen surface. Points on the object and on the image correspond to one another because they are struck by the microscope electron beam and the CRT electron beam at the same instant. Secondary electrons collected do not actually form an image, but rather intensely modulate the CRT image at one picture point. There is no need to focus the secondary electrons because those collected at any given instant come from the point where the probe has entered the specimen. Magnification with the scanning microscope depends upon the ratio of the screen raster size (approximately 4" × 5") to that of the raster scanned on the specimen.

The electron-optical column of a scanning microscope, like that of a transmission microscope, consists of an electron source (which may be a conventional heated filament or field emission gun), and a series of electromagnetic lenses that focus and demagnify the filament image onto the specimen. The electron gun and gun chamber assemblies are similar to that of a transmission instrument. The column of the SEM is shorter than that of the transmission instrument; there is no need for imaging lenses, and the entire column functions as a multiple condenser (demagnifying) lens system that demagnifies the source image into a small intense "spot" of electrons that is scanned over the specimen.

Signal Generation in SEM

When the electrons in the probe strike a thick specimen, several types of signals are generated (Figure 5). As the electrons penetrate the specimen, they lose energy and slow down. They may also be

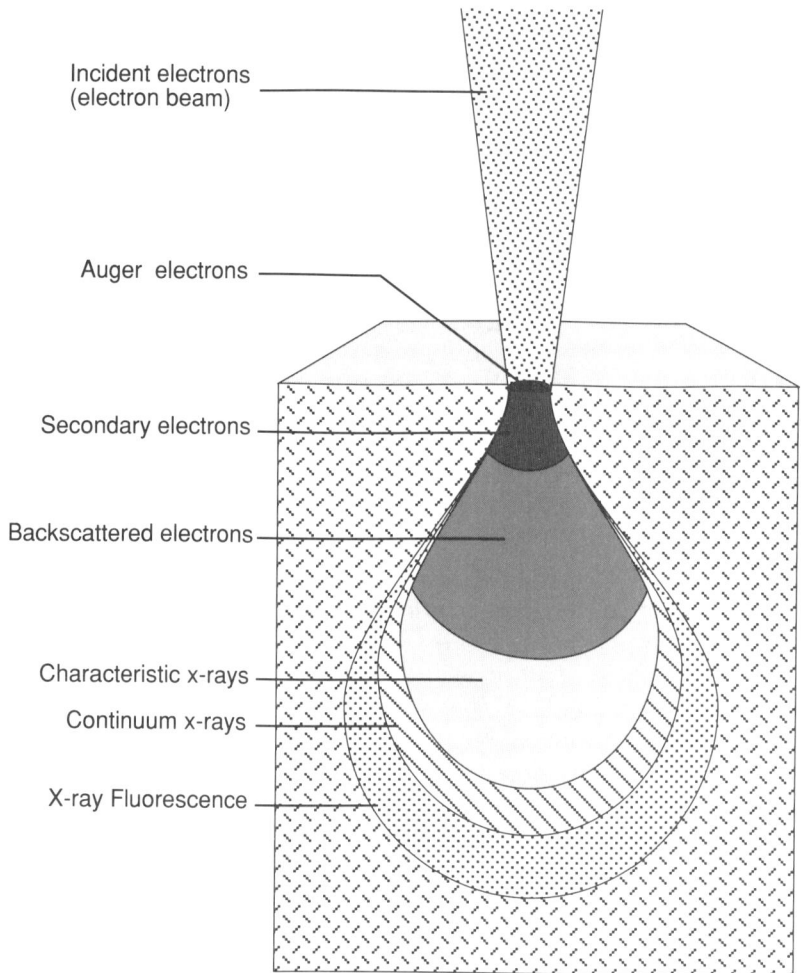

Figure 5. Signal generation in SEM.

scattered through large angles. Finally, some of the electrons may reemerge from the specimen surface, traveling in a direction unrelated to that of the incident beam. In principle, any signal generated when the beam strikes a given point in the object can be used to produce an image. Primary (beam) electrons that are reflected with relatively little loss in energy are not appreciably deflected by a few hundred volt potential difference and will not enter the secondary collector unless it lies directly in their path. These (backscattered) electrons can, however, generate secondary electrons at surfaces other than the specimen that will contribute adversely to the final signal. The probability that the secondary electrons will escape from the sample decreases exponentially as their point of generation moves away from the surface layer; this depth is 0.5 to 5 nm in metals and somewhat thicker for insulators.

As the electron beam impinges on the specimen surfaces, x-rays characteristic of the material from which they are excited are also emitted. X-rays that have an approximate range of wavelengths of 0.01 to 10 nm are produced as the rapidly moving electrons decelerate and convert their energy of motion into quanta of x-radiation. The wavelength of the emitted radiation will depend on the energy of the electrons; the greatest concern is x-rays having a wavelength of about 0.1 nm. X-rays are also emitted by certain radioactive isotopes, for example ^{55}Fe. Although such sources are convenient for testing and calibration, they have not been used for diffraction purposes.

Under normal conditions of x-ray excitation, most of the electrons are not brought to a full stop by a single collision and a continuum of radiation is formed. The minimum wavelength of this "white" radiation is determined by the accelerating voltage and may be calculated from:

$$\lambda_{min} = \frac{12.398 A}{V_{acc}}$$

The greatest intensity occurs at longer wavelengths. As the voltage is increased, not only are the cut-off and peak intensity moved to shorter, more energetic wavelengths, but also the total intensity increases even though the electron current remains the same.

The ability to perform chemical analysis of particles with a scanning microscope is thus due to the existence of a simple and unique relation between the wavelength (l) of the characteristic x-rays emitted from an element and its atomic number (Z). The origin of characteristic x-ray emission is illustrated in Figure 6. If an electron beam incident on a sample has sufficient energy to exceed the excitation potential (bonding energy) of a core electron, then that core electron can be ejected from its parent atom leaving an orbital vacancy behind. The atom is then in an excited state, and any orbital vacancies formed are filled by electronic relaxation accompanied by simultaneous emission of an x-ray photon with a finite energy level corresponding to the difference between the energy levels of the electrons.

At energies of about 10,000 eV (for elements with atomic number of <30), primary (beam) electrons can remove electrons from the

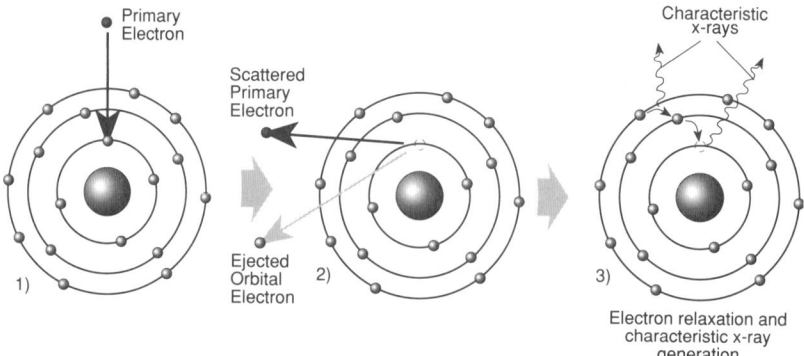

Figure 6. Generation of characteristic x-rays.

innermost (K) shell. When a vacancy in the K shell thus results, it is filled by an electron from the next higher shell (L) or the one above that (M). The decrease in potential energy as the electron goes from the higher level to the lower appears as radiation, and as the energies of the shells are well defined, each transition gives a nearly monochromatic line. The principle energy peaks are:

$K\alpha 1$, $K\alpha 2$ L→K orbital transitions
$Kb1$, $K\beta 1$ M→K orbital transitions

Once created, the x-ray photon is then either emitted from the sample or its energy is transferred to another electron, called an Auger electron, which is ejected from the atom. The fraction of electronic transitions that result in x-ray photon emission is the fluorescent yield; this will depend both on the atomic number of the element and the orbital where the ionization occurs. The characteristic x-ray spectral lines are denoted by the symbols K, L, and M, corresponding to the values of the principal quantum numbers (n = 1, 2, or 3) for the atom. The continuous (white) radiation, or bremsstrahlung, emitted in addition to the characteristic elemental x-rays when the electron beam strikes a specimen is the source of background and is a principal factor limiting analytical sensitivity (Lechene and Warner 1977).

The collection of elemental x-rays emitted by a specimen material is the basis of the electron application in combination with EDXS. The characteristic X-rays emitted are used to obtain an elemental analysis of the specimen area being scanned. If the beam is scanned in synchrony with a CRT and the x-ray signal used to modulate the brightness of the CRT spot, the instrument can be used to give a "dot map" image containing information concerning the distribution of particular chemical elements within the specimen.

The electron microprobe (wavelength dispersive) microanalyzer uses crystal x-ray spectrometers to identify and count x-rays based on their wavelength. The energy of an x-ray photon, which corresponds to the transition energy between orbital shells in the atom, can be expressed as an equivalent wavelength, $\lambda = hc/E$. The phenomenon of diffraction can be used to separate the wavelengths according to Bragg's law: $n = 2d \sin \alpha$. The principal limitation of this type spectrometer is that the geometrical requirements of x-ray focusing restrict the solid angle of x-rays from the specimen that can be analyzed. The small solid angle covered by a typical high-resolution fully focusing spectrometer combined with absorption losses in the diffracting crystals produces a total efficiency of only about 10^{-4}. Despite this drawback, the sensitivity of crystal spectrometers is greater than energy dispersive spectrometry with regard to detection limits (Farlow 1957).

The energy-dispersive spectrometer measures x-ray energy directly, producing a spectrum of counts versus energy. As each x-ray enters the detector, it produces a shower of photoelectrons that strike silicon atoms and raise bound electrons to the conduction band. Each such event requires 3.8 electron volts of energy, so that the total number of electrons freed is linearly proportional to the energy of the entering x-ray. The charge produced by each x-ray is collected by a bias voltage before the next x-ray enters the detector. In order to prevent loss of the electrons during this collection process, it is necessary to fill up any imperfections or dislocations in the silicon lattice that might trap electrons. This is done by diffusing in (drifting) lithium atoms. The EDXS detector is operated at liquid nitrogen temperatures to reduce its dark current and thermal noise and permit the accurate collection of the very low levels of current generated by x-rays striking the collector.

Energy dispersive x-ray analysis allows the detection of x-rays from the entire energy spectrum at one time as opposed to wavelength dispersive analysis, which only examines a single x-ray line at one time. This constitutes both an advantage and a disadvantage, since a single line cannot be isolated for critical analysis as with a crystal spectrometer. A further advantage of solid state detectors used for EDXS is that they are nearly 100% efficient over a wide energy range. This results in a proportionality between counts per second and the intensity of the x-ray line at a given energy, thus allowing the comparison of ratios of different lines as a means of identifying the elements in the sample.

The quantitation of electron energy also can serve as a means of particle identification, since the energy of the emitter electrons or the loss of energy from the incident electron beam by inelastic collisions is characteristic of the composition of the sample. Using the mechanism, EELS spectroscopy analyzes the decrease in energy of the incident electron beam. The EELS analysis is accomplished with detectors that selectively exclude electrons with energies below a specific value via a magnetic deflection detector, where the magnetic field can be set so that only electrons with a specific velocity and energy will be deflected to the detector. Varying the magnetic field will allow a determination of the energy spectrum of the electrons. Auger electron spectroscopy is useful for the study of the surface composition of a sample. Auger electrons are produced by the internal conversion of a characteristic x-ray, and occur with energies of up to about 4 keV. Electrons with these energies are very effectively absorbed by inelastic collisions and, as a result, only those electrons emitted from a 1–2 nm surface layer are detected, which makes this means of analysis well suited to the study of surface effects or particles.

Application of X-Ray Spectroscopy

It has long been recognized that x-ray spectroscopy in combination with SEM or TEM is invaluable to the particle analyst (Winding and Holmes 1976; Bodapatti et al. 1980; DeLuca and Bodapatti 1980). Particles less than 0.1 µm in size may be examined at high resolution and simultaneously analyzed for 1% or greater concentrations of elements of atomic number >9 (Fluorine). This analysis represents detection of subpicogram quantities of elements. One of the greatest advantages of the method is that spectrum acquisition and basic interpretation of the acquired line spectrum can be accomplished by an analyst with very limited training. The use of x-ray spectroscopy is widely used in general (Anderson 1982), and pharmaceutical particle analysis (Bollinger et al. 1978; Draftz and Graf 1974; and Oles 1978).

Particulate matter samples may be directly viewed in the scanning electron microscope without application of a conductive coating if they are a conducting material. For viewing and x-ray spectroscopic analysis such materials are simply attached to carbon specimen supports of appropriate size with some adhesive material, such as acrylic cement, and placed in the instrument. Particles can also be mounted using two-sided cellophane tape, whereby the particles are picked up from the substrate with one side of the tape or dusted on to the tape surface, and then the tape attached to the mounting post with its other adhesive side. Specimens for transmission microscopic analysis must be sufficiently thin to allow electron penetration through their whole volume. This requirement often makes the preparation for TEM involved and time consuming.

Particulate matter specimens to be analyzed in a TEM are most commonly placed on a thin film support attached to a metallic or nonmetallic grid. Consideration must be given in grid selection to the type of analysis to be performed (morphologic or x-ray spectroscopic) and the thickness of film that may be used, as this will determine the size of the grid openings used (thermal films, such as silicon require, smaller grid openings). Supporting films are usually made of plastic or carbon, though other materials may be used. Suitable solutions for film production may be made up of 2% collodion in amyl acetate or 0.5% Formvar® plastic in ethylene dichloride. Several methods may be used to produce films. The most common method involves stripping a collodion or Formvar® film from a microscope slide. A microscope slide is cleaned with a detergent solution and polished with a soft cloth without rinsing to facilitate later stripping of the film. The slide is then dipped into the Formvar® or collodion solution and allowed to drain dry. A razor blade is used to produce a scratch around the edge of the slide and the film is then floated onto a water surface. Then grids are placed on the surface of the film with a forceps and the film with the attached grids is picked up by touching it from above with a strip of masking tape or newspaper. A simple method of producing a TEM prep from a powder sample is to place a few milligrams of the powder on a microscope slide, add a drop of the suspension of Formvar® in a suitable solvent and rub the powder out on the slide with a glass rod. For films on grids, a drop of the particulate matter suspended in water may be simply placed on the filmed grid and allowed to dry.

Methods of bulk particle mounting have two undesirable features: (1) they may lead to particle agglomeration, and (2) the degree of dispersion may vary with the particle size and shape. Both of these artifacts will result in a sample that will not truly represent the original sample. Particularly when particle identification is the primary objective, it will be desirable to select and mount individual particles for analysis. A stereo microscope is used for the selection of the particle, and it is then picked up with the tip of a tungsten needle and adhered to a carbon or beryllium support with some adhesive.

After the particle has been mounted it must typically be provided with a conductive coating. Nonconducting or poorly conducting materials will accumulate a negative charge from the electron beam in typical high voltage scanning electron microscopes. The use of low voltage scanning electron microscopy (LVSEM) allows visualization of uncoated particles by using accelerating voltages of a few hundred volts. The accumulation of charge produces a potential that causes a deflection of low energy electrons and increases the artifactual emission of secondary electrons from the sample surface. This results in sporadic variations in the emissivity of the sample, poor resolution, and possible radiation damage to the sample. In general, as the energy of the electron beam increases, so does charging. This problem is overcome by coating the particle surface with a conducting material such as gold or gold-palladium to provide a conductive path for the removal of the charge that builds up on the sample surface.

Elemental Composition Analysis

Energy dispersive x-ray spectroscopy has become an invaluable tool to the pharmaceutical particle analyst over the past 15 years. In qualitative analyses a spectrum from a submicron particle on which particle identification can be based often requires less than a minute to acquire. State-of-the-art thin window detectors allow detection of carbon and oxygen with excellent resolution and sensitivity. The light element detection capability proves very valuable in analysis of many of the particles that are isolated from injectable solutions.

The first step in qualitative analysis of a sample using EDXS is to locate a major x-ray line for the element of interest. If the critical excitation energy for the element involved is less than the beam energy, then all of the characteristic lines of that element should be excited. Once a strong line has been located, say a Kα line, then the next step is to look for another line that serves to confirm the first, such as the Kβ. If the suspected element is actually present, the second line should be found and, further, the ratio of its intensity to that of the principle line should be within 10% of published data. If the second line is absent, this strongly suggests that the element is not present and that the primary line is due to some other element. If the confirming line is present but the intensity is more than 10% different from the published value, it may be caused by peak overlap and, if so, additional characteristic lines of the elements should be checked to resolve the discrepancy.

Wavelength dispersive x-ray analysis (WDXS) can also be used for particle identification and its resolution is more than an order of magnitude better than energy dispersive systems. This subject is well-covered in the referenced book by Heinrich (1981). In addition to attaining a much higher peak-to-background ratio, wavelength dispersive analysis allows the identification of elements present at lower concentration (as low as 0.1%). The procedure for qualitative analysis is generally the same as with energy dispersive systems. With the higher resolution of a wavelength dispersive system, the number of lines available for scrutiny is increased. Historically, the complexity of operation of the crystal spectrometers, and the time requirement for WDXS, caused many particle analysts to avoid the use of the wavelength dispersive instrument in favor of the EDXS mode (which is far more simplistic in use and rapid in application). Further, the level of expertise required for routine use of the WDXS in analyzing particles took much more time to acquire than most particle analysts felt justified in spending. The historical drawbacks are no longer applicable. Imaging capability of current generation, multiple spectrometer microprobes are equal to those of conventional high voltage scanning microscopes; multiple computer-driven spectrometers are applied simultaneously to scan for elements over a wide atomic number range. Despite the advances in WDXS technology, it remains doubtful whether the additional cost of wavelength dispersive capability will be justified in most cases, if an EDXS instrument is available.

Several methods for the calculation of correction factors for particle size effects have been described. These methods are useful only if computer-based calculations are used for the various steps in correcting the x-ray data to obtain elemental concentrations as the corrections become exceedingly complex. The NBS publication by Heinrich (1980) will provide a useful overview. Particle standards provide a valid way of comparing the unknown sample to a standard with the same or similar size and shape, such that particle size effects can be minimized. Particle standards can be made by pulverizing bulk materials, but it may not be possible to obtain the appropriate particle size and shape that will be suitable for a particular sample. Particle population analysis for compositional characteristics can also be performed by EDXS (Post and Buseck 1984).

The X-ray spectra of some contaminant particles encountered in pharmaceutical products are shown in Table I.

Table I. X-Ray Spectra of Pharmaceutical Contaminants

Material	Elemental Composition*
Acoustic tile fabric	**Ca**, Si, Fe, Mg, Al
Glass fibers	**Si**, Ca, Fe, Mg
Calcium phosphate	**Ca**, P
Kaolin	**Si**, Al, Ti, Fe
Gypsum	**Ca**, S, Fe
Skin cells	**S**, Ca, Na, K, P
Barium sulfate	**Ba**, S, Fe
Calcium carbonate	**Ca**, C, O
Titanium dioxide	**Ti**, O
Sand	**Si**, O, Fe
Abrasive powder	**Al**, S, Fe, Ba
Rubber (chlorobutyl)	**Cl**, S, Ca, Si
Plant fragments	**P**, S, Cl, K, Na, Fe
Rust (stainless steel)	**Fe**, Ni, Cr, O
Wear particles (homogenizer/bearings)	**Ca**, Fe, Zn, Al
Dried blood	**S**, Ca, Na, P, K, Fe
Paper	**Ti**, C, Ca, O, S
Calcium stearate	**Ca**, C
Calcium oxalate	**Ca**, C
Paint (white)	**Ti**, Si, Al, Fe
Paint (brown)	**Fe**, S, Ti
Face powder (cosmetic)	**Si**, Mg, Ti, Fe, Zn
Drug degradant (cephalosporin)	**S**, C
Amino acid residue	**S**, C

*Predominant elements are boldface; others appear in order of relative decreasing concentration.

X-ray spectroscopy is most commonly applied in a qualitative analysis mode for particle identification. In this application, the presence of specific elements and their proportional concentrations are frequently sufficient to allow the composition and source of a particle to be identified. If elemental composition is not diagnostic, comparison standards can be used in the same fashion as for microscopy and other forms of analysis. The quantitative analysis of particles is significantly more difficult.

The difficulties in quantitative analyses of particles arise primarily from the fact that the dimensions of the particle may be less than the range of the beam electrons, and that x-ray absorption effects (and fluorescence) will differ from that of a bulk sample. Hence, the classical multiplicative correction factors for atomic numbers effecting x-ray absorption and fluorescence effects (ZAF) do not apply. Most particles analyzed have rough or irregular surfaces that interfere, to greater or lesser extents, with x-ray collection geometry. Despite the theoretical complexities of qualitative analysis, good results can be obtained if particles to be analyzed are mounted on thin films of Formvar® plastic and irradiated with a raster frame slightly larger than the particle. The thin film support will minimize background (substrate) effects, and the use of a raster scan (instead of point excitation) will tend to average out density differences within the particle.

Infrared Microspectrophotometry

In the opinion of some, the most important tool of the organic analytical chemist is the infrared spectrophotometer. The addition of a microscope accessory to a current generation, state-of-the-art Fourier transform infrared (FT–IR) spectrophotometer allows the analytical capabilities of this instrument to be applied to pharmaceutical particulate matter (Long et al. 1988; Meserschmidt and Harthcock 1987). Contaminant particles can be identified by microscopical examination of their morphological characteristics, but, when unique morphology is lacking, infrared or EDXS spectral data becomes critically important for particle identification (Cotter 1987; Lacy 1982). One obvious application of infrared microspectrophotometry in pharmaceutical research is the identification of drug contaminants and degradants.

In today's pharmaceutical particle analysis laboratory, the micro FT–IR spectrophotometer powerfully complements the use of the scanning electron microscope with EDXS capability (Humecki and Muggli 1982). In combination with SEM–EDXS, this instrument has revolutionized the chemical analysis of particulate matter. The inorganic elemental constituency of an unknown particle can readily be obtained by EDXS; the FT–IR microspectrophotometer can obtain well-defined infrared absorption spectra from particles as small as 10 μm in size and provide information on organic composition. Thus, the combination of the two instruments provides for identification, or at least the structural elucidation and characterization, of the large majority of particles encountered in pharmaceutical research or troubleshooting.

Microscopic infrared analysis requires an all-reflecting (Cassegranian optical) microscope attached to an infrared spectrometer and interferometric, rather than dispersive, detection.

Interferometric detection allow the advantages of Fourier transformation to be realized and avoids overheating the sample with an intense beam of infrared radiation.

Infrared microscopes are usually used in a transmission mode, requiring the transfer of a sample to an appropriate substrate such as BaF_2, KCl, or NaCl. Reflectance optics, available on some commercial instruments, allow a double-pass transmission measurement to be made from particles, provided the sample is in close contact with a reflective surface and is not too thick. With particles, as with bulk samples, thickness and shape can have detrimental effects on infrared spectra. Fibers and irregularly shaped particles can create focusing and scattering effects, which can lead to baseline distortions and very inaccurate absorbance measurements. These problems can be of such a magnitude that spectral subtraction, a valuable method of interpreting spectra of mixtures, becomes impossible. Flattening the sample, manually or in a KBr cell, is necessary in some cases.

In general, micro FT–IR is very sensitive and is capable of recording useable spectra for nanogram sample quantities. As with bulk samples, the particle infrared spectrum is useful because it provides functional group information, and it has a fingerprint region that is specific for a given molecule. Comprehensive spectral libraries are available with most infrared data systems. The most common type of microsampling accessory uses a reflecting infrared microscope that includes a visible illumination system for the visual examination of the samples, and a dedicated or axis, small area MCT detector. The small area detector reduces the detector-induced noise, thus yielding higher sensitivity. The sampling size can range upwards from less than 10 mm in size (Cournoyer et al. 1977; Curry et al. 1985). The construction of a typical infrared microspectrophotometer is shown in Figure 7.

The sensitivity of the microsampling technique in transmission studies is illustrated by Figure 8. This figure shows the spectrum of a Dacron® (polyethylene terephthalate) fiber with the aperture set to sample at 5×25 µm area. The background necessary to produce this transmission spectrum was also recorded with the aperture set to the same dimensions. The signal-to-noise ratio of the spectrum from the fiber compares favorably to the bulk spectrum down to 1000 cm^{-1}. One would normally expect to observe diffraction effects in the fiber spectrum in the figure, as the aperture size used was comparable to the wavelength of the infrared radiation. However, most diffraction effects cancel out when the sample and the background spectra are both recorded using the same aperture opening.

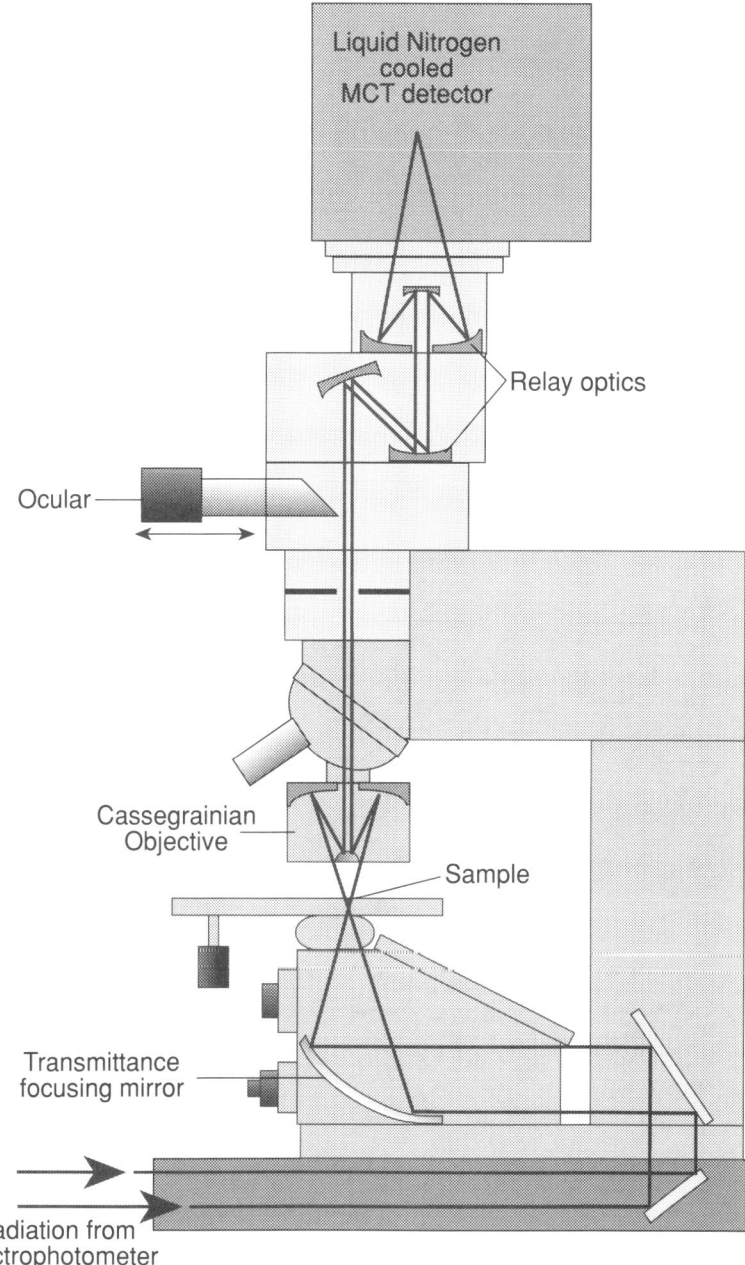

Figure 7. Infrared microspectrophotometer with solid state detector.

168 *Pharmaceutical Particulate Matter*

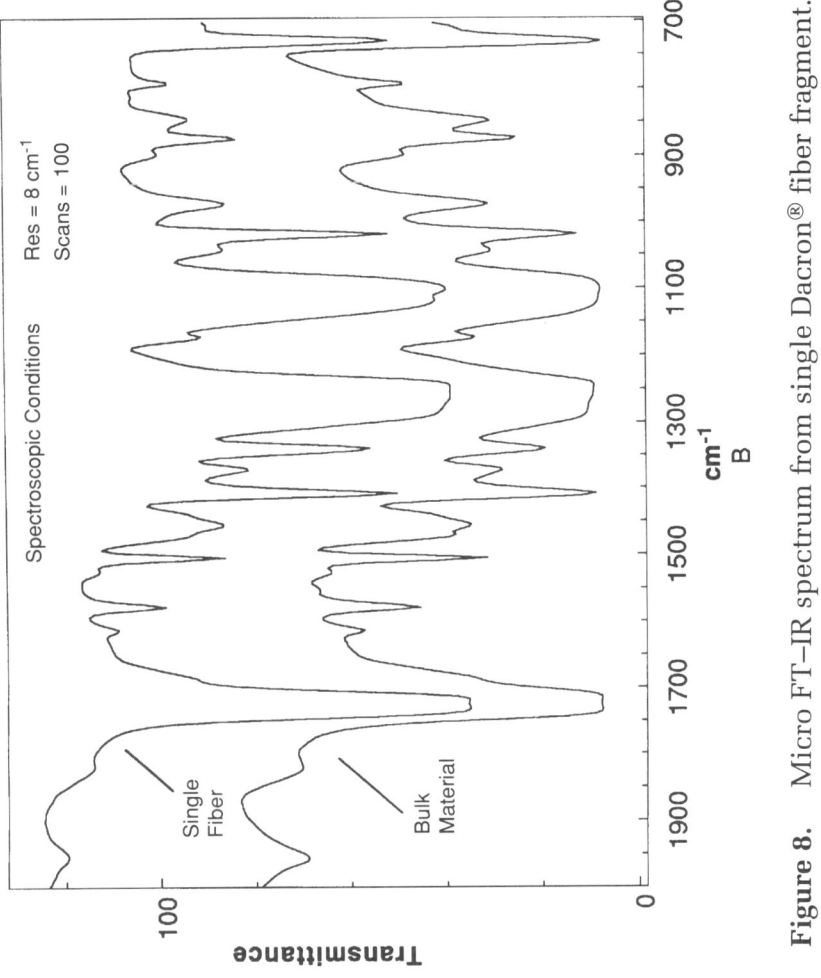

Figure 8. Micro FT–IR spectrum from single Dacron® fiber fragment.

The microsampling accessory can be adapted for use in the near infrared region by replacing the MCT detector by an InSb detector. Overtone and combination bands, and electronic transitions can be studied by using this method. When one wants to study the transmission spectra in the mid-infrared, the sample thickness must be cut down to the 10–20 micrometer range, in some case by microtoming the sample. Thicker samples can be used in the near infrared.

The application of micro FT–IR analysis is basically simplistic. The particle of interest is isolated by conventional technique (i.e., by microneedle) and transferred to a circular salt plate that is placed on the x-y stage of the instrument. The particle is then centered in the microscope field and delimited by an adjustable aperture that will restrict the area through which the IR beam passes in analyses. Once the particle is selected, Cassegranian optics are swung into place on the microscope turret and the beam passes from the optical bench of the spectrophotometer through the particle and into a solid state detector at the top of the microscope. For dichroic studies, an infrared transmitting polarizer (gold wire grid supported on KRS-5) may be inserted in the optical train above the eyepiece of the microscope. With this arrangement, the sample under study can be visually examined in the usual fashion, the sample area of interest can be chosen using the variable aperture, and the dichroic measurements can be made without disturbing the optical train.

Mass Spectrometry

Mass spectrometry can be extremely useful in characterizing or identifying particulate matter. Contemporary instruments provide high mass resolution and accuracy in mass determination for both atomic ions and complex organic species. There are a number of ways for obtaining mass spectra from particles. Probably the best, if a conventional instrument is to be used, is direct insertion on a wire probe, and desorption by heating, chemical ionization, or fast atom bombardment. This sampling method is useful for many types of samples and allows relatively small amounts of particulate matter to be analyzed in the high resolution, double-focusing mass spectrometers typically used for bulk materials. Mass spectrometry is a very sensitive means of analysis and is capable of analyzing subnanogram quantities of particulate matter. This technique does have some disadvantages, however. Mass spectrometry using thermal or chemical desorption exhibits greater sensitivity for volatile compounds, so that particles of volatile material or those with volatile components are favored in the analysis. For this reason, it is important to evaluate the residue of the sample after analysis to ensure that the spectrum seen is truly representative of the bulk of the sample and not simply a volatile component. Some particles are difficult or impossible to volatilize, thus preventing their analysis by this method.

LAMMA

The laser microprobe mass analyzer (LAMMA, Figure 9) meets many of the requirements for chemical analysis of particles,

170 *Pharmaceutical Particulate Matter*

including delimiting of the ionizing radiation to the area of a single particle. The instrument illustrated simply consists of a laser ion excitation mechanism attached to a conventional time of flight mass spectrometer. The particle(s) to be analyzed are visualized using the microscope accessory, and targeted with the pilot laser (Cotter 1987). Ions are produced by a short, powerful burst from the Nd-YAG laser. In the case of techniques, such as direct insertion, the technique is primarily limited to particles greater than 10 μm in

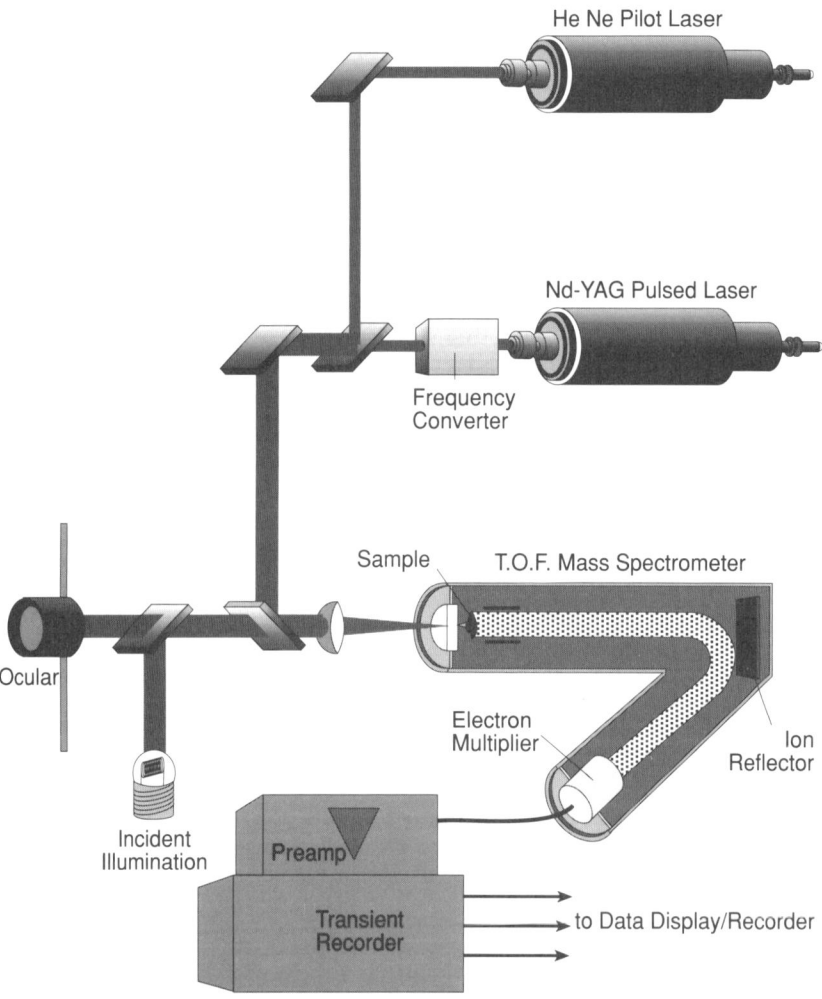

Figure 9. LAMMA.

size, but the size range amenable to LAMMA analysis starts at approximately 0.2 µm.

In the LAMMA, the microprobe objectives and other diffracting elements are made from UV-transparent material. The specimen is located underneath a thin (0.15 mm) quartz slide that serves both as a vacuum seal and optical window. This configuration permits the use of a wide range of light microscope objectives, including 100× immersion objectives. Visualization of the specimen is possible by either incident or transmitted light, including UV microscopy at 260 nm. This not only improves the imaging resolution of the microscope, but also provides for better optical classification of an inhomogeneous particle sample. During analysis, the specimen can only be seen by incident illumination because the optical condensor underneath the specimen has to be exchanged for an electrostatic ion lens. To select the area of interest, the vacuum flange that the specimen is mounted on is manually shifted in the x- and y-direction via two micrometer screw-drives, and focusing in the z-direction is achieved by a screw-drive acting on the microscope. The area of interest is indicated by focusing a red target (He-Ne) laser into the microscope field of view. The typical diameter of the analyzed area is about 0.5 µm with a 100× objective and 1 µm with a 30× objective. The pulsed YAG laser is then used to ionize the sample.

The time-of-flight spectrometer consists of an accelerating and focusing electrostatic lens underneath the specimen, a field free drift tube 1.20 m in length, an ion reflector at the end of this tube reflecting the ions to an angle of nearly 180°, and a second drift tube about 60 cm in length. A secondary electron multiplier is used as the ion detector. The ion reflector compensates for the spread of initial ion energy (0 to 50 eV). When laser light is focused on solid-state material, the predominant energy transfer process depends strongly on irradiance (i.e., the power density in the focus) and may cover classical absorption at the low irradiance end of a large variety of nonlinear optical processes occurring at irradiance $\geq 10^6$ to 10^7 W/cm^2. The total amount of energy deposited per unit volume determines the occurrence and the amount of physical parameter changes within the irradiated material, such as heating, phase transition processes, and ionization.

The primary disadvantages of the LAMMA technique are (1) the high laser beam energy, that may result in uncontrolled ionization or carbonization of an organic sample rather than a controlled generation of ions; and (2) the time-of-flight spectrometer used has rather poor mass resolution. The results obtained with LAMMA show a strong influence of sample preparation, and the geometry of the sample as well as of the laser beam. In particle analysis, there will usually be a predominance of volume evaporation. There is an upper limit of particle diameter beyond which the particle can no longer be totally evaporated by laser desorption (Conzemius and Capellan 1980). This limit is around 1 µm, if one relies on the laser beam geometry in the focus. The upper limit at which signal intensities are proportional to the volume of the particle has been found to be only in the range of 0.6 µm by Surkyn and Adams (1982) employing glass microspheres, whereas Kaufmann et al. (1980) found a limit of 1.2 µm for a 32× objective, and 3.0 µm for a 100× objective in a size-dispersive specimen of NaCl microcrystallites. If particle size exceeds these upper limits, selective or only partial evaporation and eventually redeposition of material must be taken into account. Further disadvantages under these circumstances are saturation effects on the multiplier for signals related to leading constituents, and peak deformations due to larger time and energy spreads of the produced ions.

In a short time after its introduction into particle and aerosol research, the LAMMA technique demonstrated its capability to provide many unique insights into the chemical nature of particulate materials unattainable by alternative techniques (Hillencamp and Kaufman 1982; Kruger and Scheuler 1981). While the instrument's sensitivity allows for the detection of trace contaminants in single particles, analysis time is fast enough to obtain statistically meaningful data in a comparatively short period of time; however, quantitation of resultant data is extremely difficult.

Secondary Ion Mass Spectrometry

In a simplistic assessment, the SIMS instrument consists of a mass spectrometer with a highly sophisticated excitation mechanism. In secondary ion mass spectrometry (SIMS), particles or surfaces to be analyzed are bombarded by a focused or collimated beam of high energy ions (most commonly $^{16}O^-$, $^{32}O^+$, $^{40}Ar^+$, or $^{133}Cs^+$). The primary ions acquire their high energy levels by acceleration across a potential of 5–20 kV in the "gun" area of the instrument. The most commonly used ions for analysis are $^{32}O^+$ (produced in cold cathode field emission sources) and $^{133}Cs^+$ (produced by thermionic emission). SEM images are obtained by using an electron multiplier to detect secondary electrons emitted from the sample under ion bombardment. These images may be used to precisely locate the area for ion analysis. Secondary ion images are obtained by setting the mass spectrometer to detect only the element of interest. The primary ion beam can be used to perform bulk or surface mass analyses on isolated particles of less than 10 µm in size. The instruments currently available differ both in column design and mechanism of ion detection. An instrument based on a quadrupole mass spectrometer is shown in Figure 10.

The SIMS technique constitutes a very useful nonroutine method of particle analysis. The references by Gavrilovic (1984) and Wilson et al. (1989) provide excellent overviews of the method. Two different designs of SIMS instruments (the ion microscope and the ion microprobe) are in use today. Within the ion microscope (developed by Castaing et al. 1960), a relatively large 3 µm to 300 µm ion beam strikes the sample and a magnified secondary ion image is produced through ion transfer optics. Any portion of this image can be selectively isolated, examined, and analyzed in detail for chemical composition, isotopic ratios, and so forth. The spatial resolution of an ion microscope is 1 µm or better while the mass resolution depends upon the mass spectrometer design. The ion microprobe, designed by Liebl (1967), is based upon an electrostatic ion optics system that focuses a primary ion source into a 2 µm ion beam. This primary ion beam may then be rastered over either a large or small area to generate secondary ions from the sample area of interest. The secondary ions are analyzed using a mass spectrometer.

Each of these instrument designs have advantages and disadvantages in comparison to one other. Ideally, when performing an analysis on a small particle, one would like to use a magnified secondary ion image for the location of small particles. In performing surface analysis, the quality of the light optics is not only important but essential, since (if the ion optics system is used to visualize the area of analysis) the surface layer of interest may be removed before the analysis can be performed. Unfortunately, the light optics within the ion microscope are frequently poor, thus the ion microprobe has advantages for both surface and particle analysis (Erike et al. 1980; McHugh 1975).

The ion beam sputters atoms from the surface of a solid or particle in a complex interaction. The reaction that occurs in the plasma cloud around a solid particle is complex and not entirely understood (Figure 11). Most of the sputtering occurs with 5–10 mm of the surface of the particle. Neutral atoms, positive and negative ions, and electrons are all created in the small plasma cloud above and around the small particles being bombarded. The condensation of some of the positive and negative ions formed occurs in the immediate vicinity of the particles. This phenomenon may

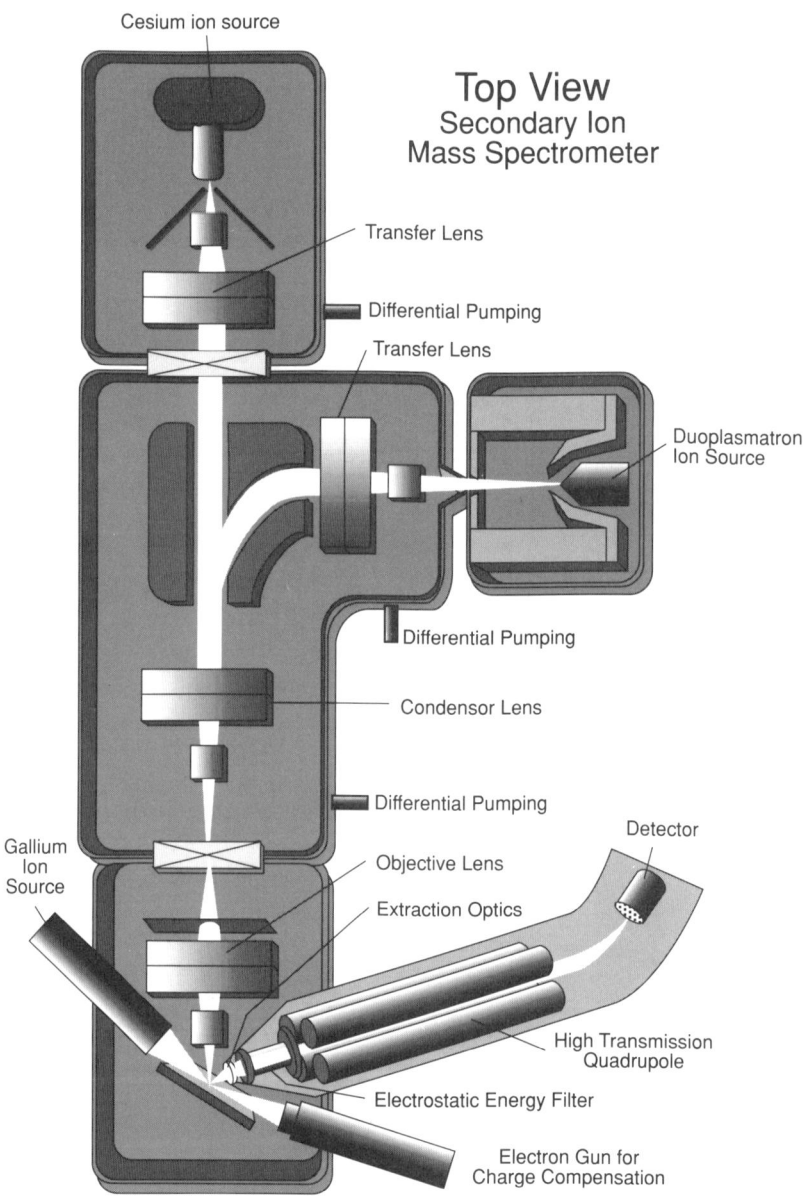

Figure 10. SIMS instrument with quadrupole mass spectrometer (courtesy of Cameca Instruments).

be important to the conduct of analysis of small particles since it provides additional material for analysis (Gavrilovic 1984).

Some of the ions generated on the sample surface are neutralized by collision with electrons, and other ions combine with each other or with the ions from the primary beam. Energies within the primary beam impact area are greater than 1000 eV, and the energies of the chemical bond of a compound on a solid surface are well below that level. In addition, the plasma temperature may be 10,000 K to 12,000 K. Therefore, the breakdown of chemical compounds on the sample surface and within the plasma cloud is

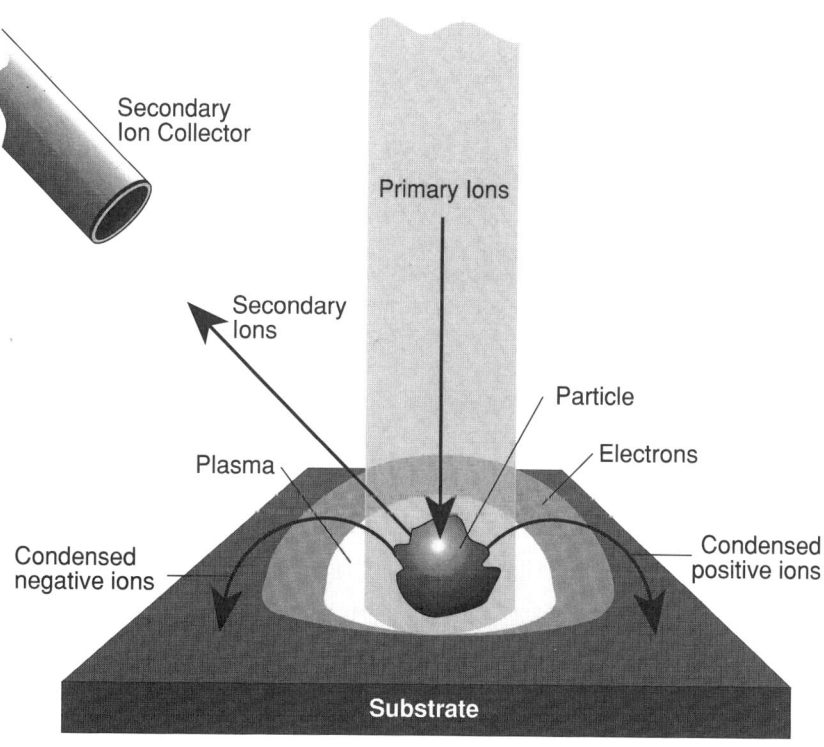

Figure 11. Interaction of ion microprobe beam with particle.

almost complete. When organic compounds are analyzed, their molecules are broken down to relatively small fragments, most of them having mass to charge (m/e) ratios below 50. Many extremely short-lived molecular fragments (such as CH^+, CH^+_2, CH^+_3, and so forth) may be detected.

As the sputtering process proceeds, the sample is gradually eroded away with the erosion rate of the small particle being dependent upon numerous factors:

- The incident energy of the primary ions,
- The type of primary ions,
- The polarity of the primary ions,
- The density of the ions in the beam (ions/μm),
- The shape and size of the particle and surface morphology, and
- The chemical composition of the sample.

Although SIMS analysis of small individual particles is ultimately restricted by particle size and the total number of atoms available, such analyses are highly practical. Assuming a 1% secondary ion yield and a 10% collection transmission for the mass spectrometer system, the number of counts that a small particle will yield at 10% consumption is such that even a submicrometer-size particle can provide a sufficient count rate for the analysis of a number of elements in a second, and the signal for an associated mass peak may reach over a million counts per second (in some cases reaching to the parts per billion range). Thus, for the bulk analysis of small particles, SIMS constitutes an extremely sensitive analytical method. This sensitivity cannot be achieved under the restricted conditions encountered in the surface analyses of small particles. In these instances, the sensitivity is severely hampered by the small sample size.

The particulate matter analyses typically performed on particles using SIMS technique may be characterized as dynamic analyses, that is, as the analysis is performed, increasingly greater amounts of the mass of the particle or particles are sequentially removed by the primary ion beam. In this mode of analysis significant amounts of material are removed in relatively short intervals of time, and a high secondary ion yield is obtained. Static SIMS is generally less applicable in particle analysis; in this mode of analysis, the surface of the sample is sputtered lightly so that only a fraction of the outermost atomic layer of the sample is removed for analysis.

Methods for preparing particles for SIMS analyses are critical. Particles exposed to high-energy ion bombardment tend to dissipate some of the absorbed energy by becoming electrically charged (by heating, etc.). This tends to render the particle unstable on its substrate. Therefore, some common methods used in mounting very small particles for other microanalysis techniques cannot be used on particles for SIMS when surface analysis is desired. In the surface analyses of small particles, it is a few monolayers that are of concern and, therefore, most of the sample is left uncontaminated and intact by the mounting technique. For surface analyses, particles larger than 10 µm are usually placed a "tacky" collodion film. With this technique, the collodion does not flow and coat the upper part of the particle. In spite of numerous limitations, SIMS is a viable analytical technique for determining the surface chemical composition of particles down to the micrometer size range. In some cases, such as the detection of minute quantities of specific elements on small particles, SIMS remains a very useful (and by far the most sensitive) surface analytical method available.

X-Ray Diffraction Crystallography

This mode of chemical analysis has a limited application in the analysis of particulate matter, but in small numbers of analyses the definitive identification of particles may be obtained by no other means. The principle applied involves the use of x-ray irradiation to produce a highly specific diffraction pattern from a crystal of the material of interest. The texts by Bloss (1961) and Stout and Jensen (1968) provide both introductory and sample-specific technical information on this technique. If particulate matter can be obtained in pure crystalline form, either through its formation as a precipitate or by selective dissolution and recrystallization, this mode of analysis will generally provide unequivocal identification. The recent development of computer databases has reduced the labor associated with the determination of crystal structures by x-ray diffraction analysis. As a result, x-ray crystallography is a powerful tool for particle analysis. The single essential criterion that a particle must meet to be amenable to this means of analysis is that it can be obtained in the form of a single crystal.

The atoms of a crystal are ordered (or packed) in a specific arrangement with the inter-atomic spacings precisely defined on 3-dimensional (X, Y, Z) axes. This arrangement is specific for each crystalline form of a given compound. A simplistic analogy is provided by the hexagonal packing by a pile of marbles or other spherical objects of equal size. To simplify crystal structure further, we may consider a planar two-dimensional point array. Such an array is illustrated in Figure 12 by regular repetition of a point image (Stout and Jensen 1965).

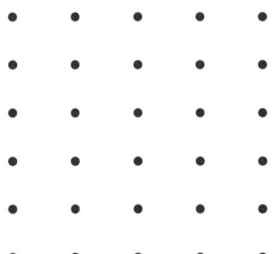

Figure 12.   Two-dimensional point array.

This array forms a two dimensional lattice or grid system. Such a grid may be depicted in a number of different ways, such as the number of ways to draw grid lines. Figure 13 shows three ways for the point array in Figure 12.

In Figure 13 the grid lines are drawn at equal intervals corresponding to repeating intervals of atoms in the array; the arrangement of atoms surrounding each line intersection is identical. Crystals of pure material exist as very uniform three dimensional arrays of atoms in the form of lattice planes. These grid systems may be extended into three dimensional arrays of lattice planes. The process of reflection of the x-ray in a collimated beam at the successive planes of a crystal lattice gives rise to the x-ray diffraction patterns that are uniquely descriptive of chemical compounds.

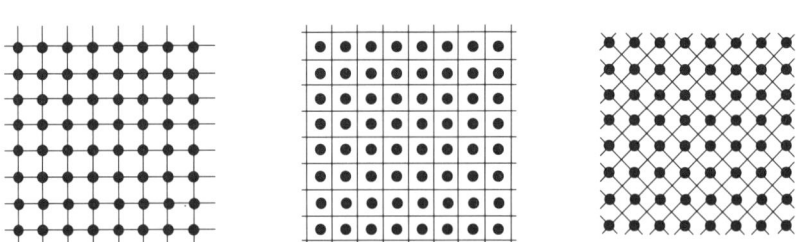

Figure 13.   Grid systems for array of Figure 12.

While engaged in experimental studies in the early part of this century, Sir Lawrence Bragg (1890–1971) noted the similarity of diffraction to reflection and derived an equation treating diffraction as a collective reflection from planes in the crystal lattice. Consider an x-ray beam incident on a pair of parallel planes P_1 and P_2 with interplanar spacing d (Figure 14). The parallel incident rays 1 and 2 make an angle θ with these planes. The x-rays reflected at O and C will have the same wave length as those of the incident beam. For that particular direction where the parallel secondary rays 1' and 2' emerge at angle θ as reflected from the planes, a diffracted beam of maximum intensity will result if the electromagnetic waves of these rays are in phase and reinforce one another.

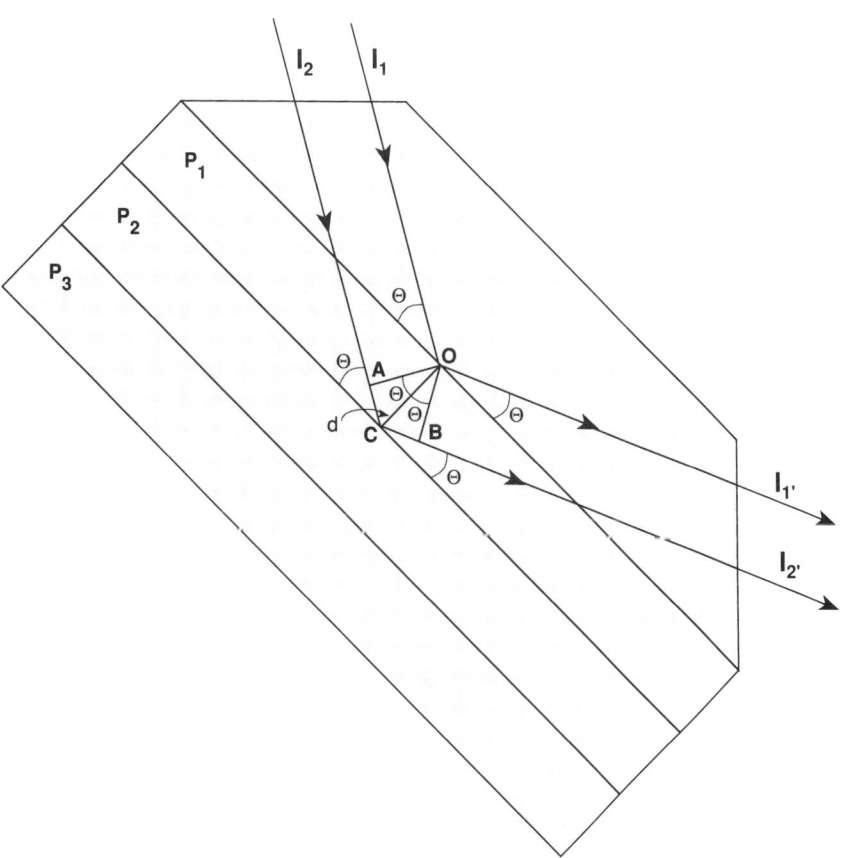

Figure 14. Diffraction of x-rays at sequential lattice planes.

By drawing perpendiculars from O to A and B, we generate the angular relationship:

$$\angle AOC = \angle BOC = \theta.$$

Hence $AC = BC$, and waves in ray 2' will be in phase (peak-to-peak) with those in 1' if $AC + CB$ (= $2AC$) is an integral multiple of the wavelength, λ. Thus,

$$2AC = n\lambda$$

where n is an integer multiple of λ. Then $AC = d \sin \theta$ and

$$2d \sin \theta = n\lambda.$$

The latter equation is Bragg's law.

The process of reflection at successive crystal planes is described above in terms of incident and reflected X-rays, each making an angle θ with a fixed crystal plane. With a fixed incident beam, reflection occurs from planes at the angle θ with respect to the incident beam and giving a reflected ray at an angle of 2θ with respect to the incident beam. An x-ray diffraction camera is shown in Figure 15. An x-ray diffraction pattern from the unknown crystal is formed as a series of dots of varying intensity with fixed angular relationships and recorded on the photographic film in the cylindrical film holder that encloses the sample; at this point the structure of the crystal becomes known, but its chemical composition remains unknown. Many diffraction patterns resulting from single crystal analysis have been cataloged for use in identification of unknowns (see IUCR list [Buerger 1960b]). In the absence of

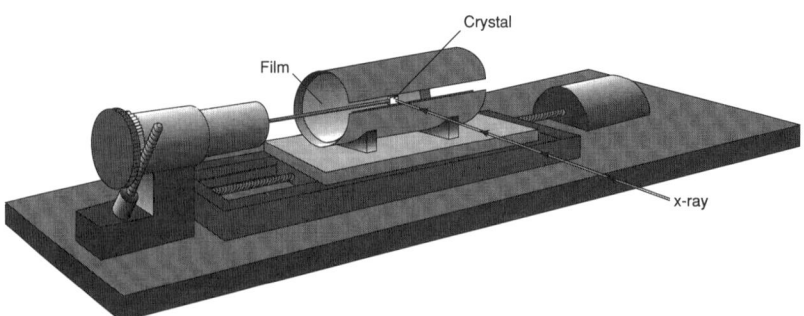

Figure 15. X-ray diffraction camera.

spectral data files, diffraction patterns may be collected from known comparison standards.

Simplistically, it is only necessary to obtain the particulate matter of interest in a pure form as a single crystal that can then be mounted in a diffraction camera to produce a diffraction pattern for comparison to reference patterns or those produced by known standards (Buerger 1960a; James 1965). This is far more easily said than done. Obtaining a well-formed crystal of the unknown will typically be far more difficult than the actual analysis; this is a nontrivial undertaking and it is at this point that the particle analyst should turn to a crystallographer and/or chemist with appropriate training for assistance. If the particulate matter consists of crystals originating from a slowly forming precipitate without mechanical disturbance in a liquid dosage, a single crystal may simply be isolated for analysis. If, in the far more likely case, the material exists as poorly defined crystals or as an amorphous material intermixed with miscellaneous extraneous particles, dissolution and recrystallation are required. This generally entails collection of a significant mass (several milligrams) of the material needed to grow a single crystal with dimensions of 0.1 mm to 0.3 mm and then redissolving the material in a solvent. One of the simplest methods of growing crystals is by allowing a saturated or nearly saturated solution to sit quietly while the solvent (slowly) evaporates. Good crystals are usually produced only when the solution is allowed to evaporate without mechanical disturbance. Solutions of some materials tend to become supersaturated. The eventual crystallization is usually so rapid that only microscopic crystals result. Supersaturation can often be prevented by mild mechanical shock or by seeding the solution with a few crystal fragments of the material to be crystallized. This is obviously a delicate procedure requiring specialized skill and knowledge.

A second method that may be employed to grow crystals from solution is slow cooling. The size of crystals formed is generally related to colling rate; cooling rates for solutions contained in common laboratory glassware are generally too rapid to produce anything but microscopic crystals. The rate of cooling may be decreased by placing the vessel containing the solution in a large container of hot water or by insulating it with some appropriate material. The process may also be carried out in a Dewar flask. Slow rates of cooling can be obtained in an oven with a solid-state temperature controller by reducing the temperature in small increments over a period of time.

If difficulty is experienced in growing crystals from individual solvents, mixtures of two or more solvents may be used. Changing the solvent may have a pronounced effect on the habit and size of crystals grown; the factors that influence crystal growth include solution density, dielectric constant, and viscosity. All of these factors can be varied over wide ranges and adjusted to the conditions required for good crystal growth.

A method that can produce good single crystals with milligram amounts of particulate matter involves crystallization from the solvent by vapor diffusion. Figure 16 illustrates this procedure. A solution of the particulate matter in a primary solvent is placed in the small Ehrlemeyer flask or in a test tube. A second solvent is placed in the closed beaker surrounding the flask. The secondary solvent is chosen on the basis of its ability to form a mixed solvent system with the primary solvent in which the material to be crystallized is of decreased solubility. If the secondary solvent is more volatile, it is possible for the volume of solution to increase during

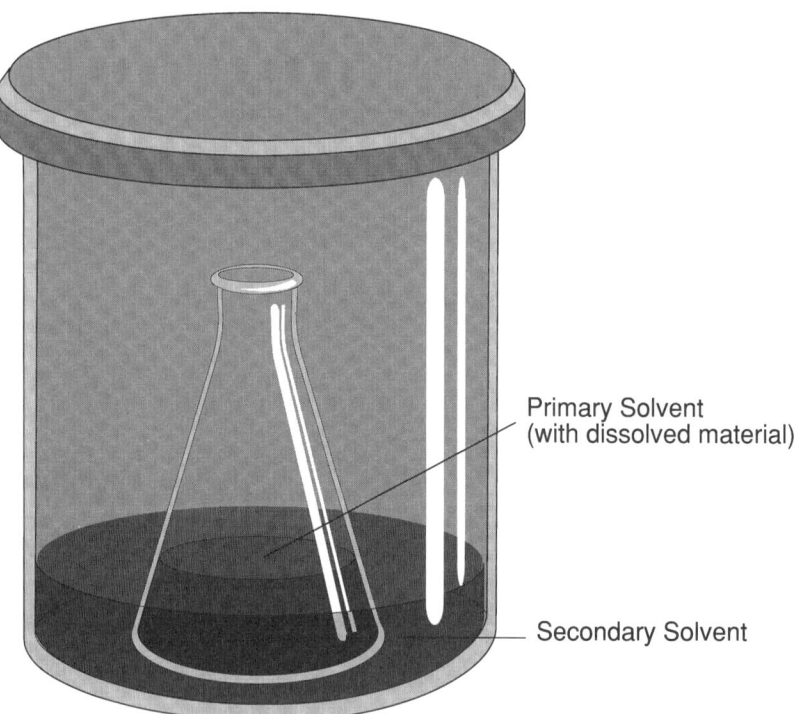

Figure 16. Crystallization by vapor diffusion.

crystallization, thus avoiding the surface "crusts" of precipitated material that often form when concentration occurs during evaporation or diffusion.

Summary

Although many techniques can yield information on the composition of particles, there is a wide variation in their capabilities. Characteristics important to the analysis of particles include spatial resolution and imaging, multielement analysis, sensitivity, and sample preparation. Classical atomic absorption and emission techniques are poorly suited to the analysis of solid samples. Furthermore, dissolution of particulate matter to yield solution samples would negate the concentrating effect achieved during particle isolation. The use of EDXS as an atomic spectroscopic technique in combination with micro FT–IR to gather molecular data represents a powerful combined approach. Mass spectrometry with laser or conventional means of excitation is also useful in a smaller number of cases. X-ray crystallography is a powerful technique with a limited range of application.

The instrumental techniques discussed in this chapter generally represent methodologies with a narrower range of applicability than microscopy and require a higher degree of specialization on the part of the operator. All are currently in wide use in pharmaceutical research facilities.

References

Aldrich, D. S. 1990. Identification of parenteral particles. In *Proc. PDA Int. Conf. on Particle Detection, Metrology and Control*, 269–282. Arlington, VA.

Anderson, M. E. 1982. Identification of pigments of artistic, forensic and industrial importance by the raman microprobe (MOLE) and scanning electron microscopy with energy-dispersive x-ray analysis. *Microbeam Anal.* 17:197–201.

Bloss, F. D. 1961. *An introduction to the methods of optical crystallography*. 1st ed. New York: Holt, Rinehart and Winston.

Bodapatti, S., L. D. Butler, S. Im, and P. P. DeLuca. 1980. Identification of subvisible barium sulfate crystals in parenteral solutions. *J. Pharm. Sci.* 69:608–610.

Bollinger, R. O., A. M. Preuss, P. R. McClain, and W. T. Hill, Jr. 1978. Study of particulate matter in carbencillin disodium using scanning electron microscopy and microbeam x-ray spectrography. *Am. J. Hosp. Pharm.* 35:312–317.

Borchert, S. J., A. Abe, S. D. Aldrich, L. E. Fox, J. E. Freeman, and R. D. White. 1986. Particulate matter in parenteral products: A review. *J. Parent. Sci. and Technol.* 40:212–239.

Buerger, M. J. 1960a. *Crystal-structure analysis.* In *Crystal-structure analysis,* ed. D. P. Shoemaker, 152–241. New York: Wiley.

Buerger, M. J. 1960b. *IUCR world list of crystallographic computer programs.* 2nd ed. A. Oosterhoek's Uitgevers Mij. N.Y., Domstraat 11–13, Utrecht, Netherlands.

Castaing, R., B. Jouffrey, and G. Slodzian. 1960. Sur les possibilities d'analysis locale d'un echantillon par utilization de son emission Ionique secondaire. *Acad. Sci.* 122 (1960).

Conzemius, R. J., and J. M. Capellan. 1980. A review of the applications to solids of the laser ion source mass spectrometry. *Int. J. Mass Spectrom. Ion Phys.* 34:197–204.

Cotter, R. J. 1987. Laser spectrometry: An overview of techniques, instruments and applications. *Analytical Chemical Acta* 45–49.

Cournoyer, R., J. C. Shearer, and D. H. Anderson. 1977. Fourier transform infrared analysis below the nanogram level. *Anal. Chem.* 49:2275–2277.

Curry, C. J., M. J. Whitehouse, and J. M. Chalmers. 1985. Ultramicro sampling in infrared spectroscopy using small apertures. *Appl. Spectrosc.* 39:174–180.

DeLuca, P. P., and S. Bodapatti. 1980. Guidelines for the identification of particles in parenterals. *FDA Guidelines* No. 3 (July).

Draftz, R. G., and J. Graf. 1974. Identifying particle contaminants. *Bull. Parenteral Drug Assoc.* 28:35–52.

Erike, A., W. Sichtermann, and A. Benninhhoven. 1980. Secondary ion mass spectrometry of nucleic acid components: Pyrimidines, purines, nucleotides. *Org. Mass Spectrom.* 15:289–296.

Farlow, N. H. 1957. Quantitative determination of chloride ion in 10^{-6} to 10^{-12} gram particles. *Anal. Chem.* 29:883–885.

Gavrilovic, J. 1984. Surface analysis of small individual particles by secondary ion mass spectroscopy. In *Particle Characterization* in *Technology, Vol. I: Applications in Microanalysis,* ed. J. K. Beddow, 32–46. Boca Raton, FL: CRC Press.

Heinrich, K. F., ed. 1980. *Characterization of particles.* NBS (NIST): Special Publication 533.

Heinrich, K. F. 1981. *Electron beam x-ray micro-analysis.* New York: Van Nostrand Reinhold.

Hillencamp, F., and R. Kaufmann. 1982. Laser microprobe mass analysis (LAMMA): A new approach in biomedical microanalysis and mass spectrometry. *Laser Applications in Medicine and Biology,* Vol. 4. ed. M. L. Wolbarsht. New York: Plenum Press.

Humecki, H. J., and R. Z. Muggli. 1982. Microsample identification with FT–IR spectroscopy. *Microbeam Anal.* 17:243–246.

James, R. W. 1965. *The optical principles of the diffraction of x-rays,* Chapters 3 and 5. New York: Cornell University Press.

Kaufmann, R., and P. Wieser. 1980. Laser microprobe mass analysis (LAMMA) in particle analysis, in characterization of particles. In *NBS Spec. Publ.* 533, ed. K. F. J. Heinrich. Washington, D.C.: U.S. Government Printing Office.

Kruger, R. F., and B. Scheuler. 1981. Organic mass spectra obtained by fission-fragment- and pulsed laser-induced desorption. *Adv. Mass Spectrom.* 718:8–20.

Lacy, M. E. 1982. Isolation and molecular identification of ultramicro contaminants by Fourier transform infrared spectroscopy. *Proc. Inst. Environ. Sci.* 28:185–188.

Lechene, S. P., and R. R. Warner. 1977. Ultramicroanalysis: X-ray spectrometry by electron probe excitation. *Ann. Rev. Biophys. Bioeng.* 6:7–85.

Liebl, H. 1967. Ion microprobe mass analyzer. *J. Appl. Phys.* 38:5277–5291.

Long, P. L., J. E. Katon, and A. S. Bonanno. 1988. Identification of dust particles by molecular microspectroscopy. *Appl. Spectroscopy* 42:313–317.

McCrone, W. C., J. A. Brown, and I. A. Stewart. 1980. Electron optical atlas and techniques. *The Particle Atlas,* Vol. 4, 2nd Ed. Ann Arbor, MI: Ann Arbor Science Publishers.

McHugh, J. R. 1975. Methods of surface analysis. In *SIMS,* ed. S. P. Wolsky and A. W. Czanderna. Amsterdam: Elsevier.

Meserschmidt, R. G., and M. A. Harthcock. 1987. *Infrared microspectroscopy theory and applications.* New York: Marcel Decker, Inc.

Oles, P. J. 1987. Particle analysis and identification in the pharmaceutical industry. *Microscope* 26:41–48.

Post, J. E., and P. R. Buseck. 1984. Characterization of individual particles in the Phoenix urban aerosol using electron-beam instruments. *Environ. Sci. Technol.* 18 (1):35–42.

Stout, G. H., and L. H. Jensen. 1968. *X-ray structure determinations.* New York: Macmillan Co.

Surkyn, P., and F. Adams. 1982. Laser microprobe mass analysis of glass microparticles. *J. Trace Microprobe Tech.* 1:79–87.

Wilson, R. G., F. A. Stevie, and C. W. Magee. 1989. *Secondary ion mass spectrometry.* New York: Wiley Interscience.

Winding, O., and B. Holms. 1976. Method for determination and elemental analysis of particulate contamination in injectable solutions. *Am. J. Hosp. Pharm.* 33:1154–1159.

Wischnitzer, Saul. 1981. *Introduction to electron microscopy,* 3rd Ed. New York: Pergamon Press.

VI

Environmental Particulate Matter Monitoring and Control

For purposes of this discussion, environmental particles are defined as those present as randomly-dispersed airborne contaminants in the ambient air of a process room or production facility. These particles range from submicron fragments of glass, plastic, metal (or human skin) to large visible fibers of paper or cotton. This particulate matter population is distinct from process- or point-generated particles that may occur at high levels in local areas due to human or machine operations. The control of environmental particles is based on three key mechanisms: (1) continuously supplying clean air to the process area by means of high efficiency particulate air (HEPA) filters; (2) removing contaminated air through return plenums; and (3) monitoring airborne particle numbers with optical particle counters (OPC).

HEPA filters fulfill critical functions in the pharmaceutical industry in a variety of ways. They are used both to prevent access of particles to product and to provide clean airflow that serves to dilute fine particle aerosols generated within the confines of a clean area where sensitive processes, such as aseptic filling, are being carried out. Often HEPA filters are used to generate laminar airflow that serves to "wash" particles away from a particularly sensitive area.

The monitoring of aerosol particles in pharmaceutical manufacturing environments is critical to maintenance of Good Manufacturing Practice (GMP) and the assurance of product quality. The primary reason for the concern with the monitoring of aerosol particles is simply that these materials can adhere to surfaces that should be clean or enter product via the container or closure. Although such particles are generally nonviable organic or inorganic materials, they may transport bacteria and conceivably could be chemically reactive. The GMP regulations enforced by the Food and Drug Administration deal specifically with monitoring in controlled environments, monitoring over filling lines, and monitoring of compressed air lines. The GMPs in some cases specify maximum particle concentration limits and provide procedural recommendations for monitoring. Particle monitoring to ensure that air quality is maintained is particularly critical in aseptic fill processes.

Most contamination control efforts concern the total numbers of contaminants within the air, but requirements also exist for specific control of bacteria, spores, viruses, or drug powder particles that are contained in the air. Airborne particles range in size from 0.001 μm to several hundred microns. Suspended particles settle onto containers, closures, and exposed surfaces at a rate that depends on the size and density of the particle. For example, according to Stokes Law, a spherical particle of 50 μm size with a unit density would take less than one minute to settle 10 feet, while a particle in the 1 μm range could take 15 or 20 hours to settle the same distance.

Before any methods of environmental control of airborne particles can be applied successfully, a decision must be made as to how critical particulate matter is to the process or operation. The allowable size and number of an airborne particles at a point within an area depends on the most critical tolerances of the process to be performed at that particular point. At the same time, the quantity of the particles of a given size that might be generated at process points within the area of concern must be considered.

Particles from sources both internal and external to the process are important. Despite filtration and other safeguards, gross atmospheric contamination and particles from surrounding areas tend to find their way into the protected environment. External contamination, such as combustion particles, may be brought in through the air-conditioning system that supplies the process room with makeup air. In addition to the air-conditioning system, contamination from adjacent areas will enter through doors and pass-throughs. The external contamination from adjacent areas to which a process is exposed is critically affected by the type of filtration used, overpressure gradients, and human access.

People and processes are the greatest source of contamination due to the fact that they continually produce and shed particles (both viable and nonviable). Shedding of skin cells generates particles in the 1 µm–10 µm range, and exhaled air contains large quantities of particles ranging from submicrometer size to several hundred micrometers. In addition to people, moving contact between surfaces creates contamination. Writing with a pencil on a piece of paper generates an aerosol cloud of fine carbon particles and paper fiber fragments. The movement of a metal part on a bearing surface sometimes generates particulate matter in the form of a fine metallic dust. Particles of dry powder drugs are notorious as an all-pervasive contaminant in powder fill facilities.

In a "clean" working environment, air movement results from people walking and operation of machinery, fans, and motors. All of these cause the air to move with random velocity and direction within the work space. Particles caught in random currents within a given work space may easily move from one area to another unless they are controlled by some means. This movement of contamination via random air currents from one part of the space to another or to adjacent areas is termed cross contamination and is a significant contributor to the general process contamination level. In this regard, unidirectional airflow can be used to eliminate cross contamination and "sweep" particles away to return ducts. Over time, contamination from all sources will build up in the process area on surfaces and in the air and reach a steady state condition with particles being added as quickly as they are removed. Depending on the type of manufacturing environment considered, the steady state count may reach as high as 100,000 particles larger than 0.5 µm per cubic foot.

Applicable Standards

Numerous standards have been generated to deal with particulate matter control in controlled environment areas (CEAs) and clean rooms. The two most widely used are Federal Standard 209-D and British Standard 5295 (Part 1). These standards specify allowable particle levels at specific sizes for various classifications (Figures 1a and 1b). Recommended practice 006 (IES) is also a useful standard and other applicable standards are given in the FS 209-D reference list.

These two standards are extremely useful in that they provide a basis for implementation of uniform procedures for particulate matter control and monitoring. The user of these specifications should avoid two misconceptions in their use. Both provide graphs

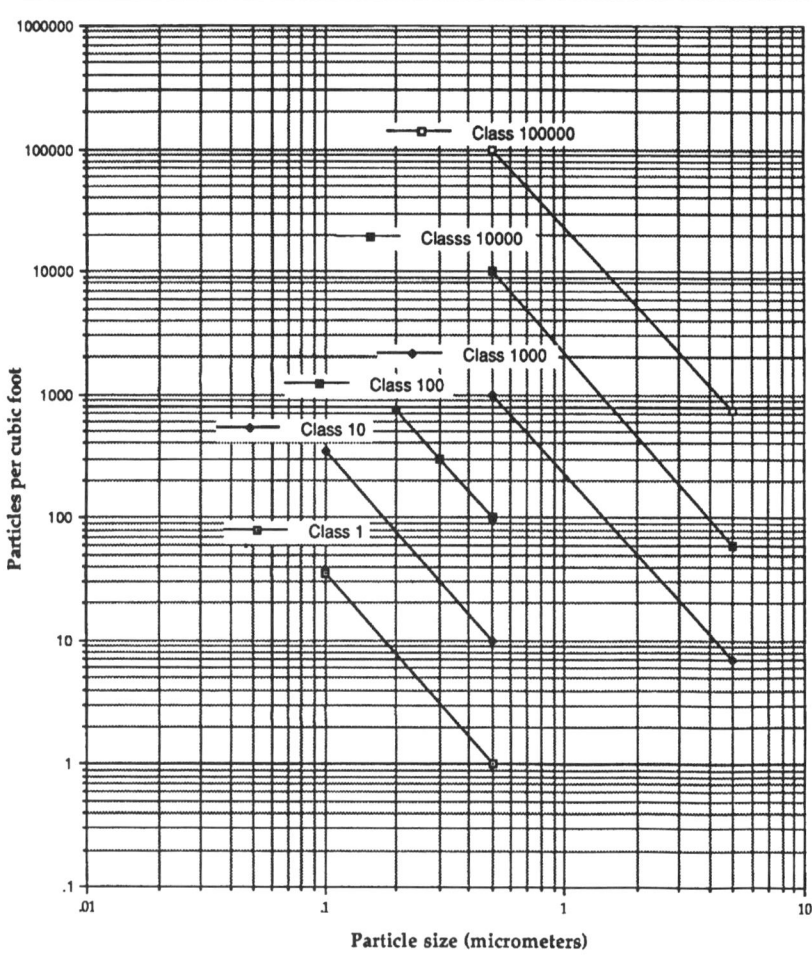

Figure 1a. Total number of particles per cubic foot equal to or larger than stated particle size per Federal Standard 209-D.

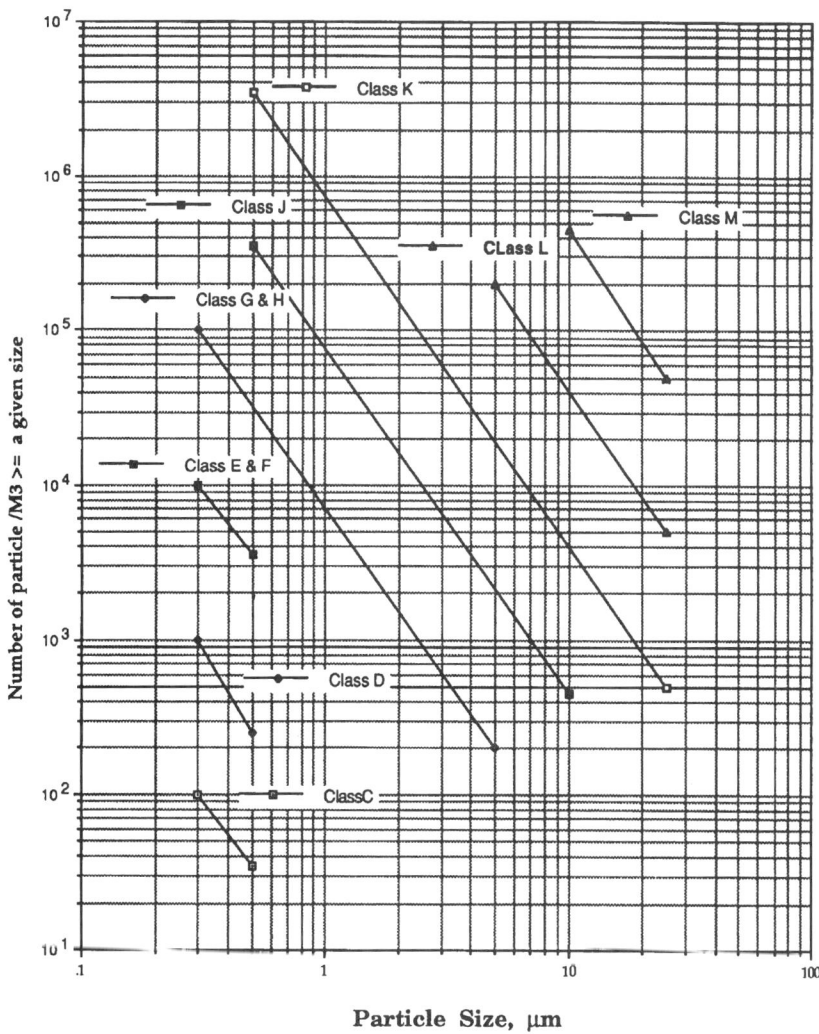

Figure 1b. Maximum number of particles per cubic meter equal to or greater than given size for designated classes (BS 5295).

showing particle distributions for various cleanliness classes. The distributions shown are, unfortunately, theoretical and have no basis in fact. Monitoring airborne counts at a single size has no implication regarding counts at other sizes. Secondly, both standards specify schemes for verifying the various classifications. The plans specified are useful, but not optimal for all areas that will be monitored. Thus, a manufacturer may devise and implement better monitoring plans than those specified without being considered out of compliance in the eyes of the Food and Drug Administration (FDA) or Department of Health and Social Services (U.K.).

Principles of HEPA Filtration

High efficiency particulate air filters are a critical control mechanism in pharmaceutical environments. Today, HEPA filters are made of glass fibers of a few microns in diameter. Despite the fact that it is constructed of glass, the HEPA medium is often referred to as "paper." These fibers are disposed randomly throughout the depth of the filter medium. In older designs the glass medium was supported by pleated or corrugated metal dividers (Figure 2); current designs often incorporate pleats or "dimples" for separation (Figure 3); HEPA filter paper does not have a controlled pore size.

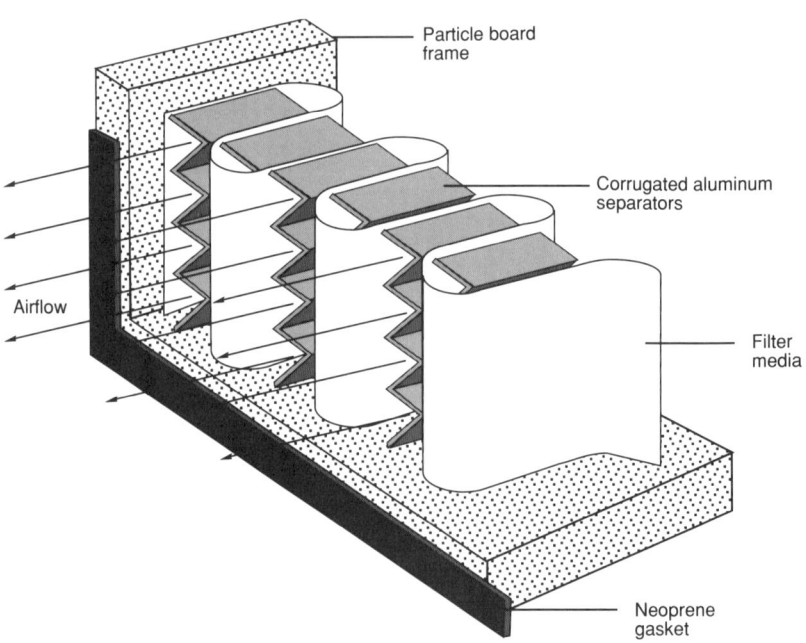

Figure 2. Historical HEPA filter construction.

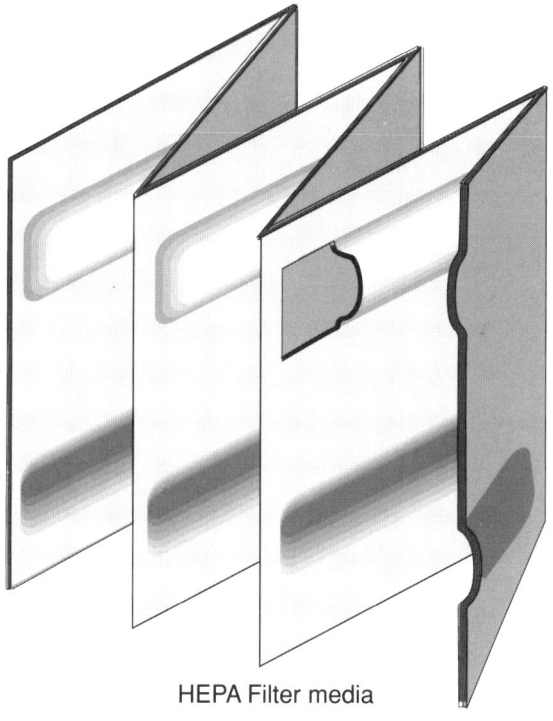

HEPA Filter media

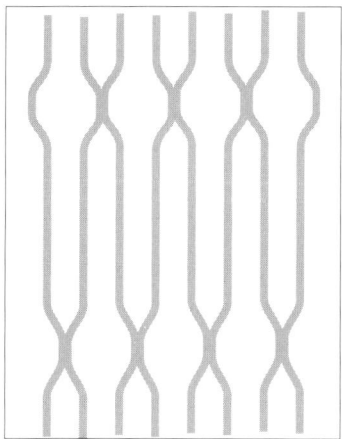

Cross section of filter media

Figure 3. Folded HEPA filter media with "dimple pleat" separation of layers (Flanders Filters, Inc.).

In fact, the spaces between fibers are most often much larger than the particles captured. As an aerosol moves through the filter paper, the entrained particles collide with the fibers or with other particles that are already stuck to the fibers. When a particle bumps into either a fiber or a particle already stuck to a fiber, strong attraction is established between the particle and the fiber or particle that has captured it. This particle, once adhered to the fibers of the HEPA filter, is unlikely to be dislodged.

All HEPA filters are constructed so that the filter paper is arranged in a large number of parallel pleats separated by some means. The pleats are narrow and relatively deep. A typical 2 ft × 4 ft × 6 in. HEPA filter contains 120 to 200 such pleats. These pleats act to align the flow paths of air molecules flowing through the filter. The resistance of HEPA filter paper to gas flow is reasonably uniform, meaning that approximately equal volumes of gas move simultaneously through each pleat of the filter. These two factors, the uniform resistance of the filter paper and the large number of parallel pleats, cause the filtered air to converge in uniform parallel flow paths 3 inches to 9 inches downstream from the HEPA filter face. This flow pattern is called laminar flow. The use of HEPA filters in a process area does not guarantee laminar airflow patterns at critical process points. Other parameters such as airflow rate and placement of equipment, such as light fixtures, must be controlled in order to maintain laminar flow (Figure 4).

Three principal mechanisms—impaction, diffusion, and interception—cause particles to contact a capture point on a fiber of a HEPA filter (Figure 5). In the process of capture by impaction, particles large enough (i.e., with enough mass) to have sufficient momentum leave the air stream as the air turns to move around a fiber and strike it. In capture by diffusion, the smaller particles (i.e., those without sufficient mass to leave the air stream on their own) move about randomly because they are constantly bombarded by other small particles and by the molecules of the gases in which they are suspended. This random motion eventually results in the smaller particles contacting the filter fibers. Larger particles that have deviated from their flow path enough to contact fibers in a "grazing" manner are captured by a mechanism known as interception. A fourth mechanism of filtration, screening or straining, can also occur in a HEPA filter. Straining simply means that the spaces between the fibers are smaller than the particles that are captured so that particles lodge in the spaces between fibers. Straining is primarily important for particles >5 μm in size.

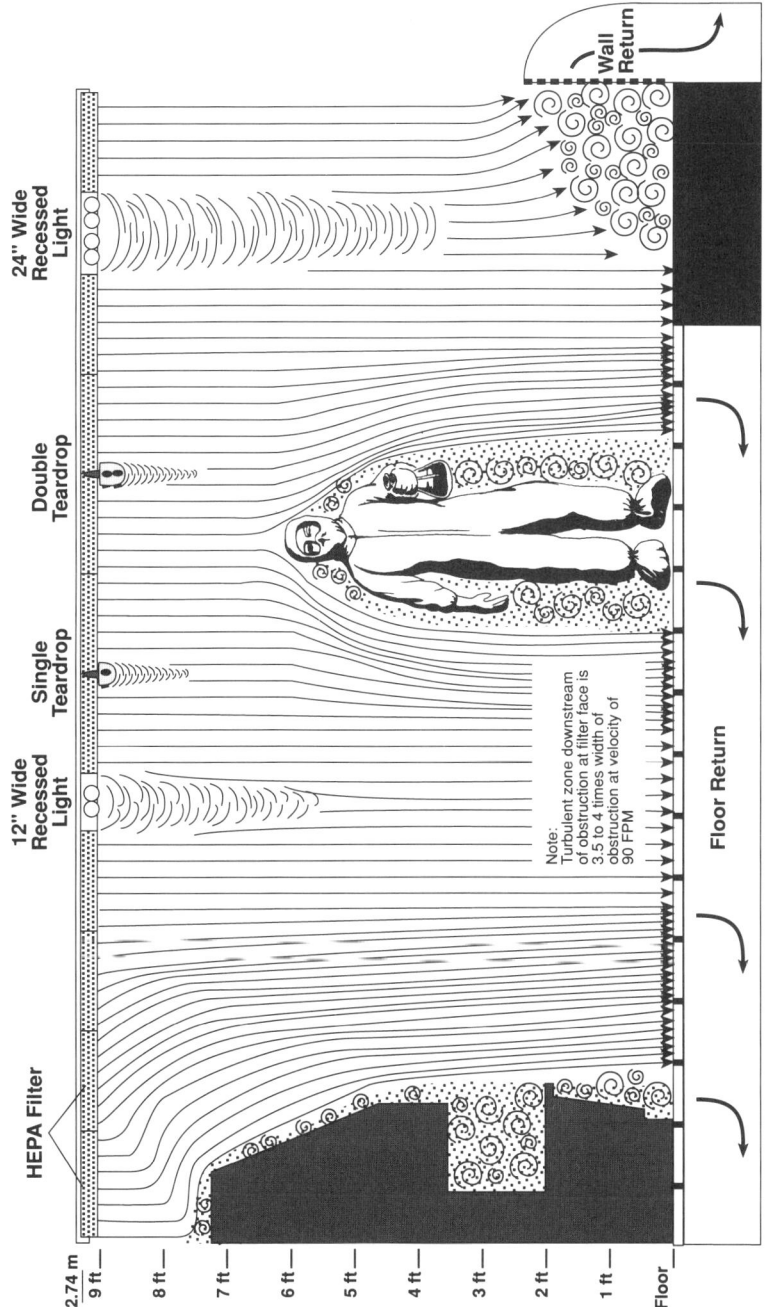

Figure 4. Laminar and turbulent flow in clean room.

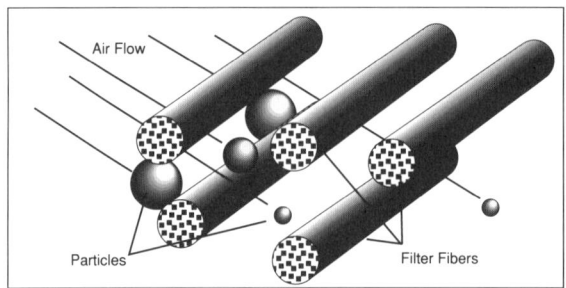
Strainer Effect

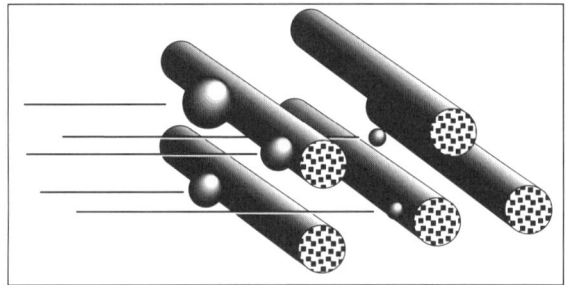
Interception

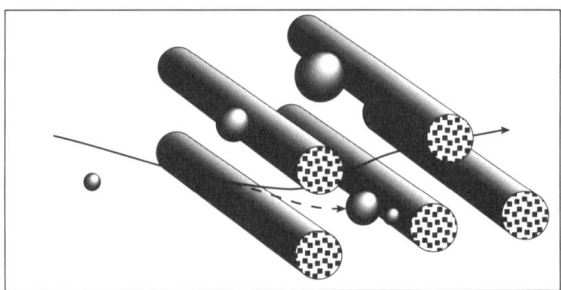
Interception aided by particle inertia

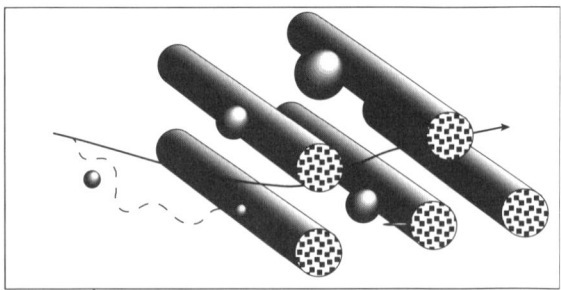
Interception aided by diffusion

Figure 5. Particle entrapment by media of HEPA filter.

HEPA Filter Particle Retention Characteristics

Filtration of small particles by fibrous filters has been subject to numerous theoretical and experimental studies during the past 30 years. As a result, the dependence of filtration efficiency on particle size is now well established. Larger particles are captured by the interception and inertial impaction mechanisms; smaller particles are collected due to diffusion. There is an intermediate particle size region between these two where both mechanisms are least effective. This is the region where the particle penetration through the filter is a maximum and the retention efficiency of the filter is at a minimum (Figure 6) (Flanders Technical Bulletin 581D 1989).

The existence of minimum filter efficiencies is well established. The minimum filter efficiency and the particle size at which the minimum efficiency occurs will vary depending on the type of filter and the flow velocity. For fibrous HEPA filters operating at relatively low filtration velocities (70–100 fpm), the generally accepted minimum filter efficiency occurs at approximately 0.3 µm. This is the basis of the widely used hot dioctyl phthalate (DOP) test for HEPA filters that makes use of monodisperse DOP particles with a distribution centered around 0.3 µm for testing the filter. The 0.3 µm minimum efficiency figure was established in the 1950s. The more sophisticated equipment available today (laser particle counters) suggest 0.09–0.2 µm may be the sizes most difficult to capture. In any case, airflow rate through the filter will impact the filtration efficiency at a given size; a higher flow rate increases capture by impaction and interception and decreases capture by diffusion, a lower flow rate works in the opposite fashion.

In-Use Testing of HEPA Filters

By definition, a HEPA filter has an average minimum efficiency of 99.97% when challenged with a thermally generated dioctylphthalate (DOP) aerosol whose droplet diameter is 0.3 µm (Flanders Technical Bulletin 581D 1989). Various standards refer to this "fog" as being monodisperse at this size, but this is not strictly true. This average efficiency is a widely accepted manufacturing standard. It is important to note that a filter's initial (clean) DOP efficiency represents only the initial efficiency of that filter. Since a filter's efficiency increases as it accumulates particulate matter in service, the initial efficiency may well be the lowest efficiency during its life. Minute areas of greater penetration, either at the edge

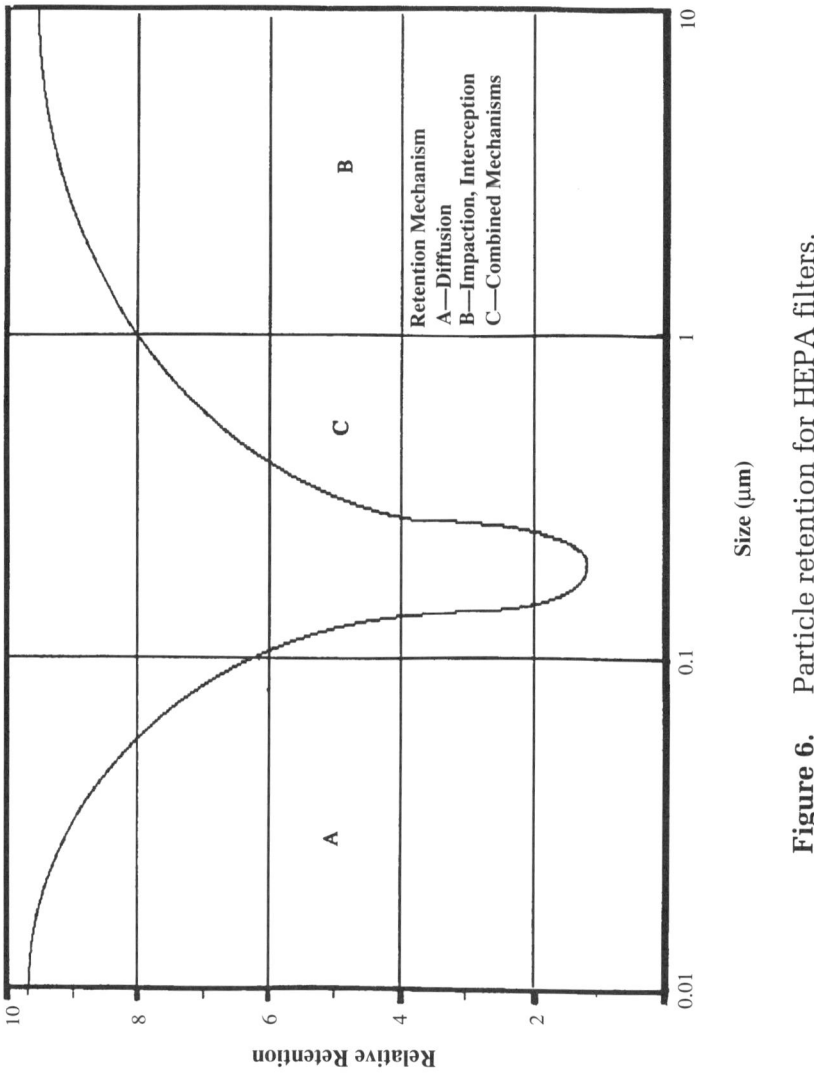

Figure 6. Particle retention for HEPA filters.

seal between the filter element and the filter's integral frame or in the paper itself, may be present when the filter is tested by the manufacturer, but particles passing through these leaks are diluted by the greater amount of clean air passing through the filter. Most pharmaceutical containment requirements are well satisfied by achieving average filter bank efficiencies of 99.95% or greater for 0.3 mm particles.

Pinhole leaks may be intolerable in laminar flow systems (such as clean work stations, clean rooms, downflow hoods) where HEPA filters are located at the end of a air supply entering the clean room or work area. In order to dilute particles from the pinhole leak with the clean air passing through the filter, either fill-in by clean air or some method of mixing (with a baffle) are required. A baffle would defeat the purpose of a laminar flow clean room. Therefore, a potential exists that the product or process requiring particulate free air during manufacture or assembly operations could be located directly downstream of a pinhole leak. Such leaks may be induced by the installation operation when the filler is set in place.

Of necessity, there are in-use field test procedures to scan or probe the downstream face of a bank of filters in a laminar flow system, not only to locate pinhole leaks in the filter element, but to determine whether the filters are properly sealed to their mounting frames. A challenge aerosol, usually a polydisperse cold DOP aerosol with a droplet size range of from 0.1 to 3.0 μm, is generated and introduced upstream of the filter bank while the system is in operation. The downstream side is then probed with a portable forward light scattering photometer. Pinhole leaks and filter-to-frame leaks must be identified and patched, typically with silicone sealant, based on the outcome of the test.

The cold DOP aerosol is generated using a device called a Laskin nozzle that is immersed in DOP. There are two sets of holes in the nozzle. One set of four holes is located directly beneath a collar around the bottom of a tube that is immersed in the liquid DOP. The second set of four holes is located in the collar itself, with each hole being positioned directly above the corresponding hole at the end of the tube. The air flowing out of the holes in the bottom of the tube causes the DOP oil to be drawn through the holes in the collar, fragmenting the liquid into an aerosol. Unlike the homogeneous, monodispersed particles generated in the hot DOP test used by the filter manufacturer, the cold DOP is heterogeneous and poly-dispersed. The cold aerosol is arbitrarily stated to have an approximate droplet size distribution as follows (IES RP–CC-001-86; IES RP–CC-006-84T):

99% less than 3.0 mm
95% less than 1.5 μm
92% less than 1.0 μm
50% less than 0.72 μm
25% less than 0.45 μm
10% less than 0.35 μm

Once a suitable test aerosol is generated, the filter is tested by scanning the filter face for leaks using the aerosol photometer. A photometer of the type used is simply a device for measuring the total light scattered by the dispersed DOP aerosol particles in its sensing volume. The light scattering effect is measured independent of particle size and the total light scattered is related to various cold DOP aerosol concentrations (µg/L) used to calibrate the instrument.

The photometer probe is connected by flexible tubing to the intake of the light scattering chamber of the photometer. To test the filter the operator scans the filter perimeter and then, using slightly overlapping strokes, and being careful not to touch the filter, probes the entire face of the filter. Most photometers sample at 1.0 CFM. Air is drawn through the chamber and any entrained particles present in the sampled air deflect the light source onto the sensitive area of the photomultiplier tube. This causes the needle on the meter to move, indicating the size of the leak by the meter reading. If the photometer reading is greater than 0.01% of the upstream challenge concentration, the leak is unacceptable and the leak must be repaired.

No alternative to the use of a cold DOP challenge for in-place tests of HEPA filters has been validated by a pharmaceutical manufacturer and presented to regulatory authorities. Two key issues that must be dealt with in the selection of any test method are the nature of the material that will be used as a challenge aerosol and certainty of leak detection with a minimum amount of time expended in testing. There is little doubt that the application of a conventional cold DOP fog at a concentration of 80–100 mg/L concentration upstream of the tested filter represents "overkill" in terms of certainty of leak detection and shortens the useful life of HEPA filters.

The condensation nucleus counter (CNC) approach, which relies on the high numbers of 0.05 µm particles in unfiltered air as a challenge, is better but it does not test HEPAs at the most penetrating particle size and is also extremely time-consuming (Greiner 1990; Cooper et al. 1991a, 1991b). One enhancement to cold DOP challenge would seem to be the use of currently available aerosol photometers that are 10–100 fold more sensitive than the older models in use by most manufacturers. These instruments will provide the same certainty of leak detection as the present test with a 10-fold lower (10 µg/L) challenge aerosol concentration upstream. Their use would serve the purpose of greatly decreasing the amount of DOP used with consequent lower filter loading and decreased human exposure. Validation of this approach would, of course, be required and a comparison of results with the historical database would be necessary, since current methods are tied into the 80–100 µg/L challenge. Another alternative that seems promising would be the use of a monodisperse (0.3 µm or smaller) thermally generated fog that would give the same certainty of leak detection with a lower total DOP concentration upstream.

Environmental Particle Monitoring

The particle monitoring technology currently available to the pharmaceutical manufacturer in 1991 is far advanced over that available only 5 years ago. Optical particle counters that are the key element of airborne particle monitoring have been greatly improved over earlier models (Szymanski and Wagner 1990; Umhauer and Bottlinger 1990). Whereas 5 years ago the most common practice for airborne monitoring included white light-based counters and manual site monitoring, many manufacturers today apply laser sensor-based OPC remote sampling or remote sensor technology with sophisticated computer-based data collection and data reduction.

Since 1977, a variety of new airborne particle counting instruments and systems have been developed. At this time, the most sensitive instruments are capable of counting and sizing 0.05 µm particles in air at a flow rate of 2.8 liters/min (0.1 CFM) (Lieberman 1988). A variety of particle counting instruments are available for measurement of particles larger than 0.1 µm at sample flow rates of 28.3 liters/min (1.0 CFM). These instruments are well adapted for rapidly verifying and monitoring areas of Class 10 to Class 100 areas. For areas rated at Class 1000 and higher, instruments with lesser sensitivity and lower flow rates can be used equally well.

Generalized function of a light scattering OPC is shown in Figure 7. Particles pass through the light beam (sensing volume) one at a time. Intensity of scattered light is measured by a photodetector. Photodetector pulses are analyzed by a pulse height analyzer (PHA). Calibration permits conversion from pulse height to particle size. Relating the pulse height data to the particle size information yields a response curve for the instrument and allows particles counted at given size thresholds to be quantitated.

The type of counter used for monitoring is extremely important (Wen and Kasper 1986). Several key considerations are pertinent to the decision-making process that a manufacturer goes through in selection or upgrading of airborne particle monitoring technology, including:

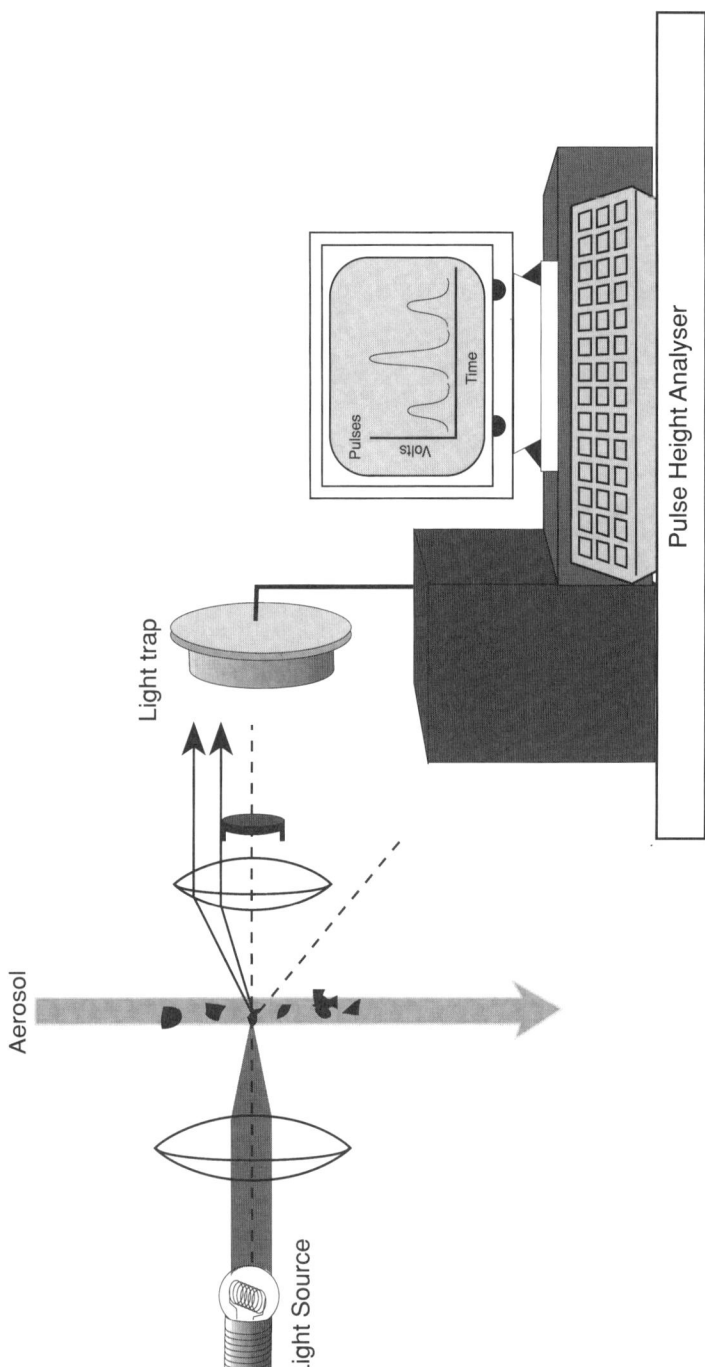

Figure 7. Operational principles of light scattering optical particle counter.

- Particle sizes to be monitored;
- Use of white light or laser light source for sensors;
- Application of remote monitoring methodology;
- Appropriate data handling techniques;
- Reconciliation of historical data base with counts collected using new technology;
- Calibration methodology;
- Validation of monitoring plans;
- Selection of instrumentation; and
- Interpretation and application of standards.

The goal of the following discussion is to help provide basic information for establishing a monitoring program in a pharmaceutical manufacturing plant. Some background information is provided toward this end, and applications and procedures are briefly discussed. Particular emphasis will be placed on the first three items listed above in an effort to assist a manufacturer who is in the process of a total or partial technology upgrade.

Laser Versus White Light Aerosol Counters

The accuracy of the size distribution measured by an OPC is dependent upon the response of the counter, which is in turn affected by the refractive index and shape of the particles as well as by the optical design of the instrument, including the light source used. Some understanding of the function of these instruments is critical to the selection of the best instrument for a given application based on its operational parameters. The reader should be aware that different models of counters as well as different counters of the same model may give significantly different count data even when samply side by side in a particular controlled environment area. A counter with better "low end" sensitivity, for example, 0.2 µm, should be suspect of giving somewhat higher counts at the 0.5 µm size used to define Federal Standard 209-D classifications than one stated by the manufacturer to have a 0.5 µm lower sensitivity limit. Despite the statistical advantage of counting at smaller sizes in Class 100 or Class 10 areas, the 0.5 µm size is still the size most frequently monitored in pharmaceutical manufacturing based on the FDA guidelines for aseptic filling (1987).

The basic, most critical differences between single particle OPC marketed today involve source illumination (laser or white light) and the geometry of scattered light collection (forward, near forward, or wide angle) (Liu et al. 1985; Montague and Sommer 1989, 1990). A white light sensor with wide angle collection geometry is shown in Figure 8. With white light counters, quartz-halogen bulbs are typically used as a light source. Laser counters may use He-Ne hard-seal lasers or a solid state laser diode. Other factors being equal, sensitivity (i.e., the smallest particle that may be sensed and counted) will be dependent on intensity of the illuminating radiation and its wavelength range. A hard-seal laser used in the active cavity mode gives an essentially monochromatic light with an extremely high photon density and results in the best sensitivity available (0.05 µm). Generally, more intense illuminating radiation results in a greater amount of scattered light for particles of a given size. A functional drawing of a contemporary laser-based OPC is shown in Figure 9. A key feature of this design is diode array detection of scattered light (Knollenberg 1970). The signal-to-noise ratio for light scattered by a particle of given size is increased due to a particle's scattering (signal) being concentrated on a single array element while the molecular ensemble scattering (noise) is shared among all elements.

The response of an OPC to aerosol particles is a complex relationship between functional properties of the instrument and physical and optical properties of particles in question (Horvath et al. 1990; Hovenac 1990). The critical factors of the instrument in this regard are sensor design, type of illumination, electronic amplification, and noise. Particle size, shape, and refractive index also have a significant effect on how a particle is sized.

Importantly in this consideration, counters calibrated by different methods or of different design must be expected to yield different counts for the same particle populations (Bemer et al. 1990; Buettner 1990). Particle population distribution information from different counters, particularly, may be expected to show wide variation. The response curve of OPC is typically nonmonotonic for particles that have different sizes and refractive indices; the shape of the response curve may also differ dependent upon whether the collection optics used are of near-forward, wide angle, or off-axis design (Figure 10). At sizes <1 µm, particles of different sizes with different shapes and refractive indices can in many instances give the same pulse height and thus appear the same size. While counter pulse height response generally increases with particle diameter, resonances in the response curve may result in very different

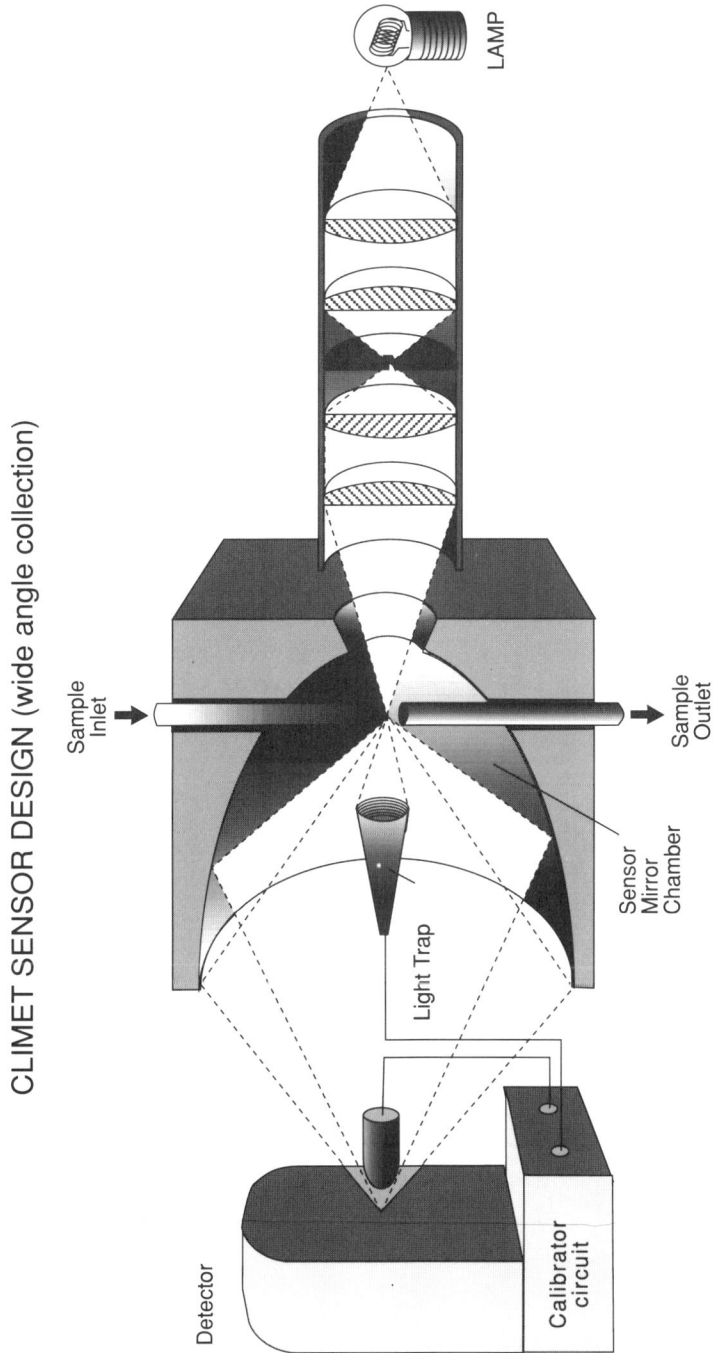

Figure 8. White light-based OPC with ellipsoidal mirror collection optics.

206 *Pharmaceutical Particulate Matter*

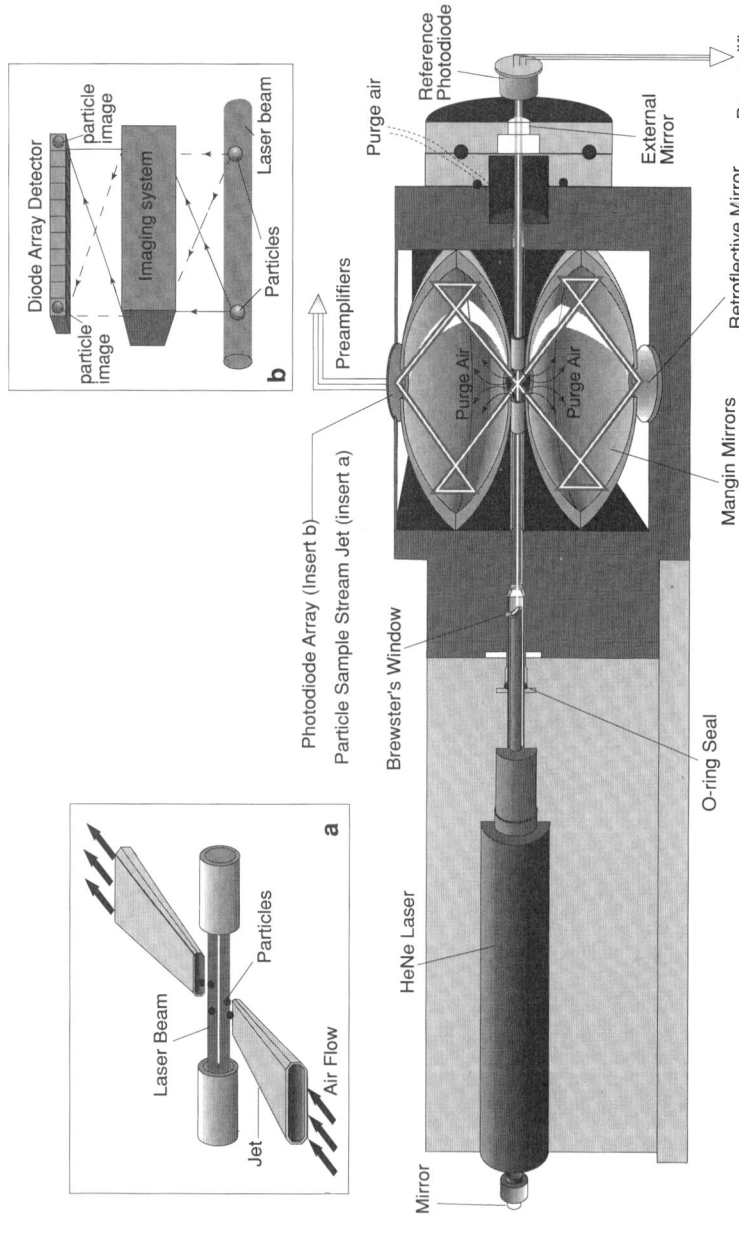

Figure 9. Active cavity laser OPC sensor with strip photodiode detector (Particle Measuring Systems, Inc.).

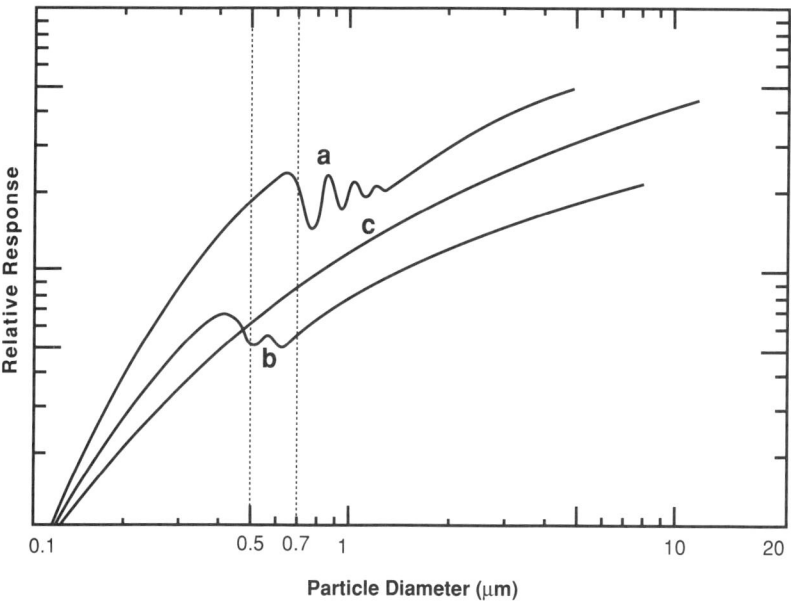

Figure 10. Generalized response curves for counters of different optical design.

responses for particles of closely similar sizes (Caldow and Blesner 1989).

Shape and orientation of nonspherical particles also affect the counter response (Cooper and Grotzinger 1989; Sommer 1989). If particles have dimensions less than the wavelength of illumination, the measured size may be considered equal to the volume equivalent diameter. For particles with dimensions above the wavelength of illumination, the measured particle size approximates the projected area equivalent diameter for instruments with wide-angle collecting optics. Refractive index differences between particles of the same size may cause an OPC to see them differently (Knollenberg 1989). The refractive index of a particle is described by a complex number. The real (scattering) and imaginary (absorption) components of this number are both functions of the wavelength, λ. Both components of the refractive index affect the response of an OPC.

A key concern for the manufacturer in upgrading OPC technology is the high count levels that may be obtained with some current generation counters versus their older counterparts (Sommer and

Montaque 1990; Sommer 1990). The situation may arise whereby a new counter, applied in a Class 100 area would indicate out-of-limits conditions whereas counts with an older model were well below 100 particles ≥ 0.5 µm per cubic foot (Liu and Szymanski 1987), even when both are calibrated per ASTM F328-80. In this regard, a comparison calibration procedure may be conducted per ASTM F649-80. The purchaser is well advised to: (1) thoroughly test new units prior to purchase; (2) become familiar with operational principles and calibration techniques; and (3) ensure that the older units to which new ones will be compared are in calibration and are not operating at decreased sensitivity due to their age and long use.

Remote Particle Monitoring

Remote monitoring of airborne particulate matter with remote sensors or by the use of tubing to transport samples to a counter transport is widely applied in the pharmaceutical industry today. This is particularly true in the case of aseptic fill operations that are typically conducted in Class 100 (or better) areas. Remote systems have many advantages over the manual sampling of preselected sites that was prevalent at the beginning of the 1980s (Lieberman 1979a, 1979b). The implementation of a remote system is a nontrivial undertaking and requires a considerable expenditure of funds, careful planning, and thorough validation. Suitable counters and other equipment is offered by Climet, Particle Measuring Systems, Met-One, and other vendors.

The following is an important consideration for the manufacturer contemplating purchase and installation of a system for remote monitoring of an aseptic fill area. The FDA is extremely sensitive to the function of particle control measures in aseptic fill areas. Inspectors will not necessarily be impressed by the use of space-age technology in monitoring endeavors, but will rather inspect for the manufacturer's adherence to the principle of the guidelines for aseptic filling (1987). The actual means of monitoring is secondary to minimizing intrusion of particulates into the clean room and through the primary barriers (e.g., air curtains) that shield the point at which the sterile powder is placed in sterile vials. Thus, in aseptic fill areas, the manufacturer should ensure that whatever means of monitoring is used must be integrated with the philosophy of maintaining acceptable cleanliness in critical process areas. Importantly, inspectors will consider particle counts in the immediate vicinity of unprotected products to be of equal or greater importance than those above the process.

Generally, four approaches are used for the monitoring of particle concentrations in pharmaceutical CEAs or clean rooms.

1. **Intermittent (Manual) Sampling:** Particle counting equipment is placed on a laboratory cart and wheeled into a clean area to perform point monitoring of the concentration. Portable counters sampling at 0.1–0.2 CFM (such as the Climet 4100 and Hiac/Royco portable model) may also be used in classifications above 10K or in lower classification areas if their sensitivity is <0.5 µm. The method has low initial capital requirements, but is labor-intensive, and yields data of limited value. It is most suitable to high class (i.e., 10K–100K) where frequent counts are not required.

2. **Multiplexed Air Sampling** (Figure 11a): In this technology a particle counter is mounted in a single location outside or within a clean room. Remote sampling is accomplished by adding an attachment (manifold) that will select from a number of sample tubes that draw air from various points in a clean room. This method has fairly modest capital requirements and allows sampling in several different areas in a clean room according to a preset schedule. However, only one location can be measured at a time, and critical information from some areas may be missed. In addition, the transport of air through tubing carries with it the potential for particle loss.

3. **Continuous/Multiplexed Air Sampling** (Figure 11b): This approach also uses tubing transport of the sampled air. Two particle counters are used. One measures an aggregate sample from a number of sample tubes, and the other measures the particle concentration from a specific tube. The advantage claimed for this approach is that the mixed sample can be used to detect a problem area, on the basis of elevated counts, and the specific location of the elevated counts can then be found by rapidly scanning specific tubes. The obvious disadvantage here is that counts at a single point may be significantly elevated without effecting the overall mean count. Also, a spike of high counts may evade the scan that is initiated when the aggregate count becomes momentarily elevated.

4. **Multiplexed Sensors** (Figure 11c): Here, a number of particle sensors are distributed in critical areas in a facility, and the signals are multiplexed and processed by a central computer. The advantages of this system are the ability to

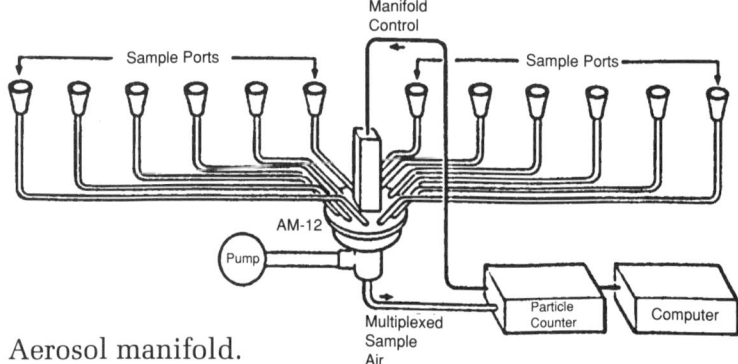

a. Aerosol manifold.

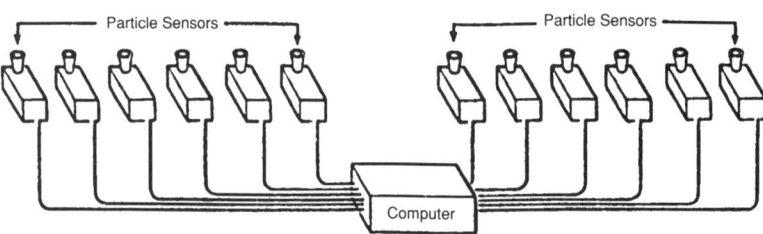

b. Continuous/multiplexed aerosol manifold.

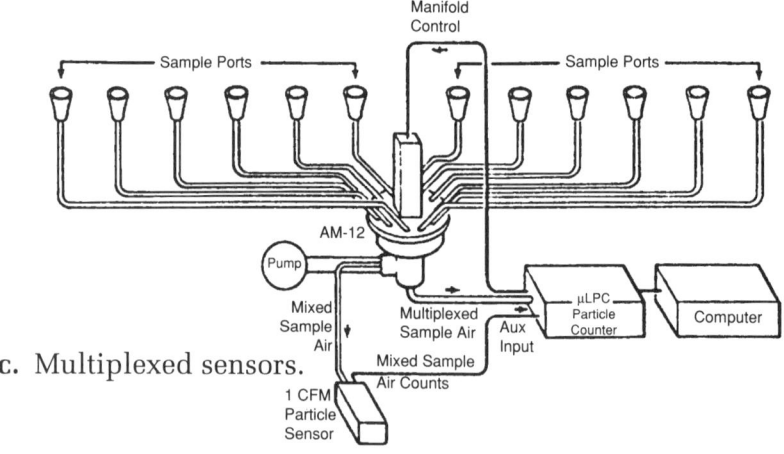

c. Multiplexed sensors.

Figure 11. Remote monitoring systems (courtesy of Particle Measuring Systems).

measure continuously and the elimination of any possible bias introduced by sample tubing (Keady et al. 1990). The large capital investment required is a real disadvantage that must be offset by the criticality of counts in the areas monitored and the value of product made there. It is also necessary to ensure that all of the sensors used have closely similar counting efficiency.

With regard to remote sampling, generally one must choose between (1) multiplexing sample air from a number of sample points into a single particle counter or (2) providing a sensor at each sampling location. The multiplexing approach, is less expensive than installing a sensor at each point to be monitored, but it has some limitations involving sample transport, with the attendant possible loss of larger particles in the tubing. The most serious objection to using an aerosol manifold system is that the particle counter must divide its attention between the sample points, rather than monitoring each continuously.

Monitoring each point with an individual sensor allows continuous simultaneous monitoring, but this approach also has limitations. Even with the introduction of lower cost sensors, high cost is still the most frequent objection to this approach. In addition to the initial cost of the sensors, installation and maintenance costs are often significantly higher. Another problem with the multiple sensor approach is obtaining agreement between the sensors. If two or more sensors are used to monitor different points in the same process, the quality of the data will be problem unless the sensors have closely matched calibrations. Yet another limitation of the individual sensor concept is obtaining a sample that is representative of the conditions near the sample inlet point. While the manifold samplers commonly used have a nominal flow rate of 1 CFM per sample point, individual remote sensors most often have a flow rate of 0.1 CFM. This factor of three- to thirty-fold difference in sample collection volume affects the number and spacing of sample points, and therefore is a significant factor in total system cost. Further, the user must carefully evaluate the affect of sample size on the strength of the estimate of particle burden obtained by remote monitoring of 0.1 ft^3 sample volumes. Low counts for this sample volume in clean areas may necessitate counting for 5–10 minutes or more to collect meaningful data. As with any other computer-based system, validation of remote sampling systems will be important. Vendor assistance in this regard should be evaluated before purchase.

It must be kept in mind during the planning and design phases of a remote particle counting system that the counting of environmental particles constitutes only one of the components of environmental monitoring that may be required for compliance with GMP guidelines. Other areas of concern include pressure gradients, directional airflow, air velocities, temperature, humidity, and possibly microbial counts. Some available facilities' monitoring systems offered by vendors of airborne particle counting equipment have the capability for handling data from a wide range of sensors that might be used in monitoring those other parameters as well as storing the different types of data acquired. Thus, a consideration of a total system may be a sensible approach and the use of a central computer based data handling system for all environmental monitoring activities may offer savings both in terms of initial capital outlay and manhours required for operation.

Application of Federal Standard 209-D

The general impression among pharmaceutical manufacturers is that Federal Standard 209-D is poorly suited to application in our industry. This is not surpirising, considering the document's being drafted as a generally applicable standard, not one pertinent to specialized requirements such as those of the pharmaceutical industry. First, there is a concern with the emphasis placed on verification of the count levels in an as-built controlled CEA or clean room. The in-use condition is of overwhelming importance in pharmaceutical manufacture, and monitoring rather than verification is thus of greatest importance. Federal Standard 209-D was written with the aerospace and electronics industries in mind and fails to address properly many issues that are important to pharmaceutical manufacturing (Munson and Sorenson 1990). The document gives class limits for clean areas (Table I) and specifies the minimum sampling volumes for various air classifications (Table II).

Table I. Class Limits in Particles per Cubic Foot

	Measured Particle Size (μm)				
Class	0.1	0.2	0.3	0.5	5.0
100	NA	750	300	100	NA
1,000	NA	NA	NA	1,000	7
10,000	NA	NA	NA	10,000	70
100,000	NA	NA	NA	100,000	700

Table II. Minimum Volume per Sample in Cubic Feet

Class	Measured Particle Size (μm)				
	0.1	0.2	0.3	0.5	5.0
100	NA	0.1	0.1	0.2	NA
1,000	NA	NA	NA	0.1	3.0
10,000	NA	NA	NA	0.1	0.3
100,000	NA	NA	NA	0.1	0.3

The particle size distribution curves shown in 209-D have caused problems for manufacturers. There has been an unfortunate tendency on the part of some users to "pick and choose" to find a size at which an area consistently met the class limits, then count for record at that size (e.g., 0.2 μm, 0.5 μm, or 5.0 μm). This is unacceptable to the FDA, and untenable on the basis of the technical principles involved, since the counts at the different particle sizes specified in FS 209-D cannot be shown to have any definable relationship to a specific environmental particle population (Munson and Sorenson 1991). The FDA aseptic processing guidelines state that "air in the immediate proximity of exposed sterilized containers/closures and filling/closing operations is of acceptable particulate quality when it has a per-cubic-foot particle count of no more than 100 in a size range of 0.5 μm and larger (Class 100) when measured not more than one foot away from the work site during filling/closing operations." Any monitoring plan that measures at particle sizes other than 0.5 μm to circumvent the requirement to supply air as clean as possible to the area where aseptic drug products are assembled will likely be the subject of an adverse inspectional observation.

For Class 100, measuring at 0.5 mm, the minimum volume per samples is 0.2 cubic feet (per Table II). In the FDA view, this sample volume is not adequate to assess aseptic processing facilities. For critical areas, the agency viewpoint is that, based on a minimum of two sampling locations, and on the use of an OPC with a flow rate of 1 CFM, the sampling time should be 5 to 10 minutes at each sampling location, to give a total sample of 10 to 20 cubic feet. This is not, obviously, an absolute criterion, and other valid sample plans may be devised (Whyte 1983). The intent is to collect a large enough sample so that valid assessments may be made based on the small numbers of counts that will be collected and the variability between repeated samples.

The statistical handling of data prescribed in 209-D also causes problems for the pharmaceutical manufacturer (Bzik 1986). Remember that the FDA philosophy and the principles of aseptic fill stress product protection and minimal levels of particles in areas where product is unprotected. The acceptance criteria in FS 209-D requires that the average concentration at each sample point be within the Class limit and that the mean of these averages meet the Class limit with a 95% confidence limit. Varying numbers of samples can be collected at each sampling point, and an area can meet Class 100 although some sample point readings exceed the Class limit.

The obvious defect in this plan, that has also been a problem for microelectronics producers, is that an area can pass even though the individual sample point readings vary widely. For example, consider that three counts at an individual sample point in a Class 100 area are 159, 102, and 9. The average value for this point is 90 counts. This point meets the criteria for being within the Class limit, but contains two out-of-limits values. If the vendor samples at five locations, all showing this same spread of data, the area could still conceivably be within 209-D limits. The extreme spread of values at the sample point is obviously not in keeping with the aseptic fill guidelines and indicates an out-of-control condition. A pharmaceutical manufacturer operating under these conditions would in fact be out of compliance with the regulatory guidelines. The FDA would find this situation unacceptable. This example demonstrates the inadequacy of applying the 95% confidence limits to the count averages at each location. It would be more appropriate to apply these statistics to the readings at each sampling point or to all of the count values obtained to demonstrate that the clean area is, in fact, under control and uniformly meets the appropriate Class limits.

Another problem with the 209-D method of particle count calculation is that an area that is under control and operating within Class limits can fail because of statistical manipulation. Some areas in an aseptic fill room will be much cleaner than others, and this may be entirely in keeping with the principles of product protection. For instance, samples collected in an area just below HEPA filters could be quite clean, with counts of 0 to 10 per cubic foot. Other areas sampled near the filling nozzles might be in the range of 40 to 50 counts. Areas near vials that contact each other on moving conveyor belts may have counts in the 50 to 100 range. Although the averages at these sample points might vary only slightly, the room may still fail based on 209-D criteria when statistical treatment is applied to the sample point average. Ironically, if some critical areas have higher counts, the 209-D statistical test may result in the area passing.

It must be emphasized that the number of sampling locations specified in FS 209-D, one per 25 square feet, or the square root of the Class, whichever is less, is a minimal number. If a fraction remains, the number derived from this calculation must be rounded up. Special equipment/protection in some pharmaceutical controlled environment areas configurations dictate the use of more sample points. For example, although the area under a laminar flow module over a linear fill process may be less than 50 square feet, the length of the module, equipment placement, and multiple points of entry may dictate that more than the minimum two sampling locations should be used in the area. Sampling locations should be indicative of worst case conditions at the point of fill. All values at each sampling location should meet the Class limit and all readings taken must demonstrate consistent control of particulate matter within Class limits. If aseptic filling of powder material precludes sampling in some areas during filling, particle counts in these areas must be rigorously validated under "in-use" conditions with no powder present.

Federal Standard 209-E

This standard will be the successor to Federal Standard 209-D that is currently in force. The final draft of the new document should be issued in late 1992; drafts are currently available from the General Services Administration. The factors that combined to make the earlier standard generally unsuitable for application in the medical products industry (most notably the emphasis on general air cleanliness rather than point-generated or personnel-generated particles that can have severe effects on product quality), are still present. There are a number of changes in the new document that may make it even less suitable than 209-D for application in pharmaceutical manufacture, including:

1. A somewhat confusing presentation of a combined classification based on the metric and English systems;

2. Somewhat more complex statistical considerations involving sample size, number, and location, and reduction of count data;

3. Elimination of the graphical presentation of particle numbers at different sizes within specific cleanliness classes;

4. Introduction of the concepts of optional ultrafine particle measurement and sequential sampling, that are generally not applicable in pharmaceutical manufacture;
5. Failure to include any provision for waiving verification of clean zones and clean rooms based on historical counts and product particle burden, that is, acceptance of class level as demonstrated by monitoring data.
6. Inclusion of a statistical plan directed primarily at decreasing through sampling plans count variability at a given test point rather than eliminating the cause of the variability;
7. Allowance of remote sampling based on tubing transport without adequate discussion of tubing materials and other technical factors;
8. Generally inadequate discussion of implications of counts taken in clean areas under "as built," "at rest," or "operational" conditions;
9. Failure to provide for smaller numbers of sample points in high count areas with non-unidirectional airflow, where air mixing may allow assessment of average counts with less sampling; and
10. Provision for counting at any of a large number of different particle sizes that might encourage a "count until it passes" approach.

Some of the technical information included in 209-E is useful in terms of providing general background regarding airborne counting (e.g., isokinetic sampling). Still, it is difficult to determine any way that the new standard represents an improvement over the old for those responsible for airborne monitoring in pharmaceutical environments. Part of the reason for the generation of the new standard would appear to be a perceived urgency on the part of the Institute of Environmental Sciences regarding the generation of standards for international use: "If we don't generate a new standard, ISO will." Indeed, a standard generated by an international agency such as ISO would be more problematical than 209-E. The new standard may be a necessity in terms of the world evolution into a common economy and marketplace. To remain competitive the U.S. must participate in the generation of internationally acceptable standards and practices. The use of standards as trade barriers is not new, and the consequences of a lack of U.S. standards in specific areas may be more serious in the future (Fitch 1992).

The presentation of class limits is made in Table 1 of 209-E. This is reproduced as Table III. While it is stated that classes as specified in 209-D remain acceptable, confusion results from the use of the two systems results, and the implicit principle of a change to different measurement units suggests complex issues to be dealt with in the future.

One of the most problematical components of 209-D, the separation of criteria for monitoring and verification activities, remains in 209-E. Verification is intended to ensure that the clean room functions as intended with regard to the assigned classification. Importantly, the number of sample sites specified for verification activities does not apply to monitoring. The regression for monitoring, or on-going testing (to ensure that the environment remains within class limits) simply specifies that a monitoring plan must be in place that is based both on the degree of cleanliness control necessary for product protection within the room(s) in question, and the airborne particulate matter cleanliness class. The monitoring requirement allows manufacturers of medical products considerable latitude in establishing monitoring plans as long as the following are specified:

- Frequency of testing;
- Operational conditions during which testing is performed;
- Method of counting;
- Sample location;
- Sample number;
- Sample volume; and
- Method of data interpretation.

The new standard allows both microscopic and instrumental counting to be performed for particles ≥5 µm in size, but results from the two methods cannot be combined.

A word of caution is in order regarding the size of particles to be counted for classification purposes. The data in Table III indicate that, dependant upon classification of the area considered, particles from 0.1 mm to 5.0 mm in size are specified for all cleanliness classes if sampling times are to be kept within reason (except in the case of low classification area where counts at the smaller sizes provide a distinct statistical advantage). Counts at the 5.0 µm size should generally be avoided, due to the low numbers of particles encountered and the unfavorable sampling dynamics for

Table III. Airborne Particulate Cleanliness Classes (FS-209E)

(Class limits in particles (p) per unit volume (μm^3 or ft^3) of size equal to or greater than particle sizes (μm) shown.*)

Class**		0.1 μm		0.2 μm		0.3 μm		0.5 μm		5 μm	
SI	Former FS 209-D	(p/m³)	(p/ft³)	(p/m³)	(p/ft³)	(p/m³)	(p/ft³)	(p/m³)	(p/ft³)	(p/m³)	(p/ft³)
M 1		350	9.91	75.7	2.14	30.9	0.875	10.0	0.283	—	—
M 1.5	1	1240	35.0	265	7.50	106	300	35.3	1.00	—	—
M 2		3500	99.1	757	21.4	309	8.75	100	2.83	—	—
M 2.5	10	12400	350	2650	75.0	1060	30.0	353	10.0	—	—
M 3		35000	991	7570	214	3090	87.5	1000	28.3	—	—
M 3.5	100	—	—	26500	750	10600	300	3530	100	—	—
M 4		—	—	75700	2140	30900	875	10000	283	—	—
M 4.5	1000	—	—	—	—	—	—	35300	1000	247	7.00
M 5		—	—	—	—	—	—	100000	2830	618	17.5
M 5.5	10000	—	—	—	—	—	—	353000	10000	2470	70.0
M 6		—	—	—	—	—	—	1000000	28300	6180	175
M 6.5	100000	—	—	—	—	—	—	3530000	100000	24700	700
M 7		—	—	—	—	—	—	10000000	283000	61800	1750

*The class limit particle concentrations shown are defined for class purposes only, and do not necessarily represent the size distribution to be found in any particular situation.
**In naming and describing the Classes, SI names and units are preferred, but the units formerly used in earlier editions of FS 209-D are also acceptable.

particles of the size with OPC. Microscopic testing should be avoided except where absolutely necessary, such as in areas where water vapor or similar interferences exist. If counting at 5 µm is resorted to by either microscopic or instrumental measures, the reason for the variance in technique should be documented. Any indication that a monitoring plan allows for a "count until it passes" or a sliding scale with regard to the size chosen for counting can be expected to raise a flag for a regulatory investigator—and rightly so.

The discussion of interpretation of counts in aseptic fill areas in the preceding sections on 209-D also pertain with regard to 209-E. The critical consideration in aseptic filling is the maintenance of cleanliness at vertical process points rather than in the room environment away from the process. Further, single counts at a sample point that exceed the class limit must be considered to indicate inappropriate conditions even if the average count at a sample point is within limits. A useful consideration of sampling statistics for low classification areas is provided in the paper by Cooper (1990). Interestingly, 209-E allows areas in CEA's that have lower particle limits that the general room environment.

Isokinetic Sampling

The new standard contains some considerable discussion of isokinetic and anisokinetic sampling (see Hinds 1982). Briefly, the principle of interest here is that sampling velocity and flow rate of the air being sampled in directional airflow must be matched if the best precision of particle counts is to be attained. The effects of isokinetic and anisokinetic sampling probe velocities are shown in Figure 12. Importantly, the drawing of Figure 12 assumes that flow is isoaxial, that is, the probe faces directly into the air stream sampled.

Generally, if the sample probe velocity is subisokinetic, some of the smaller particles approaching the sample probe opening will be entrained in the streamlines passing around the probe and avoid the nozzle so that an error due to disproportionately elevated counts of larger particles (3 µm to 5 µm) will result. If velocity through the probe is greater than that of the air approaching the probe, small particles will be drawn into the nozzle opening from streamlines beyond the probe opening diameter. This results in count errors of the type shown in Figure 13, whereby the proportional presence of large particles is decreased. In the opposite case, if the probe velocity is lower than ambient, relative numbers of

220 *Pharmaceutical Particulate Matter*

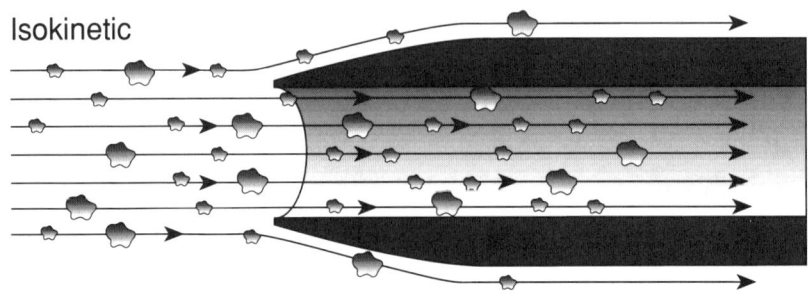

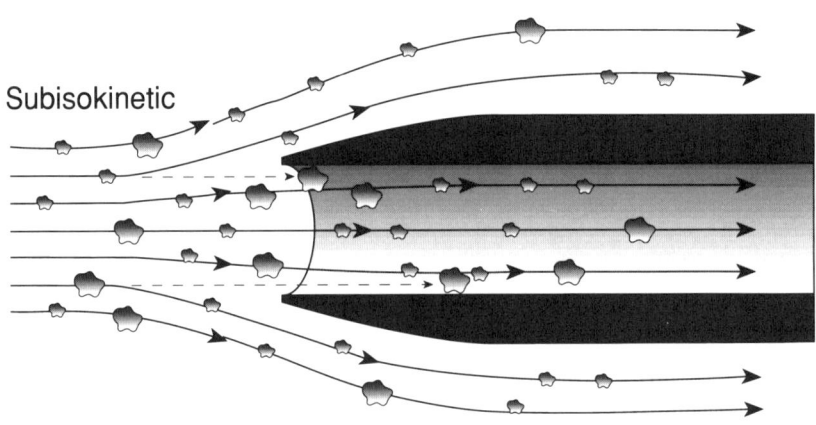

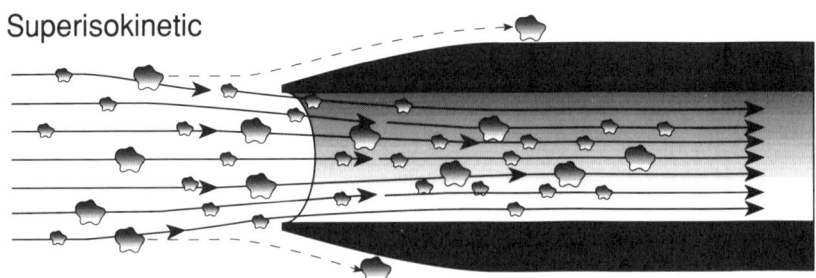

Figure 12. Flow lines at probe nozzle for various relative stock and probe velocities.

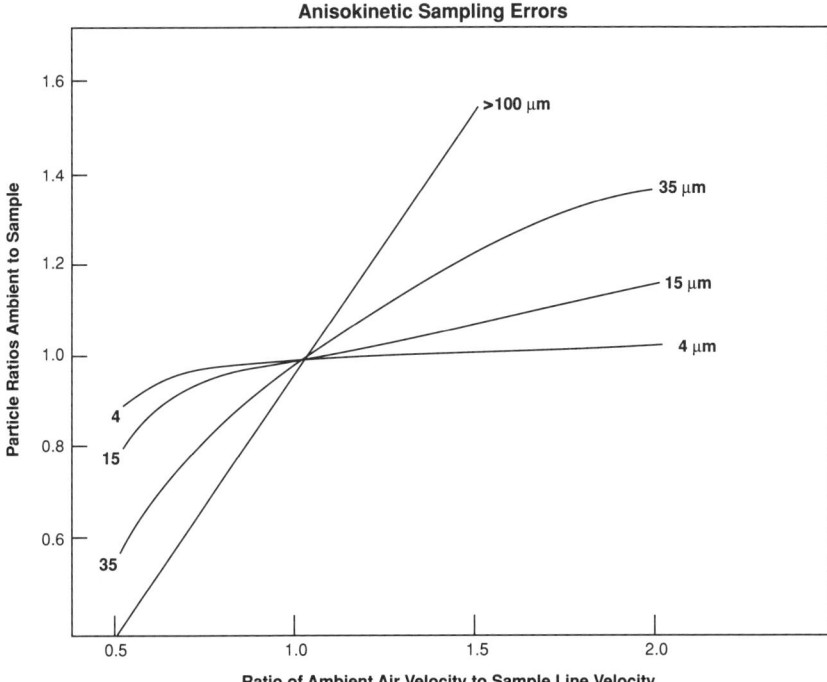

Figure 13. Ratio of ambient air velocity to sample line velocity.

---

large particles are increased. The detrimental effects of nonisokinetic sampling pertain primarily to particle counts at larger sizes (≥3 μm). Probe velocity can vary significantly (20% to 40%) from that of the ambient air flow without causing any appreciable error for particles of 0.5 μm and less.

Obviously, a requirement for isokinetic sampling might lead to very complex manipulations if probe velocity had to be matched to the velocity of the air being sampled in all situations. A simplified widely-used sampling technique usually suffices to give suitably accurate results. The velocity of unidirectional airflow that is most often sampled is the 90 ft/minute ±20% that is delivered by HEPA filters. All manufacturers of OPCs market "isokinetic" probes that serve to match up the 1 ft^3/minute airflow of a counter with the velocity of HEPA airflow. These are typically conical probes of 25 mm to 30 mm in diameter that serve to collect a volume of air from the HEPA airflow that is equivalent to the counter sample flow rate, and smoothly accelerate particles of all sizes into the sample tube. It is interesting to consider in the light of this discussion, that when OPCs are used to sample ambient air, probe flow patterns are always superisokinetic.

The situation shown in Figure 14 is pertinent with regard to sampling of turbulent air (Lieberman 1992). In the figure, S_t is the

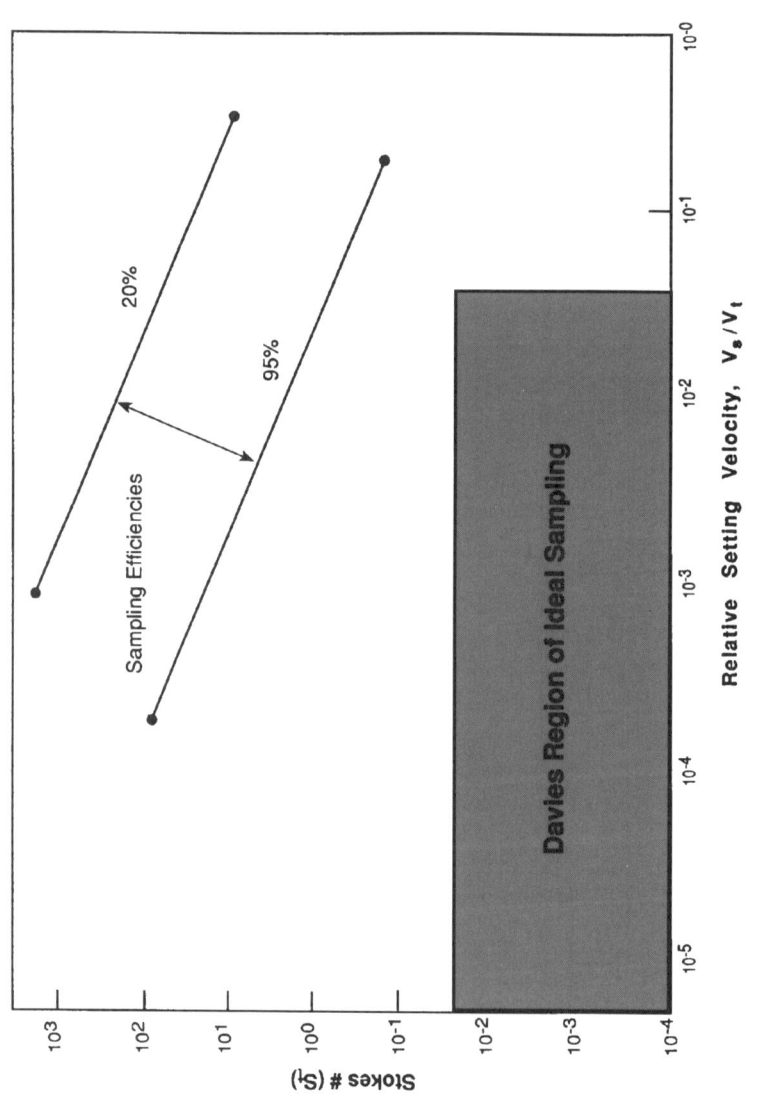

Figure 14. Sampling efficiency curves for various combinations of S_t and V_S/V_τ.

Stokes number. The Stokes number is the product of the particle relaxation time (time for a particle to respond to a change in air velocity and/or direction), and the particle velocity divided by the diameter of the sample tube inlet, or

$$S_t = \frac{\tau w}{R}$$

where   t = particle relaxation time
                w = free stream gas velocity
                R = radius of probe

If the relative settling velocity of a particle (V_s/V_τ, where V_s is the particle setting velocity and V_τ is the inlet sample tube velocity) is plotted against the Stokes number, a family of sampling efficiency curves can be developed for particles with specific characteristics (Stokes number). Generally, as probe radius increases and particle relaxation time and velocity decrease, sampling efficiency increases such that representative sampling can be carrried out over a wide range of V_s/V_τ ratios. As described by Davies (1964), a zone of "perfect" sampling exists for V_s/V_τ ratios of 10^{-5} to 0.004 and S_t numbers of 10^{-4} to 0.032.

Sampling of Compressed Gases

Isokinetic sampling is also highly desirable if compressed air or other gases are to be sampled from a line. The historical methodology used, with an in-line pressure reducer, is less than ideal (Figure 15). In this situation, the sampling effectiveness (E) is defined as the percentage of the true count for a particle of a given size that is displayed by the counter. (For this exercise, counter efficiency is assumed to be 100%.)

In Figure 15, the pressure reducer is of simple design, serving only for reduction of the line pressure to ambient, so that the pump of the counter can collect an unpressurized sample. This general design incorporates a number of undesirable features including tubing bends, a butterfly valve, and large diameter supply tubing that allows an excessive volume of compressed gas to enter the chamber with resultant turbulent impaction, and loss of particles. Valves in line between the gas stream to be sampled can both generate and trap particles, and are especially problematical. Obviously, with this type of sampling, it is essential that the sample tubing, valve, and expansion chamber are purged before counts are recorded. Adequate purging is indicated by low variability between successive

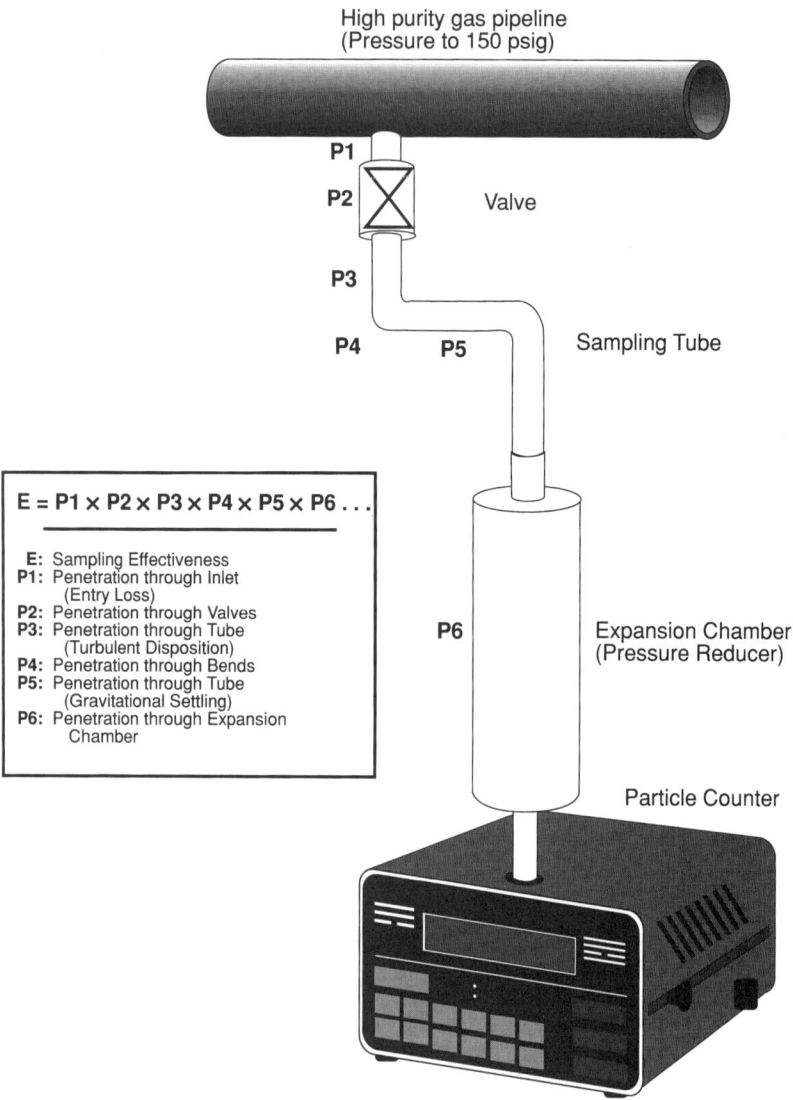

Figure 15. Sampling of compressed gas line.

counts. The potential for particle generation or entrapment in this type of sampling outweighs the effects of anisokenetic sampling. Care must also be taken that ambient air is not drawn into the exhaust ports of the pressure reducer at low sample flow rates.

More refined pressure reducers incorporate a sonic flow restriction (critical orifice) at the orifice plate or a capillary orifice (Figure 16). The orifice-type pressure reducer makes use of a thin orifice plate to reduce the pressure while the capillary-type reducer makes use of a capillary tube. The evaluation by Rubow et al. (1990) showed that the orifice-type reducer gives much lower background counts than the capillary-type reducer, due to the much smaller surface area that the high purity gas comes into contact during expansion through the devices. Particles are sampled by a sample extraction tube located at the axis of the chamber, with the excess gas flow exiting through a 90 bend or through lateral buffer or holes. The pressure reducer typically reduces the absolute pressure

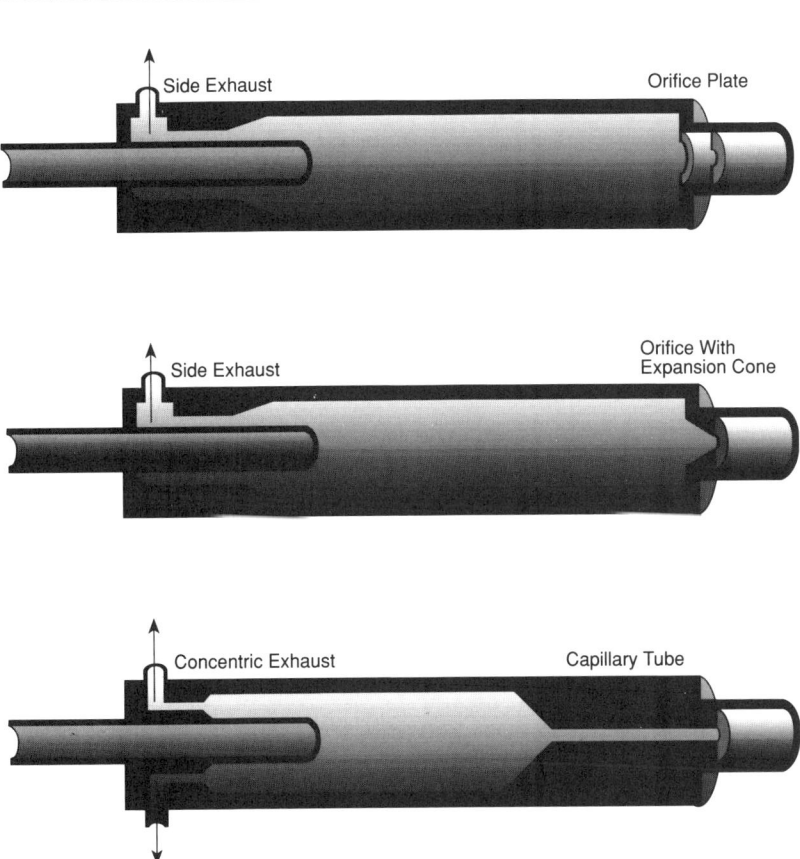

Figure 16. Design concept of pressure reducers for isokinetic sampling.

from above 100 psi in the high purity gas line to an ambient pressure of 14.7 psi. The pressure ratio exceeds the critical ratio and a sonic flow is therefore formed at the orifice.

The efficiency of penetration through all of these reducers is very good for particles up to 20 µm in size. Since the 0.5 µm particle size is of primary concern, these general types of pressure reducers are entirely adequate for pharmaceutical compressed gas sampling.

One caution in the use of pressure reducers for compressed air or gas sampling regards adiabatic cooling and the condensation of moisture from the air to form water droplets. This condition should be suspected when flow of air into the pressure reducer at full line pressure of 80 psi to 105 psi results in counts that are tenfold or more higher than those observed when the pressure in the reducer is decreased by one half or one third. Care must also be taken to keep reducers clean, given the low count limits generally placed on compressed gas.

Tubing Transport of Particulate Matter Samples

The use of tubing to transport samples to OPC from remote sample sites has historically raised concerns regarding particle loss and/or segregation. Federal Standard 209-E indicates that both the probe and transit tube should be configured so that the Reynolds number is between 5000 and 25,000. For particles in the range of 0.1 µm to 1 µm and for a flow rate of 0.028 m^3/min (1.0 ft^3/min), a transit tube of up to 30 m long may be used per the standard; for particles in the range of 2 µm to 10 µm, the transit tube should be no longer than 3 m. Under these conditions, losses of small particles by diffusion and of large particles by sedimentation and impaction are predicted to be no more than 5% during transit through the tube. This transport efficiency is entirely adequate for the great majority of situations that will be encountered in airborne particle monitoring in pharmaceutical production.

The Reynolds number is a dimensionless descriptor of flow characteristics in tubing, piping, or flow channels. It is calculated for airflow in tubing as:

$$R = \frac{VDp}{u}$$

where V is the tubing airflow velocity, D is the diameter, p is the density of air, and u is the viscosity of air. Representative values of R for different flow rates and tubing diameters are shown in

Table IV. Generally, Reynolds numbers in excess of 2000 are deemed sufficient to produce turbulent flow characteristics in the flow channel.

Table IV. Reynolds Numbers for Various Sampling Conditions (Courtesy of Climet Instruments, Inc.)

Flow Rate (CFM))	Tube ID (inches)	Tube Length	Velocity (ft/sec) (feet)	Residence Time* (seconds)	Reynolds Number
0.1	0.125	25	19.56	1.28	1274.88
0.25	0.125	25	48.49	0.51	3187.20
1	0.125	25	195.57	0.13	12748.78
0.1	0.25	25	4.89	5.11	637.44
0.25	0.25	25	12.22	2.05	1593.60
1	0.25	25	48.89	0.51	6374.39
0.1	0.375	25	2.17	11.50	424.96
0.25	0.375	25	5.43	4.60	1062.40
1	0.375	25	21.73	1.15	4249.59
0.1	0.125	50	19.56	2.56	1274.88
0.25	0.125	50	48.89	1.02	3187.20
1	0.125	50	195.57	0.26	12748.78
0.1	0.25	50	4.89	10.23	637.44
0.25	0.25	50	12.22	4.09	1593.60
1	0.25	50	48.89	1.02	6374.39
0.1	0.375	50	2.17	23.01	424.96
0.25	0.375	50	5.43	9.20	1062.40
1	0.375	50	21.73	2.30	4249.59
0.1	0.125	100	19.66	5.11	1274.88
0.25	0.125	100	48.89	2.05	3187.20
1	0.125	100	195.57	0.51	12748.78
0.1	0.25	100	4.89	20.45	637.44
0.25	0.25	100	12.22	8.18	1593.60
1	0.25	100	48.89	2.05	6374.39
0.1	0.375	100	2.17	46.02	424.96
0.25	0.375	100	5.43	18.41	1062.40
1	0.375	100	21.75	4.60	4249.59

*FS-209D specifies a residence time of 5 seconds or less; this requirement has been deleted in FS-209E.

Two factors (static charge attraction and inertial impaction) are responsible for most particle loss in transport tubing (Liu et al. 1985). As suggested by FS-209E, losses in 150 feet of 3/8" flexible tubing, at 1.0 CFM air flow rate have been empirically shown to be 4.2% at 0.5 µm and much greater (25%) in the 3.0 µm to 5.0 µm range (Zweers 1983). Tubing losses generally remain constant throughout the working life of the tubing, however, and do not vary nearly as widely as do OPC electronic sensor outputs over time. Particle losses at 5.0 µm in tubing are large but the measurement error is not significant considered in the light of the poor statistical validity of the few 5.0 µm particles present in the usual one minute/one cubic foot sample. Particle problems are almost invariably indicated by generation of 0.5 µm or smaller particles.

Static losses in tubing are a function of tubing diameters, flow rates within the tube, tube materials, as well as particle size. Minimum particle losses are sustained in a tube when turbulent flow exists. A Reynolds number in excess of 2000 will assure turbulent flow and minimize static particle loss. Laminar flow, resulting in increased static losses, will occur in 1/2" diameter tubing at 1.0 CFM air flow; lower air flows (e.g., 0.25 CFM) result in even lower Reynolds numbers for equivalent diameter tubing, leading to more severe losses of particles 0.5 µm to 5.0 µm in size.

Flow rate variation may occur because of differing pressure drops in different lengths of tubing. By minimizing variation in tubing length, the facility planner can effectively minimize differences in pressure drop and sample volume. This effect is generally not significant. For instance, between a five foot length of 1/4" tubing and a fifty foot length of 5/16" diameter, the pressure differential is less than 0.5 psi. The resultant air flow will be of the order of 1–2% at 1.0 CFM. Again, such variances in air flow are generally not significant when related to normal variances between individual electronic OPC sensors that are often 10% or greater.

Another parameter of interest to the facility planner is the particle residence time in tubing (see Table IV). Alternatively, a sample tube volume calculation can be quickly calculated for any tube/diameter combination. For example, calculations at 1.0 CFM air flow on a 100 foot length of 3/8" diameter tubing show the tube to be completely cleared in less than 5 seconds. Manifold systems should, therefore, include a short delay time (5 seconds as a minimum in the preceding example) to purge the tube of the prior sample. Commonly, 2–3 volumes are purged to assure a representative sample.

The designer of a remote sampling system will also need to consider the physical aspects of the tubes to include materials, installation attitude, Port placement, bend radius, and cost. Table V lists commonly used materials in ascending order of relative particle loss (i.e., stainless steel minimum losses, aluminum maximum losses). One cost-effective, efficient, and easy to install material is polyester; conductive carbon-impregnated EVA tubing lined with polyethylene is also available. Suppliers of this type of flexible tubing include DuPont Chemical (Wilmington, DE 19880) and Thermoplastic Scientifics, Inc. (Warren, NJ 07060) under the tradename Bev-A-Line®. Stainless steel, at about ten times the cost per foot of polymer tubing (not including installation) will reduce losses at 0.5 µm by only a fraction of a percent. However, it may be the material of choice in clean room situations utilizing steam sterilization techniques. Flexible tubing, of course, allows the planner more latitude to reposition the tubes to meet changing manufacturing needs. The user of PVC tubing should keep in mind that heating of this tubing can result in the escape of plasticizer vapor that will impact particle count data at the 0.5 µm size.

Table V. Tube Material Selection

Stainless Steel
Conductive Plastic
Polyester
Polyurethane
Polyethylene
Copper
Glass
Nylon
Tygon (PVC)
Aluminum

Large Particle Monitoring

The rate at which large particles (10 µm–100 µm) settle onto surfaces in a process area may also be measured using electronic particle counters. Because the numbers of particles in this size range are far lower than total numbers of airborne particles ≥0.5 µm, the statistical strength of the data collected will be decreased. Results obtained in different portions of a process area or for samples taken at different times of a day may also be expected to show higher variation (Borden et al. 1989). One such device is the Model 11A fallout sensor marketed presently by Hiac/Royco. This device is shown in Figure 17. It consists of a laser particle detector mounted below a stagnation column. The stagnation column (sampling tube), which is simply a cylindrical tube 2" high and 1" in diameter, sorts settling particles from the particles drifting with air flow. The settling particles are then counted with a laser light scattering detector. The column and bottom cover create a dead air space around the detector, which is located in the sensor body. The entire sensor fits on a mounting base with dimensions of only 5" × 3".

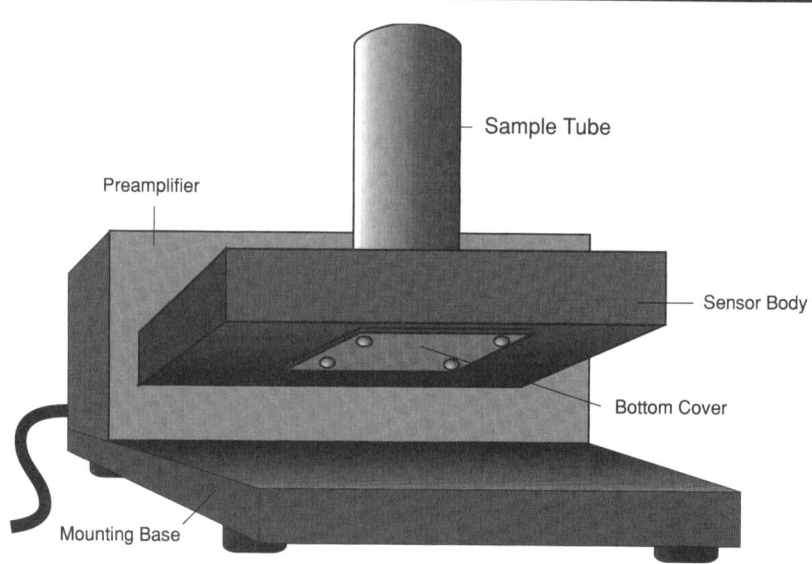

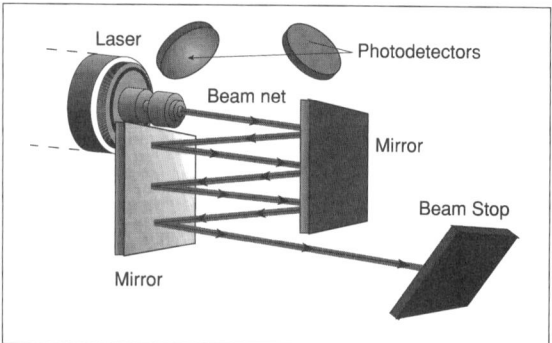

Figure 17. Electronic real-time fallout monitor (Hiac/Royco).

Figure 17 also shows the optical configuration of the sensor mounted under the stagnation column. It is similar to particle detectors used in vacuum process equipment for the microelectronics industry, but it is detuned to reduce its sensitivity to particles smaller than about 10 microns in diameter. It consists of a laser diode source and lenses that project a 30 mW laser beam at a 780 nm wavelength back and forth between two mirrors. This creates a "net" of light under the stagnation column. Particles settling through the beam scatter light onto twin photocells mounted above the mirrors. This creates electrical signals that are amplified in a preamplifier and then sent to a control unit up to 100' away for processing. I should observe that use of this type of device in place of witness plates should be preceeded by an assessment of counting efficiency.

Personnel Monitoring

Personnel are the largest single source of particles in a clean room. Most of the particles shed by people are skin cells, that have been identified as a source of bacterial contamination and fibers. There is an extremely high level of sensitivity to human contamination in our industry and within regulatory agencies. The viable and nonviable particles that are shed from people has been described as "human dust" that is continually being shed by personnel at a rate of 10^5–10^7 cells/day. The skin cells that make up most of this "dust" transport microbes that are present in significant numbers on the human body. No monitoring program for aseptic fill areas is complete unless there are provisions for personnel testing (Dixon 1990). This monitoring provides information both on the effectiveness of gowning procedures and employee aseptic practices.

Monitoring should be performed monthly or at more frequent intervals on workers in an aseptic fill area; as with the clean room itself, action and alert limits should be established. Each area of overgarments worn should have different limits based on proximity to the critical area during filling manufacturing. Gloves must have the lowest limits, while boots have the highest limits. Although the ultimate goal of personal protection is to have zero counts, action and alert limits must be set at realistic levels; the goal is simply to keep contamination at a minimum and under control. If results for an individual exceed limits or if a trend is indicated, the person may be counseled or required to take a review course in gowning and aseptic practices. Importantly, personnel testing data can sometimes be correlated with the failure rate of media fills performed to validate aseptic fill processes.

The pharmaceutical industry (like the microelectronics industry) uses overgarments specifically designed for clean rooms to protect the aseptic environment from the viable and nonviable particles shed by personnel. The use of overgarments equates to enclosing the worker in filter medium to "filter out" the particles that they generate. These must be designed to cover the entire body from head to toe, including the face and eyes ("bunny suit" design). Any exposed area of skin will generate particles. The head covering, gloves, and boots should be sealed to the coverall in such a way as to prevent the spread of particles by compression and expansion of the overgarment as the person moves about. The face should be completely covered, since viable particles can be shed from the face, or the worker inadvertently touching the face with the sterile gloves. The protection offered by protective garb is only as good as gowning techniques and aseptic procedures practiced by the personnel. Garments may be made of tightly woven polyester, Tyvek® or (more recently) Gore-Tex®, Fluropore®, and TF®. Tyvek® garments are available in both disposable and reusable types and feature extremely good control of particles shed by a worker, but are not "breathable" and are thus somewhat less comfortable to wear than garments of other materials.

Summary

Implicit in the foregoing discussion is the premise that HEPA control of the environmental air particulate matter burden and monitoring of airborne particle counts ≥0.5 µm are key elements in the manufacture of pharmaceutical products. Such is indeed the case. It must be kept in mind that neither of these measures have any significant effect on either large particles that occur randomly in the process environment and are not effectively controlled by HEPA filtration, on processes- or human-generated particles that occur in intimate proximity to the product, or on particles adherent to containers as received.

The forces that adhere particles to surfaces are a significant issue when particles up to 50 µm are considered, and the velocity of HEPA airflow is insufficient to remove particles once they have adhered to a container or device. Large particles are not effectively entrained by HEPA airflow and are difficult to remove from surfaces. Airborne particulate matter monitoring is ineffectual in enumerating particles of larger size that occur randomly or may be generated by container or product contact with humans or machines. Airborne particle counting is a statistical process and counts obtained are meaningful only when particles that occur in significant numbers are considered. The next chapter of this book deals with control and enumeration of process-generated particles occurring at point sources and particles related to the product itself.

References

Bemer, D., J. F. Favries, and A. Renoux. 1990. Calculation of the theoretical response of an optical counter and its practical usefulness. *J. Aerosol Sci.* 21 (5):689–700.

Borden, P., J. Munson, D. Bartelson, and M. McClellan. 1989. Real time monitoring of large particle fallout for aerospace applications. In *Proc. Ann. Meeting Inst. Env. Sci.,* 394–396.

British Standard BS5295. 1989. Environmental cleanliness in enclosed spaces. Part 1. Specification for clean rooms and clean air devices. London: British Standards Institution.

Buettner, H. 1990. Measurement of the size of fine nonspherical particles with a light-scattering particle counter. *Aerosol Sci. Tech.* 12 (2):413–421.

Bzik, T. J. 1986. Statistical management and analysis of particle count data in ultraclean environments, Part I. *Microcontamination* (May):89–90.

Caldow, R., and J. Blesner. 1989. A procedure to verify the lower counting limit of optical particle counters. *J. Parenteral Sci. and Technol.* 43 (July/August):174–179.

Cooper, D. 1990. Particle statistics for contamination control: An introduction. In *Proc. PDA Int. Conf. on Particle Detection, Metrology and Control,* 183–208. Washington, D.C.

Cooper, D. W., and S. J. Grotzinger. 1989. Comparing particle counters: cost vs. reproducibility. *J. Environmental Sci.* 35 (5): 32–34.

Cooper, D. W., R. J. Miller, and J. J. Wu. 1991a. Comparing three condensation nucleus counters and optical particle counter in the measurement of small particles. *Microcontamination* 9 (4):19–26.

Cooper, D. W., R. J. Miller, and J. J. Wu. 1991b. Measurements with condensation nucleus counters and an optical particle counter in a cleanroom. *J. IES.* (July/August):702–711.

Davies, C. N. 1964. The aspiration of heavy airborne particles into a point sink. *Royal Society London Proc. (Series A)* 279:413–428.

Dixon, A. M. 1990. Human contamination issues in cleanroom manufacturing. In *Proc. PDA Int. Conf. on Particle Detection, Metrology and Control,* 65–81. Washington, D.C.

Federal standards for clean room and work station requirements, controlled environment. 1989. *Fed. Standard* 209–D.

Fitch, H. D. 1992. Federal Standard 209-E: Its evolution and role. *Clean Rooms* 6 (September):92.

Flanders Technical Bulletin No. 581D. 1989. *HEPA Filters and Filter Testing,* 3rd Ed. Washington, D.C.: Flanders Filters Inc.

Food and Drug Aministration. 1987. *Guideline on sterile drug products produced by aseptic processing.* Rockville, MD: Food and Drug Administration.

Greiner, J. 1990. HEPA filter leak testing using the particle counter scan method. *Clean Rooms* 4 (9):36–39.

Hinds, W. C. 1982. *Aerosol Technology.* New York, Wiley, p. 289.

Horvath, H., R. L. Bunter, and S. W. Wilkison. 1990. Determination of the coarse mode of the atmospheric aerosol using data from a forward scattering spectrometer probe. *AS&T* 12 (4):964–980.

Hovenac, E. A. 1990. Scattering from non–spherical particles. In *Proc. 2nd Int. Congr. Optical Particle Sizing,* 108–117. Tempe, AZ.

IES Recommended Practice IES RP–CC-001-86 HEPA Filters. 1986. Mt. Prospect, IL: Institute of Env. Sci.

IES Recommended Practice IES RP–CC006-84T. 1984. Mt. Prospect, IL: Institute of Env. Sci.

Keady, P. B., P. A. Nelson, and J. Blesner. 1990. State-of-the-art in sensor technology for multipoint monitoring. *ICCCS* 90:32–35.

Knollenberg, R. J. 1970. The optical array: An alternative to scattering or extinction for airborne particle size determination. *J. Appl. Meteorology* 9:86–103.

Knollenberg, R. G. 1989. The measurement of latex particle sizes using scattering ratios in the Rayleigh scattering size range. *J. Aerosol Sci.* 20 (3):331–345.

Lieberman, A. 1992. Personal communication.

Lieberman, A. 1988. A new 0.05 m 0.1 CFM optical particle counter. In *Proc. 20th DOE/NRC Nuclear Air Cleaning Conf.,* 1137–1143. Boston.

Lieberman, A. 1979a. Free air monitoring of non-viable aerosol particles, Part I. *Pharm. Technol.* (February):71–77.

Lieberman, A. 1979b. Free air monitoring of non-viable aerosol particles, Part II. *Pharm. Technol.* (March):61–66.

Liu, B. Y. H., and W. W. Szymanski. 1987. Counting efficiency, lower detection limit and noise level of optical particle counters. In *Proceedings Meeting of Inst. of Env. Sci.* 417–421. Mount Prospect, IL: Inst. Env. Sci.

Liu, B. Y. H., W. W. Szymanski, and K. O. Ahn. 1985. On aerosol size distribution measurement by laser and white light optical particle counters. *J. Environ. Sci.* (May/June):19–24.

Montague, W., and H. Sommer. 1990. Reliability and count accuracy of optical counters. *IES* (May/June):131–139.

Montague, W. and H. T. Sommer. 1989. Performance parameters of optical aerosol particle counters. *Filt. News* (Nov/Dec):26–30.

Munson, T. E., and R. L. Sorenson. 1990. Environmental monitoring: Regulatory issues. In *Sterile Pharmaceutical Manufacturing: Applications for the 1990s,* 163–184. M. J. Groves, W. P. Olson, and M. H. Anisfeld, Eds. Buffalo Grove, IL.: Interpharm Press.

Rubow, K. L., J. Lee, D. Y. H. Pui, and B. Y. H. Liu. 1990. Performance evaluation and comparative study of pressure reducers for aerosol sampling from high purity gases. *Proceeding of 10th International Symposium on Contamination Control* (September).

Sommer, H. T. 1989. Resolution, sensitivity, counting efficiency and coincidence limit of optical aerosol particle counters. In *Proc. Fine Particle Soc. Conf.* (Aug 21–25, Boston) (per Hiac/Royco, Silver Springs, MA).

Sommer, H. T. 1990. Optical sizing of single particles (Hiac/Royco laser). In *Proc. 2nd Int. Congr. Optical Particle Sizing,* 612–618. Tempe, AZ (per HIAC, Silver Springs, MA).

Sommer, H. T., and C. F. Harrison. 1991. Aerosol size concentration measurements from scattered light signals. In *Proc. Conf. Sensor '91,* 14–16 May, Nurnberg, Germany (per Hiac/Royco, Silver Springs, MA).

Sommer, H. T., and C. E. Montague. 1990. Design and performance of optical aerosol particle counters with different light sources. In *Proc. 3rd Chinese Aerosol Conf.,* 28 September 28, Beijing, China (per Hiac/Royco, Silver Springs, MA).

Standard practice for determining counting and sizing accuracy of an airborne particle counter using near-monodisperse spherical particulate materials. 1989. *ASTM Standard Practice F328-80.*

Standard practice for secondary calibration of airborne particle counters using comparison procedures. *ASTM Standard Practice F649–80.* Available from American Society for Testing and Materials, 1916 Race St., Philadelphia, PA 19103.

Szymanski, W. W., and P. E. Wagner. 1990. Absolute aerosol number concentration measurement by simultaneous observation of extinction and scattered light. *J. Aerosol Sci.* 21 (3):441–451.

Technical Bulletin No. 581D. *HEPA Filters and Filter Testing,* 3rd Ed. Washington, D.C.: Flanders Filters, Inc.

Umhauer, H., and M. Bottlinger. 1990. The effect of particle shape and structure on the results of single particle light scattering analysis. In *Proc. 2nd Int. Congr. Optical Particle Sizing,* 425–434. Tempe, AZ.

Wen, H. Y., and G. Kasper. 1986. Counting efficiencies of six commercial particle counters. *J. Aerosol Sci.* 187 (6):947–961.

Whyte, W. 1983. A multicentered investigation of cleanroom requirements for terminally sterilized pharmaceuticals. *J. Parent. Sci. Technol.* 37 (4):184–197.

Zweers, J. R. 1985. Personal communication.

VII

Process- and Product-Related Particles

Particulate matter burden, sterility, and pyrogens are the three most critical factors in production of injectable products. This chapter is directed at the elimination of particles from parenteral dosage forms. The intent of this chapter is not to provide a comprehensive listing of sources of particulate matter in parenterals. Rather, I have attempted to provide examples of sources of particulate matter and outline general approaches for troubleshooting and particle source elimination that will serve as a starting point in these endeavors. The book by Akers (1985) is a valuable reference in this regard and provides a very useful discussion of particulate matter in relation to overall product quality. Other key references include Aldrich (1985), Borchert et al. (1986), Ernerot (1985), McCollum et al. (1984), Sharp (1985), and Backhouse et al. (1987).

The monitoring and control of environmental particles, discussed in the preceding chapter, constitutes only one component of the control of particles that may enter and contaminate parenteral products. The total particulate matter burden of a product is determined, in fact, by the contribution of particles from five sources.

1. The environment,
2. Packaging materials,

3. Solution and formulation components,
4. Product-package interactions, and
5. Process point-generated particulates.

Items (2)–(5) on this list are typically categorized as nonenvironmental particle sources and their control and their elimination frequently is more important than control of environmental particulates. The control of particles from these sources typically requires more diverse control measures than does the control of dispersed environmental (airborne) particulates, and an uncontrolled situation with regard to these particles typically will have a more serious effect on product quality than particles from the general environment.

Within the four general categories of nonenvironmental particles listed above, the following sources of particles have historically been of significant concern:

- Human activity,
- Container and closure-related contaminants,
- Filling operations,
- Particles arising at specific process points,
- Degradation of drug materials,
- Product-closure interaction, and
- Extraction of materials from containers.

In a general sense, all particles that occur in injectables will come from one of two sources. The majority of such particles, certainly with regard to distinct types, typically originates from extraneous sources. Extraneous sources include container components, various process points, filling machinery, and human contact—to name a few. Lower numbers of particles generally originate from the formulation itself, but precipitates, degradants, or particles related to a detrimental interaction of the formulation with its container may result in very high numbers of particles in isolated instances. In the following discussion, I will use the two categories (extraneous and formulation or product-related) as a basis for my discussion rather than "intrinsic" and other terms that are adequately descriptive, but may be somewhat confusing in different contexts.

Extraneous particulate material may enter the final product as the result of insufficient cleaning or product assembly issues such as particle generation by a filler. Formation of particles in the product is a much more complex phenomenon, and can involve degradation, aggregation, agglomeration, precipitation, crystallization, and/or sedimentation reactions. Personnel activity and equipment design and maintenance are critical factors, since point-generated particles arise from these sources. Ideally, nonenvironmental particulates are eliminated by process design rather than process troubleshooting. Process design incorporates not only the consideration of process machinery, environmental cleanliness, and filtration, but of container and closure cleanliness as well. Currently available process technology for both small volume injection (SVI) and large volume injection (LVI) product incorporates the potential for significant reduction of product nonviable particle burden.

Process design with regard to elimination of particles must begin when a facility is on the drawing board so that exclusion of particulate matter from the product can be built into the manufacturing line. As we all know, this opportunity is not often presented in the real world. Too often we are faced with the problem of reducing particulate matter levels inherent in an "old" process that started running a decade or more ago when higher levels of process-related particulate matter were acceptable. Often progress in process design–based particulate matter control must be made stepwise, as new lines or facilities that will use an existing process are built, or as process lines are upgraded.

Particles reflect the quality of product including both design and execution. Particles may occur in parenterals because they gain access during assembly, or they may form during product shelf life. To minimize access of extraneous particles to product particle, controlled assembly procedures with high quality packaging components is essential. Control of particle formation is often more complex than control of extraneous particles from the process or environment, involving both raw material and rigorous formulation compatibility/stability testing. On occasion, particles are readily identified; in other cases, a comprehensive multidisciplinary approach is required. This approach must include an understanding of the morphology and physical and chemical characteristics of the particle. Efforts to eliminate particles from the product do not begin with highly controlled filling environments; R&D efforts that identify the best container components, diluents, and packaging components are essential to ensure product quality. Particle identification efforts are an integral part of the quality process. Identification of the particulate matter allows location of its source, hence its elimination.

Extraneous product-related particles occurring in parenteral products may provide negative indications regarding:

- The level of raw material control,
- The stability of the formulation (physical stability),
- Process design,
- Process execution, and
- Potential sterility problems (for aseptic fill process).

Particle elimination, in general, results in an improved manufacturing process and the manufacture of more product at lower cost. Thus, manufacturers make increasing efforts to decrease product particle burden (Davis and Turco 1971; Davis et al. 1970).

Packaging Materials

Containers and closures constitute an important source of particulate matter; this contamination is diverse in composition due to the complex nature of containers and stoppers (Aldrich 1985). The most obvious and perhaps simplest examples of extraneous materials present in the parenteral product are foreign material introduced into the container before and/or during filling, or resulting from inadequately cleaned packaging materials. These are also classified as process-related particles, since they originate from the preparation, manufacturing, and filling environments. Glass, metals, biologicals, fibers, and machine fragments are not the only types of process-derived particles, but represent common materials that fall into this category.

The elastomeric stoppers used to close vials and bottles can also release particles and extractables, especially when steam sterilized (Dolcher 1990, 1991). Such soluble extractables may then react with the solution to produce insolubles. The first rubber stoppers for parenterals were made from sulfur-cured natural rubber. This material has a relatively high permeability, is prone to release high concentrations of extractables, absorbs drug materials and preservatives, and contains plant proteins and other undesirable materials. It has been largely replaced by the halobutyl rubbers (bromobutyl and chlorobutyl). These two rubber formulations are compatible with most solutions, and can be cured by mechanisms not involving sulfur. They are less likely to release significant amounts of leachables. Stoppers are now available that have silicone resin, Teflon®, polyethylene, or other materials of low reactivity coated onto their inner surfaces. These coatings and improvements in the environmental conditions during stopper manufacture have resulted in significant reductions in particle contamination from closures.

Many pharmaceutical closures are lubricated with silicone oils. The reconstitution of lyophilized parenterals can be affected through the use of excessive oil levels. Moreover, excessive levels can cause: (1) elevated "particulate matter" counts via light extinction methods; (2) incidence of visible "particles" via schlieren effects; (3) occurrence of slowly-dissolving lyophilized cake fragments, due to encapsulation of the cake by the oil. The treatment of stoppers with silicone oil or emulsions is a necessary evil, if butyl stoppers are to be used in automatic stoppering machinery. Alternatives to coating with silicone may be found in proprietary surface treatment of the halobutyl rubber stoppers or through the use of baked on silicone coatings. Some drugs (e.g., cephalosporins) are reactive with rubber so that an inert coating such as Teflon® is required on the product contact surfaces of stoppers used.

If a closure elastomer contains low molecular weight ingredients (accelerators, plasticizers, etc.) that bloom out of the surface during molding, sterilization, or storage, there will be a potential source for particles in the product. Mercaptobenzothiazole (MBT), an accelerator once widely used in stopper formulations, was notorious in this regard (Peterson et al. 1981; Tchao et al. 1977). Even after an efficient washing cycle that cleans the surface, these ingredients may bloom out after a time (weeks or months) and completely cancel out the effect of the previous washing treatment (Nishida 1985; Nishimura et al. 1979). It is of the utmost importance that rubber used in stoppers have a high chemical purity. Decreasing the number of ingredients (i.e., control of physical properties with formulations rather than additives) gives a decreased particle release and also guarantees a broader compatibility range. Fillers and rubber fragments constitute other important stopper-related particles; filler materials may be caused to segregate at the surface of rubber parts by some molding processes and are subsequently washed off by the product. Extraneous particles that may be added by packaging or handling of the closure must be controlled. Ideally, washing should be required to remove only a small number of particles left by the total process (Hayashi 1980a, 1980b).

Closure-related particle problems may relate to fragments of the closure itself. In one specific instance, large volume solution product showed elevated particle counts due to large, dark-colored particles (25–100 µm)—rubber closure fragments. Microscopic examination of the closures used in these units showed fragments of closure material were on the cut surface of the closure. In addition, pitting and fissures were found in the body of the closure. Nondefective units in adjacent batches contained closures of normal morphology. The problem was determined to be caused by a combination of a dull cutting die used by the vendor and incompletely cured stoppers.

Another potential risk of particulate matter generation related to stoppers may occur due to coating materials present on stoppers when they are received from the vendor. This involves the chemical combination of materials present as a coating on the stoppers with dry powder material or with dissolved drug. This has occurred several times in the author's experience. One occurrence was due to the presence of traces of mold release agent that was incompletely removed by washing, on the product contact surface of stoppers. A second involved the presence of a reactive impurity in the silicone emulsion used to lubricate the stoppers. In both cases, the particulate matter formed was an amorphous or gelatinous material that formed indistinct spots or smears on membrane filters, and imparted a hazy appearance to the solution. Both materials gave EDXS spectra containing silicon as the predominant detectable element, allowing investigations to focus on the stoppers as the most likely source of other problems. The mold release agent was identified by a computerized FT–IR spectral file search. The reactive impurity in the silicone emulsion was also identified by FT–IR. In this case, conversations with the supplier of the silicone emulsion indicated the material to be a known contaminant of their material.

Containers are made of a wide range of types of glass and plastic (Luscher 1985). Reasonably, stoppers with a larger surface area can be expected to generate more particles than smaller surface area stoppers of the same rubber. Plastic solution containers almost invariably give lower particle counts than glass, since they do not have stoppers and are typically manufactured so that there is a decreased chance of contamination from the environment (Whitlow et al. 1974; Yakowitz 1966). In some cases, they are made from tubular extrusions and the container surface never is exposed to process-generated or environmental contaminants. Blow molded plastic bottles may be filled immediately after forming so that there is minimal chance of environmental contamination. The ratio of container surface area to solution volume is often a key determinant of particle burden. Plastic containers are frequently used for larger volumes of solution so that there is less particle contamination per volume of fluid.

Glass containers for pharmaceutical products are typically made from two types of glass (Abendroth 1985). These are soda lime glass with a surface treatment (Type II) or borosilicate glass (Type I). Type I glass containers typically are cleaner when received from the vendor and are more readily cleaned by washing than are Type II bottles. Contamination of glass containers often occurs during manufacturing, packaging, or transportation of bottles. General cleanliness is most often dependent on the effectiveness of cleaning measures immediately prior to filling. Large volume glass bottles are likely to bear high levels of particles on their inner surfaces prior to washing. Despite this higher initial level of particulate matter, it is sometimes easier to attain a given level of cleanliness with a large container than a small one and this may partly explain why smaller units may contain relatively more particles than large ones. As the volume of the container decreases, the area of the stopper and the walls of the container to which particles can adhere also will not decrease proportionately, allowing more surface area for the release or generation of particles (Green et al. 1979). Ampoules are relatively easily cleaned, but may contribute significant numbers of particles on opening (Korbl et al. 1967; Ernerot and Mellstrom 1969; Ernerot and Dahlinger 1969) or on solution removal with any size (DeLuca and Kowalsky 1972).

Much of the particulate matter in glass containers is found to be particles of glass or contamination from extraneous sources that are introduced during manufacture, packaging, and storage, but not removed by washing prior to filling (Brewer and Dunning 1947). The amount of particle contamination in plastic containers is dependent on the type of plastic and method of container fabrication. Sterilization may alter the particle burden in both glass and plastic containers.

Solution and Formulation Components

The paper by Speed (1985) provides interesting insight into this issue. Precipitation or crystallization has historically been a source of particulates in parenteral solutions. Some particulates may be the result of precipitation of one of the components of the parenteral formulation (Hasegawa et al. 1982). Generally, products are not intentionally formulated near or above the solubility limits of the components, but this is a possibility that must not be overlooked. Control of solubility as a function of pH and excipient concentration in preformulation studies provides little protection against drug or excipient precipitation that is a result of temporary storage at cold temperatures. Sodium phosphate buffers may produce the relatively insoluble $Na_2HPO_4 \cdot 12H_2O$ at refrigerated temperature (Borchert et al. 1986; Hasegawa et al. 1982). The presence of a contaminating species that has been leached from a closure or inadvertently introduced prior to filling can also result in precipitation; this type of contaminating material always has the potential to interact with solution components to form insoluble compounds.

Crystallization is not uncommon in LVP solutions of concentrated dextrose, dextrans or similar materials that may be formulated near the solubility limits, particularly if the products see low temperatures. Pharmacy-produced admixtures frequently develop precipitates due either to a marginal formulation with regard to solute concentration or through degradation of admixture components (e.g., the formation of calcium oxalate from degradation of ascorbic acid). Drug solutions may contain crystallized particulates related to a small amount of impurity that precipitates on storage of a solution of the drug. Penicillinoic acid thiolactones in penicillin SVIs are an example of this phenomenon. In addition to oversaturation conditions, precipitation requires the existence of nucleation sites. Thus, the introduction of nucleation centers, such as contact with a closure surface, a glass defect, or a syringe needle, may cause the sudden formation of large numbers of particles. Extremely small amounts of materials can be responsible for a problem level of precipitates. An example is the combination of trace levels of calcium and aluminum from phosphate-containing pH-adjusting reagents to give a precipitate. Precipitation reactions may also be highly variable between units; it is not uncommon to see units containing readily visible particles and unaffected units in the same batch. Similarly, individual units from the same batch may contain crystal precipitates of distinctly different morphology.

The surfactant nature of many parenteral products can cause unique effects with regard to particle formation. Some drugs are ampiphilic in nature (i.e., the drug molecules exhibit both polar (hydrophilic) and nonpolar (lipophilic) characteristics). This behavior is characteristic of the general class of detergent molecules. Behaving as detergents, some drugs form micelles in solution. Micelles also serve to solubilize lipophilic molecules. There is a critical concentration above which surfactant added to a solution enters micelles and the concentration of monomeric surfactant remains essentially constant. This concentration is called the critical micelle concentration (CMC). At surfactant concentrations above the CMC, the solubilization capacity for nonpolar materials generally increases with the surfactant concentration. Surfactant-emulsified microdroplets are readily counted by light extinction particle counters and may be responsible for compendial count failures. Surfactants, especially when present at concentrations above the CMC, can dramatically influence the solubility of some formulation ingredients. The nonpolar environment in the interior of micelles can act as a distinct solution phase in which hydrophobic molecules can dissolve. Dissolved materials in an SVI may precipitate following dilution into an infusion solution if the dilution brings the surfactant concentration below the level necessary for emulsification (Yalkowsky and Valvani 1977). Alternatively, a seemingly insignificant increase in the level of an impurity might lead to the precipitation of another species dissolved in the micellar phase if the impurity alters the solubilizing ability of the micelles. Sodium methylprednisolone succinate is an example of a micellular drug (White 1985). At high concentrations of the sodium salt, solutions of this material contain a large number of micelles. These can dissolve nonpolar materials, such as the free alcohol form of methylprednisolone. With age, methylprednisolone succinate hydrolyzes to methylprednisolone, a nonpolar compound. This both reduces the number of micelle-forming molecules and increases the number of water-insoluble molecules that need to be solubilized. As this reaction proceeds, the equilibrium solubility of the drug may be exceeded, in that case a precipitate results.

In addition to precipitated material or particulate matter related to surfactant activity, some drugs and carbohydrate or amino acid solutions may contain amorphous (noncrystalline) material related to a small amount of degradation of a solute ingredient. Cephalosporin antibiotics frequently contain amorphous or gelatinous particles from this source (Rebagay and DeLuca 1976). The tendency of dextrose solutions to contain amorphous or gelatinous fragments of 5-hydroxymethyl furfural is acknowledged by the USP, which allows for assay of dextrose-containing solutions by light extinction counting rather than microscopy. A similar brown amorphous material can occur in amino acid or protein-containing drugs due to tryptophan degradation.

On occasion, complex particulate matter problems arise with drug material that may require application of a wide range of instrumentation and expertise. In the study by Ashline et al. (1990), a degradation product of penicillin drug powder required the use of nuclear magnetic resonance, mass spectrometry and X-ray crystallography for identification. This problem was first observed as high instrumental and microscopic particle counts in aqueous solutions of sodium nafcillin and sodium oxacillin. The moiety responsible, a thietan-2-one, was observed to form by precipitation in solutions of the drugs held at room temperature, and particles increased in number with increasing time of storage.

Some of the particulate matter problems that arise during storage of liquid formulations are related to adsorption phenomena. Materials present in solution may be concentrated on surfaces. This is true for trace impurities or contaminants present in solutions stored in glass vials or in plastic containers. While the concentration of a reactive impurity in solutions may be insufficient to result in particle formation, surface concentration of the material may result in generation of particles. In one example of a problem of this type, low concentrations of bismuth were present in a solution that contained bisulfite as a preservative (antioxidant). The combination of the bismuth with sulfide ions to form particles was evidenced by a brown ring that appeared on the surfaces of the glass bottles and polyethylene airway straws at a depth of approximately 1 mm beneath the solution-headspace interface. The brown particles of BiS and BiS_2 formed were identified using EDXS; the metal contaminant was then traced to one of the raw material components of the dosage using inductively complex plasma (ICP) spectroscopy.

Dry Powder Drug Materials

The reduction or elimination of extraneous particulate matter in dry powder dosage forms is a critical and complex undertaking (Ernerot and Mellstrom 1969). In powder filling operations particulate matter from whatever sources present in the bulk raw material used cannot be excluded from the product, and the particle burden of the powder in a final product vial will be directly related to the particle burden of the raw material. Lyophilized or spray-dried powders typically will have a lower particle burden than crystallized powders due to the application of filtration prior to drying operations. These preparations, however, may be affected by the presence of impurities that form amorphous particles on drying, or form particles that do not dissolve on reconstitution. In the case of extraneous insoluble particles in powder-filled material, elimination of particles may be simple and straightforward; elimination of drug-related soluble impurities that can pass through filters to form particulate matter at some later time may call for high-level problem solving and involved procedures for particle identification.

In the case of crystallized powders that are obtained in bulk and processed by aseptic powder filling, the most important potential sources of particulate matter are the processing equipment where crystallization and drying takes place, and in the packaging process for the bulk powder. The situation is made more complex by virtue of the fact that many powdered materials, for example, penicillins, may be available from a number of different vendors who may apply a wide range of particulate matter control measures. Similarly, a single vendor may employ different processes for the same drug manufactured at different facilities. Some vendors of dry powder drug materials may produce different "grades" of raw material based on particulate matter content, and supply product with more or fewer extraneous particles to more or less discriminating customers.

The best course of action for the manufacturer of powder dosage forms is to routinely perform particulate matter assays on raw material lots prior to filling. Conducted appropriately, inspections of the candidate raw materials will prevent filling of a powder with an unacceptably high particle burden, and the consequent inability to release. Ideally, all three types of compendial assays will be applied to the raw material (visual inspection, microscopy, and light-extinction counting). The light-extinction assay will serve to detect immiscible materials as well as small (≥ 2 µm to ≥ 10 µm) particles, but it is of little or no value for detection of particles that may be a problem with regard to visual inspection later on. Microscopy is of great value due to its provision of data not only regarding particle number and size, but identity as well.

Lyophilized materials should be subjected to acceptance inspections as well. In the case of either type of powder, however, freedom from insoluble particles on dissolution does not necessarily give an indication that the material is free of soluble impurities that may form precipitates at a later date. An example of this type of particle problem is provided by the penicillinoic acid thiolactones that may be present in penicillin powders. Extremely low levels of this impurity can form subvisible insolubles over the shelf life of product, that in the worst case may necessitate product recall. The only sure protection against this type of defect is a thorough knowledge of the chemical constituency of the raw material; this knowledge is most easily obtained from the manufacturer of the drug. Of particular concern is that a single drug may be manufactured by a number of different processes. As those manufacturers working with generic antibiotics have discovered in the recent past, different synthetic pathways and extraction procedures can yield compounds that are identical chemically, but have significantly different levels of impurities. Generally, one does well to beware of vendors of raw materials who do not have a comprehensive knowledge of their product as indicated by efficient process execution and extent of testing. Similarly, reluctance or inability of a vendor to supply information in depth regarding trace materials present in the raw material may be a reason to seek another supplier.

Product-Container Interactions

Probably the best known product-container interactions that result in particle generation relate to interaction of products with the elastomeric closures of glass containers (Damme 1970; Danielson et al. 1983). As an example, cephalosporin drug powder antibiotics can react with uncoated butyl or halobutyl stoppers to generate particulate matter due to extraction of stopper components into the drug. As discussed earlier, the composition of a rubber stopper can be quite complex and, besides the elastomer, may include some or all of the following ingredients: a vulcanizing agent, a filler, an accelerator, an activator, an antioxidant, a pigment, a plasticizer, and a lubricant. In addition to fragments of the elastomeric formulation, a variety of closure extractables can thus result in haze or particulate matter formation. Some of the extractables may not be soluble in the parenteral solution and others can react with another component to form an insoluble material. Volatiles from stoppers may also cause haze formation in freeze-dried parenterals.

The interactions of products and containers are frequently complex, and extremely small mass quantities of insoluble material can cause particulate matter problems. Copper or other metals such as iron found at 1 part per million in solutions may cause precipitates (White 1985). The solubility of iron is about 5 ppb in high pH (7.8) solutions due to the formation of insoluble iron hydroxide $Fe(OH)_3$. The kinetics of formation of insoluble iron hydroxides is complex, unpredictable, and may occur at slow rate. Species such as $Fe(OH)^{++}$, $Fe(OH)_2^+$, and $Fe_2(OH)_2^{+++}$ are also involved. At sufficiently high pH, the iron is somewhat more soluble due to the formation of higher hydroxides. The presence of silicon is often detected in particles; this most often results from the silicone oil used as a closure lubricant. The presence of sulfur in particles in SVI is often an indicator of the presence of MBT, a vulcanizing agent used in stoppers. This material can combine with soluble metal ions present in trace amounts to form a metal-organic complex, or it may be observed as isolated particles.

Another example of particulate matter from product-container interactions involves barium sulfate (Aoyama and Horioka 1987). This material has very limited solubility. Subvisible particles of this material have been identified in a wide range of products. It is important to note that although most barium sulfate particles that have been identified in various solutions are subvisible, their size may vary significantly. The crystals typically are symmetrical, which is typical of slow crystal growth via nucleation reactions. The $BaSO_4$ particles are frequently formed by the reaction of the Ba^{++} ions that may be extracted from glass ampoules or vials with SO_4^{--} ions that originate from the anion of drugs and/or the bisulfite ion of the antioxidant (Bodapetti et al. 1980). One remedy to this problem is use of borosilicate glasses that do not contain barium. Some elastomeric closures contain a barium sulfate filler that may segregate at the stopper surface during molding.

In addition to barium, other soluble extractables such as aluminum and calcium (Borchert et al. 1989; Borchert and Aldrich 1990) may come from glass. There are also other sources of these elements, including drugs, excipients, and buffers. Besides particulate matter that is the result of soluble extractables from glass containers, glass flakes occur in some parenteral products (Roseman et al. 1978). Generally these particles result from erosive attack of glass by basic solutions (pH 7.6 and above). Most of this material is highly transparent and very thin, although some may appear as white, fluffy particles. Even though most of the flakes are quite thin (<1 µm), they are often detected under visual inspection conditions because of their reflective nature.

Process Point-Generated Particles

These are extraneous particles resulting from any manufacturing step in which packaging components are manipulated or handled, including the formation of the container, as well as the fill process. The following are some typical sources:

- Fill nozzle misalignment,
- Capper misalignment,
- Stopper feeder,
- Vial or ampoule turntable,
- Handling of container or closure,
- Cutting the neck of blow-molded containers, and
- Machinery wear fragments.

Additionally, any human handling of product containers is liable to add particles. The literature has numerous references to colorless, transparent, ovoid, flake-like particles that are, in fact, human skin cells. Powdered gloves are a potential source of starch, talc, or calcium carbonate particles. Powder-free gloves are the only recommended types to be used in product filling areas.

Extraneous particulate matter from these sources must be carefully controlled. Despite filtration, it must be assumed that any contaminant particle present in the solution mix tank of an LVI fill process or in a drug solution that will be lyophilized is a potential contaminant of the final product. Similarly, particles originating in process equipment, such as solution lines or fillers, will have a detrimental effect on product quality if they are not denied access to the final product. Control of particulates from extraneous sources is, therefore, dependent both upon control of particulate matter sources related to every process component that touches the product and final filtration; the latter is often overemphasized at the expense of the former. While process filtration is extremely important, its emphasis too often leads to a philosophic disregard of particulate matter sources within the process that occur downstream of filters and can lead to product contamination. In any consideration of particulate matter elimination in the fill process, contribution of the fill path and fill equipment must be given careful consideration.

With regard to fill equipment, the following are important considerations:

- Existence of pockets or dead-legs in fill line circulation;
- Number and nature of joints and welds in the fill line;
- Type of pumps used;
- Filler characteristics (diaphragm vs. piston, etc.); and
- Length and nature of fill line path downstream of line filters and filler.

The elimination of pumps from the fill line whenever possible and the use of gravity or pressurized solution fill has many benefits. Centrifugal pumps are highly efficient, but invariably contribute wear particles (gasket, bearing, and seal materials) to a process line. Due to the high rotational speed and close tolerances at which such pumps operate, slight misalignment of the rotors can generate very high levels of particles by abrasion. Similarly, simple piston-type fillers are an inevitable source of wear particles and contemporary diaphragm or time-pressure fillers with nonparticle shedding valves are far superior with regard to particle generation. Minimally, filters should be used between the last piece of equipment in the fill line that has moving parts and the fill nozzle; the length of the flow path downstream of the final filter must be kept at an absolute minimum. This, of course, suggests the use of filling head filters. Filling nozzle contact with the neck of an ampoule or vial is notorious for the production of glass or metal fragments. Fill processes, including placement of the fill needles or nozzles, are designed to be very uniform. Thus, misalignment of vials or the filler may result in almost every unit in a batch being affected by this defect.

Filtration is of obvious extreme importance. The book by Meltzer (1986) provides a detailed discussion of all critical aspects of filtration as it relates to pharmaceutical manufacture. It must be kept in mind that filter housings shed particles and the microporous (spongiform) media of most process filters has the potential for particulate matter generation through fragmentation. Thus, the simple placement of a filter in a process line does not ensure that particle-free solution will be filled. Filters placed in the fill tubing downstream of the filler may be effective in eliminating particles that originate in the fill mechanism, but must also be able to reliably withstand the constant pressure surges of the filler. Rupture of a nozzle filter with release of retained particles and filter fragments can lead to tragically high levels of particles in product. Cartridge filters for pharmaceutical solutions marketed today by the major vendors are designed to be extremely efficient in particle removal, to have low particle shedding characteristics, and to be inert to the solutions filtered. Construction of a typical process filter is shown in Figure 1.

Although solution filtration is often viewed as a simplistic process, it is, in reality, quite complex. Particles are removed from liquids by different mechanisms dependent upon the type of solution being filtered, the material of the filter, the filter retention rating (pore size) and the size of the particles of interest. The sieve retention mode of particle capture occurs whenever a particle is too large to pass through a filter pore. This type of particle capture is largely independent of filtration conditions, including any reasonable pressure. Sieve retention is also generally independent of the particle challenge level. If a sieving mechanism is considered, regardless of the number of particles contacting the filter, all the particles above a given size will be retained. Additionally, sieving particle retention will be independent of the suspending liquid vehicle with regard to its ionic strength, pH, surface tension, temperature, viscosity, and presence or absence of surfactant.

The membrane type filters used in parenteral production can be viewed as either depth or sieve filters depending on the particle sizes of interest. Generally speaking, the production cartridge filters

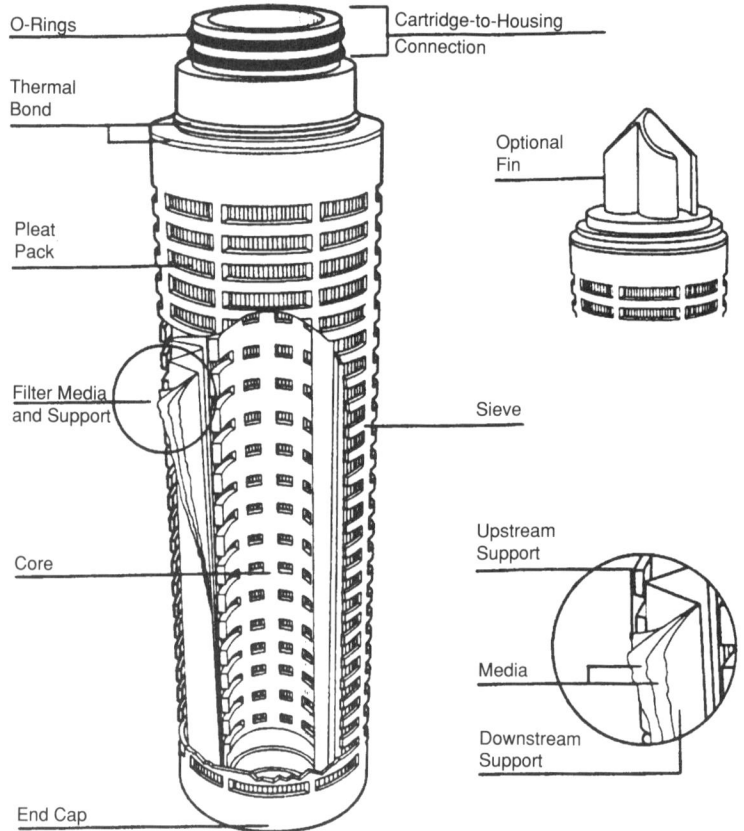

Figure 1. Cartridge filter of current design for application in pharmaceutical manufacture (Gelman Sciences).

used for pharmaceutical solutions will affect not only the removal of particles above the retention rating, but also large numbers of smaller particles. Particles below the filter retention rating may be removed by adsorptive contact within the filter matrix; this mode of particle capture is less important than sieving if particles greater than 1 μm in size are a consideration, since the filters used in parenteral solution production will most often have a 0.22 μm or 0.45 μm retention rating (Brock 1983). Particles smaller than the retention rating will not necessarily pass through a filter. Generally, both electrostatic and van der Waals forces are active in attracting particles below the pore size to the filter medium and adhering them. Most filters possess a negative charge when wet and negatively charged fine particles will be more likely to pass through the filter than positive ones. Surface retention on a fluid filter may also result in exclusion of particles smaller than the nominal pore size of the filter.

Filters applied to protect products from extraneous solid particles may contaminate the product filtrate with immiscible contaminants. Phthalates present in cellulose ester filters have historically been implicated in this regard. In an occurrence reported by Aldrich (1985), the problem material was poly-(diethyleneglycol) isophthalate (PDEGI) that was not related to the product. The material was traced to a bulk drug isolation filter used to harvest the crystallized drug, which was composed of Dacron®, and contained small quantities of PDEGI. In order to maximize yields, the process involved collection of additional drug from the initial filtrate. Filling of the product through 0.2 µm sterilization filters did not diminish the content of the polymer in the formulation. Due to the high concentration of the drug relative to the polymer and slow formation of the polymer-related particles, the problem was not immediately detected. Further production of the drug without the culprit isolation filter yielded polymer-free material.

Filling machines constitute a class of production machinery that have a significant impact with regard to product particle burden. The filling of liquid product into a sterile container is complicated by the flow of air around the mouth of the container during the fill cycle. In the past, filling heads were often set onto bulky supports that controlled the vertical movement of the filling needles. Such structures, overhanging the filling line, disrupt the laminar HEPA air flow resulting in eddies and turbulence in a portion of the critical area. Typically, in machines of current design, solution metering is by diaphragm valves or pinch clamps. A design approaching the ideal suspends the filling needles from a slender post that moves up and down, or has only small diameter tubing overhanging the vials being filled. The machinery of a filling machine should ideally be below the opening of the final container, and below the continuous belt or endless screws that move the bottles.

Particulate Matter Problem Solving

Isolation and identification of particles is invariably a critical step in this regard. The identification of the chemical composition of particles may require ingenuity in addition to sophisticated instrumentation. Light optical microscopy is the starting point for most identifications and is followed by x-ray analysis, infrared spectroscopy, and microchemical testing. Once the identity of the particles is known, it is usually possible to form a hypothesis regarding their source. This hypothesis must then be tested and confirmed or, if necessary, modified until a solution to the problem is achieved.

An understanding of the mechanism of particle formation is often based on simple chemistry. Gross problems generally manifest themselves in either unsatisfactory visual inspection or subvisible particle count results. If a given product has consistently shown a reject rate of <2%, a sudden increase to 10% or higher must result in investigation and corrective action. The use of light extinction counting in monitoring product typically provides a more sensitive indication of problems than human visual inspection and is far less variable. If the number of 10 micron diameter particles per mL increases from a "historic" 5 to 35, we must assume that something is amiss even if visual inspection results are not drastically affected. Elevated subvisible particle counts often precede visible inspection problems.

Documentation must accompany all problem-solving efforts. The first question invariably asked should be whether or not the particulate matter inspection or monitoring procedures have changed. Formulation adjustments, changes in cleaning procedures or detergents used, substitutions in processing equipment and/or filter vendors, changes in water systems, and so forth, often result in particle problems, especially if validation of the changes was not carefully performed. The impact of any and all process changes must be evaluated. Even though raw materials and packaging components are released for use only after passing established tests, purchasing from a new vendor or process changes by a vendor can still result in particle problems and this source must be considered as a contributor to a problem under investigation.

The identity of particles in most cases gives a good indication of their source, and thus provides a basis for a rational approach to solving a given problem. Isolation and scrutiny of individual process steps including samples taken before and after a suspect step of the process will generally confirm a given source, so corrective action can be taken immediately. A rational approach to sample collection will invariably narrow down the range of possibilities. With solution products, it is sometimes possible to isolate a causative mechanism by separately evaluating suspected components through substitution of different stoppers, bottles, or control solutions such as water. As an example, absence of a contaminant in fluid collected into a flask at the filling nozzle suggests container, drug, or closure problems. Absence of particles when containers are filled with filtered water or detergent solutions instead of product and stoppered as usual would suggest that drug-related problems are involved. If the economics of the problem are significant, the use of consultants and/or outside laboratories is generally justified in an attempt to find a quick solution. A flow chart for a generalized attack on a particulate matter problem is shown in Figure 2 (Ernerot 1985).

Philosophical Considerations

The foregoing discussion seems to imply that point-generated extraneous particles are much more important than airborne environmental particles. This is true in a sense, since point-generated or container-related particles are always in the immediate vicinity of the product and have a high probability of gaining access to the final container (Schoen 1968). One must remember that HEPA filters and directional airflow will not, in fact, remove particles from product. As particles decrease in size, the force required to dislodge them from a surface to which they adhere is increased dramatically due to boundary layer effect, static electrical charge attraction, and van der Waals forces that bind the particles to the substrate.

Laminar airflow itself simply serves to provide directional airflow away from product. However, should larger particles become airborne, the laminar airflow will serve to restrict their float time in the air and restrict access to product at a remote process point. Larger particles (≥ 10 µm) tend to settle much more rapidly than a smaller ones. A 50 µm particle (spherical radius) settles at a rate in the range of 50 feet/minute. If the particle is elongated or fibrous, the time required may be decreased tenfold; in the absence of directional airflow, a particle 1–10 µm in size may be suspended indefinitely. Protection of product by HEPA filtered laminar airflow must be carefully designed and monitored if product is to be effectively protected.

It is essential to make containers as clean as possible; it is not practical to count on cleaning or washing to give a minimal particle burden. A glass vial is sterile and free from particles at the moment it is made from molten glass. If the cooling process, packing, handling, and transportation are carried out in such a way that no contamination reached the inside of the vial, there is less concern about washing or sterilization before filling. If vials are handled in a clean environment from the time of manufacture and wrapped in plastic film, it is a much simpler task to clean the vials than if they

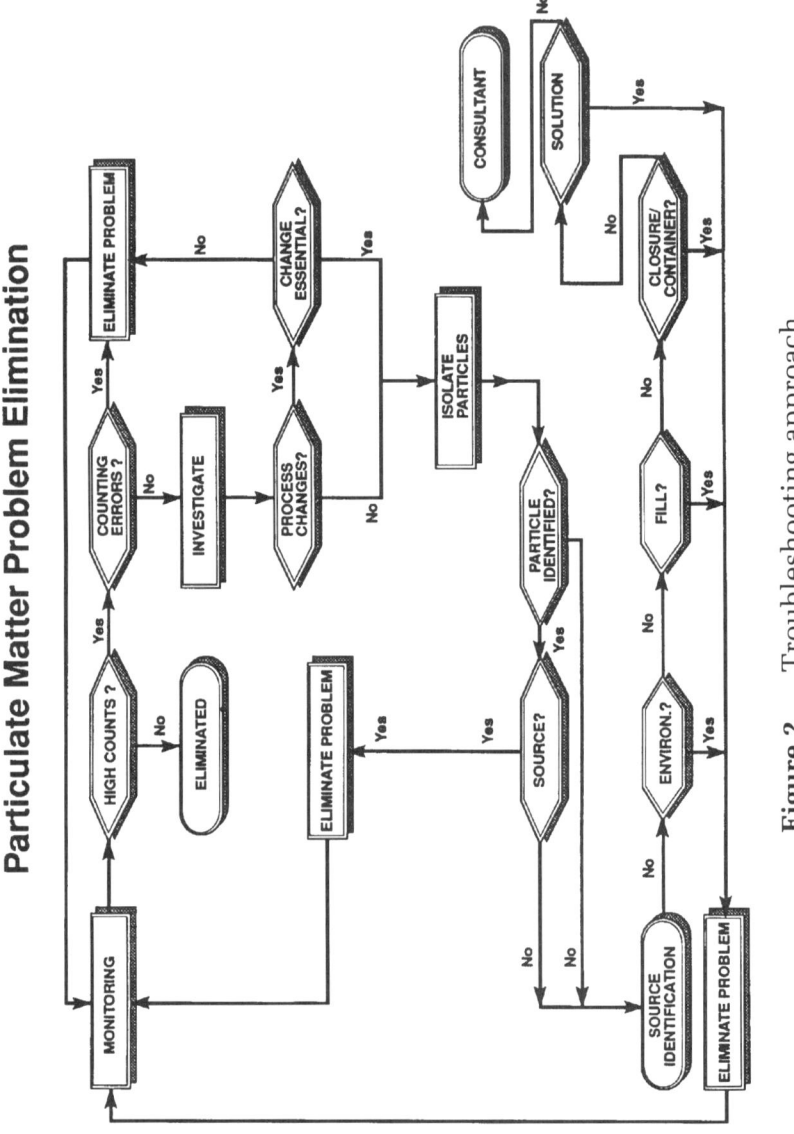

Figure 2. Troubleshooting approach.

are packed open in cardboard boxes. Modern ampoule product contains extremely low numbers of particles. Ampoules are made from clean tubular glass, and annealed at 500–600°C. Organic materials, such as fibers and oil droplets, should be destroyed in this process.

Since no one has yet been able to open an ampoule without the solution being contaminated by glass particles, a small number of glass particles in an ampoule are probably not a significant practical issue (Brewer and Dunning 1947; Davies and Smart 1982; Alexander and Veltman 1985).

Monitoring and inspection procedures are very important (Ernerot 1985). If a normal, noncritical visual inspection removes about $2/3$ of the units that contain visible particulate matter, by definition $1/3$ are not detected. (Some units will also be rejected even if there are no particles present.) Thus, if the true reject rate is 3%, inspectors will pick up 2% of the true rejects and leave about 1%, some of which will be detected by the customer. Therefore, it is not possible to reach a total quality level by visual inspection. As long as the inspected material has some rate of occurrence of visible particles, human inspectors will always release some items that should have been rejected. Increasing the speed of inspection will result in inspectors rejecting less defective product, with more time they will reject falsely at a higher rate. The same general considerations pertain to machine inspection.

Washing may be an effective means of decreasing particle burden (Hallock 1971). Filtered water for injection with a low particulate matter burden should be used as the final rinse for any glass container. Once vials are washed, the transfer of stoppers or vials from the washing area to the sterilizing tunnel through turbulent air must be carefully protected. Whenever possible, containers must be made clean and shipped and stored clean rather than relying on washing to remove contamination. The interaction between particles and containers must often be altered with surfactant if contamination is to be effectively removed. These methods remove one kind of contamination but may add others. Ultrasonic treatment, as widely practiced in Japan, is very useful, but time consuming. The best solution is to have a glass that is as clean as possible when it enters the washing machine. Again, the smaller a particle is, the more difficult it is to remove by washing (Hayashi 1980a, 1980b).

With regard to production of aseptically-filled SVI vial product, the outlet from wash tunnels or pass-throughs into the process room is generally less critical than the inlet since the outlet typically that enters a clean area is Class 100 or better (Federal Standard 209-D). Laminar flow protection between the tunnel and the filling machine remains important; however, although it is always difficult to avoid a buildup of vials between the tunnel and the filling line, this should be kept small. Turntables where vials are rotated before filling should be carefully monitored at all times.

Clean, sterile glass surfaces, when they are rubbed together, will generate particles that will find their way into the vials or result in out-of-limits airborne particle counts (Schoen 1968).

Stoppers are often manufactured under dirty conditions, and grease and extractables must be washed away (Dolcher 1990, 1991). As I have discussed, it may also be necessary to add silicone oil to the rubber surface to achieve "machineability." Here, modern, closed cycle washing machines can remove debris, add silicone, and sterilize in the same operation and finally feed the stoppers aseptically into particle-free nylon bags or directly into a turn-key integrated SVI filling machine. One solution to the SVI particulate matter problem that may enhance solution cleanliness in the future is the use of plastic ampoules. Plastic granules, typically polyethylene, are used for form, fill, and sealing processes. One example of this technique is the Automated Liquid Packaging (ALP) Bottle-Pack System that is currently used for IV fluids, irrigation solutions, and eye drops. This technique approaches an absolutely clean process; it significantly decreases both particle levels and microbial contamination of vials.

As discussed earlier, personnel continuously and significantly contribute to particulate matter issues. They are the primary contamination source in any "clean area." The benefits of removing personnel from critical areas are seen as cleaner products and lower costs. "Clean" garments dramatically reduce the shedding of particles, but the effect of cleaning the clothing is often forgotten and this procedure must be done carefully. Fibers from the washing or rinsing water may contaminate washed garments and may be found in product. Disposable garments provide one answer to this problem. Automated and robotic processes that minimize human exposure to product are undeniably the way of the future.

The Japanese execution of process design to eliminate contaminating particles is interesting. The majority of the LVI solutions (Hiraoka 1990b) sold in Japan are marketed in blow-molded (blow-fill-seal) polyethylene bottles. The processes for blow molding and filling of these units are designed to totally exclude environmental particles (Hiraoka 1990a). Process-generated particles are low in number due to the specific design of the process machinery and the use of laminar airflow enclosures of the type typically used in Western countries for aseptic filling. The polyethylene containers also incorporate stoppers that are made from rubber with extremely low levels of leachables. For product in these containers and in glass, vendors are required to furnish stoppers that are extremely clean and, in many cases, ready for use.

The Japanese design for filling and product handling machines incorporate minimal potential for particle generation. Filling machines are operated under manufacturing conditions before delivery and particulate matter generation is monitored. The filling machinery used for LVIs incorporates a high level of container protection from particulate matter.

Sampling for Large Particles

Airborne particle counters, as were discussed in Chapter 6, provide an excellent means of monitoring particles <0.5 µm in size. These particles typically occur in high numbers in most environmental particle populations and are readily transported into the counter sensor. Unfortunately, there is little correlation between airborne particle classifications and large particle fallout or point-generated particles. In fact, the actual particle populations in a process room often show size distributions quite different from the Federal Standard 209-D or the British Standard 5295 classification. If one takes into account that the airborne classification is largely determined by particles of between 0.5 µm and 5 µm and that surface contamination is due to particles of over 5 microns, it can be seen that product cleanliness may not necessarily correlate with airborne particle measurements.

Monitoring of large particles present in low numbers in controlled environment areas requires special techniques. Surface contamination can be measured by time-consuming microscopic counting and sizing, and for nonaccessible surfaces, one can use tape sampling methods. There are also camera-based techniques. Surface cleanliness levels can also be measured using scanning laser light scattering devices. In electronics manufacturing, these may be used directly for the critical product itself, for example, silicon wafers or chips.

Yet another method of cleanliness monitoring is an indirect method based upon microscopic evaluation of "witness plates" that have been exposed to the same environment as the product. Automated devices for reading witness plates are available, and the exposed plates are readily examined manually with a simple light microscope. The technique is extremely valuable in that it provides a means of quantitating the large particles that are poorly represented in any instrumental count data.

Witness plate samplers may be constructed using one of the following materials:

- Double-sided vinyl tape,
- Agar,
- Filter membranes, or
- Glass or aluminum mirrors.

The tape method is most widely used. A 1" square of black double-surfaced vinyl tape is placed in a petri slide® container. The tape surface is washed in 0.2 µm filtered water and dried in HEPA airflow. Following drying the tape section is examined microscopically for cleanliness. Exposure of the plate for appropriate intervals allows all types of large particles with a significant settling velocity to be collected. The number of particles settling on the tape in a given time gives the fall-out rate. Numbers of these plates placed in different process areas are used to map a controlled environment area for cleanliness.

Summary

In the final analysis, the control of nonenvironmental particles demands a knowledge of both process and product. Although simple science will often suffice, the use of a comprehensive analytical capability is often required. A key factor in most situations will be particle identification. Despite the frequent need for analytical services, those skilled at practical aspects of process particulate matter control can often perform critical problem solving.

I will always remember a lesson learned from one such person regarding process particle sources. Vibratory feeder bowls are notorious sources of particulate matter. A problem had arisen whereby a plastic container closed by a small natural rubber port was contaminated by fibrous particles. Variability of product received from the vendor was blamed. The shift supervisor insisted the vendor was not the cause, but the feeder bowl. This was greeted with a great deal of skepticism. The feeder bowl was under laminar flow HEPA filtered air. To address the unbelievers, the supervisor added a bag of the parts to a cleaned feeder bowl and allowed them to vibrate for intervals of 5 minutes, 10 minutes, 30 minutes, and 1 hour. His test system consisted of 500 mL bottles of water for injection. He opened these and dropped groups of about 30 parts into the bottle. The bottles were then closed, vigorously agitated, and visually inspected. The parts as received from the vendor had few particles; those that had been in the feeder bowl for 1 hour had many large fibers. It further developed that the personnel from one shift frequently let parts vibrate in the feeder bowl over lunch break. Problem solved! Greatness in solving process-related particle problems is where you find it.

References

Abendroth, P. 1985. Development of a USP Type 1 glass for the pharmaceutical industry. *J. Parenteral Sci. and Technol.* 39:112–113.

Akers, M. J. 1985. *Parenteral quality control: Sterility, pyrogen, particulate and package integrity testing.* New York: Marcel Dekker Inc., p. 253.

Aldrich, D. S. 1985. Particulate formation as a result of packaging. In *Proc. Europ. Conf.on Visible and Subvisible Particles in Parenteral Products,* 261–279. European Org. Q.C.

Alexander, D. M., and A. M. Veltman. 1985. Particulate contamination in ampoules. *J. Pharm. Pharmacol.* 37:53–55.

Aoyama, T., and M. Horioka. 1987. Barium sulfate crystals in parenteral solutions of aminoglycoside antibiotics. *Chem. Pharm. Bull.* 35:1223–1227.

Ashline, K. A., R. P. Attrill, E. K. Chess, J. P. Clayton, E. A. Cutmore, J. R. Everett, J. H. Naylor, D. E. Pereira, W. J. Smith, J. W. Tyler, M. L. Vieira, and M. Sabat. 1990. Isolation, structure elucidation, and synthesis of novel penicillin degradation products: Thietan-2-ones. *J. Chem. Soc.* (Perkin Trans. 2):1559–1566.

Backhouse, C. M., P. R. Ball, S. Booth, M. A. Kelshaw, S. Potter, and C. N. McCollum. 1987. Particulate contaminants of intravenous medications and infusions. *J. Pharm. Pharmacol.* 39 (4):241–245.

Bodapatti, S., L. D. Butler, S. Im, and P. P. DeLuca. 1980. Identification of subvisible barium sulfate crystals in parenteral solutions. *J.* Pharm. Sci. 69:608–610.

Borchert, S. J., A. Abe, S. D. Aldrich, L. E. Fox, J. E. Freeman, and R. D. White. 1986. Particulate matter in parenteral products: A review. *J. Parent. Sci. and Technol.* 40:212–239.

Borchert, S. J., and D. S. Aldrich. 1990. Glass container contributions to parenteral particulates. In *Proc. PDA Int. Conf. on Particle Detection, Metrology and Control,* 132–154. Washington, D.C.

Borchert, S. J., M. M. Ryan, R. L. Davidson, and W. Speed. 1989. Accelerated extractable studies of borosilicate glass containers. *J. Parent. Sci. Technol.* 42:187–194.

Brewer, J. H., and J. H. F. Dunning. 1947. An in *vitro* and *in vivo* study of glass particles in ampoules. *J. Amer. Pharm. Assoc. (Sci. Ed.)* 36:289–293.

Brock, T. A. 1983. Membrane filtration: A user's guide and reference manual. *Science Tech.* Madison, WI.

Damme, P. A. 1970. Effect of rubber on injection solutions, foreign particles. *Pharm. Act. Helv.* 45:564–667.

Danielson, J. W., G. S. Oxborrow, and A. M. Placencia. 1983. Chemical leaching of rubber stoppers into parenteral solutions. *J. Parent. Sci. Technol.* 37 (3):89–92.

Davies, P. J., and J. D. Smart. 1982. Particulate contamination in small volume ampoules. *Int. J. Pharm. Tech. and Prod. Mfg.* 3:53–58.

Davis, N. M., and S. Turco. 1971. A study of particulate matter in I.V. infusion fluids–phase 2. *Am. J. Hosp. Pharm.* 28:620–623.

Davis, N. M., S. Turco, and E. Sivelly. 1970. A study of particulate matter in I.V. infusion fluids. *Am. J. Hosp. Pharm.* 27:822–826.

DeLuca, P. P., and R. J. Kowalsky. 1972. Problems arising from the transfer of sodium bicarbonate injection from ampoules to plastic disposable syringes. *Am. J. Hosp. Pharm.* 29 (3):217–222.

Dolcher, D. 1990. Material and process environment related particles from elastomeric closures. In *Proc. PDA Int. Conf. on Particle Detection, Metrology and Control,* 103–132. Washington, D.C.

Dolcher, D. 1991. Particles on rubber closures. *Pharm. J.* 246:267.

Ernerot, L. 1985. Particulate matter problems during manufacture of parenteral products; A manufacturer's experience. In *Proc. Europ. Conf. on Visible and Subvisible Particles in Parenteral Products,* 49–58. European Org. Q.C.

Ernerot, L., and L. Dahlinder. 1969. The contamination of ampoules in connection with opening. *Act. Pharm. Sueccica* 6:401–406.

Ernerot, L., and G. Mellstrom. 1969. Foreign particles in powder ampoules and vials. *Act. Pharm. Sueccica* 6:283–286.

Federal standards for clean room and work station requirements 1989. Controlled Environment, *Fed. Standard* 209-D.

Green, H., J. McNelis, and S. Steinman. 1979. The container size/volume relationship in particulate contamination. *J. Parent. Drug. Assoc.* 33:319–324.

Hallock, W. K. 1971. Cleaning techniques for rubber closures. *Bull. Parenteral Drug Assoc.* 25:65–67.

Hasegawa, K., K. Hashi, and R. Okada. 1982. Physicochemical stability of pharmaceutical phosphate buffer solutions. II. Complexation behavior of Al (III) with Additives in Phosphate Buffer Solutions. *J. Parent. Sci. and Technol.* 36:168–173.

Hayashi, T. 1980a. Relationship between the compositions of rubber closures and occurrences of particulate matter in parenteral solutions. *Yakuzaigaku* 40:68–73.

Hayashi, T. 1980b. Studies on the particulate matter in small volume injections. 3. Evaluation criteria on quality of particulate matter in small-volume injections. *Yakuzaigaku* 40:133–136.

Hiraoka, K. 1990. Particle control in form/fill/seal systems. In *Proc. PDA Int. Conf. on Particle Detection, Metrology and Control,* 626–635. Washington, D.C.

Korbl, J., E. Kraus, and F. Tomicek. 1967. Cleaning of injection ampoules and the detection of particles in injection solutions. In *Proc. 24th Congr. Pharm. Sci. 1965*, 291–301. Butterworths, London.

Luscher, R. 1985. Glass components for sterile products. In *Proc. Europ. Conf. on Visible and Subvisible Particles in Parenteral Products,* (October):1–3. European Org. Q.C.

McCollum, C. N., S. Booth, S. R. Potter, M. A. Kelshaw, P. R. Ball, and G. D. Low. 1984. Particulate contamination and sources. *Proc. Sym. Interphex* 84:51–57.

Meltzer, T. H. 1986. *Filtration in the pharmaceutical industry.* New York: Marcel Dekker, Inc., p. 1091.

Nishida, S., T. Muraki, and S. Ichiyoshi. 1985. Ultra-clean pharmaceutical rubber stoppers. In *Proc. Europ. Conf. on Visible and Subvisible Particles in Parenteral Products,* 73–86. European Org. Q.C.

Nishimura, R., J. Kishimoto, Y, Nishida, Y. Noguchi, and S. Imai. 1979. A novel system for washing parenteral rubber closures individually. *J. Parent. Drug. Assoc.* 33:96–103.

Peterson, M. C., J. Vine, J. J. Ashley, and R. L. Nation. 1981. Leaching of 2-(2-hydroxyethylmercapto) benzothiazole into contents of disposable syringes. *J. Pharm. Sci.* 70:1139–1143.

Rebagay, T., and P. P. DeLuca. 1976. Residues in antibiotic preparations, II. Effect of pH on the nature and level of particulate matter in sodium cephalothin intravenous solutions. *Am. J. Hosp. Pharm.* 33:443–448.

Roseman, T. J., J. A. Brown, and W. W. Scothorn. 1976. Glass for parenteral products: A surface view using the scanning electron microscope. *J. Pharm. Sci.* 65:22–25.

Schoen, D. R. 1968. Practical experience with particle problems. *Bull. Parent. Drug. Assoc.* 22:24–30.

Sharp, J. 1991. Particulate contamination of injections. In *Good manufacturing practice: Philosophy and applications,* 59–70. Buffalo Grove, IL: Interpharm Press.

Speed, W. 1985. Prospective analysis of packaging/formulation interactions with regard to particulate formation and product stability. In *Proc. Europ. Conf. on Visible and Subvisible Particles in Parenteral Products,* (October):87–146. European Org. Q.C.

Tchao, T., J. P. Merceille, and G. Rumpler. 1977. Study of the contribution of rubber stoppers to the particle contamination of large volume parenteral solutions. *R. Sci. Techn. Pharm.* 6:207–230.

White, R. D. 1985. Mechanisms of particulate formation. In *Proc. Europ. Conf. on Visible and Subvisible Particles in Parenteral Products,* (October):195–223. European Org. Q.C.

Whitlow, R. J., T. E. Needham, and L. A. Luzzi. 1974. Generation of particulate matter in large-volume parenteral containers. *J. Pharm. Sci.* 63:1610–1613.

Yakowitz, M. L. 1966. Problems associated with the manufacture, storage and use of large volume parenteral solutions. In *Proc. Sym. on Safety of Large Volume Parenteral Solutions,* 3–5. Washington, D.C.: FDA.

Yalkowsky, S. H., and S. C. Valvani. 1977. Precipitation of solubilized drugs due to injection of diluent. *Drug Intelligence and Clinical Pharmacy* 11:417–419.

VIII

Particle Population Analysis

In discussions of particulate matter in pharmaceutical products, the control, identification, and elimination of extraneous particles is often emphasized at the expense of any consideration of particle population analysis. Population analysis consists of characterizing the size/number distribution of particles in samples such as powders, suspensions, emulsions, and aerosols. Aerosols were considered in Chapter 6—environmental particles; I will limit the present discussion primarily to dry powders or solid materials suspended in liquids.

The definition that we assign to particle populations depends to some extent on how we describe an isolated, single particle. A particle is a fragment of material that is small in relation to the volume of system in which it exists. Thus, the electrons in shells around the nucleus of an atom, grains of sand on a beach, erythrocytes in whole blood, or the planets in a galaxy are particles. A prerequisite of this description is that each particle possesses a discrete boundary that separates it both from the medium in which it is suspended and its fellow particles. A particulate matter system is composed of a dispersing or suspending phase and a dispersed phase—the particles themselves. The particles may be solids (powder), liquid (emulsion), or gases (foam). A group of particles existing in a specific system is referred to as a population. Dry powders, smokes, sponges, the foam on beer, paints with pigment granules, fogs, smogs, xerography toners, and mayonnaise are examples of materials that are amenable to study as particle populations. Each member of the population of particles in such materials has a definable relationship to other particles in the system. Scientific interest in particle populations is not new. In the year 218 B.C., Archimedes addressed the mathematical reckoning of numbers of sand grains in spheres of different sizes in a treatise to Gelo, the eldest son of Hiero.

Understanding the size distribution of particles in a dispersed system may be of great importance in pharmaceutical science. The bulk properties of a powder material depend on the particle-size distribution, that is, on the relative numbers of particles of each size that make up the material. Thus, the behavior of a powder can often be studied and predicted from the distribution data. Size, surface area, and surface-to-volume ratio of a particle can be related to the physical, chemical, and pharmacologic properties of a drug. Stability and dissolution rate of drug powders are dependent on their particle-size distribution, and the formulation of suspensions, emulsions, and tablets also depends on the particle size of the dispersed material involved. In dry powder filling, control of particle size is essential in achieving the necessary flow properties. Tableting processes depend on the size distribution and dispersion of the excipient, the binder, and the active ingredient. Particle size measurement techniques have thus become important tools both for pharmaceutical quality control and product development.

This field of particle analysis is complex, and a wide variety of analytical methods are available. These are described in the texts by Allen (1990), Lloyd (1987), and Veals (1972). The text by Martin et al. (1983) contains an excellent description of particle population analysis in the chapter on micromeretics. The approach I have used in this book will hopefully provide the reader with an understanding both of the basic principles and requirements of population analysis, and of the instruments that are most commonly applied in the analysis of pharmaceutical particle populations. This information should serve a useful starting point for the investigator in this area, and should also be useful to those technically responsible for the application of this type of analysis in the laboratory.

Particle population analysis involves three critical parameters: (1) particle size; (2) particle shape; and (3) particle number. Measurements of each of these characteristics may be expressed in many different ways based on the type of instrumentation applied, how data reduction is performed, and the goal of the investigation being conducted. Importantly, neither of these descriptors is a unique property of either a single particle or a population; each will be a function of the means of measurement applied. Similarly, there is no such thing as "accuracy" with regard to the true size of a particle or correct particle number; precision of a measurement of size or number is the only valid term. The result most often required in this type of analysis is a determination of numbers of particles within certain size ranges over the width of the particle population of interest. As an example, many researchers are concerned with the particle-size distribution of pharmaceutical emulsions. Emulsified oil droplets in these emulsions may range from <50 nm to >10 μm or larger in size. For some purposes it may be necessary to separate these particles into size bins or channels of 100 nm width over a distribution width of 5000 nm or greater. Two or more instruments using different measuring principles may be required to cover this range.

Importantly, anyone working with the analysis of particle populations must realize that the parameters of size, shape, and number are interrelated to such a degree that they are very difficult to consider as separate characteristics. The method of measurement will define how size is measured. Shape of a particle will determine how it is sized, with particles that depart from a spherical or cuboid shape often being a size that is somewhat poorly representative. Numbers of particles placed in a given size class by the method of choice will obviously depend on how the size measurement is made. Even though the discrimination between size, shape, and number is difficult to make, I will discuss these parameters separately in order that the specifics of each may be better understood. The classic book by Herdan (1960) remains an excellent reference regarding particle measurement in general, and for particulate matter statistics.

Particle Size

Useful discussions of particle-size analysis are found in *Remington's Pharmaceutical Sciences* (Osol 1980; Gennaro 1990), the texts by Carstensen (1977) and Fayed and Otter (1984), and the book edited by Stockham and Fochtman (1979). Any definition of a particle population in terms of a size-number relationship will be arbitrary, based on the type of instrument used to obtain the size distribution data. Commonly used terms such as fine and coarse or large and small, are relative with regard to particle populations, and have different meanings when used in different contexts. Historically, particles have been classified into size ranges corresponding to specific measurement methods. As an example, the conventional sieve size range consists of particles larger than about 40 μm, which is the size of the opening in the finest wire-mesh sieves in common use in the pharmaceutical industry.

Analytical methods based on microscopy and light extinction analysis have a sensitivity down to about 1 μm. Thus, a range of sizes based on these means of analysis has been designated the subsieve range (1 μm–50 μm). Variation in particle-size distribution within this size range can critically influence the behavior of drug powders (e.g., stability, dissolution rate, bioavailability). Some specialized pharmaceutical particle population analyses (liposomes, emulsions) are directed at particles in the size range of 0.1 μm to 10 μm. The size range extending from 1 μm downward is called the submicron range. Analytical methods applied in this range include electron microscopy, gas adsorption, centrifugal sedimentation, and various types of light scattering analysis.

A useful general classification of particles based on their size is as follows:

Coarse powders	>1000 μm (1 mm)
Conventional powders	50 μm–1000 μm
Fine particles	1 μm–50 μm
Very fine (submicron) particles	0.1 μm–1 μm
Ultra-fine particles	<0.1 μm

As discussed earlier in the chapters on instrumental particle counting and microscopy, particle size can be expressed in a number of ways. Microscopy allows the analyst to characterize a particle according to several linear or circular measurements. Light scattering, light extinction, and electrical zone sensing methods relate particle size to an equivalent spherical diameter based on an area or volume. With aerosols, one is often interested in the aerodynamic behavior of the particle and the Stokes diameter is used.

A number of equivalent spherical diameters may be used as descriptors of particle size. These are described as follows (Air Pollution Manual 1968; Stockham 1979; Edmundson 1967):

Equivalent spherical diameter, d_{es}, (or ESD) is the diameter of a sphere producing the same response in a specific measuring instrument as the particle of interest. This term is of wide use, since many particle counting instruments relate the size of a particle to that of a spherical calibrant producing the same response.

Volume diameter, d_v, is the diameter of a sphere with the same volume as the particle of interest. This parameter is readily measured by means of the Coulter or Elzone counter. Threshold readings of this instrument are proportional to particle volume or d_v^3.

Projected diameter, d_p, is the diameter of a sphere with the same projected area as the particle at rest on a horizontal surface and viewed vertically. It is determined microscopically by allowing the particle to settle on a filter and comparing the area of the magnified image with the area of circles on a graticule.

Surface diameter, d_s, is the diameter of a sphere with the same surface area as the particle. Its use is limited because calculation of surface areas from linear measurement is possible only if the particles have a uniform shape.

Volume-surface diameter, d_{vs}, is the diameter of a sphere that has the same ratio of surface area to volume (i.e., the same specific surface) as the particle in question. This term is most frequently used in reference to an average diameter for a collection of particles.

Sieve diameter, d_{si}, is the diameter of the largest sphere that will pass through the same sieve opening as the particle. It is equal to the size of the smallest square apertures that will pass the particle and is, therefore, related to the particle's width rather than its length.

Stokes diameter, d_{st}, is the diameter of a sphere with the same density as the particle and the same free-falling velocity in a given fluid medium. Sedimentation and centrifugation methods are most frequently used to make this measurement.

The size of a spherical particle is uniquely determined based on its diameter. Other size descriptors for a sphere, such as surface area and volume, are dependent on the diameter:

$$\text{Surface area of a sphere} = \pi d^2$$

$$\text{Volume of a sphere} = \pi d^3/6$$

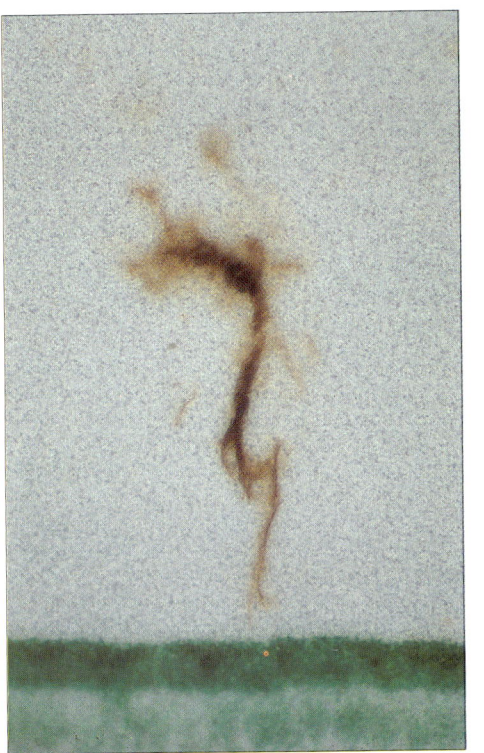

Exhibit A. Amorphous material.

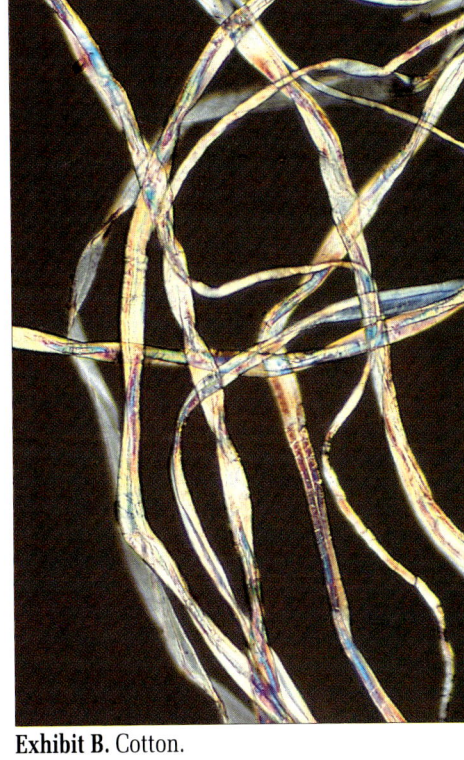

Exhibit B. Cotton.

Exhibit C. Polyester (Dacron®).

Exhibit D. Diatoms (from diatomaceous earth).

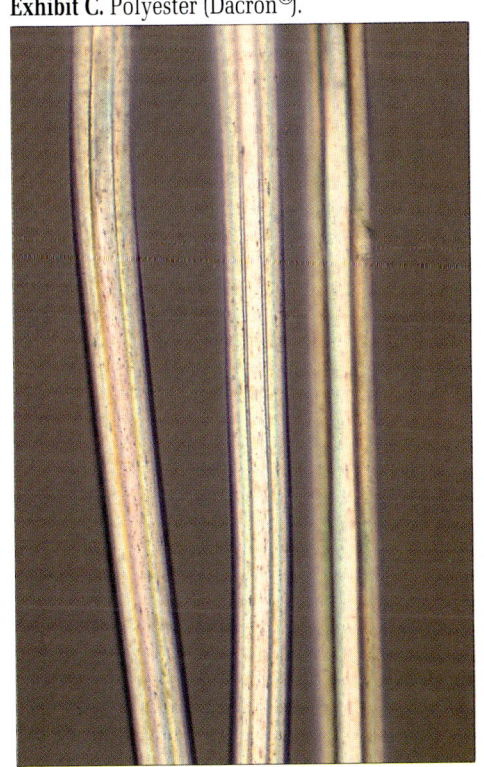

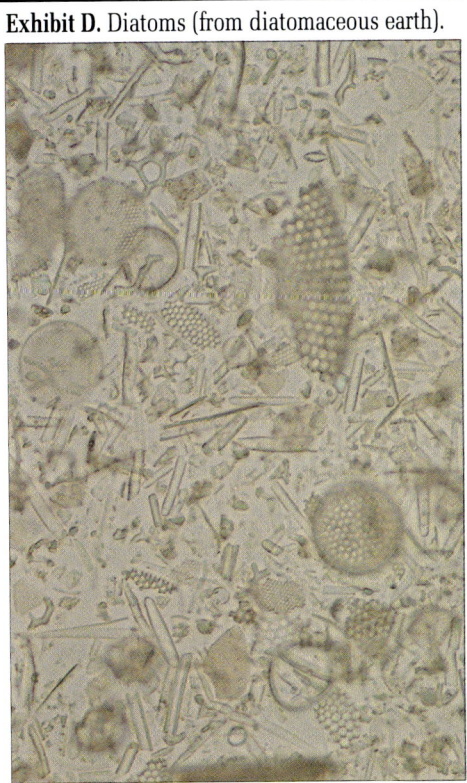

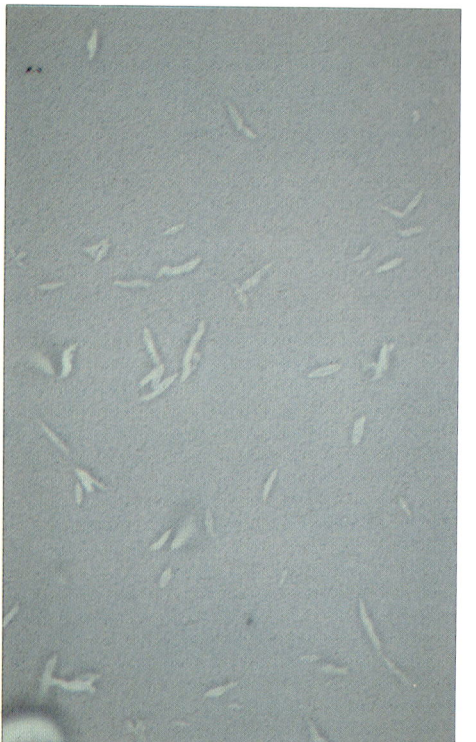
Exhibit E. Filter Fragments.

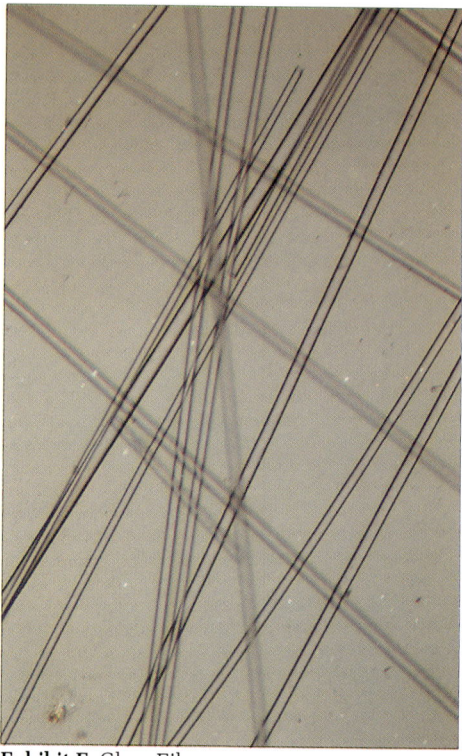
Exhibit F. Glass Fibers.

Exhibit G. Hair (Human, Caucasian, blond).

Exhibit H. Polyamide (Nylon).

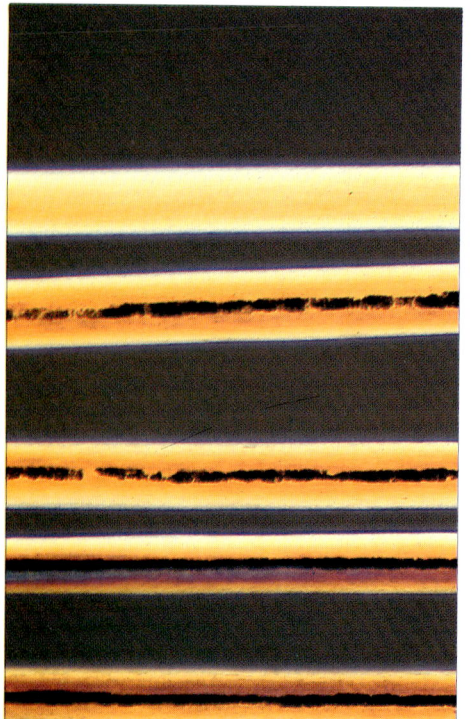

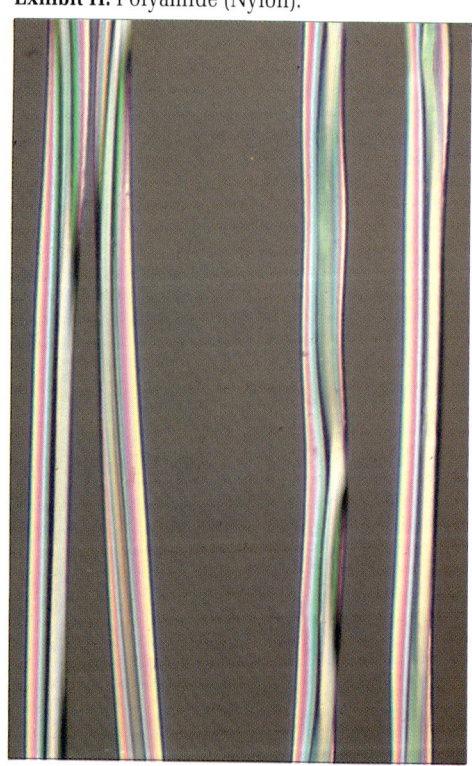

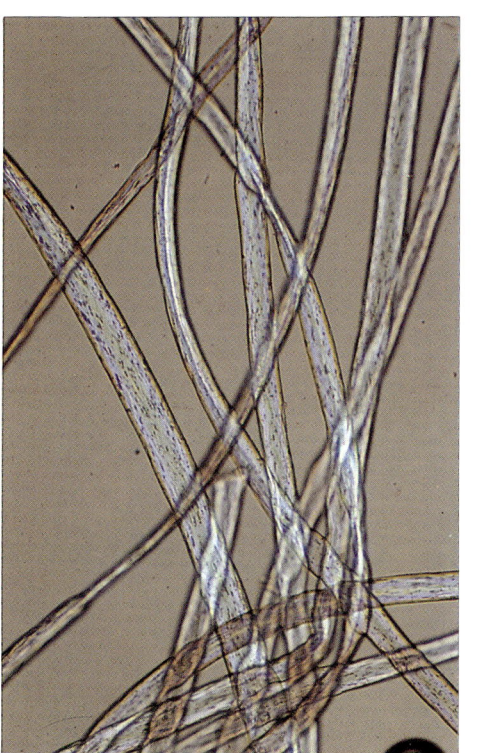

Exhibit I. Acrylic (Orlon®, delustered).

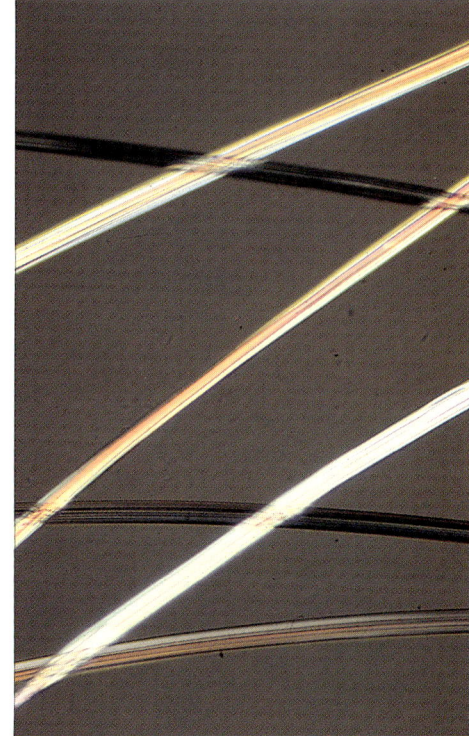

Exhibit J. Rayon.

Exhibit K. Iron Oxide.

Exhibit L. Epithelial cells (skin fragment).

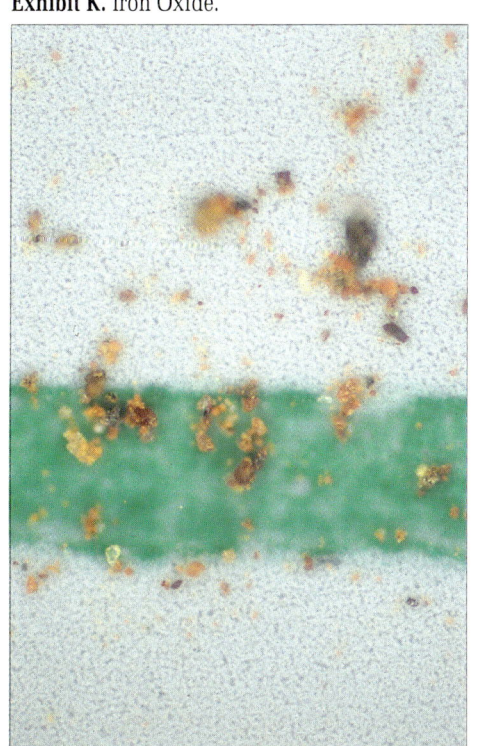

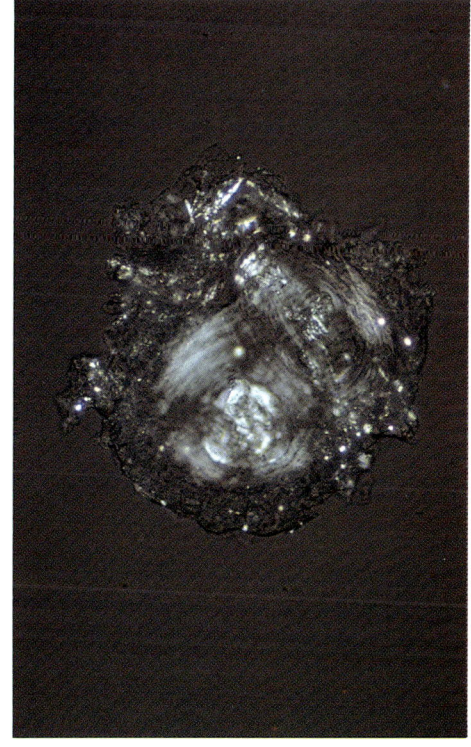

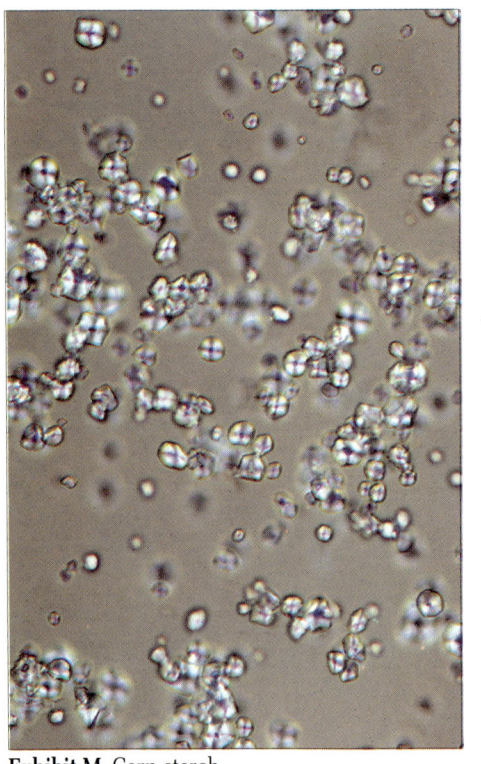

Exhibit M. Corn starch.

Exhibit N. Talc.

Exhibit O. Hardwood chemical fibers.

Exhibit P. Softwood chemical fibers.

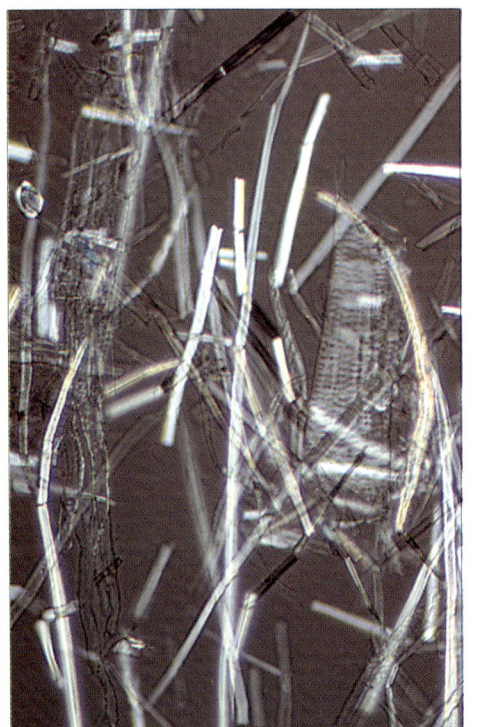

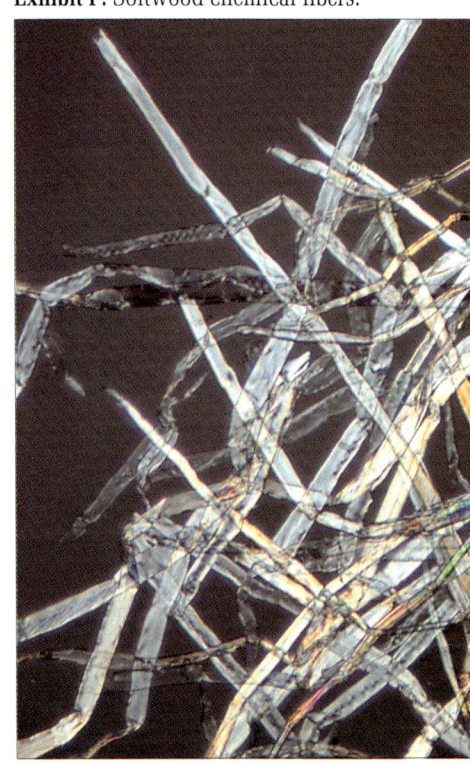

A nonspherical particle also has a specific surface area and volume, but its apparent length will vary with its orientation. Thus, in addition to the spherical diameters, there are also the microscopically determined diameters.

Perimeter diameter, d_c, is the diameter of a circle having the same perimeter as the projected outline of the particle.

Feret's diameter, d_F, is defined as the mean value of the distance between pairs of (typically vertical) tangents parallel to the perimeter of the particle.

Martin's diameter, d_M, is the linear measurement (typically horizontal) that divides particles into two equal halves.

Equivalent circular diameter, d_{ec}, is the diameter obtained by estimating the projected area of the particle and comparing it with circles of known diameter in a microscope graticule.

Unrolled diameter, d_r, is the mean chord length through the apparent center of gravity of a fibrous particle.

In summary, the size of a particle is the descriptor that characterizes its dimensions in relation to other particles in a population. For a spherical particle, the diameter is a single dimension that can be readily used as an unequivocal descriptor of size. Particles of irregular shape can be sized in various ways, but no single linear measurement exists that provides a universal size description of irregular particles. Fibers are a special case (Davies et al. 1975). Different methods may be used to determine different size-dependent properties, such as volume, surface area, or light-scattering. Thus, sizes reported may be volume weighted, area weighted, and so forth. The particle sizing technique applied in a given study should be selected based on what characteristic of a particle is being used to assign a size. For instance, if the volume represented by particles of different sizes in a population is the critical determination to be made, an electrical zone sensing counter is often the method of choice. In any investigation of particle size based on either microscopic or instrumental measurements, one must understand the particle dimension that is being reported, and how that dimension relates to the properties of the system being studied.

Particle Shape

Particle shape is difficult to define for nonspherical particles. The instruments applied in population analysis provide a range of operational definitions of the population, each of which is based on the operating principles of the instrument. Most of these data outputs do not take particle shape into account. As discussed above with respect to particle size measurement, some instruments perform a shape-independent conversion of a particle's size to that of an equivalent sphere (i.e., a sphere of a size that produces an instrumental response equal to that of the nonspherical particle). Different instruments obtain this diameter by measuring the particle mass, its projected area, or its effective volume. Many light scattering instruments produce a response related to particle volume, then provide the user with extrapolated data relating to particle diameter. This extrapolated data is limited in accuracy since the basic measurement will almost invariably be heavily biased toward larger particles. The microscope alone provides critical descriptors of particle shape and even this instrument has limitations due to the two-dimensional image that is formed.

The selection of an instrument to be used in a specific study should be based on what aspect of shape is most important. An analysis that allows measurement of maximum surface (a microscope) might be chosen in dissolution studies, while instruments that give a measure of length would ideally be used for fibers. In some instances, a particle's irregular shape is simply a source of artifact that leads to a level of error in the accuracy of the results obtained. In other cases, the ability of an instrument to differentiate differences in shape is essential.

Simple "cognitive" shape descriptors, such as spherical, cylindrical, acicular, irregular, and angular, are easy to apply. They can be readily applied, and for many purposes adequately describe the general shape of the particle (Figure 1, Table I).

Table I. Descriptions of Particle Shape (British Standard 2955)

Acicular	Needle-shaped
Angular	Sharp-edged or having a sharply polyhedral shape
Crystalline	Angular geometric shape
Dentritic	Branching
Fibrous	Regularly or irregularly thread-like (aspect ratio ≥10:1)
Flaky	Plate-like, flattened
Granular	Having approximately an equidimensional irregular shape (equant)
Irregular	Lacking any readily definable symmetry
Modular	Having a generally rounded, irregular shape
Spherical	Sphere-shaped

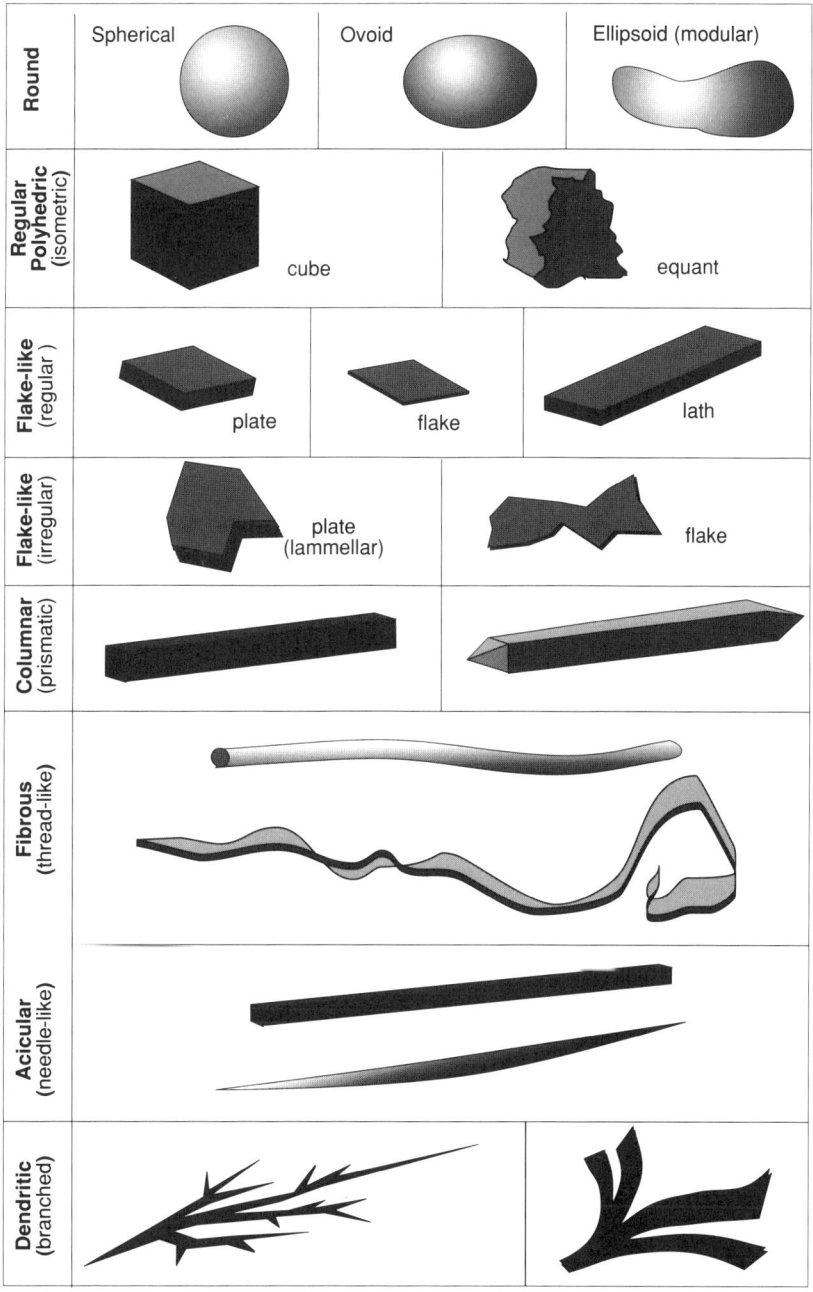

Figure 1. Description of particle shapes in common terminology.

As implied in the previous discussion, there are two points of view regarding the assessment of particle shape. One is that the actual shape is unimportant, and all that is required for a comparison of populations is size-number data. The opposing view is that it should be possible to accurately reconstruct the original particle shape from measurements made. Any quantitation, related even to such simple descriptive terms as those in Table 1, is extremely difficult in cases of all but spheres and cubes; complex equations may be required to define the shape of irregular particles. Pioneering work in this area was performed by Wadell (1932), Hatch and Choate (1929), and Heywood (1947, 1973). Most recently, the work of Beddow (1980), Beddow and Meloy (1980), and others has provided a precise methodology regarding the mathematical description of particle shape.

A basic term used in the description of particle shape is the degree of sphericity (ψ or $\emptyset w$). As defined by Wadell (1932), the term relates d_v, the diameter of a sphere of equivalent volume, to d_s, the diameter of a sphere of equivalent surface.

$$\text{Sphericity } (\psi) = \frac{\pi dv^2}{\pi dv^3} \text{ or } \left(\frac{dv}{ds}\right)^2$$

Approximate ranges of values of ψ for some typical particle types are given in Table II.

Table II. Range of Values of ψ for Various Materials

Type of Material	ψ
Rounded particles such as sand grains or pebbles	.65–.82
Angular particles such as gravel or crushed rock	.55–.65
Flake-like particles: skin cells, glass chips	.41–.63
Thin flakes: mica, delaminated glass	.21–.30
Acicular particles of high aspect ratio	.18–.25

Heywood (1937, 1947) developed a number of the principles of particle shape description that are in use today. It is of interest that much of the pioneering work in this field was done by mechanical engineers concerned with the efficiency of crushing and grinding machinery and by geologists concerned with the properties of comminuted rock or gravel, and sand. Heywood studied rock fragments that were viewed in their position of maximum stability on a flat surface. He then defined the thickness (*T*) as the minimum distance between two parallel planes tangential to opposite surfaces of the particle, with one plane as that of maximum stability. The breadth (*B*) was defined as the minimum distance between two parallel planes that are perpendicular to the planes defining the thickness and tangential to the opposite sides of the particle. The length (*L*) was described as the distance between two parallel planes that are perpendicular to the planes defining thickness and breadth, and also tangential to the opposite sides of the particle. Heywood emphasized the minimum width (i.e., breadth) as a key dimension because it relates directly to the minimum sieve opening through which the fine particle can move (Figure 2). On this basis,

$$\text{Elongation Ratio} = \frac{\text{length}}{\text{breadth}}$$

and

$$\text{Flakiness Ratio} = \frac{\text{breadth}}{\text{thickness}}$$

The Heywood indices are based on measurements made with respect to three mutually perpendicular axes. Indices based on three-dimensional measurements are on this historical basis sometimes referred to as triaxial shape indices, or simply shape indices.

In a study of sand, Heywood (1947) derived the following, more complex equation for describing particle shape:

$$f = 1.57 + c \, \frac{k^{4/3}}{m} \, \frac{(n + 1)}{n}$$

where f = surface coefficient ($fda^2 = \pi ds^2$);
k = volume coefficient ($kda^3 = \pi dv^3$);
n = length/breadth = elongation ratio;
m = breadth/thickness = flakiness ratio; and
c = coefficient of geometric form.

One of the simplest ways in which a shape factor can be applied to routinely examined materials, such as a drug powders, is shown in Figure 3. In this hypothetical case, 500 particles of a drug powder have been examined by microscopy and sized by maximum length and elongation ratio. The result indicates that larger

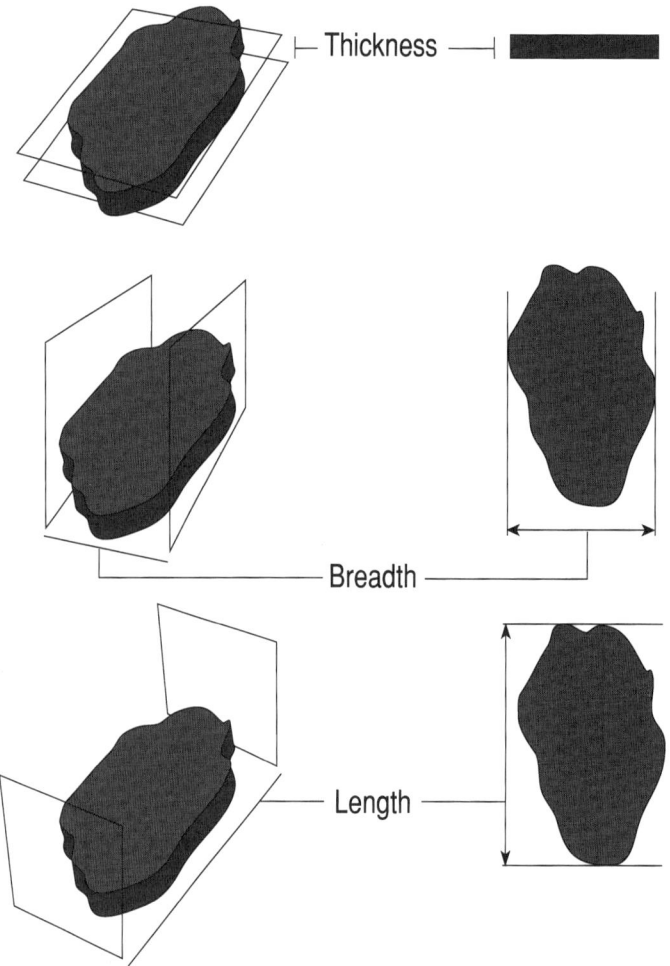

Figure 2. Thickness, breadth, and length measurements.

particles tend to have a greater index of elongation. This allows a general assessment of particle shape in the population to be arrived at in a very simple manner.

The numerical definition of particle "size" is obviously critically dependent on particle shape. In today's particle analysis literature, the term *shape factor* is somewhat loosely used to define any parameter correlating a linear dimension of a fine particle to some other property (such as the surface area), or to some

Particle Population Analysis 277

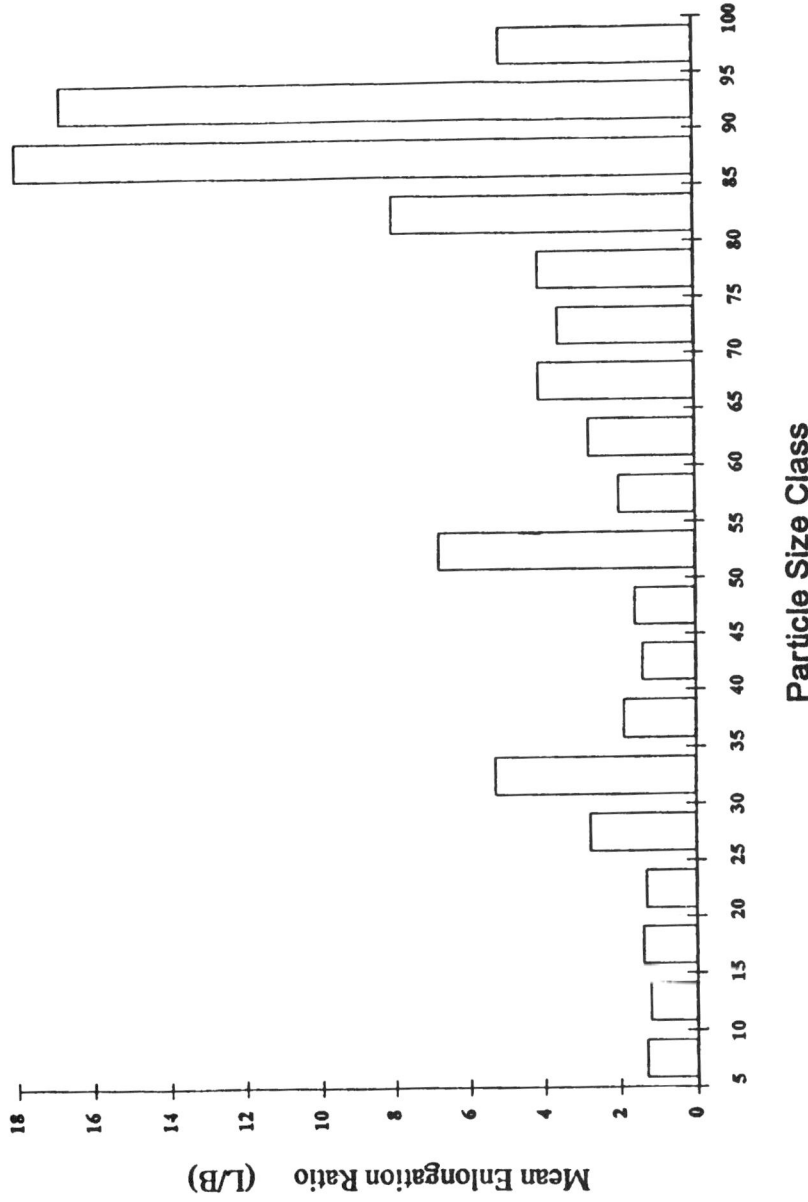

Figure 3. Frequency-shape factor plot for drug powder.

functional property of the fine particle (such as its power in a paint film), or to describe the variation in behavior of a particle with respect to the equivalent behavior of a spherical particle of similar mass.

In recent years there has been an increased interest in particle shape analysis using computer-based pattern recognition techniques in which input data from microscopic measurements of particles are categorized into descriptive classes. The reader interested in the area is referred to the work of Beddow (1980, 1983), Beddow and Meloy (1980), and Luerkins (1991) for detailed information. This mode of shape analysis relies on computer processing of particle images collected by light microscope-based image analysis systems. Dependent on the application of appropriate calculations, shape factors are assigned based on the geometric (morphological) properties of particles. As an example:

$$\text{Sphericity, } \theta = \frac{\text{surface area of equivalent volume sphere}}{\text{actual surface area of particle}}$$

$$\text{Circularity, } \theta = \frac{\text{circumference of circle of area equal to particle projected area}}{\text{actual perimeter of circle}}$$

$$\text{Rugosity, } \gamma = \frac{\text{perimeter of particle profile including minor irregularities and corrugation}}{\text{perimeter of smooth curve circumscribing particle profile}}$$

$$\frac{\theta}{\gamma} = \text{Circularity, including effects of Rugosity}$$

A powerful, and certainly the most complex, computer-based type of shape factor analysis is fractal analysis (Kaye 1981). In fractal analysis the particle edge is approximated by a polygon with all but the closing side of the same length. Particle ruggedness is inferred from increase in polygon perimeter as the length of polygon sides is reduced. A simple example is shown in Figure 4. The concept of fractal analysis is not new. In theory, it relates to the method used by Archimedes in determining the value of pi (π). Archimedes determined the value for pi by measuring the perimeters of inscribed and exscribed polygons of increasing numbers of

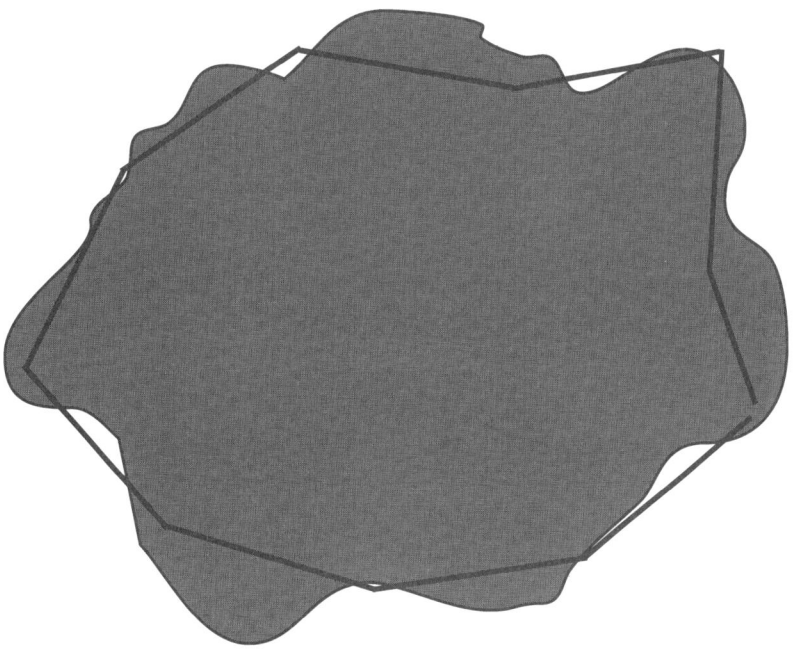

Figure 4. Fractal analysis.

sides. This random walk procedure allowed him to place the value for the factor between $3^{1}/_{7}$ and $3^{10}/_{71}$ (Fink 1966).

The discussion up to this point has been directed at primary particles that represent individual units that cannot be separated into smaller particles except by physical comminution. Particulate matter can also exist as secondary particles. These are groups or clumps of primary particles held together in agglomerates by weak electromagnetic forces, van der Waals forces, or friction; and in aggregates and comglomerates by strong bonds resulting from sintering, cementation, or chemical bonding (Figure 5). Agglomerates are formed when fine powders are handled, shaken, rolled, or stored in a single position. Aggregates are typically formed when powders are heated, compressed, or dried from suspension.

Fine particle agglomerates formed in aqueous systems (flocs or clusters) may have densities much lower than that of the solid material, due to their high porosity, even when heavy metal compounds are considered (Table III) (Kaye and Boardman 1982).

280 *Pharmaceutical Particulate Matter*

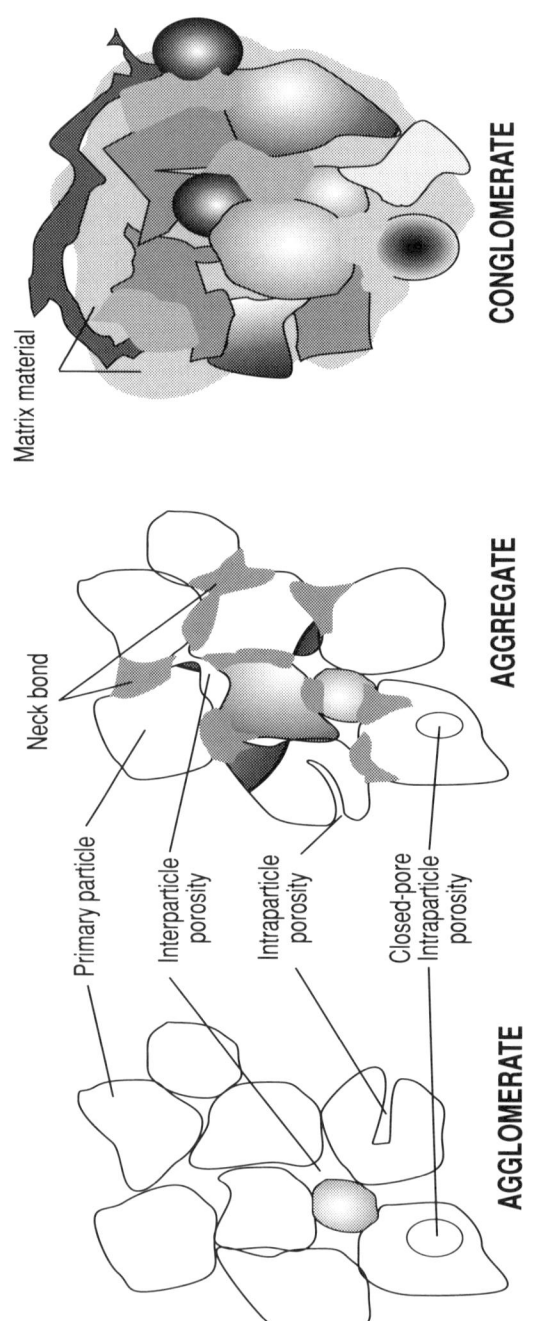

Figure 5. Aggregate and agglomerate structure.

Table III. Approximate Density of Particle Agglomerates of 80% Water by Volume

	Particle Density	Agglomerate Density
aluminum oxide	5.6	1.91
cadmium oxide	6.5	2.10
lead monoxide	9.4	2.67
magnesium oxide	3.6	1.53
mercuric chloride	5.5	1.89

Particle-Size Distributions (Particle Number)

When the number of particles within given size ranges is plotted against size range, a frequency distribution curve is obtained. An example is shown in Figure 6. Such plots give a visual representation of the distribution that is superior to a numerical description. Graphical presentations of particle distribution data are widely used, and important to the understanding of distributions. It is possible, for instance, to have two samples with the same average diameter but totally different distributions. Also, the particle-size classification in which the largest number of particles occurs is readily apparent. (See Martin et al. 1983.)

It should be observed that the Gaussian particle size and number data shown for illustration in Figure 6a is atypical. Such a population distribution might be produced by a chemical process (such as emulsion polymerization) or might represent a biological particle population (such as bacteria or blood cells). The plot of this figure is called a line plot, or a smoothed bar plot. This curve is commonly derived by the simple expedient of connecting the midpoints or geometric means of the bars of a bar plot or histogram with a superimposed density curve. If, for some reason, unequal size class intervals are determined in an analysis, the graphical presentation of Figure 6b may be used. In this presentation, the area of a bar is proportional to the number of particles in the class interval. In the opinion of the author, this type of plot is of limited usefulness, and population analyses should be run whenever possible with equal size class intervals or counter channel widths. Smoothed bar plots can also be derived mathematically from the

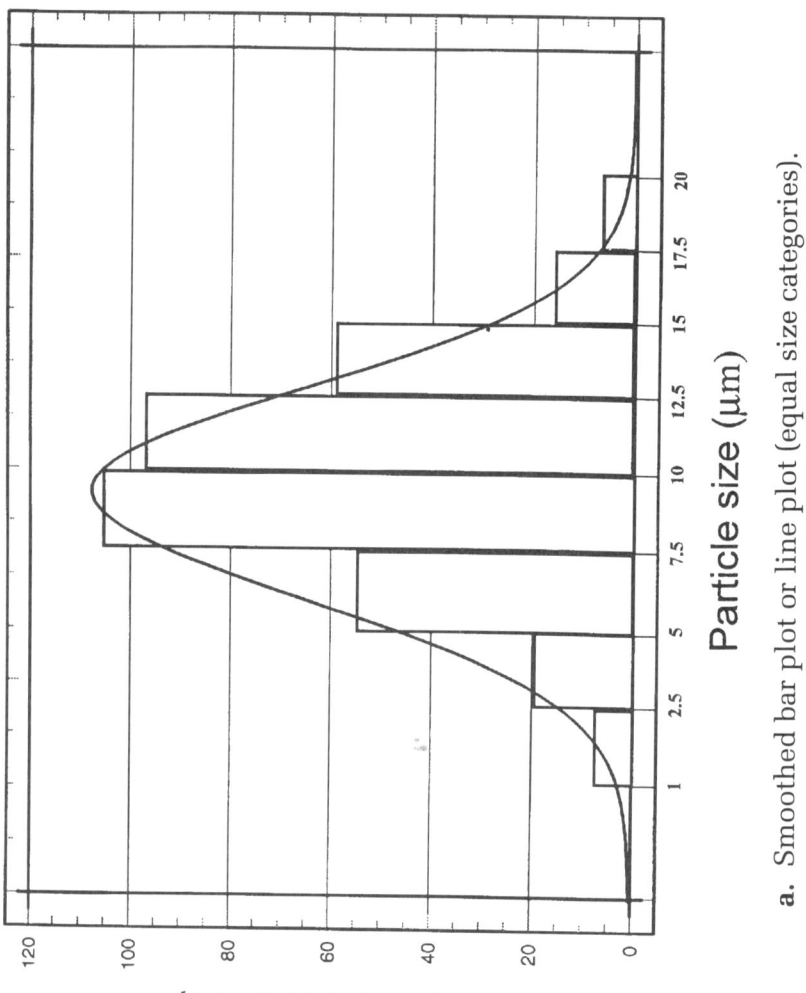

Figure 6. Size frequency distributions.

plot of Figure 6b using the geometric mean of the size class as a point for the plot, and adjusting the area of the size class around the geometric mean. This type of plot cannot be readily compared to one obtained using a different sample size, or a different number of particles, or different class intervals.

The population distribution analysis of pharmaceutical powders often involves the determination of the central tendency of a

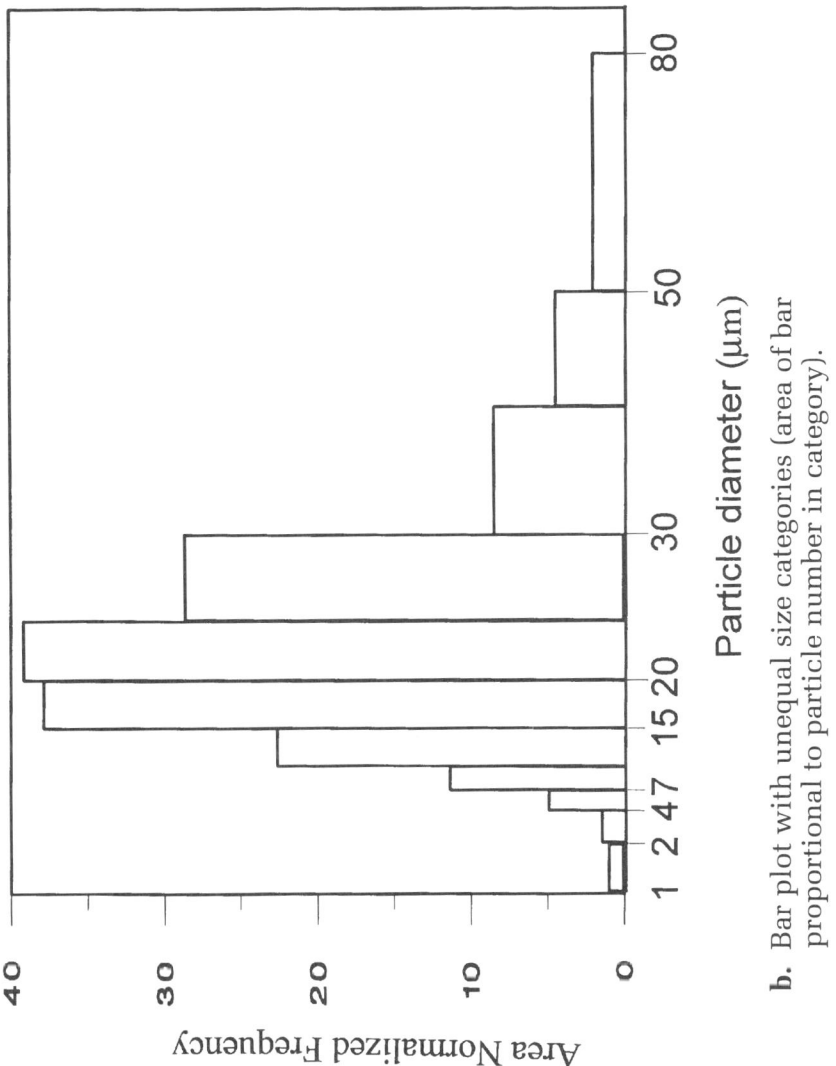

Figure 6. Size frequency distributions.

population. There are three simple measures of central tendency for any distribution. According to Stockham (1979), these are:

1. arithmetic mean (d_{av});
2. median ($d_{1/2}$); and
3. mode (d_o).

The arithmetic mean of the frequency distribution, d_{av}, is the numerical average size. The mean is affected equally by all sample values and thus is significantly affected by extremes or outliers. The median, $d_{1/2}$, divides the frequency distribution into two equal areas. The mode of a frequency distribution, the value that occurs most frequently, is rarely used in describing particle-size distributions due to the fact that (1) it may not be a unique value, and (2) the actual distribution of the sample mode is unknown. For a Gaussian distribution, these three values are the same.

Other key parameters used in particle distribution analysis describe the distribution of observed values about the population mean or median. The standard deviation (symbolically s or σ) is the most useful descriptor of distribution about the central tendency. These values are derived from the variance of the sample or population respectively:

$$\text{Population} \rightarrow \sigma^2 = \frac{\Sigma(X_i - \mu)^2}{n}$$

$$\text{Sample} \rightarrow \sigma^2 = \frac{\Sigma(X_i - \mu)^2}{n-1}$$

In a Gaussian distribution, 99.7% of the population lies within $\pm 3\sigma$ of the mean. In texts and publications relating to pharmaceutical particle population analysis, σ is often used, albeit incorrectly to describe population variability, even though the estimate of σ is based on a small number of samples, and s would be more appropriate.

Most fine particle systems, whether formed by comminution of a bulk solid material or resulting from agglomeration and/or precipitation, have particle-size distributions that obey a non–Gaussian distribution function. When particle size is plotted as a function of the number of times each size occurs, a skewed (leptokurtic) particle-size distribution is obtained, as illustrated in Figure 7. Like Gaussian distributions, non–Gaussian distributions may also be characterized by the parameters that measure the central tendency of the distributions, and the dispersion about that central tendency (Figure 8). The central tendency of a skewed frequency distribution is generally more adequately represented by the median size rather than the mean. As shown in Figure 8, measures of central tendency based on mass are heavily biased toward larger particles present in small numbers in a distribution. Measures of central tendency based on mass represent center of mass values or mass balance points for the population.

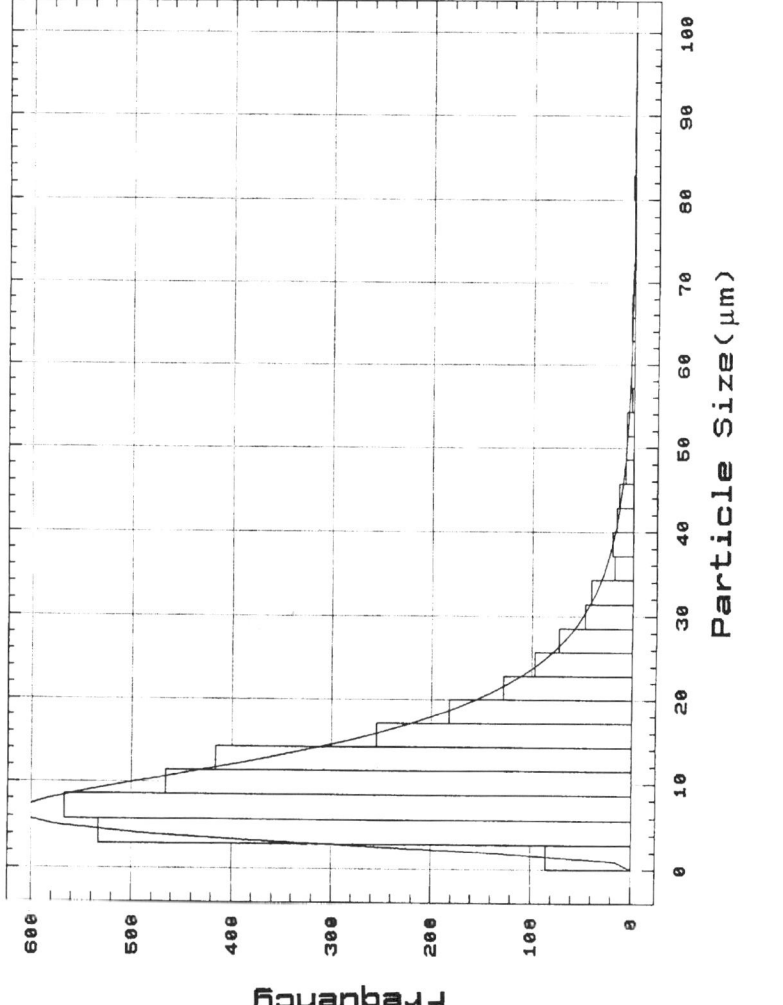

Figure 7. Skewed particle-size distribution of powder material.

The distribution shown in Figure 7 may be replotted using the logarithms of the particle-size classifications. The skewed curve is transformed into the bell-shaped curve of Figure 9. Negative values may be avoided by the use of log+1 on the abscissa. Populations for which this transformation may be made are said to be log normal. This transformation is of utmost importance because after transformation, the resulting distribution is amenable to all the statistical

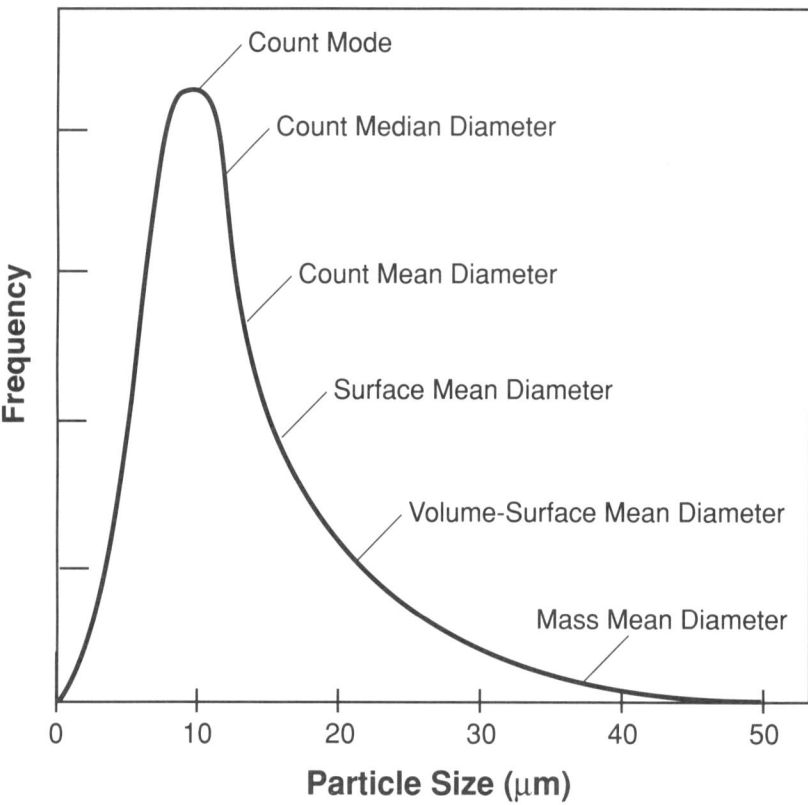

Figure 8. Comparison of particle-size average.

procedures developed for the normal (Gaussian) distribution. For the transformed log-normal distribution plotted in this fashion, the mean, the median, and the mode also coincide.

The reader is cautioned that, although some texts on particle analysis consider all skewed distributions to be log normal, this may not be the case. Other skewed distribution functions (such as negative binomial or Poisson) have the same general shape. The Poisson distribution has an interesting and useful property in that s or σ approximates the mean. The actual distribution represented by the data can be determined using statistical software, such as STAGRAPHICS® to test the fit of the data to a mathematically defined curve. A general observation in this regard is that population size versus number data based on large numbers of counts may

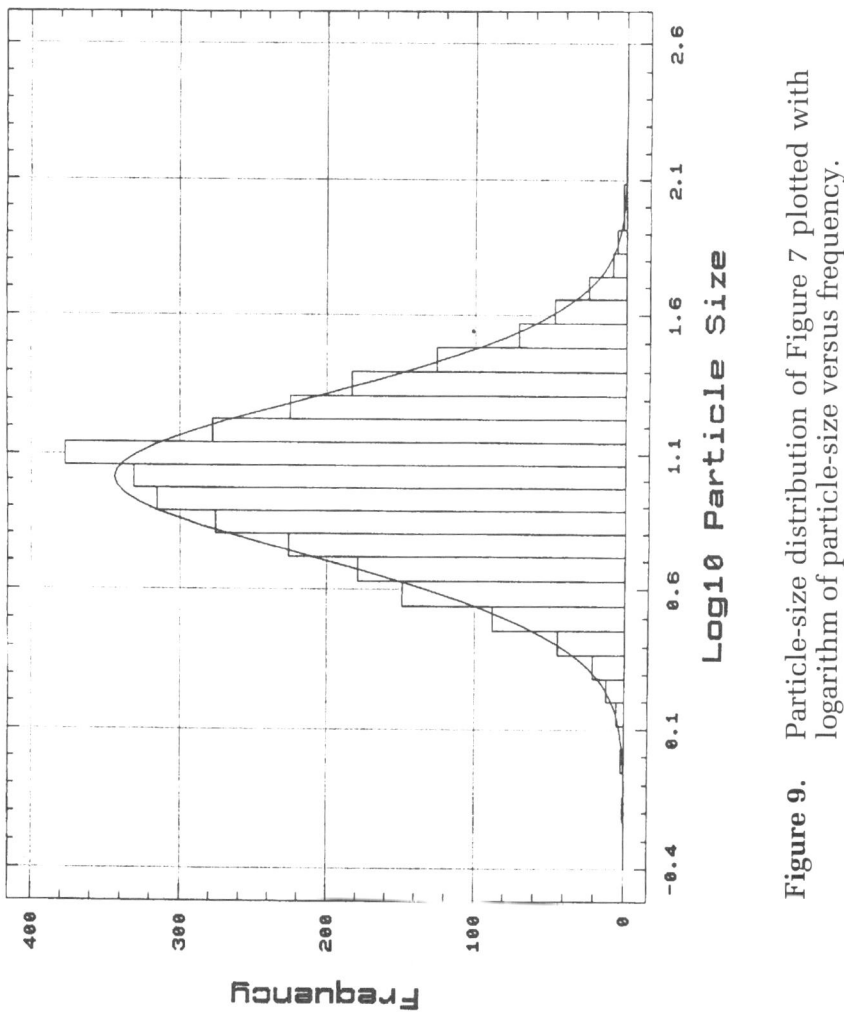

Figure 9. Particle-size distribution of Figure 7 plotted with logarithm of particle-size versus frequency.

approximate log normality, but count data for the small numbers of extraneous particles in a parenteral solution unit at the 5 µm, 10 µm, and 20 µm sizes (plotted against frequency of occurrence) is more likely to be distributed as a Poisson variable.

A most useful central tendency estimate for a log-normal distribution is the geometric median particle size (d_g), and the related measure of variability is the geometric standard deviation (σ_g or s_g)

These two values provide a description of a log-normal particle-size distribution; as do the same parameters for an arithmetic distribution. An assessment of a log-normal distribution function can be tested, and the values of d_g and s_g derived, by plotting cumulative frequency data on logarithmic probability graph paper or using the appropriate software. If the particle distribution is log normal, a straight line will be obtained on the log-probability (log-probit) plot (Figure 10). Here d_g is equal to the 50% greater than or less than point of the distribution, and s_g is equal to the ratio of the 84% size to the 50% value or the 50% value divided by the 16% value. Stated another way, the geometric mean and standard deviation can be calculated by taking the logs of the original data, calculating the arithmetic median and standard deviation, and then taking their antilogs.

The key criteria of the log-normal distribution of particle size have been summarized by White (1963) and Stockham (1979).

1. The distribution is completely specified by the two parameters, the geometric median particle size, d_g, and the

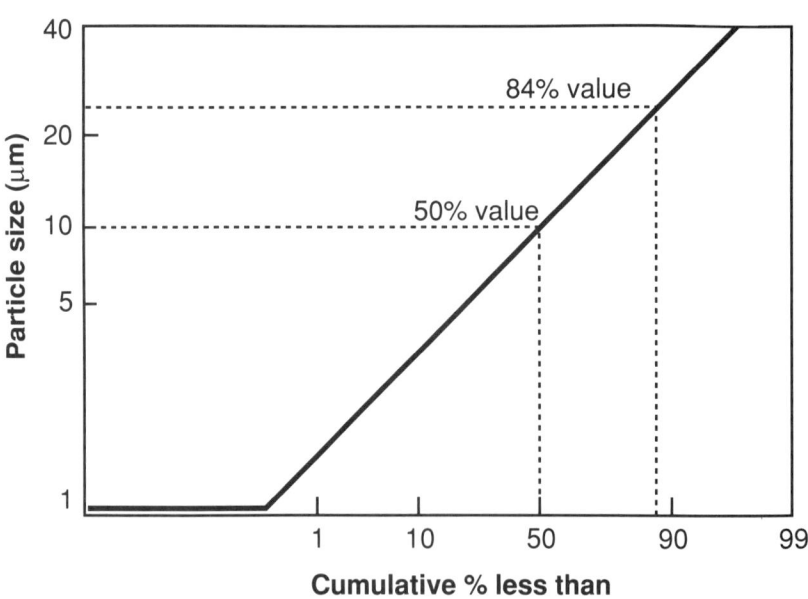

Figure 10. Cumulative-log-probability curve for log-normal distribution.

geometric standard deviation, σ_g. For a log normal distribution, the coefficient of variation (CV) or relative standard deviation is equal to and is constant regardless of the mean.

$$CV = 100 \frac{SD}{mean}$$

2. Conversions among the various particle-size parameters and statistical diameters may be expedited mathematically and graphically by use of transformations, notably those of Hatch and Choate (1929).

3. The geometric standard deviation is identical for all methods for specifying the particle-size distribution, whether by particle number, surface, mass, or any other quantity of the form kd^n where d is the diameter and k is a parameter common to all particles. Plots of the cumulative distribution on log-probability paper are then parallel straight lines for number, mass, or surface.

4. Values for the arithmetic mean, median, and mode are easily calculated.

$$d_{av} = \text{mean diameter} = \text{antilog}$$
$$(\log d_g + 1.1512 \log^2 \sigma_g)$$
$$d_{1/2} = \text{median diameter} = d_g$$
$$d_o = \text{mode diameter} = \text{antilog}$$
$$(\log d_g - 2.303 \log^2 \sigma_g)$$

5. The geometric mean diameter, d_g, and the geometric standard deviation, σ_g, may be found by a simple graphical procedure as illustrated in Figure 10.

6. The geometric mean diameter, d_g, is equal to the median or central value of the distribution.

Table IV presents numerical data relating to a hypothetical log normal distribution. The data of Table IV can be plotted in frequency distribution graphs as shown in Figure 11. Here the number and weight distributions, respectively, are plotted against frequency.

Another method of representing particle population data of this type, is to plot the cumulative percentage either over or under a particular size versus particle size. This has been done in Figure 12 using the cumulative percent undersize. A sigmoidal curve results,

Table IV. Number Distribution and Weight Distribution for Log-Normal Particle Population

(1) Size Range (μm)	(2) Geo. Mean Size (d) (in μm)	(3) # of Particles in Each Size Range	(4) % n	(5) Cumulative % Frequency Undersize (#)	(6) nd	(7) nd²	(8) nd³	(9) Weight % nd³	(10) Cumulative Weight Frequency Unders
0.0–2.0	1.4	1	0.3	0.3	1	2	3	—	—
2.0–4.0	2.8	36	10.9	11.2	101	282	790	0.3	0.3
4.0–6.0	4.9	87	26.4	37.6	426	2089	10235	3.8	4.1
6.0–8.0	6.9	71	21.5	59.1	490	3380	23324	8.7	12.9
8.0–10.0	8.9	54	16.4	75.5	481	4277	38068	14.3	27.1
10.0–12.0	11.0	39	11.8	87.3	429	4719	51909	19.5	46.6
12.0–14.0	13.0	21	6.4	93.6	273	3549	46137	17.3	63.9
14.0–16.0	15.0	11	3.3	97.0	165	2476	37125	13.9	77.8
16.0–18.0	17.0	6	1.8	98.8	102	1734	29478	11.0	88.8
18.0–20.0	19.0	3	0.9	99.7	57	1083	20577	7.7	95.5
20.0–22.0	21.0	1	0.3	100.0	21	441	9261	3.5	100
		Σ = 330	100		2546	24,032	266,907	100	

Particle Population Analysis 291

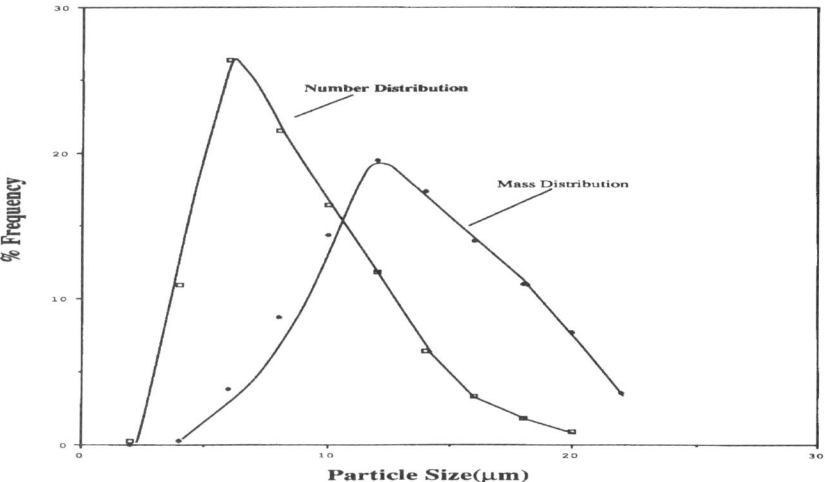

a. Arithmetic distribution.

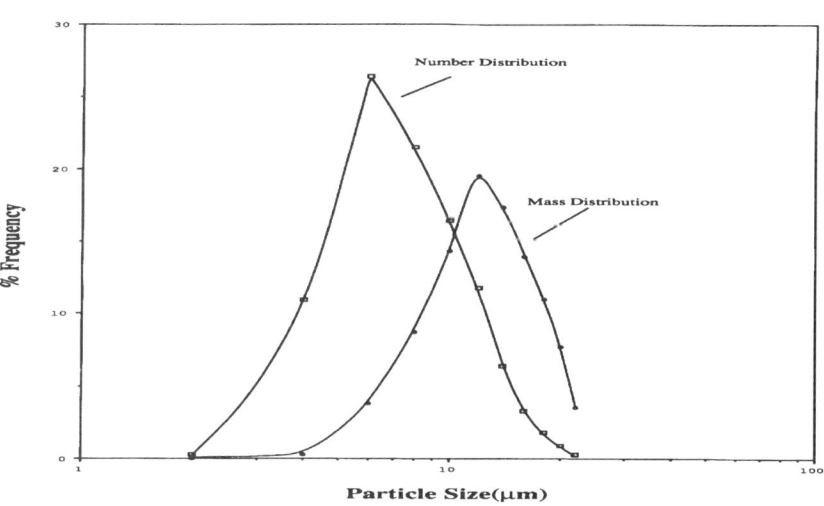

b. Log distribution.

Figure 11. Frequency distribution plots of data in Table IV.

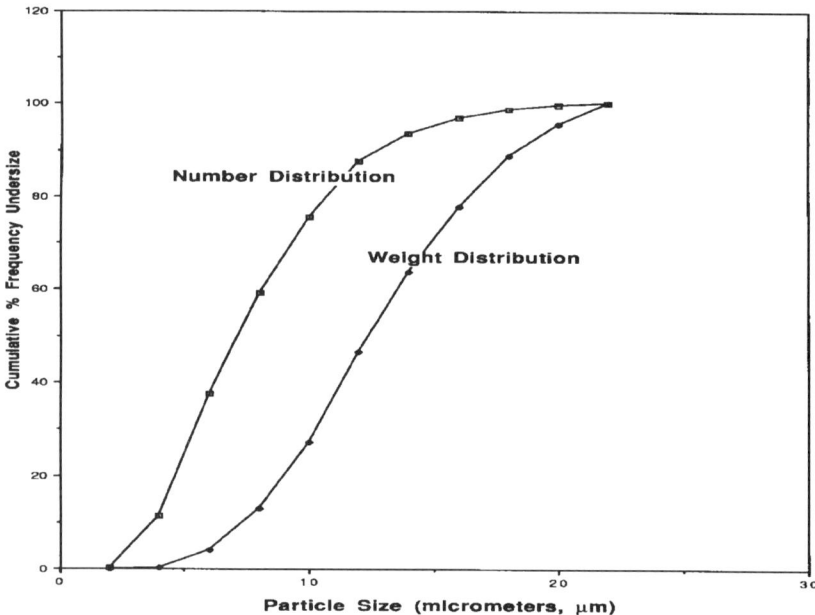

Figure 12. Frequency distribution plot of data in Table IV showing log-normal relation.

with the mode being that size at the greatest slope. If both weight and number distributions are plotted, a closed curve resembling a hysteresis loop results.

A log probit plot (percent less than) of the data from Table IV is shown in Figure 13. The reference point used is the logarithm of the particle size equivalent to 50% on the probability scale, that is, the 50% size. This is the geometric mean diameter, d_g. The slope is given by the geometric standard deviation, σ, which is the ratio

$$\frac{50\% \text{ size}}{16\% \text{ undersize}} \text{ or } \frac{84\% \text{ undersize}}{50\% \text{ size}}.$$

The data in Table IV are shown as a size-number distribution. Frequently, the analyst may be interested in obtaining data based on a weight, rather than a number, distribution. This can be done using a technique such as sieving, but it will often be more convenient to simply convert the number distribution to a weight distribution. Two approaches to obtain this data are available. In Table IV, such an estimate of the weight distribution has been obtained

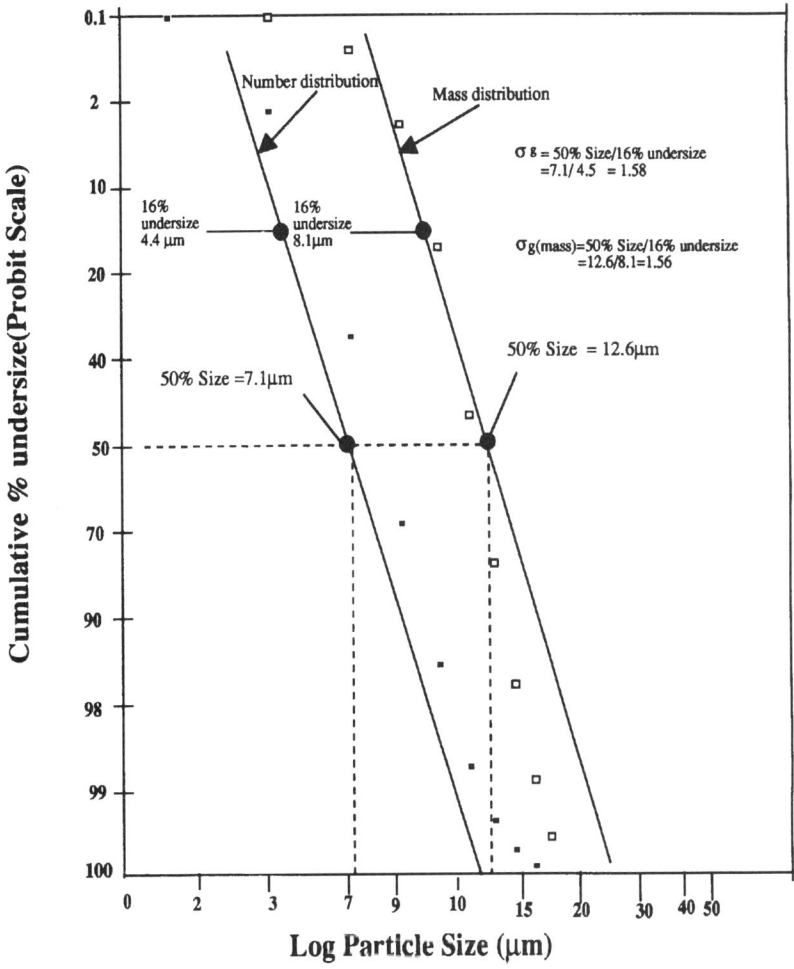

Figure 13. Log-probability plot of distribution given in Table IV.

by calculating the values shown in columns 9 and 10. These are calculated from the nd^3 values in column 8.

It is worthy of mention at this point that a number of commercially available software packages for use with microcomputers are extremely useful for "number crunching" related to particle population analysis and graphing results (see vendor listing). These programs have the great benefit of allowing analytical functions to be routinely performed, since the time required for obtaining a numerical or graphical result is a small fraction of that required if a calculator is used. Examples of such software include *STA-GRAPHICS®, Lotus,* and *EXECUSTAT®*.

Distribution of Extraneous Particle Counts

As discussed in the introduction, the size-number data for particle populations (in products such as parenteral solutions) sometimes follows a log-normal distributions. In some cases, two or more extraneous particle populations may be present (e.g., starch grains and wear fragments from machinery). The generally heterogeneous nature of extraneous particle populations would reasonably be expected to result in distributions less uniform than those of the particle of homogeneous material, such as drug powder. With regard to extraneous particle populations, it is often of more interest to know the distribution of counts at a specific size in a number of tested units rather than the population distribution. The former data may allow prediction of the probability that a given number of units in a batch will exceed limits values. This is shown in Figures 14 and 15. In these figures, the distribution of ≥ 10 µm counts (as determined using a light extinction particle counter to test a large number of units) is plotted against frequency of occurrence of a given count. The majority of units tested will have relatively low numbers of counts, 5–10. Higher counts are found at a much lower frequency. Conversion to a log scale on the abscissa (x-axis) results in a normal curve. A similar manipulation may be performed by plotting the frequency at which a given count (e.g., 10 particles/mL) occurs versus particle size. If a sufficient number of size channels are available on a counter, this plot can often be shown to fit a log-normal or Poisson distribution.

Average Diameters

As discussed above, log-normal particle-size distributions can be described by the values d_g and σ_g. These values, while describing the distribution, have little significance regarding various physical properties of the population. As a result, other average values have been derived to assist in determining or predicting physical properties of populations. An average diameter is the diameter of a hypothetical particle that in some way represents the total number of particles in the sample. Mean diameters representing length, surface area, volume, and specific surface may be determined. Some of the most commonly used average diameters are defined in Table V.

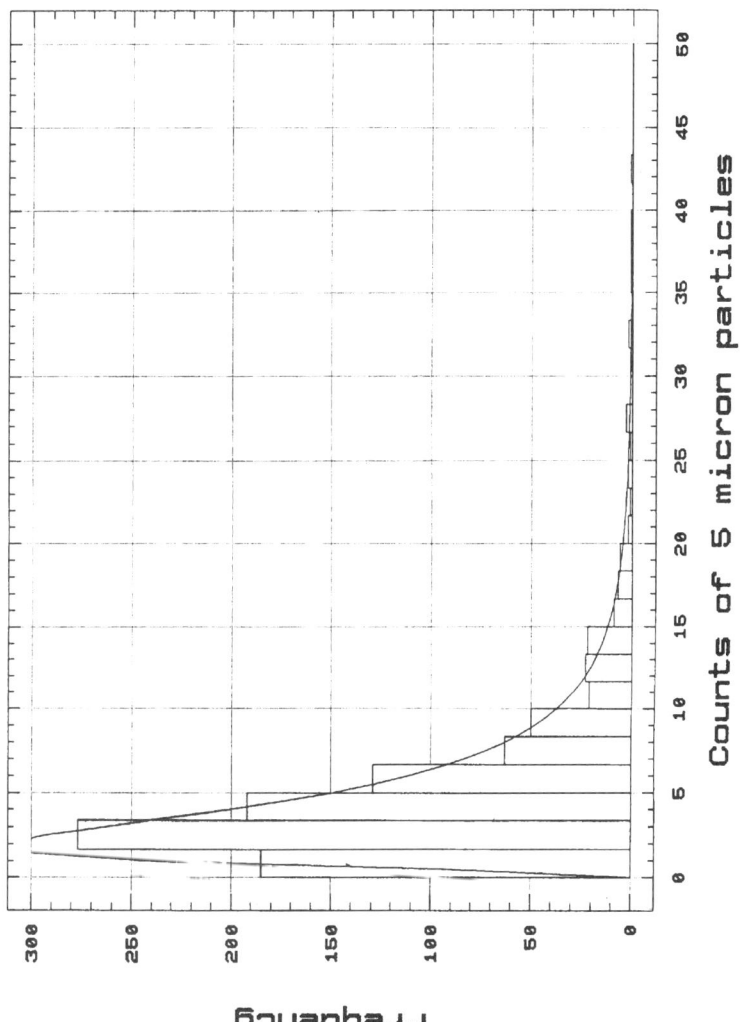

Figure 14. Skewed particle-size distribution: 10 μm counts in a parenteral solution with log-normal curve fit.

These mean measurements are based on instrumental or microscopic measurement of single particles. The notations refer to the mean measurement rather than that of a single particle. A wide variety of descriptive names, symbolic notations, and mathematical expressions are found in scientific and engineering literature for mean particle diameters. Those presented in Table V represent

296 *Pharmaceutical Particulate Matter*

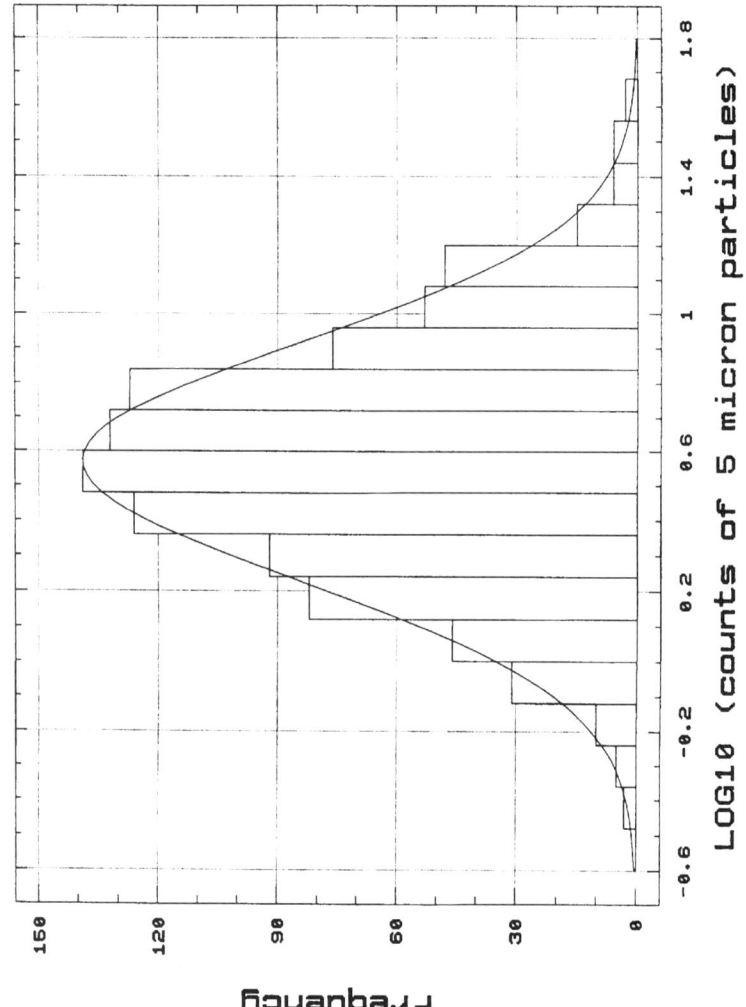

Figure 15. Log conversion data from Figure 14.

Table V. Mathematical Definition of Average Diameters (after Edmundson, 1967)

Average Diameter	Symbol	Mathematical Description	Definition
Length number mean	d_{ln}	$\dfrac{\Sigma nd}{\Sigma n}$	The sum of all diameters divided by the total number of particles
Surface mean diameter	d_{sn}	$\sqrt[2]{\dfrac{\Sigma nd^2}{\Sigma n}}$	The diameter of a hypothetical particle having average surface area
Volume Number mean	d_{vn}	$\sqrt[3]{\dfrac{\Sigma nd^3}{\Sigma n}}$	The diameter of a hypothetical particle having average volume and weight (also called the mass median diameter)
Geometric number mean	d_{gn}	anti log $\dfrac{\Sigma n \log d}{\Sigma n}$	Geometric mean diameter based on count frequency
Volume-surface mean diameter	d_{vs}	$\dfrac{\Sigma nd^3}{\Sigma nd^2}$	The average size based on the specific surface per unit volume
Volume-weighted mean diameter (also DeBroucker mean)	d_{wm}	$\dfrac{\Sigma nd^4}{\Sigma nd^3}$	The average size based on the weight of the particles

some of the more frequently used diameters. The presentation of these diameters by Edmundson (1967) is probably the most easily understood. The calculation of the various diameters from a set of data is illustrated in Table VI.

$$d_{ln} = \frac{\Sigma nd}{\Sigma n} = 11.9 \ \mu \qquad d_{vs} = \frac{\Sigma nd^3}{\Sigma nd^2} = 26.9 \ \mu$$

$$d_{vn} = \sqrt[3]{\frac{\Sigma nd^3}{\Sigma n}} = 17.9 \ \mu \qquad d_{sn} = \sqrt[2]{\frac{\Sigma nd^2}{\Sigma n}} = 14.6 \ \mu$$

$$d_{gn} = \text{anti log} \ \frac{\Sigma n \log d}{\Sigma n} = 9.7 \ \mu \qquad d_{wn} = \frac{\Sigma nd^4}{\Sigma nd^3} = 39.8 \ \mu$$

The volume-surface mean diameter, d_{vs}, is one of the most important averages in pharmaceutical particle population analysis. It will usually fall between other means that emphasize the small or large particle contribution to a sample, and it is inversely proportional to the specific surface of the sample. The specific surface of spherical particles (Edmundson, 1967) is:

$$S_w = \frac{\text{total surface area of particles}}{\text{total weight of particles}}$$

The usefulness of a term relating surface area to volume in pharmaceutical powders is obvious, since the surface area per unit weight of drug materials will frequently be a key factor in determining their activity.

Instrumentation and Methods

The instrumentation applied for particle-size distribution analysis of particle populations can generally be divided into two types (Weiner and Fairhurst 1989). Microscopes, light extinction counters, and Coulter counters deal with particles as discrete entities; in the microscope particles are sized and counted singly and in these two types of counters, each individual particle is represented by a single electronic pulse. Other types of light scattering instruments, such as photon correlation spectrometers, laser diffraction instruments, and nephelometers (Knollenberg 1990; Lieberman 1990), measure collective or interactive particle

Table VI. Calculation of Average Diameters

Particle Size interval μ	Geo. Mean, μ d	Freq. of Occurrence n	Cumulative Frequency of n, %	nd	n log d	nd²	nd³	Cumulative Frequency of nd³ %	nd⁴
1.0–1.5	1.2	3	0.3	4	0.2	4	5	—	6
1.5–2.0	1.7	5	0.7	9	1.2	14	25	—	42
2.0–3.0	2.4	20	2.5	48	7.6	115	277	—	664
3.0–4.0	3.5	85	10.3	298	46.3	1041	3644	—	12755
4.0–6.0	4.9	110	20.3	539	75.9	2641	12941	0.1	63413
6.0–8.0	6.9	200	38.5	1380	167.8	9522	65702	0.3	453342
8.0–12.0	9.8	275	63.5	2695	272.6	26411	258828	1.3	2536512
12.0–17.0	14.3	175	79.4	2502	202.6	35786	511736	5.4	7317828
17.0–22.0	19.3	120	90.3	2316	154.3	44699	862686	13.6	16649856
22.0–30.0	25.7	70	96.6	1799	98.7	46234	1188222	27.6	30537293
30.0–38.0	33.8	24	98.8	811	36.7	27419	926747	60.8	31324060
38.0–60.0	47.7	10	99.7	477	16.8	22753	1085313	78.1	51769446
60.0–80.0	69.3	2	99.9	139	3.7	9605	665625	88.7	46127820
80.0–100.0	98.4	1	100.0	89	2.0	7992	714517	100.0	63877818
		1100		13106	1086.4	234236	6296268		250670856

properties and provide no discrete count data. Sieves, sedimentometers, mobility analyzers, and porosimeters also fall into this second category. For discussions of the various methods of population analysis, the reader may consult the texts by Allen (1990), Kaye (1981), and the paper by Knapp and DeLuca (1988). Some of the more commonly used instruments, and means of population analyses are summarized in Table VII. The paper by Allen

Table VII. Particle Population Analysis Methods

	Nominal Range (μm)	Size Determined
Sieving		
• Dry	<0	Breadth
• Wet	2–74	
Microscopic		
• Optical	0.5–500	Martin's, Feret's, or equivalent circle diameter
• Electron	0.002–15	
Electrical Zone Sensing	0.05–500	Volume weighted diameter
Light Extinction	1–500	Equivalent circular diameter
Photon Correlation Spectroscopy	0.003–3.0	Volume-weighted mean diameter
Laser Diffraction	0.1–600	Volume-weighted mean diameter
Elutriation		Equivalent spherical diameter (ESD)
• Laminar flow	3–75	
• Cyclone	8–50	
Centrifugal Classification	0.5–50	ESD

(1990) provides an interesting and readable summary of the performance of different types of instruments.

The situation with regard to population analysis reminds one of the fable about the blind men and the elephant. Numerous instruments are available that perform an analysis involving different aspects of a population, and provide different "pictures" of the population.

	Nominal Range (μm)	Size Determined
Mercury Intrusion	0.01–200	Pore size
Centrifugal Sedimentation		
• Mass accumulation	0.05–50	ESD
• Photo-extinction	0.05–100	ESD
• X-ray	0.01–5	ESD
Gravity Sedimentation		
• Pipettes and hydrometers	1–100	ESD
• Photo-extinction	0.5–100	ESD
• X-ray	0.2–65	ESD
Hydrodynamic Chromatography		
• Packed column	0.03–2	ESD
• Capillary column	0.1–60	ESD
Cascade Impactors	0.05–30	Aerodynamic diameter
Gas Permeability	0.01–40	Mean surface weighted diameter
Gas Adsorption	0.005–50	Mean surface weighted diameter
Nephelometry	>0.1	Total light scattering (size dependent)

The methods in Table VII include both direct and indirect methods of measuring particle size. Direct methods comprise those in which the response of a sensor of some type responds to a phenomenon related to an individual particle or particles. This classification includes both the single particle counting instruments and those that produce "ensemble" measurements (e.g., diffraction instruments). Instruments that measure particle size indirectly, producing data in some form other than a particle size or average size (i.e., nephelometers, porosimeters, or adsorption devices) also produce this collective type of assessment of the population.

The means of analysis in Table VII may also be classified according to the parameter of particle size that they measure. Sieving and microscopy measure a maximum particle dimension (length). Sedimentation methods measure mass. Light extinction and light scattering methods (e.g., laser diffraction, photon correlation spectroscopy) produce data dependent upon the area and volume of the particle intersecting the illuminating radiation, with the amount of light removed from the beam by extinction phenomena dependent both upon scattering and absorption. Coulter-type counters measure particle volume based on a change in electrical resistance. Gas adsorption measurements provide estimates of mean particle size based on surface area.

The following critical definitions pertain to the operational characteristics of instruments that may be used in population analysis:

- **Accuracy:** Defines how close an experimental value is to the "true" value.

- **Precision:** Describes the variation in repeated runs.

- **Resolution:** Measures the minimum detectable differences between features in a size distribution.

- **Reproducibility:** An assessment of the extent of variation between different instruments, sample preparations, operators, and so forth.

- **Dynamic Range:** The range of measurement (typically particle size in microns) over which an instrumental response proportional to the measured particle size is produced.

The factor of dynamic range is a critical consideration in selection of an analytical method for use in population analysis. With sieving, the dynamic range of the analytical procedure is simply a function of the number of sieve screens used, and the range of opening sizes applied. The consideration is not as simple for instrumental forms of analysis. Single particle counters, such as the Coulter and Elzone counters, and light extinction counters, employ aperture tubes and sensors with a finite particle size range over which the pulse response produced is proportional to the particle ESD. The same kind of dynamic range limitation holds generally for light scattering sensors and instruments that generate count data based on diffraction methods. The skewed nature of many small particle distributions can cause problems even if the entire width of the distribution falls within the dynamic range of the instrument. The large numbers of smaller particles present may necessitate dilution of the sample to stay within instrument concentration limits; large particles may be diluted out of the sample and may not represented in the correct proportions in data collected. Issues regarding dynamic range and/or heavily skewed distributions may be dealt with by using a combination of methodologies or sensors.

In a common application of combined techniques, sieving may be used to fractionate a population prior to application of an instrumental analysis. Consider the case in which it is necessary to use a light extinction counter to analyze a drug powder with a size range of 0.5 µm to 100 µm. A laser diode sensor of that dynamic range is available, but the concentration limit is only 20,000 particles/mL. Above this concentration limit, counts from 0.5 µm to 10 µm particles begin to "swamp out" the sensor so that the larger particles that comprise a significant fraction of the mass of the powder cannot be adequately represented in the sample. In this case, air jet sieving may be used to separate size fractions of >10 µm, >20 µm, and so forth, which can then be analyzed separately, and the data combined to characterize the population. Similarly, sieving may be used to prepare fractions for analysis with different sensors. Sensors or means of analysis with widely differing dynamic range may also be used to effect a fractionation of the population. Careful attention must always be paid to what happens to the "uncounted" pulses from particles not within the dynamic range of a specific sensor, and coincidence effects must be kept in mind. If different counter types are to be applied, the operational principles and counting efficiencies of each should be well known to the operator.

Nephelometry

Nephelometry provides the most widely used means of measuring the combined light scattering properties of a particulate matter suspension. Particles dispersed in a liquid (or gaseous medium), whatever their size, scatter light. When a collimated light beam is directed into a particle suspension, the intensity of the light beam viewed directly through the suspended medium is diminished. Some portion of the light is scattered at various angles away from the axis of the beam path. Measurement of the scattered light intensity is the basis of nephelometry (Hausdorff and Coates 1982; Van de Hulst 1981). It is important to appreciate that the scattering associated with nephelometry involves no net loss in radiant power; only the direction of light propagation is affected. The intensity of radiation appearing at any angle is dependent upon the number of particles, their size and shape, the relative refractive indexes of the particles and the medium, and wavelengths of the radiation. The relationship among these variables is complex. A theoretical treatment is feasible, but because of its complexity, it is seldom applied to specific analytical problems. In reality, most nephelometric and turbidimetric procedures tend to the highly empirical (Drewel et al. 1990).

The intensity of light scattered at any particular angle is a function of the concentration of scattering particles, of particle size and shape, of the wavelength of light, and of the difference in refractive indices of the particle and the medium (Kerker 1969). For a particle that is small compared to the wavelength of the light, the scatter depends upon the area intercepting the beam, and so is proportional to the square of the effective radius of the particle. The total scatter from a number of particles, assuming no multiple scattering interactions, is simply the sum of the individual scattering, and the net absorbance of the system is directly proportional to the concentration of particles. For particles with a size approximating the wavelength of the incident radiation, the intensity of scatter is inversely proportional to the fourth power of the wavelength of the light.

A (ratio) nephelometer of contemporary design is shown in Figure 16. This figure represents a simplified diagram of the instrument's optical configuration. A beam of light is directed through the test sample. Detectors are placed to measure the 90-degree scatter, the forward-scattered light, and the light transmitted through the sample. Excellent linearity and color rejection are attained by electronically comparing the ratio of the output of the 90-degree detector to the sum of the other two detectors. The design of the optical system makes the effect of stray light negligible.

Particle Population Analysis **305**

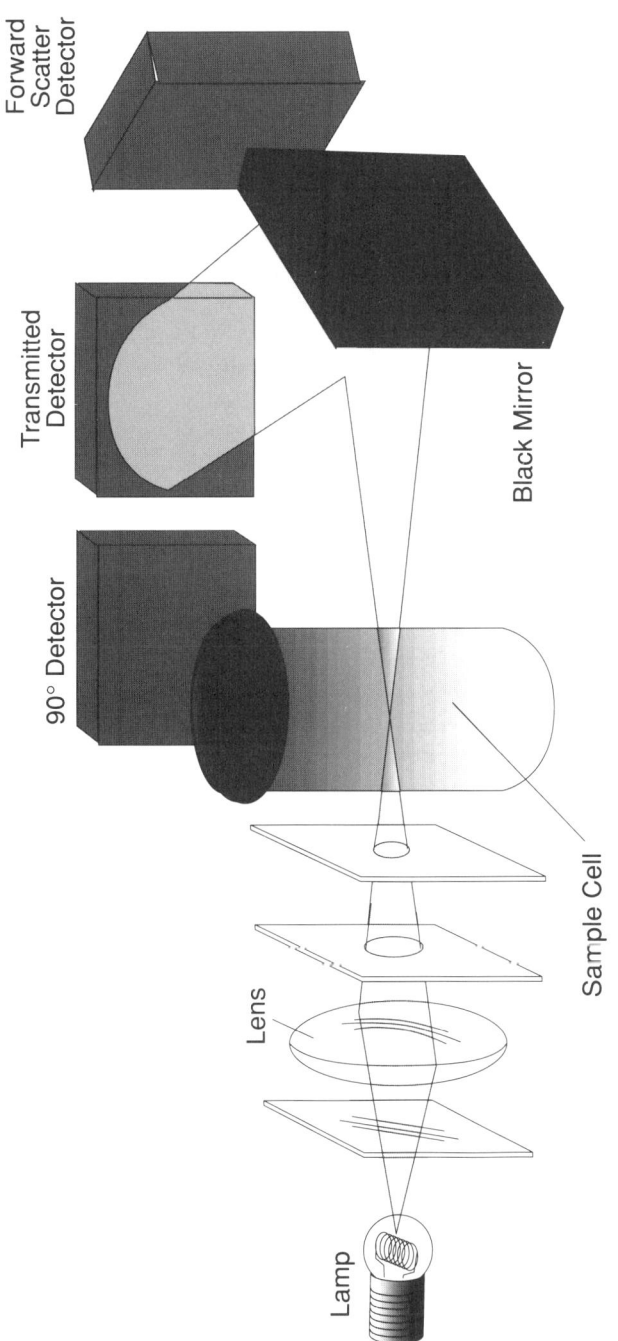

Figure 16. Ratio nephelometer (Hach Company).

Laser Diffraction

This technique is sometimes called Fraunhofer diffraction, but instruments operating on the principle of laser diffraction may not be based purely on Fraunhofer theory (Elias 1972). The Malvern MasterSizer instrument is probably the most widely used of this type. In this instrument, as shown in Figure 17, the light from a 1 mW He-Ne laser is passed through a dispersion of particles in some suspending medium. The diffracted light is focused onto a multiple-element annular ring detector. For a particle of given size in the range 0.2 µm to 600 µm, the intensity maxima in the diffraction pattern will be size-determined, so that the light intensity at different radii on the detector serve as a measure of particle size. The measurement thus obtained for the components of a population are volume dependent to a first approximation. The data from these instruments are highly reproducible and rapidly obtained (Dodge 1984) and operational calibration is rapid and reproducible (Hirleman 1987). The instrument is widely applied in the measurement of particle-size distributions of powders dispersed in air or water (e.g., drug powders or emulsions). The paper by Meury (1987) provides an excellent perspective regarding use of this instrument for pharmaceutical powders.

The term *Fraunhofer diffraction* applied to these instruments is somewhat misleading. First, the principle of Fraunhofer diffraction functions only above about 1.5 microns. These instruments attempt to use classical/Mie scattering theory to approximate the size distribution below that point. This is done typically by measuring the absolute scattering intensity at several "large" angles, far from the near-forward direction (where the Fraunhofer diffraction rings occur for diameters larger than 1.5 microns). This technique is difficult and by no means guarantees reasonable accuracy below 1.5 microns. For example, photon correlation spectroscopy instruments are typically much more accurate in this size range (provided there are not significant numbers of larger particles present, which would disturb the baseline of the autocorrelation function and, therefore, its deconvolution and the subsequent particle-size analysis. Furthermore, Mie scattering cannot be used for particle diameters smaller than about 0.12 micron (120 nm), below which there is essentially no angular dependence of the scattered intensity. There is usually poor resolution of these instruments in the Mie region.

Secondly, in the larger-particle region where Fraunhofer diffraction occurs, there is also generally poor resolution with these instruments. Bimodal distributions must generally by substantially

Particle Population Analysis **307**

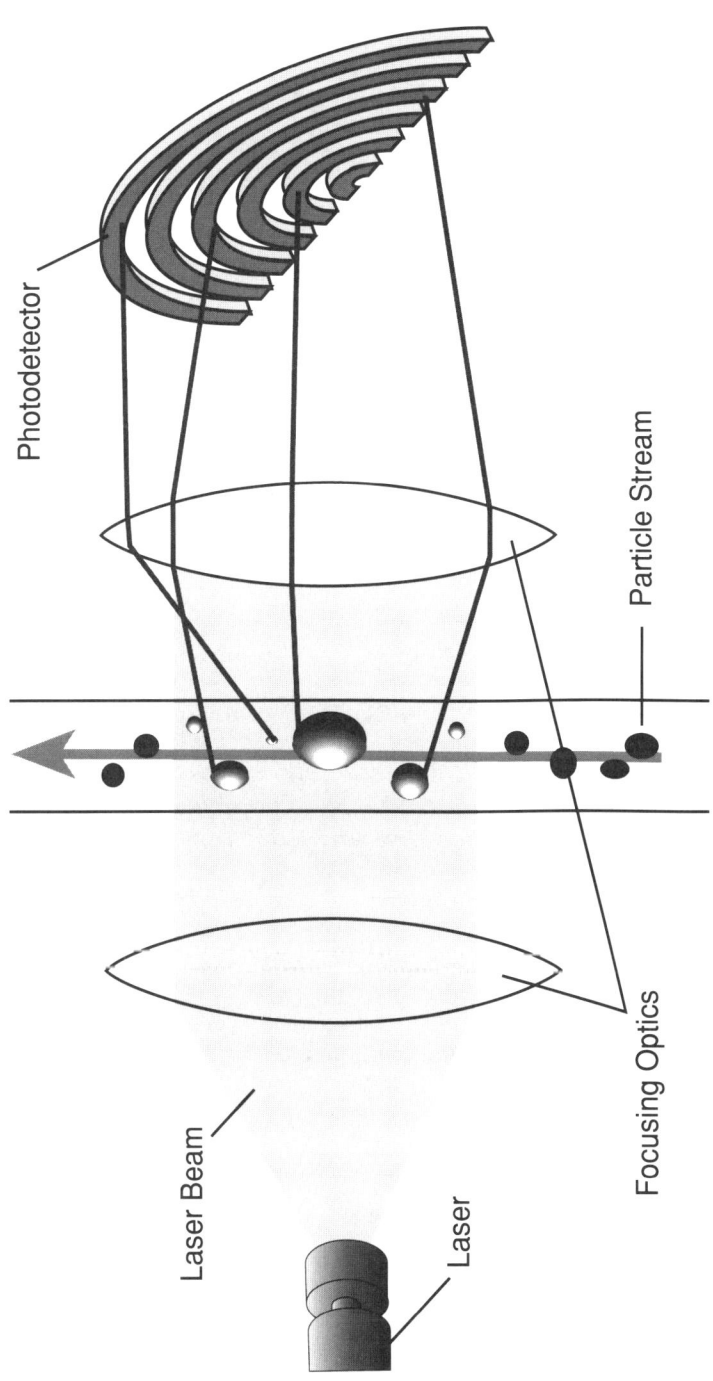

Figure 17. Laser diffraction analysis.

separated to insure detection; otherwise, a single, very wide peak would result. This limitation is particularly relevant in the case of pharmaceutical applications, where one frequently wishes to quantitate the existence of a "tail" of larger particles at the high end of an otherwise simple, single-peak distribution. This tail may consist of a relatively small number of particles, where the total mass or volume of that tail is very small compared to the rest of the distribution. Fraunhofer-based instruments generally do a very poor job of characterizing that tail, in either quantitative or qualitative terms. In fact, because of the nature of the data inversion employed, it is frequently the case that completely spurious peaks will occur in the computed distribution, "driven" by the presence of the large-particle tail. Fraunhofer-based instruments are ideal for monitoring the manufacturing process—approximate mean diameter and approximate polydispersity, which are highly reproducible from day to day, sample to sample. These instruments are not suited to making decisions based on subtle quality issues, such as the number of particles larger than a certain size, for the reasons stated above.

Terry Allen (1990) has carried out an extensive study over the past several years, comparing the absolute accuracy (precision) and reproducibility of several sizing technologies, including: Fraunhofer diffraction, sedimentation (both under gravity and centrifugal force fields), disk centrifugation (Joyce Lobel and Brookhaven), and resistive pore (Coulter). Four types of BSR quartz standards, having relatively narrow, log-normal type size distributions, where the four mean diameters vary from about 1.5 microns to 100+ microns were used.

Allen found that the Fraunhofer instruments all have the best reproducibility on a mass- or volume-weighted basis. (Interestingly, the difficulty with any single-particle counting/sizing instrument, whether "Elzone"-type or light-extinction type, is that the addition of a single large "dirt" particle is enough to compromise the volume-weighted performance on a comparative basis. That single particle, if large enough, can contribute a large amount of volume, and therefore hurt the reproducibility of distributions on a volume-weighted basis. Of course, the number-weighted distributions are essentially perfect.)

These studies also showed that the absolute accuracy of the Fraunhofer instruments is the worst of all the types considered, with deviations as large as 35–40% (i.e., in the mean diameter) observed. Furthermore, these deviations will vary widely from instrument to instrument for a given BSR size standard (because of differences in the algorithms for inversion of the diffraction data:

intensity vs. angle), as well as from standard to standard, for a given instrument (again, algorithm related). It was also demonstrated that the best instruments, in terms of absolute accuracy, are the electrical zone sensing or light extinction counters. This, of course, is not surprising, because no inversion algorithms are required to obtain the distribution. Light extinction instruments should show very similar accuracy.

Photon Correlation Spectroscopy

Conventional (static) nephelometry provides no measurement of the sizes of particles involved in the total scattering interactions (Hirleman 1990). Dynamic light scattering or photon correlation spectroscopy (PCS) is, in essence, a dynamic nephelometry whereby the size-dependent Brownian motion of particles (3 nm to 3 µm) is used to perform a population distribution analysis. This mode of analysis has also been termed Quasi-elastic light scattering (QELS) and intensity fluctuation spectroscopy (IFS) (Fairhurst and McFadden 1989; Weiner and Tscharnuter 1987). These instruments (Malvern, Nicomp, Coulter, Brookhaven) all operate according to the same general physical principle shown in Figure 18 (Swithenbank et al. 1977). A laser beam is focused into a cell containing suspended particles. A small fraction of the incident light is scattered by the particles and collected at some angle φ (usually 35–90°) by a sensitive photodiode or photomultiplier tube (PMT) detector. Each particle illuminated by the laser beam produces a scattered light wave whose phase at the detector depends on the position of the particle in solution. For a population of particles, the total scattered intensity at the PMT is the result of the superposition of all the individual scattered waves. The Brownian motion of the particles causes the relative phases of the light waves scattered from different particles to vary, which in turn causes the intensity at the detector to fluctuate in time.

The stationary detector records fluctuations in the scattered light intensity as particles undergo Brownian motion. These intensity changes occur within a millisecond or less, depending on particle size. Small particles produce fast fluctuations, while large particles produce slower fluctuations. Although individual fluctuations occur randomly, there is a well-defined time for their buildup and decay, roughly equal to the average time required for a pair of particles to change their separation by one-half the laser wavelength λ. To perform the analysis, one computes electronically the autocorrelation function $C(t)$ of the scattered intensity $I(t)$,

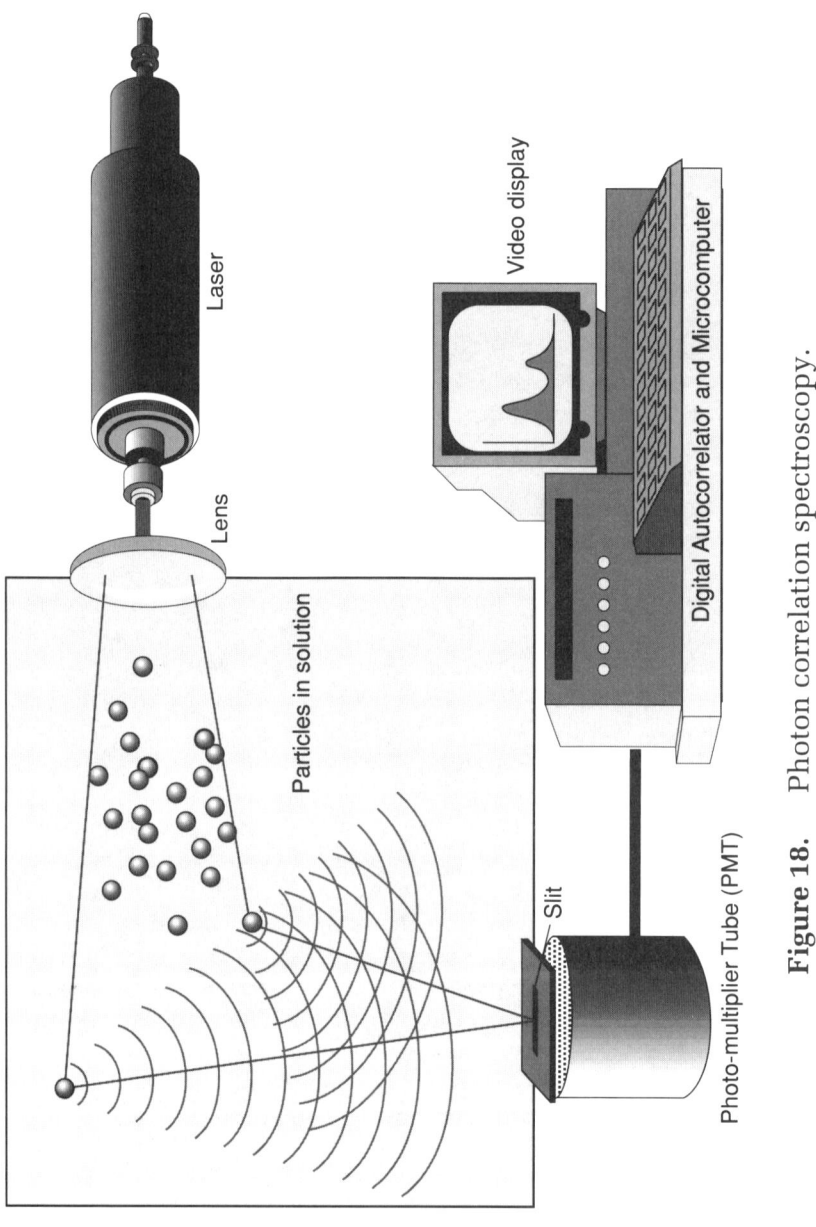

Figure 18. Photon correlation spectroscopy.

$$C(t) = <I(t') \times I(t'-t)>$$

This function is constructed by computing the product of the scattered intensity at an arbitrary time t' with the value at the earlier time $t' - t$. The symbol <> indicates a sum of such products taken at different times t'. A sufficient number of pairs of intensities are sampled (e.g., 10^5–10^7) to yield a reliable statistical average of $C(t)$. These data are used for the calculation of the population distribution of the scattering particles (Hirleman 1990). A digital autocorrelator is used to define the function $C(t)$ for many values of t, resulting in a smooth quasi-continuous function (curve or histogram).

While the physical construction of these instruments is quite similar, the programs by which they compute the autocorrelation function and distribution analysis are not (Weiner 1979; Elias 1972). A simple test for how well the autocorrelation function works is to evaluate the instrument in which one is interested using monosized and mixed latex sphere standards. The instrument that performs the analysis of standards the quickest with the highest accuracy, and the resolution of which provides the best estimate of the known distribution is probably the most suitable instrument for purchase.

The principle advantage of the PCS technique for particle sizing is that it yields an absolute measurement; that is, a PCS-based instrument is inherently self-calibrating, requiring no particle-size standard per se. The calibration is determined by the wavelength of a laser, the period of a crystal-controlled clock, the scattering angle, and physical parameters of the suspending medium (viscosity and index of refraction), all of which can be determined. A PCS measurement of particle size is immune to normal analog-type drifts, such as changes in laser power or detector sensitivity. Furthermore, the measured diffusion coefficient is unaffected by either the composition of the particles or their concentration, provided the suspension is sufficiently dilute that interparticle interactions are negligible. Additional advantages of the PCS technique include its speed (a typical measurement requires only a few minutes) and the fact that it does not in most cases disturb the system under investigation. This latter feature is especially important for emulsions and suspensions whose particle properties are a sensitive function of concentration and/or solvent composition (e.g., micelles and microemulsions). Most PCS instrumentation is relatively simple mechanically, possessing no moving parts or sophisticated optics that require careful alignment.

A further refinement of the dynamic light scattering measurement is found in instruments that use Doppler anemometry to measure particle size. Instruments of this type are typically applied in research rather than in collection of data on a routine basis, but they may be useful in specialized pharmaceutical applications. The Phase/Doppler principle is an extension of the Doppler principle, which is used in laser Doppler anemometry for determination of flow velocity. The Doppler principle is based on the fact that light scattered from moving particles will be of a different frequency than the light illuminating the particles, with the frequency or Doppler shift being proportional to the velocity. If a standard laser Doppler anemometer is combined with a second photodetector, the phase difference between the photo detector signals is (under certain conditions) a direct measure of the particle size. A third photodetector may be included to extend the dynamic range.

Microscopy and Image Analysis

Particle populations may also be analyzed using microscopic counting and sizing techniques as described in the chapter on microscopy. The reader is directed to the texts by Beddow (1980, 1983) and Beddow and Meloy (1980) for basic detailed descriptions of this mode of analysis. All of the counting techniques assume an even distribution of particles on a filter or an even distribution of a representative powder sample on a glass slide. The number of microscope fields to be counted is determined by the number of particles per field and the number of fields at a given magnification. As the number of particles per field decreases, the number of fields counted must increase in order to comply with the statistical strength required for the data. In common practice, the number of particles per field is adjusted to between 20 and 30 either by sample preparation or by changing the magnification. Under such conditions, it is sufficient to count 20 to 30 fields in order to achieve a reasonable level of confidence in the data obtained. The number of particles to be measured in a sample in order to obtain accurate and representative data also depends on the variety of sizes and the diversity of shapes. If the particle shapes are highly irregular or if there is a wide diversity of sizes, it may be necessary to count several thousand particles. On the other hand, if the samples are regular in shape and not too diverse in size, only 100 or so particles may be sufficient.

Measurement of size distributions by microscopy differs from the measurement of individual particles in several important aspects. It is essential that the sample contain representative particle types and numbers and that those particles counted be also representative. As with other forms of population analysis, it is particularly important to adequately represent the larger particle sizes, since most of the weight of the sample may be found in a relatively small number of large particles. It is also essential that sufficient particles be counted for good sampling in all size ranges and that samples be prepared so that all sizes are represented in the correct relative numbers. Generally measurement accuracy of the diameter of a single particle when a particle population is being analyzed does not require the highest level of precision, as errors due to defining the particle boundary or measurement will be offset by random errors. The time requirement is the major limitation of manual microscopic procedures for particle-size distribution measurement. Automated microscopy, on the basis of time required and precision, is generally far superior to manual microscopy for particle-size distribution analysis.

The British standard method for determining particle-size distribution utilizes the projected area diameter (Figure 19). Particles are sized by comparing their projected areas with the areas of reference circles on a standard graticule in the ocular (British Standard 3406, 1963; British Standard 3625, 1963). Each particle is assigned to a size class defined by two adjacent circles, which represent the size limits of that class. Thus, the distribution of sizes is obtained

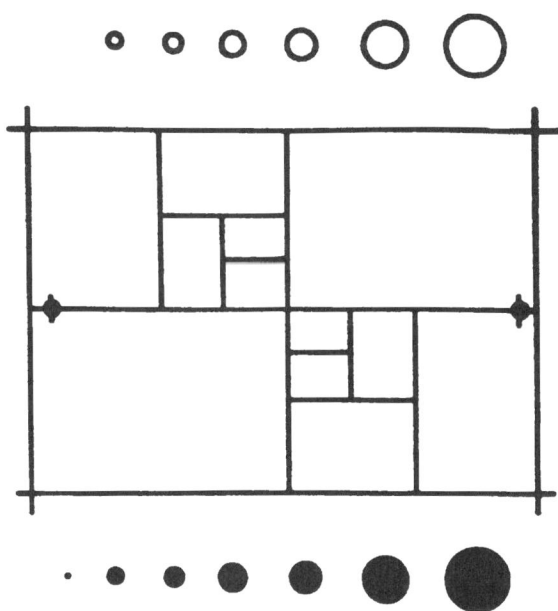

Figure 19. British standard graticule.

in terms of the diameters of circles having the same projected areas as the particles.

The circle areas double progressively, and the diameters increase by $\sqrt{2}$. The microscope method covers particles with diameters between 0.8 and 150 µm; thus, it may be necessary to change the objective magnification during a size determination. The rectangular grids of the graticule are used to relate the magnifications used to define the size and number of fields of particles to be counted and sized.

Particles collected from the environment or from a solution onto a filter membrane may also be enumerated by scanning electron microscopy (SEM). The techniques used in SEM counting are similar to those used with light microscopy. A membrane filter on which the sample has been collected is placed in the SEM and a minimum of 300–500 particles are counted. Image analysis systems are widely applied in this type of analysis. The preferred collection filter for SEM counting is a Nuclepore®-track etched filter membrane with a pore size no larger than 1/2 the diameter of the smallest particles to be counted. This type of filter membrane is preferred for SEM work because particles are easily visualized on the smooth surface. The pore size criterion ensures that the particles will be on the membrane surface, thereby allowing effective counting.

The filter with surface-adherent particles must be coated with an electron-dense element prior to SEM analysis if a high voltage instrument is to be used. Contemporary low-voltage scanning microscopes are capable of visualizing uncoated samples. Gold coating is preferred for optimum image resolution, but will interfere with the elemental analysis. Carbon coating is suitable for elemental analysis, but generally yields poorly defined images in a conventional instrument. Therefore, a two-step procedure is recommended if both particle identification and counting are to be performed on the same collection filter. First, the filter is coated with carbon for elemental analysis, then recoated with gold for SEM counting.

The scanning microscope is most frequently used to perform analysis of small particles (<5 µm). The simplest approach to particle sizing using the SEM is to take a micrograph of each field at appropriate magnification. The advantages of using micrographs for this purpose include the following:

- Operator fatigue is greatly reduced.

- Results can be independently verified by a second technician.

- Small particles are more easily measured.

- There is a permanent record of the results is obtained.

As an example of the use of this method provided in the Millipore handbook for *Detection and Analysis of Particulate Contamination* (1991), 25 random fields are recorded at a given magnification. These fields should cross the microscope field of view from left to right and top to bottom. Four additional randomly selected fields are recorded at the periphery of the four quadrants created by the first fields. Magnification is adjusted so that a total of 800 to 1000 particles are counted. The number of particles counted along with the number of fields are used in the formula shown below to determine the total number of particles on the filter.

$$\frac{I^2 \, AN \times 10^8}{m^2 \, LWn} = \text{total particles}$$

where N = number of particles counted;
  m = calibrated length of the micron marker, in μm;
  I = actual length of micron marker on the print, in cm;
  A = filtration area of collection filter, in sq. cm;
  L = length of micrograph, in cm;
  W = width of micrograph, in cm; and
  n = number of micrographs counted.

A calibration grid of known dimensions is then placed in the SEM. A micrograph, with a micron bar superimposed on it, is taken of the standard at the magnification used for counting. The length of the marker imprinted by the instrument is then compared to the standard. Adjustments to the micron bar are made if necessary. The size of the particles is then established by measuring the largest dimension of the particles with a ruler or magnifier and comparing this measurement with the micron bar of the micrograph. Recommended magnifications for specific particle sizes are shown in Table VIII.

Table VIII. Magnifications for Counting of Particles by SEM

Particle Size	Magnification sq. cm.	Size of Field (sq. cm.)	# of Fields
.200–.250	10,000×	1.0×10^{-6}	9.9×10^5
.150–.200	15,000×	4.5×10^{-7}	2.2×10^6
.100–.150	20,000×	2.5×10^{-7}	3.9×10^6
.075–.100	35,000×	8.3×10^{-8}	1.2×10^7
.025–.075	50,000×	4.0×10^{-8}	2.5×10^7

Image analysis (IA) is a generic term referring to any use of a computer-based system to process and analyze digitized images. An image analyzer interfaced to a light or electron microscope (Figure 20) can perform enumeration and sizing of particulate matter collected on a membrane filter to provide a result that is generally consistent with that obtained by manual microscopic analysis. To perform such an automated analysis, a microscopic field containing particulate matter is scanned by a television camera and digitized or broken down into electronically defined individual picture elements (pixels). The digitized image is a numerical representation of the original image that can be processed like any other data stored in computer memory. Each pixel gives an indication of the local image contrast or the gray level. The image formed is then segmented into features of interest (particles) and background (filter) based on user-established gray level thresholds. Finally, the particulate matter of interest is measured and results are printed out in the desired format, such as a particle number versus particle-size histogram.

Image analysis systems have been evaluated in the past with regard to their applicability to enumeration of particulate matter in parenteral solutions (Barber et al. 1989). In some studies, the correlation of IA data with that obtained by other counting methods has been generally poor. These results are attributable to the morphologic heterogeneity of particulate matter found in parenteral solutions and the fact that any particle count assay, microscopic or instrumental, incorporates positive and/or negative biases with regard to particles of different morphologies. Further, optimally configured IA systems were not available when earlier studies were conducted.

Particle Population Analysis 317

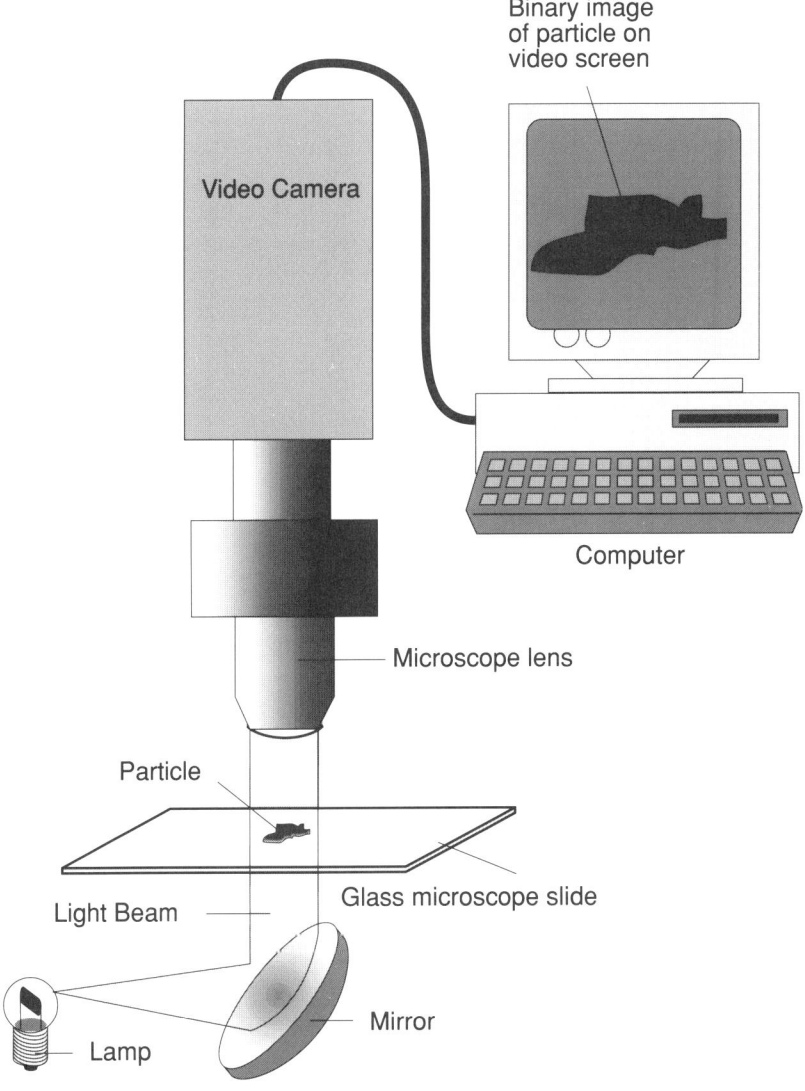

Figure 20. Light microscopic image analysis system.

Experience in image analysis and knowledge gained in evaluating currently available instruments suggests that image analysis has significant potential as a referee methodology for analysis of contaminants in parenteral solutions. An IA-based methodology appears capable of resolving difficulties with the manual microscopic compendial test and eliminating the error effects in light extinction particle counting. Laboratory technical personnel familiar with manual microscope operation can readily be trained to operate IA systems at the user level. Factors that must be carefully weighed prior to purchase include the relative complexity of the instrumentation, cost, and the required level of technical expertise for optimizing and maintaining the system purchased. Hardware is available on most SEMs that allows semiautomated counting and sizing of particles on a collection filter. If this automatic equipment is used, extreme care is required to ensure that the collection filter is very flat in the SEM. Otherwise, some of the particles will be out of focus and sizing errors will result.

Sieving

Sieve analysis is one of the simplest, most widely used methods of particle analysis, covering the approximate size range of 50 µm to 10 mm using standard woven wire sieves. A number of international and national standards are in place for sieves. The ASTM sieve range covers sizes from 635 mesh (20 µm openings) to 5/inch (ASTM specification E11-87). The apertures for the 400 mesh are 38 µm, and the wire thickness is about 26.5 µm. The USP specified sieve series (General Chapter <811> Powder Fineness) is shown in Table IX.

Table IX. Opening of Standard Sieves

Sieve Designation		Sieve Designation	
Nominal Designation No.	Sieve Opening	Nominal Designation No.	Sieve Opening
2	9.5 mm	45	355 µm
3.5	5.6 mm	50	300 µm
4	4.75 mm	60	250 µm
8	2.36 mm	70	212 µm
10	2.00 mm	80	180 µm
14	1.40 mm	100	150 µm
16	1.18 mm	120	125 µm
18	1.00 mm	200	75 µm
20	850 µm	230	63 µm
25	710 µm	270	53 µm
30	600 µm	325	45 µm
35	500 µm	400	38 µm
40	425 µm		

Wire mesh sieves are made from sieve cloth that is woven from wire, and the cloth is soldered and clamped to the bottom of open cylindrical frames. Although the apertures of woven sieves are described as square, they deviate from this shape due to the three-dimensional structure of the weave. Heavy-duty sieves for mechanical agitation are sometimes made of perforated metal plates with circular holes. Various other aperture shapes, such as slots for sieving fibers, are also available. Fine sieves are usually woven with phosphor bronze wire, medium with brass, and coarse with mild steel. Special purpose sieves are also available in stainless steel.

When division of a powder into multiple sieve fractions is desired, sieves are typically arranged in a stack of about five or more, with the coarsest at the top. A carefully weighed sample of the powder is placed on the top sieve. After the sieves are shaken for a predetermined period of time, the powder retained on each tared sieve is determined. Machine sieving is also carried out by stacking the sieves in ascending order of opening size, and by placing the powder on the top sieve. A closed pan (a receiver) is placed at the bottom of the stack to collect the fines, and a lid is placed at the top to prevent loss of powder. The stack is then vibrated for a fixed time and the residual weight of powder on each sieve determined. Results are usually expressed in the form of a cumulative percentage (greater than) in terms of the nominal sieve aperture. It is generally recommended that if losses during sieving exceed 0.5% of the original weight of powder, the test should be rejected. Preliminary hand sieving of the sample on the finest sieve may be carried out for the removal of dust prior to weighing; this dust will otherwise pass through the whole nest of sieves and prolong the sieving time, or percolate between sieves in the stack and increase weight loss.

The USP makes two important observations regarding the use of sieves: (1) For practical reasons, sieves are the preferred means of measuring powder fineness for most pharmaceutical purposes. However, their applicability does not extend into the particle size range of increasing interest with respect to attainment of prompt and complete gastrointestinal absorption of administered drugs. For the measurement of particles less than 100 µm in nominal size, devices other than sieves may be more useful. (2) The efficiency and speed with which particles pass through sieves varies inversely with the number of particles in the charge. The effectiveness of separation falls off rapidly when the depth of the charge exceeds a layer of 6 to 8 particles.

According to the USP method for determining powder fineness, a specific mass of sample is placed on the proper sieve in a mechanical shaker. The powder is then shaken for a specific period of time. The material that passed through one sieve and was retained on the next finer sieve, is collected and weighed. A sieved powder may then be assigned the mesh number of the smallest screen through which it passed, or that of the screen on which it is retained. Another convention is to assign the particles on the lower level the arithmetic or geometric mean size of the two screens.

Micromesh sieves are available from the Buckbee Mears Company (Minneapolis, MN) in aperture sizes from 5 µm to 150 µm (Figure 21). Other aperture sizes are available. The percentage open area decreases with decreasing aperture size, ranging from 2.4% for 5 µm aperture sieves, to 31.5% for 40 µm aperture sieves; extended sieving times can be expected for the smaller aperture sieves. These sieves are produced by a photoetching procedure. Basically, the photoetching process is performed as follows: A degreased metal

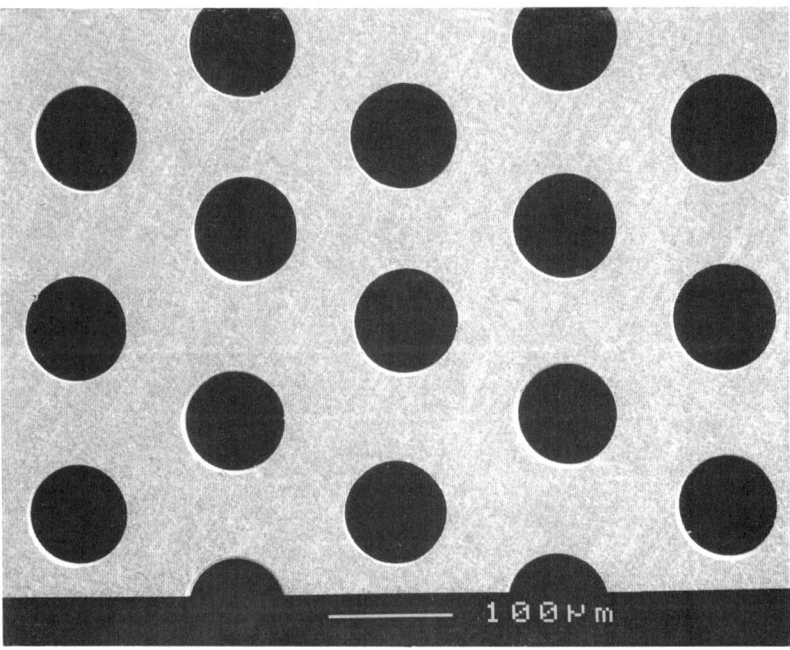

Figure 21. Photoetched metal microsieve (Buckbee-Mears, Inc.).

sheet is covered on both sides with a photosensitive coating. The desired hole pattern is then applied photographically to both sides of the sheet. Subsequently, the sheet is passed through an etching machine and the exposed metal is etched away. Finally, the photosensitive coating is removed. A supporting grid is made by printing a coarse line pattern on both sides of a sheet of copper foil coated with photosensitive enamel. The foil is developed, and the copper metal between the grid lines is etched away. The precision of this method gives a tolerance of ±2 µm for apertures up to 500 µm.

Sieving of finer particle powders may be enhanced by ultrasound. The Allen-Bradley sonic sifter is produced both in laboratory and industrial models. It is able to separate particles in the 20 µm to 20 mm range for most materials. It combines two motions to provide particle separation, a vertical oscillating column of air and a repetitive mechanical pulse. The oscillating air sets the sample in a periodic vertical motion that reduces sieve blinding and breaks down agglomerates.

Wet sieving may be used to obtain size fractions of a material suspended in a liquid or facilitate the separation of particles of a material that tends to agglomerate or cake when sieved dry. The simplest application consists of suspending the powder to be sieved in a liquid in which it is insoluble and pouring the suspension onto the top sieve of a stack, followed by washing the powder with more liquid while agitating the sieve stack by hand. Sieving devices are available that agitate and add the washing fluid automatically. In most of these methods, a stack of sieves is filled with a liquid and the sample is fed into the top sieve. Sieving is accomplished by rinsing, vibration, reciprocating action, vacuum, ultrasonics, or a combination of these influences. Commercial devices are also available in which the sample is placed in the top sieve of a nest of sieves and sprayed with water or other suspending liquid while the nest is being vibrated.

Manual wet sieving may be accomplished by moving single or multiple sieves up and down in a beaker filled with the sieving liquid, so that the direction of flow of the liquid through the sieve openings is continually reversed. This helps to prevent blocked apertures and disperse agglomerates. Depending on the type of sieve and the resistance to breakage of the particles during sieving, intermittent ultrasonic vibration may be used. Wet sieving may prove the only applicable method for some drug powders that form persistent agglomerates when dry sieved despite the application of intense mechanical vibration. The liquid will serve both to eliminate static charge and set up viscous shear forces that disperse agglomerates. For materials with high water solubility, apolar hydrocarbon liquids may be used as the suspending agent, but the analyst must beware of creating a fire hazard with flammable solvents used for this purpose.

The more recently introduced technique of jet sieving eliminates many of the problems of conventional sieving, including incomplete separation and agglomeration effects. This means of analysis uses a rotating air jet to fluidize the powder on the sieve, and may be applied to effect separation of particles at sieve cuts as small as 5 µm with some powders using precision sieves (Figure 22).

The principle of operation of the air jet sieve involves drawing air upwards through a sieve from a rotating slit, so that material on

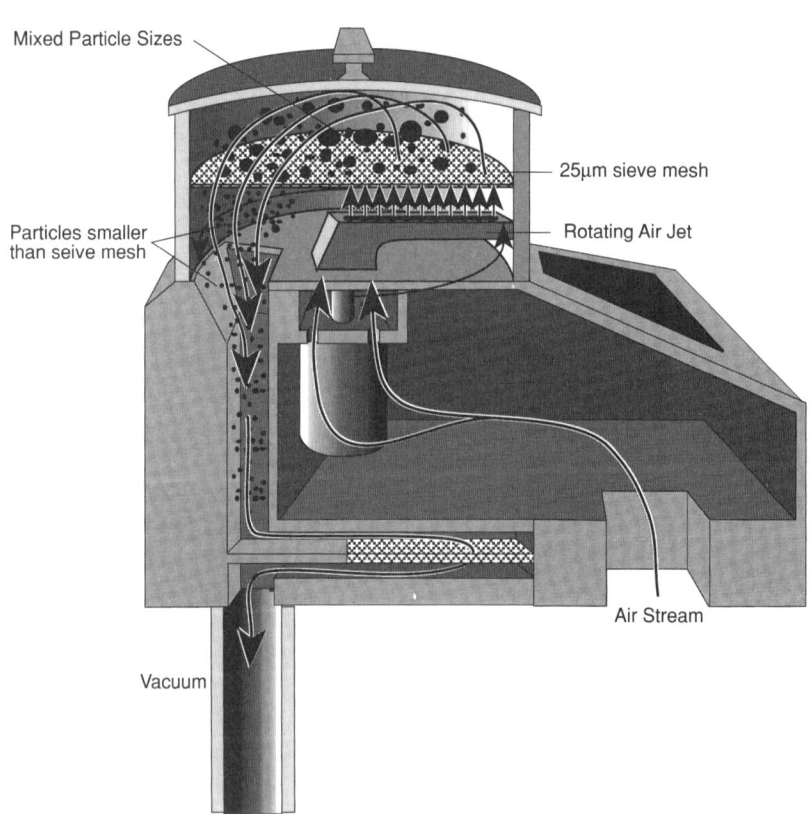

Figure 22. Micro jet sieve (Hosakawa Micron Inc.).

the sieve is fluidized. At the same time, a negative pressure is applied to the bottom of the sieve that removes fine particles to a collecting device (a filter paper) or to a vacuum cleaner. With this technique, there is a reduced tendency to blind the sieve apertures. The action is very gentle, making it suitable for brittle and fragile powders. Sieving is possible with some powders down to 5 µm. The reproducibility is much better than by hand or conventional machine sieving. Size analyses are performed by removal of particles from the fine end of the size distribution using a series of sieves of sequentially increasing size.

Most problems encountered in sieving have been known for many years and solutions have been proposed, but good reproducibility is sometimes not achieved in practice due to the failure to take steps to deal with these problems. Variation of sieving results can arise from a number of factors, including sieve loading and duration and intensity of agitation, particle agglomeration, and the presence of fines (or dust particles that are held up on screens in a manner unrelated to their size). Sieving can cause attrition of fragile granular materials such as drug powders. Care must be taken to ensure that reproducible techniques are employed, so that observed different particle-size distributions between batches of material are not due simply to different sieving conditions. Elongated particles, however, do not pass through sieve apertures as readily as cuboid ones.

Light Extinction Counting

As discussed in the chapter on instrumental counting, this method has become an indispensable technique in the analysis of extraneous particles in pharmaceuticals, owing to its ability to detect and accurately size individual contaminant particles down to 0.5 µm (Knapp and DeLuca 1988; Knapp and Abramson 1990). Areas of application include pharmaceutical solutions, semiconductor process liquids and hydraulic fluids. For these and other applications, extinction instruments are used for the ultimate purpose of excluding particles from products or materials. Light extinction counting also possesses several inherent characteristics that are ideal for measuring population distributions of a wide variety of particle suspensions, emulsions, and dispersions. These characteristics include relatively high resolution, wide dynamic range, high sensitivity, and reasonable precision.

To date, the light extinction technique has seen only limited application in the general field of particle-size distribution analysis. The principal reason for this limitation has been the need to perform extensive, often repeated, manual dilutions of a highly concentrated sample in order to avoid particle coincidence in the sensor, while still achieving an acceptable count rate to ensure adequate statistical strength of the data obtained. Application of light extinction counting in combination with autodilution (Nicoli and Elings 1991) and pulse height analysis (PHA) allows the multiple advantages of this mode of counting to be realized in particle-size distribution analysis (Nicoli et al. 1992). An instrument of this type currently available (Acusizer 770, Particle Sizing Systems Inc., Santa Barbara, CA) consists of five subsystems: autodiluter, optical sensor, pulse-height analyzer/counter (PHA), a system computer/processor, and a software controller (Figure 23). The autodiluter performs a continuous dilution of the concentrated sample suspension prior to its passage through the sensor. The PHA module continuously monitors the pulse rate during autodilution; when the particle concentration falls below the coincidence limit of the sensor (typically about 10,000/mL for commonly used sensors), the

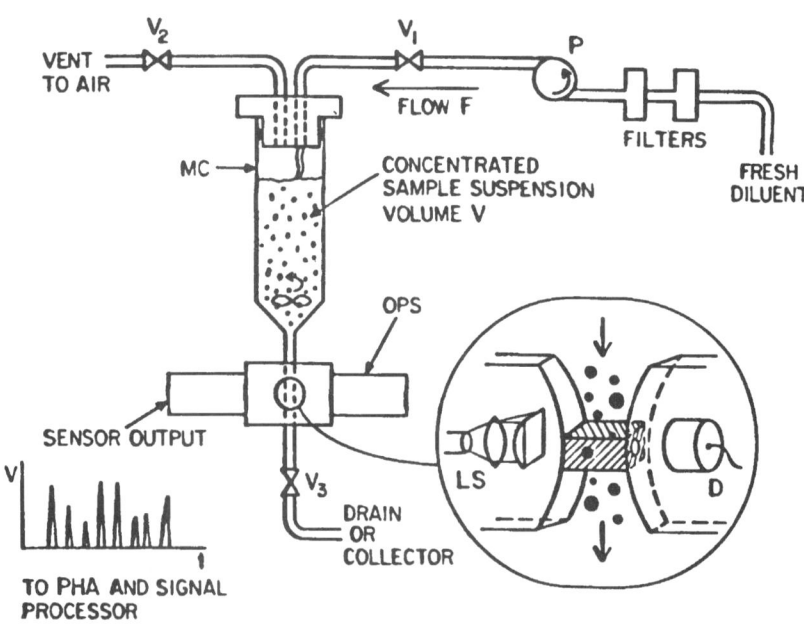

Figure 23. Autodilution mechanism for light extinction counter.

PHA unit begins collecting data. The resulting high-resolution particle-size distribution data can be displayed in real time on a display monitor as absolute particle counts versus diameter for each diameter channel (8 to 512), logarithmically spaced over the total size range covered by the optical sensor (e.g., 1.5 to 400 microns). Additional derived distributions (both differential and cumulative), based on number-, area-, and volume-weighting, are calculated from the measured population distribution with the caveats discussed earlier.

In use, a few drops of concentrated liquid suspension or several grams of dry powder are manually introduced into the mixing chamber of the instrument. The sample particles are mixed with diluent in the mixing chamber by means of a small magnetic stirrer. Under computer command, filtered diluent flows into the mixing chamber by means of a variable-speed, precision gear pump; the resulting positive pressure causes some of the suspension to exit the chamber and flow through the sensor, at a rate (typically 25 to 100 mL/min) that can be adjusted to an accuracy of better than ±10% using a precision flow gauge. The particle concentration, c, in the fluid entering the sensor decreases exponentially with time, t, according to:

$$c = c_o \exp(-t/\tau)$$

where c_o is the initial concentration of the particles in the chamber (assuming adequate mixing with diluent) prior to addition of fresh diluent, and τ is the characteristic decay time of the autodiluter. The latter quantity is given by V/F, where V is the volume of the liquid in the mixing chamber (typically 50 cc to 100 cc), and F is the flow rate (cc/sec) of diluent. The pulse rate is continuously monitored; as soon as the particle concentration falls below the coincidence limit of the sensor, data acquisition begins. Parameters for a representative analysis might be as follows:

Suspension volume in chamber	$V = 50$ cc
Diluent flow rate	$F = 60$ cc/min
Autodilution time constant	$\tau = 50$ sec
Assumed measurement time	$T = 1$ min
Assumed initial concentration	$c_o = 12{,}000$ particles/cc

The resulting total number of particles, N, which flow through the sensor and are sized is given by

$$N = c_o V[1 - \exp(-t/\tau)] = 419{,}283$$

which represents 70% of the total number of particles (equal to 600,000) present in the mixing chamber at the start of the measurement. If the measurement time is increased to 2 minutes, 90% of the particles will have been sized. Hence, in a relatively short time the system is capable of counting and sizing a very large number of particles, insuring excellent statistical accuracy and, therefore, reproducibility.

The attractiveness of the autodilution light extinction approach to particle-size distribution analysis can be best appreciated by comparing its result with those of alternative instruments based on "collective" techniques, in which a large number of particles of different sizes contribute simultaneously to the measured signal. The most popular instruments in this category are the widely used laser diffraction devices. Particle sizing instruments based on collective techniques are inherently limited in accuracy, precision, and resolution. The reader is again reminded that my use of the word *accuracy* pertains only to standards; any "accuracy" statement must be dependent on the means of analysis used. The raw detected signal must be mathematically "inverted," using an appropriate analysis algorithm, in order to estimate the distribution. In effect, these instruments must assume a shape for the distribution, using a relatively small number of parameters, and then minimize the error between the measured data and a calculated fit by adjusting the parameters.

This limitation is especially evident in the case of complex, polydisperse distributions, where a population of agglomerates or abnormally large particles lie above the main population of primary particles. In the case of an oil-in-water emulsion, this large size component may be caused by incomplete emulsification or fusion of primary droplets due to colloidal instability. In the case of powders, this large-particle "tail" in the particle-size distribution may be the result of incomplete grinding or milling, or agglomeration of primaries caused by poor dispersion.

Representative results obtained from the application of this analysis are shown in Figure 24. This sample consisted of a pharmaceutical oil-in-water emulsion. This product contains a large number of particles of submicron size that typically interfere with analysis of large (5 µm) particles that must be enumerated to assess the emulsion stability. Approximately $1/4$-million particles were sized during the 30-second period of autodilution and data acquisition. This particular sample is obviously well behaved, having a negligible "tail" due to agglomerates or abnormally large primary particles. The data for three successive 30-second intervals were

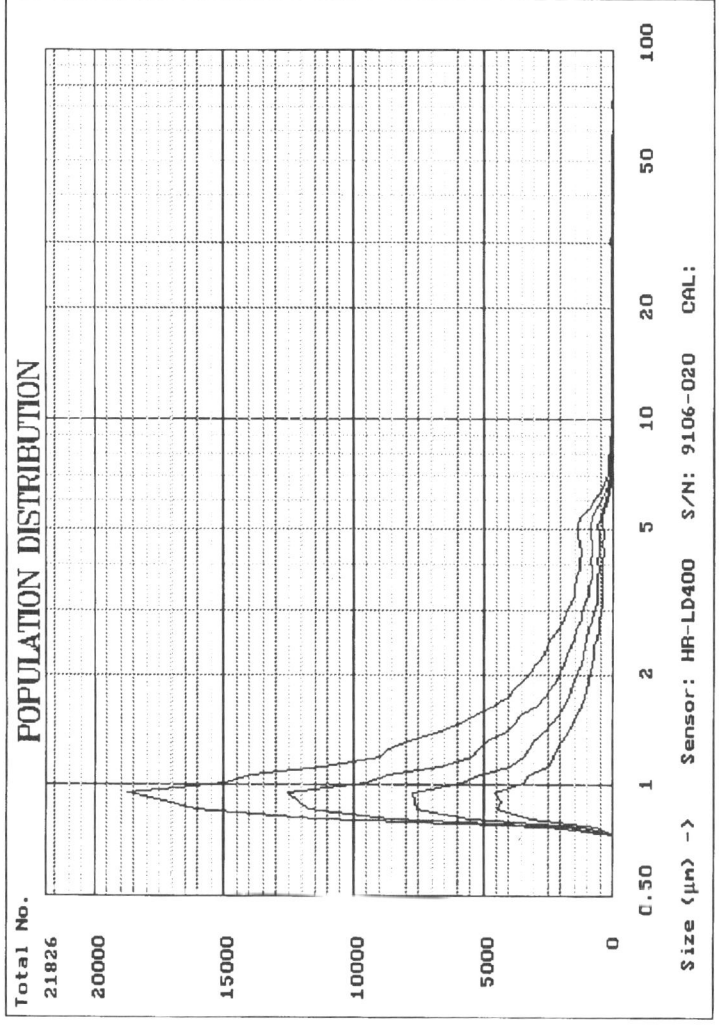

Figure 24. Particle-size distribution with sequential dilution.

acquired automatically during continuous autodilution of the starting suspension. There is a significant decrease in the number of particles counted for each diameter value with the passage of time as the concentration decreases. The number-weighted distributions for each of the three consecutive runs are nearly identical. This demonstrates the excellent reproducibility of the system. The discrepancies are obviously greatest where the number of (large) particles counted is smallest, owing to statistical fluctuations (proportional to the square root of the total count).

Sedimentation

Particle size may be indirectly determined by measurement of the rate of sedimentation in a gravitational field. George Stokes first elaborated a theoretical description of the motion of a sphere falling under the influence of gravity. The basic statistical equation on which sedimentation measurements are based is

$$d_{st} = \sqrt{\frac{18n \cdot \mu}{(p_q - p_L)g}}$$

where: d_{st} = diameter of the particle,
P_p = density of the particle,
P_L = density of the suspending fluid,
n = viscosity of the suspending medium,
g = acceleration due to gravity, and
μ = terminal velocity of the particle.

The equation holds only for spheres falling freely without hindrance at a constant rate. The law is applicable to irregularly shaped particles of various sizes, if one realizes that the diameter obtained is a relative particle size equivalent to that of a sphere falling at the same velocity as that of the particle under consideration. The particles must not be aggregated or clumped together in the suspension, since such clumps would fall more rapidly than the individual particles, and erroneous results would be obtained. Agglomeration, of course, as a source of artifact is not peculiar to this method. A deagglomerating agent must be found for the sample that will keep the particles free and separate as they fall through the medium. For Stokes' Law to apply, a further requirement is that the flow of dispersion medium around the particle as it sediments is laminar or streamlined. In other words, the rate of sedimentation of a particle must not be so rapid that turbulence is set up, since this in turn will affect the sedimentation rate.

Historically, the sedimentation principle has been applied in a number of analytical instruments, such as the Joyce-Loebl and LADAL disc centrifuges. The current technology used frequently involves a disc centrifuge with X-ray, white light, or laser light attenuation used to measure the concentration of the suspended particle ractions with time of centrifugation (Figure 25). The use of

Particle Population Analysis 329

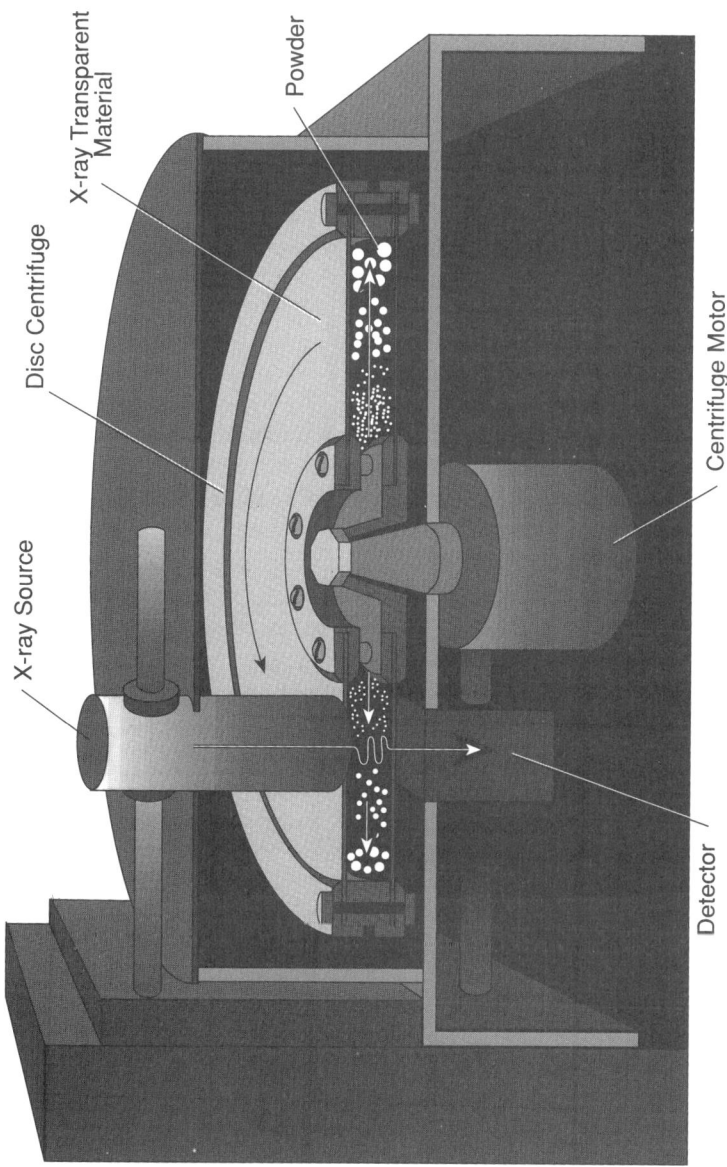

Figure 25. X-ray disc centrifuge.

X-ray detection is limited to materials that are capable of adsorbing X-rays efficiently enough to allow measurements to be made (e.g., oxides, ceramics). Organic materials of common interest in the pharmaceutical industry require the use of light extinction (Weiner et al. 1991; Coll 1991). The attenuation of the light or X-ray beam is proportional to the concentration of the suspension at the measurement radius (i.e., the concentration of particles at the size being present in the beam falling upon the X-ray detector). The largest size present in the beam may be calculated using Stokes' equation. This mode of analysis represents a somewhat specialized technique with regard to the analysis of particle populations of interest in pharmaceutical science; current generation instruments are compact, user friendly, and simplify the technique through the application of computer-based data collection (Figure 26).

Adsorption and Porosimetry

This section provides only a summary discussion of the principle of these methods. More detailed information may be obtained from the books by Allen (1990) and Kaye (1981) or the text by Gregg and Sing (1981). Both modes of analysis constitute indirect measurements of the characteristics of particle populations, gas adsorption (typically with nitrogen) providing a measure of surface area of a powder, and porosimetry (using mercury or nitrogen gas) giving an estimate of numbers of pore openings at various sizes in compacted or compressed materials. In some cases the information obtained by these two forms of analysis is not attainable by other means. The

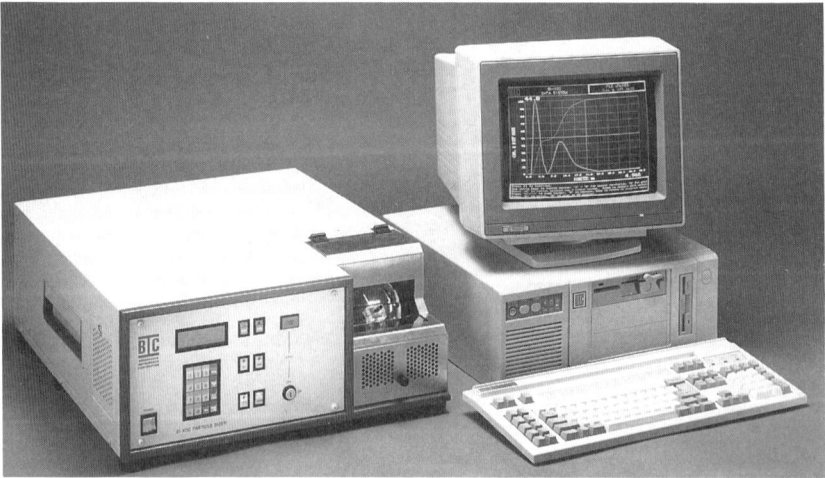

Figure 26. Contemporary sedimentometer (courtesy Brookhaven Instruments).

pore size of particles of a powdered drug, their surface area, and the porosity of compacted powders each have critical influence on the pharmaceutical properties of a material.

Physical adsorption measurements are based on the behavior of gases in contact with a surface. When a solid is exposed to a gas, the gas molecules impinge upon the solid and may reside upon the surface for a finite time. This phenomenon is called adsorption as opposed to absorption, which refers to penetration into the solid body. The amount of gas adsorbed depends upon the properties of the solid (adsorbent) and the gas (adsorbate), and the pressure at which adsorption takes place. Nitrogen, argon, and krypton may be used as surface probes for this purpose. Gas molecules, which leave the bulk of gas (even for a short time) to adsorb onto a surface, cause the average number of molecules in the gas to decrease with an attendant decrease in pressure. By calculations based on this decrease in pressure, the temperature of the gas, and the volume of the system, it is possible to determine the number of molecules adsorbed (static volumetric method). In a dynamic or flowing gas method, a blend of gases (e.g., helium, N_2) is passed over the cooled sample surface and the proportional reduction of nitrogen in the gas mix is measured. When the number of adsorbed gas molecules is known, it is possible to calculate the surface area of the tested material. This assay is typically conducted on a powder sample that has been degassed by a combination of vacuum, elevated temperature, and/or exposure to a purge gas that is not adsorbed (e.g., helium). The amount of gas adsorbed can be calculated by determining the increase in weight of the solid.

At low relative pressures, gas molecules first form a monolayer on the powder surface. As the pressure is increased, multiple layers of adsorbed molecules and pores are filled. The upper limit of this means of measurement is about 3000 Å or 300 nm. The graph of the amount of gas adsorbed (V), at constant temperature, against the adsorption pressure (P) is called the adsorption isotherm. A commonly used method of determining the specific surface of a solid is to deduce the monolayer capacity (V_m) from the isotherm. This is defined as the quantity of adsorbate required to cover the adsorbent with a monolayer. Usually, a second layer may begin to form before the monolayer is complete, but V_m is determined from the isotherm equations irrespective of this fact. The process of physical adsorption is illustrated in Figure 27.

Adsorption processes may be classified as physical or chemical, depending on the nature of the forces involved. Physical adsorption, also termed van der Waals adsorption, is caused by molecular

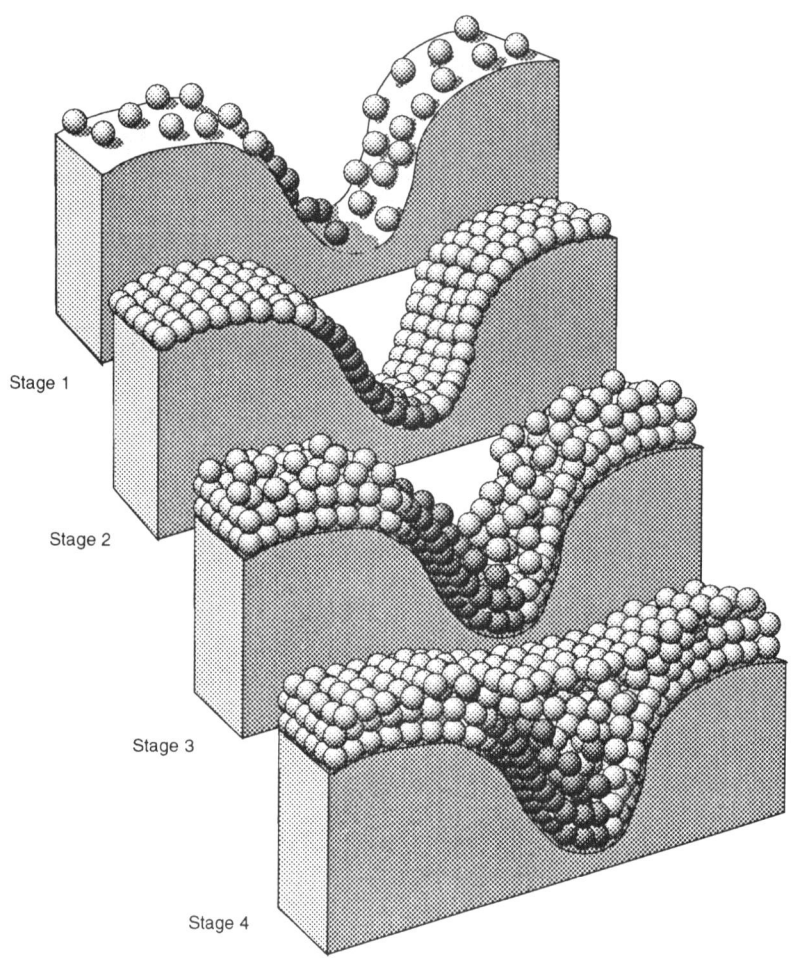

Figure 27. Sequence of steps in adsorption analysis (courtesy of Micromeretics, Inc.).

interaction forces; the formation of a physically adsorbed layer may be likened to the condensation of a vapor to form a liquid. This type of adsorption is of importance only at temperatures below the critical temperature for the gas. Not only is the heat of physical adsorption of the same order of magnitude as that of liquefaction, but physically adsorbed layers behave in many respects like two-dimensional liquids. Chemical adsorption (chemadsorption) involves some degree of specific chemical interaction between the adsorbate and the adsorbent and, correspondingly, the energies of adsorption may be quite large and comparable to those of chemical bond formation.

The principle of the devices used for this purpose, whether simple or sophisticated, is essentially the same (Figure 28). The pressure, volume, and temperature of the adsorbate is first calculated. After contact with a known mass of previously degassed

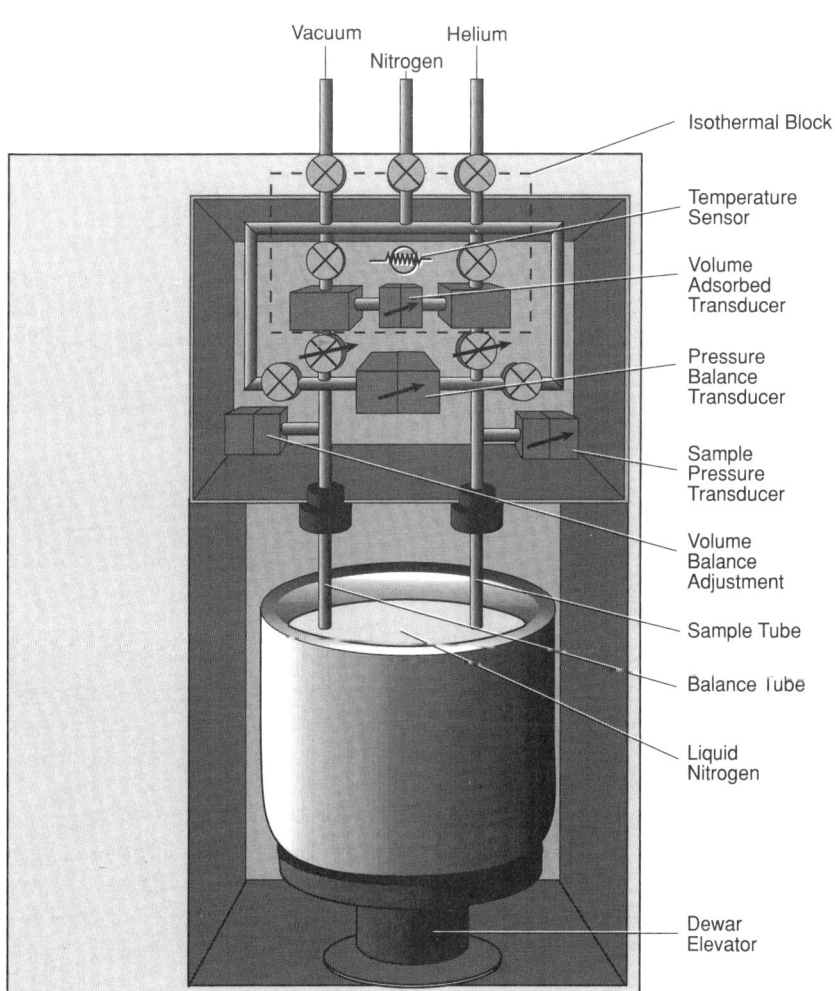

Figure 28. Gas adsorption measurement apparatus (courtesy Micromeritics, Inc.).

powder, and the collection of data regarding volume of gas adsorbed at increasing relative pressures, the volume of unadsorbed gas is again calculated. Following correction for the void volume of the powder, surface area (specific surface) of the powder can be calculated. As with many measurements made on particle populations, this measurement is of greater value for comparative purposes, that is, comparing one powder to another, rather than as an absolute value.

Adsorption studies may be extremely important in the case of micronized drug powders or other finely divided materials, since they allow the analyst to determine particle characteristics that are not apparent from the results of studies performed using microscopy or instrumental particle counting. The usefulness of the method is illustrated by the classic study of Crowl (1963) who investigated paint pigments using light and electron microscopy and gas adsorption. By light microscopy, Prussian blue and red oxide pigments appeared to have the same particle size, but by nitrogen adsorption he discovered that particles of the blue pigment seen by microscopy were actually aggregates of much smaller primary particles (0.05 µm). This finding was confirmed by electron microscopy.

Porosimetry

Pore size as well as surface area and particle-size distribution have significant effects on a wide range of properties of drug powders. Practical measurements of pore size cannot be made by adsorption, since the gas that intrudes into pores of >300 nm in size remains unadsorbed (is part of the free gas volume). Due to this limitation, pore size measurements on a sample of the compacted or compressed powder of interest are frequently made using intrusion porosimetry with mercury as the intrusion medium. A number of other means of making this measurement have also been described (Allen 1990). Pore surface area is generally accepted as being the difference between the area of the surface envelope of the particle and its total surface area. The pores may be made up of fissures and cavities in the particle; they may be V-shaped (i.e., wide-necked) or "ink-bottle" pores (i.e., narrow-necked). In order that their volume distribution may be determined using intrusion porosimetry, it is necessary that they are not totally enclosed, and that the material used for measurement purposes may enter through the neck.

Mercury intrusion porosimetry is based on a simple physical phenomenon involving the equilibrated intrusion of a nonwetting, nonreactive liquid into a porous material at selected pressures. A sample is evacuated, immersed in mercury, and the mercury pressure on the sample is isostatically increased, causing mercury to intrude into pores, with the size of the pores penetrated being inversely proportional to the applied pressure. This permits a direct measurement of pore size and volume, and provides the basis for calculation of descriptive data on the porosity of particles. The reverse process of extrusion allows additional data to be acquired providing characterization of pore complexity. A diagramatic representation of a porosimeter is shown in Figure 29.

The method is based on the capillary rise phenomenon, whereby an excess pressure is required to cause a nonwetting liquid to climb up a narrow capillary. The pressure difference (Δp) across the interface is given by the equation of Young and Laplace. Its sign is such that the pressure is less in the liquid phase than in the gas phase if θ is greater than 90°, and more in the liquid phase

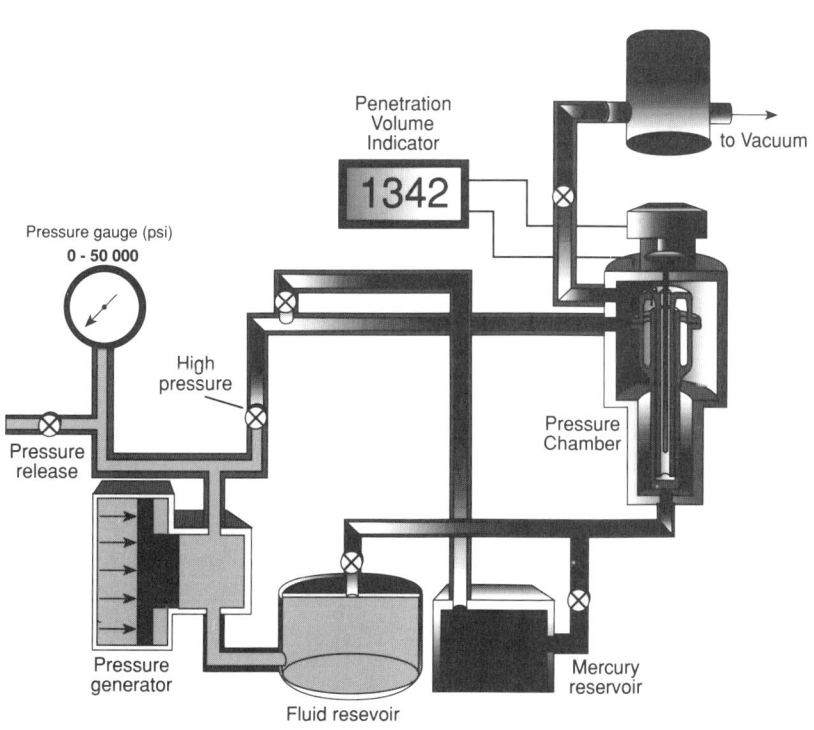

Figure 29. Mercury porosimeter.

than in the gas phase if θ is less than 90°. This relationship is expressed as

$$\Delta p = \gamma \left[\frac{1}{r_1} + \frac{1}{r_2} \right] \cos \theta$$

where γ is the surface tension of the liquid, r_1 and r_2 are mutually perpendicular radii, and θ is an angle of contact between the liquid and the capillary walls measured within the liquid. If the pore is circular in cross-section, and not too large in radius, the meniscus of the intruding liquid will be approximately hemispherical. The two radii of curvature are thus equal to each other and to the radius of the capillary.

Pore diameter and volume data are obtained from the equilibrated pressures where mercury intrudes into a given size pore. The inverse relationship between pore diameter and pressure is the Washburn equation. It may be written

$$D = \frac{-4\gamma \cos \theta}{p}$$

where D is pore diameter when p is the applied pressure. The surface tension (γ) and the interfacial contact angle (θ) of mercury are assumed to remain unchanged during an intrusion or extrusion segment of analysis. For routine calculation γ = 485 dynes/cm and θ = 130° are normally used. For ultimate accuracy, an accurate value of the contact angle between mercury and the solid sample surface must be used in the equation.

In conducting the analysis, a weighed sample of powder is placed in the sample cell and the sample cell is placed in a thick-walled pressure chamber that will withstand the high pressures of the analysis. The sample is then placed under vacuum to remove adsorbed gases. Degassing may be enhanced by heating the sample. Following drying, mercury (sufficient to fill the sample cell) is introduced into the sample cell in contact with the powder. Following raising the sample pressure to atmospheric, the pressure circuit is filled with hydraulic oil and pressure is incrementally applied to cause intrusion of mercury into pores of the sample. Readings of mercury intrusion at various pressures that will be related to penetration of various sized pores is collected.

The equipment used for mercury intrusion must possess the facility to evacuate the sample, surround it with mercury, and generate sufficiently high pressures to cause the mercury to enter the voids or pores while the pressure and the amount of intruded mercury are precisely monitored. Thus, the volume of pores at a specific size may be calculated. In almost all porosimeters, the amount of mercury penetrating into the pores is determined by the fall in level of the interface between the mercury and the hydraulic fluid, correction being applied for compression of the mercury and distortion of the interface. Remote read-out devices of varying degrees of sophistication are incorporated into commercial instruments. One means of measuring intrusion used by a commercial device (Micromeritics) involves reading the change in capacitance related to the shortening of the mercury column in a glass tube as the liquid moves into the powder.

Application of Adsorption and Porosimetry

An illustration of the combined application of these methodologies is provided by the following case study. The experimentally determined dissolution kinetics of a drug material of interest, composed of individual oval or spherical particles 100 µm to 200 µm in size (Figure 30) are not those expected based on the particle morphology. The particles dissolve at the expected rate initially, followed

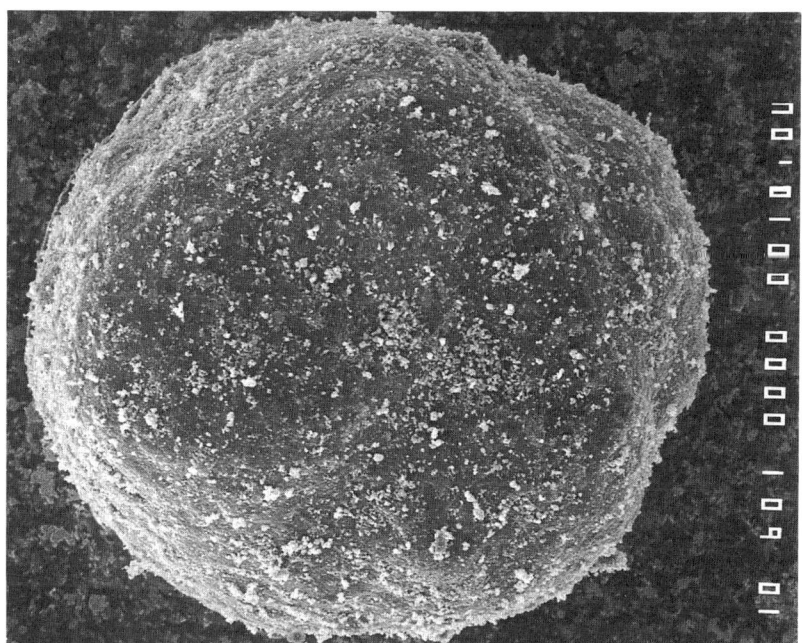

Figure 30. Granular drug powder material (600×).

by a more rapid dissolution inconsistent with particle size, shape, and calculated surface area.

The adsorption isotherm (volume of gas adsorbed versus partial pressure) indicates a much larger surface area than would be expected. This data is also reflected in a plot of surface area versus pore diameter (Figure 31), which reflects an extensive adsorption at very small pore sizes within the compressed powder sample, which was unexpected for the granule morphology.

The data obtained from mercury intrusion porosimetry is even more instructive (Figure 32). A first derivative plot of differential intrusion versus pore diameter shows peaks at 0.02 μm to 0.03 μm and at 50 μm pore diameters. While the intrusion at the larger pore diameter is explicable based on the inter-granule spaces in the packed powder sample, the intrusion in the submicron range is unexpected based on the size of the particles as determined by microscopy, light extinction counting, and laser diffraction.

These findings lead to further analysis using SEM. Comminution of the granules results in the visualization of a complex internal morphology. The drug granules are internally microporous with an internal matrix consisting of an intricately convoluted array of sheet-like or scrolled laminae that are responsible for the higher-than-expected adsorption and the smaller pores measured by intrusion (Figure 33). In the analysis, adsorption and intrusion data have yielded specific morphologic data as well as comparative information.

Aerosol Population Analysis

The USP actually contains only a small number of particulate matter requirements. In addition to the overwhelming importance of <788>, general chapter <601> addresses the analysis of drug aerosols. The USP Advisory Committee on Aerosols has recently generated a proposal to update this requirement (*Pharmacopeial Forum*, March–April 1991). The revision proposal is interesting reading and provides an insight into how pharmacopeial aerosol populations may be analyzed using cascade and single stage impactors and light microscopes.

The interest in aerosols in this context is that only particles of less than 10 μm in aerodynamic size can penetrate and deposit the drug in the deep airways of the lung. Particles of greater than 10 μm are deposited in the upper respiratory tract; particles <0.5 μm are exhaled. It is possible that, in two different manufacturers' inhalers containing the same amount of active ingredient in the discharged

Particle Population Analysis 339

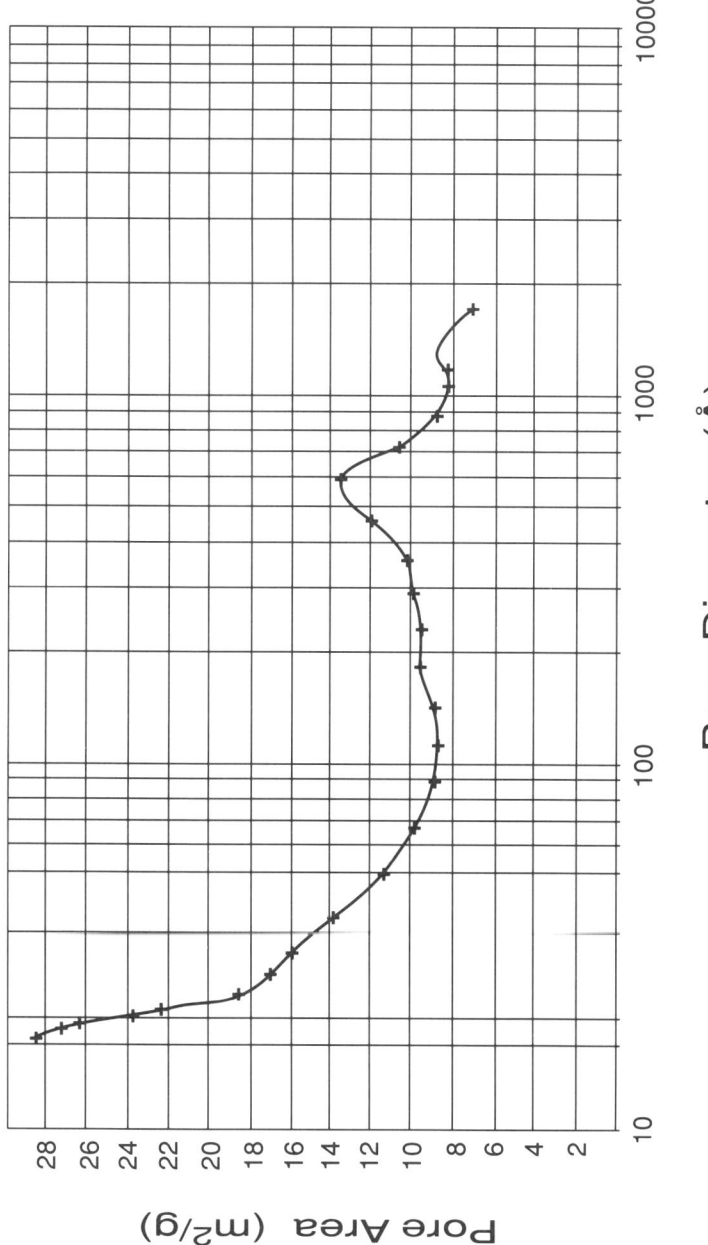

Figure 31. Adsorption versus pore diameter for drug sample.

340 Pharmaceutical Particulate Matter

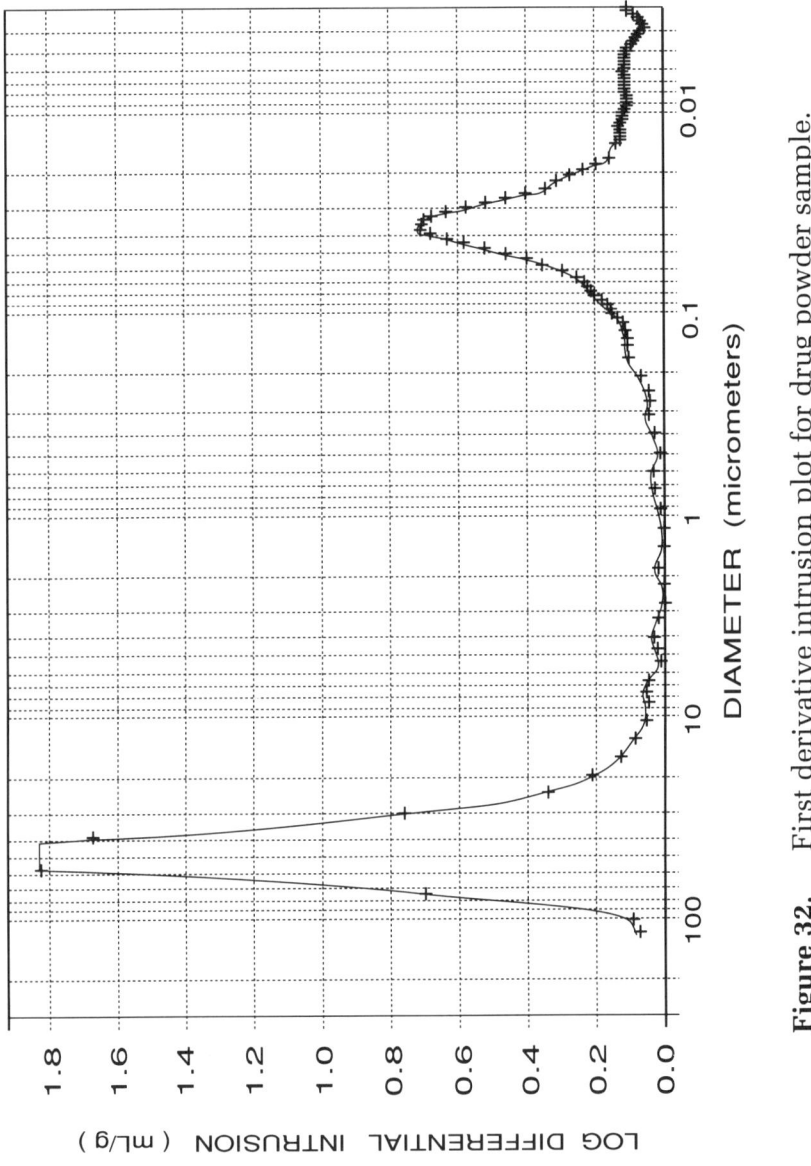

Figure 32. First derivative intrusion plot for drug powder sample.

aerosol cloud, significant differences in particle-size distribution could influence the capability of the active ingredient to reach the site of action. There is thus a need to specify methods for determining the small particle-size distribution throughout the whole of the

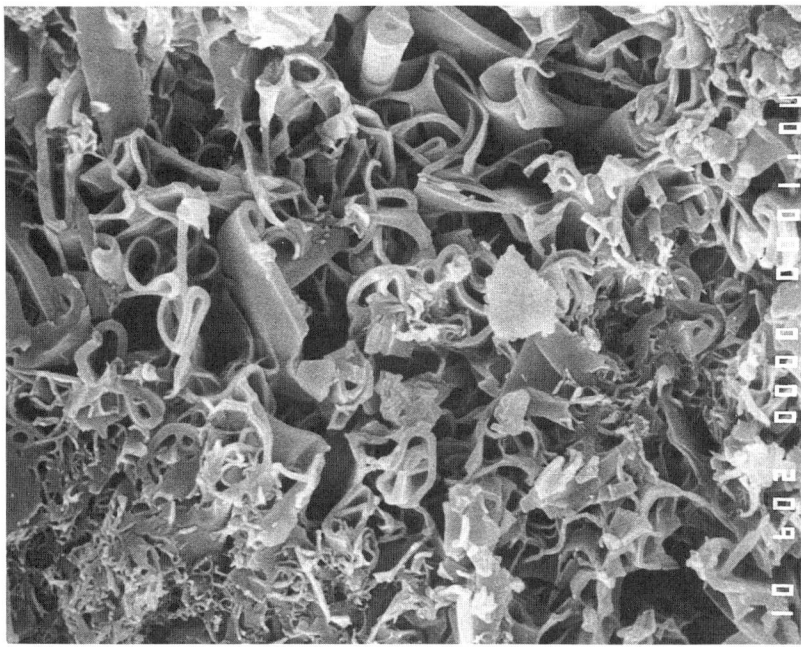

Figure 33. Finely porous internal matrix of powder granules (6000×).

---

discharged aerosol. The intent of <601> is to specify limits for metered-dose inhalers designed to treat pulmonary conditions, such that particles of the appropriate size to penetrate the alveoli are present (with respect to the active ingredient in the discharged spray). In this context, the relationship of drug activity to different particle-size fractions is also critical. Aerodynamic particle-size distribution is a major factor governing the effectiveness of the aerosol cloud discharged from the metered-dose inhaler in achieving its primary purpose of delivering the drug to the lung. The book by Allen (1990) contains a comprehensive treatment of the analysis of aerosols of different types (dusts, atmospheric particles, and ambient aerosol dispersions) in different environments.

The 1990 edition of *Remington's Pharmaceutical Sciences* (Gennaro 1990) (chapter 92) provides an excellent summary of the formulation, manufacture, and application of aerosol dosage forms. With regard to particulate matter dispersion, the goal is generally to produce a population of powder or liquid particles with a size range of 0.5 µm to 10 µm, with a mass median diameter of 5 µm to 6 µm. This distribution insures that the mass of the dosage form is transported into the alveoli and deposited out rather than being exhaled (particles <0.5 µm) or deposited in larger airways (particles ≥10 µm). In this analytical application, analysis by impactors or microscopy as described in the USP <601> requirement constitute time consuming somewhat laborious method; aerodynamic particle sizing provides a uniquely well-suited instrumental method.

Aerodynamic particle counting/sizing is somewhat unique in that it measures the size of a particle based on its aerodynamic properties rather than on light scattering, mass, or volume; the aerodynamic diameter of a particle has significant impact with inhalation therapy, aerosol dry administration, or inhalation toxicology. Commercially available time-of-flight instruments provide rapid, reproducible measurement of aerosol particles 0.5 µm to 30 µm in size. The principle of operation of these instruments is straightforward and provides advantages over other types of measurements for special-sized aerosol application.

Consider two particles falling through the air. One is a perfect sphere with a smooth surface and a density of 1 g/cm^3. The second is not necessarily spherical, does not necessarily have a smooth surface, and has an unknown density. If both particles fall with the same velocity, they have equal aerodynamic diameter. The diameter of the unit density sphere is the aerodynamic diameter of both particles. Thus, the aerodynamic diameter of a particle is defined as the physical diameter of a unit density sphere that settles through the air with a velocity equal to the velocity of the particle in question. Stated another way, the aerodynamic behavioral characteristics of a nonspherical, irregularly shaped airborne particle determines the aerodynamic size of the particle. The measurement of aerodynamic size or diameter automatically compensates for complexities of shape, surface irregularity, mass, and refractive index, and provides a measure of particle size based on one parameter characteristic that is important in many measurement programs:

- They have similar probabilities of penetrating a filter, an impactor, or other particulate matter removal device.
- They tend to deposit in similar locations of the human respiratory system.
- They have similar airborne lifetimes in the atmosphere and in most other aerosol systems.

- They have similar probabilities of entering into a particle sampling system.
- They have similar probabilities of penetrating a pipe, tube duct, or channel.

In the TSI instrument of this type (Figure 34), an integral vacuum pump draws airborne particle samples at a flow rate of 5 L/min through a flow nozzle, producing a precisely controlled, accelerating, high-speed aerosol jet. At the flow nozzle exit, the aerosol jet is constrained by sheath air that has passed through a filter and a thermal flow chamber pressure of 31 kPa (125 cm of water) below the ambient inlet pressure maintains the maximum air velocity through the nozzle—the output of a pressure transducer—and the vacuum pump regulates the pressure drop. A second thermal flow meter measures the total air flow. Depending on size, shape, and mass, individual particles accelerate within the jet at varying rates. Consequently, particle velocity at any given point relates inversely to a particle's aerodynamic size characteristics—smaller particles accelerate rapidly, while larger particles accelerate more slowly.

A two-beam laser velocimeter, using a 2-mW He-Ne laser, measures the time of flight of individual particles. A calcite plate splits the laser beam by polarization, and the remaining focusing optics

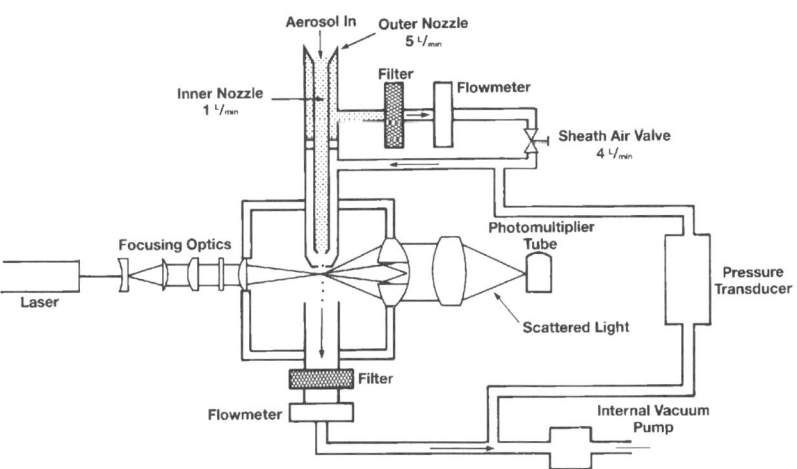

Figure 34. Aerodynamic particle sizer (courtesy TSI Inc.).

form two flat beams with rectangular cross-sections approximately 120 μm apart and about 200 μm downstream of the nozzle orifice. As aerosol particles pass through the two beams, a lens system collects near-forward scattered light and focuses it onto a photomultiplier tube. A particle passing through the two beams produces a pair of electrical pulses. The time between pulses in each pulse pair obtained from a small particle is measured by a high-speed digital clock with 2-nanosecond resolution. A 0.5-μm diameter particle produces a pair of pulses approximately 800 nanoseconds apart. For large particles, up to 30 μm, pulses can be as much as 5000 nanoseconds apart. The measurement of sizes greater than 15 μm results from the system's high speed circuitry which uses a 66.67 nanosecond resolution clock. This circuitry reduces the effect of coincidence at larger particle sizes.

Each measured transit time passes to a multichannel accumulator (MCA) within the sensor, where the counts within a "bin" spanning the measured transit time increase by one. The MCA has a total of 1024 bins, each capable of storing up to 10 million counts. At the end of the sample period, the sensor calculates the aerodynamic particle-size distribution using a previously stored calibration curve. It then transmits size distribution information via a serial port to a microcomputer for data analysis and display. Calibration of the sensor is routinely accomplished by measuring various monosized solid polystyrene latex (PSL) spheres spanning the measurement range. Calibration may also be adjusted for monotypic particles of known mass. For both native aerosols and particles resuspended from collection filters, aerosols exceeding the instrument's concentration limit of $1.0 \times 10^6/\text{ft}^3$ may be suitably diluted.

Summary

The particle size, shape, and numbers in any population will be totally dependent upon the means by which the analysis is performed. Each method of analysis produces an answer that is unique to that method. Agreement of data between methods will range from poor to adequate. The particle numbers determined in various size categories for a population will be inextricably related to the means of particle sizing applied.

Characterization of a particle population is not only heavily dependent upon the means of analysis but also upon the means of data reduction used. There are a number of measurements of the central tendency of a population based on linear measurements, using mass, volume, surface area, or a ratio of these parameters. To apply population analysis in a meaningful way, the analyst must understand the particle size parameter most critical to the bulk property of interest (e.g., chemical stability, compressibility, flowability) and the relationship of the analytical result to the parameter of interest.

References

Air pollution manual: Part II, control equipment. 1968. Detroit: American Industrial Hygiene Association.

Allen, T. 1990. An industrial perspective on optical particle sizing. In *Proceedings of the 2nd International Congress on Optical Particle Sizing.* Department of Mechanical and Aerospace Engineering, Arizona State University.

Allen, T. 1990. *Particle size measurement,* 4th Ed. New York: Chapman and Hall.

ASTM Standard E11-87. 1987. *Standard specification for wire-cloth sieves for testing purposes.* Philadelphia: American Society for Testing and Materials, p. 4.

Barber, T. A., M. D. Lannis, and J. G. Williams. 1989. Method evaluation: Automated microscopy as a compendial test for particulates in parenteral solution. *J. Patent. Sci. Technol.* 43(1):27–41.

Beddow, J. K. 1983. *Particulate systems, technology and fundamentals.* New York: Hemisphere Publishing Corporation.

Beddow, J. K. 1980. *Particle science and technology, Vol. II.* Boca Raton, FL: Chemical Publishing Co., p. 265.

Beddow, J. K., and T. Meloy. 1980. *Testing and characterization of powders and fine particles.* London: Heydon & Son Ltd.

British Standards Institution. 1963, 1985. Methods for determination of particle size distribution. *Optical Microscope Method* (4):3406. British Standards House, 2 Park Street, London, U.K.

British Standards Institution. 1963. *Specification for eyepiece and screen graticule,* 3625. British Standards House, 2 Park Street, London, U.K.

Carstensen, J. T. 1977. *Pharmaceutics of solids and solid dosage forms.* New York: John Wiley and Sons.

Coll, H., and C. G. Searle. 1987. Particle size analysis with the Joyce-Loebl Disk Centrifuge: A comparison of the line-start with the homogeneous-start method. *J. Coll. Int. Sci.* 115:121–131.

Crowl, V. T. 1963. *Determination of state of division of paint pigments.* Toddington, London: Paint Research Station No. 326.

Davies, R., R. Haruhn, J. Graf, and J. Stockham. 1975. Measurement of fiber size distribution in parenteral solutions. *Bull. of Parenteral Drug Assn.* 29 (2):110.

Detection and analysis of particulate contamination, #AD030. 1991. Bedford, MA: The Millipore Corp.

Drewel, M., J. Ahrens, and K. Schatzel. 1990. Suppression of multiple scattering errors in particle sizing by dynamic light scattering. In *Proc. 2nd Int. Congr. Optical Particle Sizing,* 130–138. Tempe, AZ.

Dodge, L. E. 1984. Calibration of the Malvern particle sizer. *Applied Optics* 23:2415.

Edmundson, I. C. 1967. Particle-size analysis. In *Advances in Pharmaceutical Sciences,* Vol. 2, 95–179. London: Academic Press.

Elias, H. G. 1972. The study of association and aggregation *via* light scattering. In *Light Scattering from Polymer Solution,* ed. M. B. Huglin, 397–457. London: Academic Press.

Fairhurst, D., and P. McFadden. 1989. Particle sizing by photon correlation spectroscopy—A tunnel at the end of light? *International Labmate* XV (7):187–190.

Fayed, M. E., and L. Otter Eds. 1984. *Handbook of powder science and technology.* New York: Van Nostrand Reinhold.

Felton, P. G. 1981. Measurement of particle/droplet size distributions by a laser diffraction technique. *2nd European Symposium on Particle Characterization Conference Papers,* p. 662.

Fink, D. G. 1966. Computers and the human mind. *Science Study Series* 43. Garden City, NY: Anchor Books.

Gennaro, A. R., ed. 1990. *Remington's Pharmaceutical Sciences.* Easton, PA: Mack Publishing Co., p. 1694–1712.

Gregg, S. J., and K. S. Sing. 1982. *Adsorption, surface area and porosity.* New York: Academic Press.

Hatch, T., and S. J. Choate. 1929. Relationship Among Particle Statistical Diameters. *J. Franklin Inst.* 207:369.

Hausdorff, H. H., and V. J. Coates. 1982. Microspectrophotometer for small-sample analysis. *Microbeam Anal.* 17:233–237.

Herdan, G. 1960. *Small particle statistics.* 2nd Ed. London: Butterworth's Publishers.

Heywood, H. 1937. Particle shape coefficients. *J. Imp. Coll. Eng. Society* 15:149–154.

Heywood, H. 1947. Symposium on particle size analysis. *Institute for Chemical Engineers Supplement* 25:14–31.

Heywood, H. 1973. *Harold Heywood Memorial Lectures.* Loughborough, UK: Loughborough University Press.

Hirleman, E. D. 1987. On-line calibration technique for laser diffraction droplet sizing instruments. *ASME* 83-GT-232.

Hirleman, E. D. 1990. A general solution to Fraunhofer diffraction particle sizing in multiple scattering environments: Theory. In *Proc. 2nd Int. Congr. Optimal Particle Sizing,* 159–168. Tempe, AZ.

Kaye, B. H. 1981. *Direct characterization of fine particles.* New York: Wiley Interscience, p. 398.

Kaye, B. H., and R. P. Boardman. 1982. Cluster formation in dilute suspension. In *Proc. Symposium on Interaction Between Fluids and Particles,* 17–22. London: Inst. of Chem. Eng.

Kerker, M. 1969. The scattering of light and other electromagnetic radiation. New York: Academic Press.

Knapp, J. Z., and P. P. DeLuca. 1988. Review of commercially available particulate measurement systems. *Supplement to J. Paren. Sci & Tech.* 42 (Jan–Feb):1.

Knapp, J. Z., and L. R. Abramson. 1990. A systems analysis of light extinction particle detection systems. In *Proc. Int'l Conf. on Particle Detection, Metrology and Control,* 283. Arlington, VA.

Knollenberg, R. G., and R. C. Gallant. 1990. Refractive index effects on particle size measurement in liquid media by optical extinction. In *Proc. Int'l Conf. on Particle Detection, Metrology and Control,* 154. Arlington, VA.

Lieberman, A. 1990. Light scattering systems for particle counting and sizing. In *Proc. Int'l Conf. on Particle Detection, Metrology and Control*, 353. Arlington, VA.

Lloyd, P. J. 1987. *Particle size analysis*. New York: John Wiley.

Luerkins, D. W. 1991. *Theory and application of morphological analysis of fine particles and surfaces.* Ann Arbor, MI: CRC Press.

Martin, A., J. Swarbrick, and A. Cammarata. 1983. Micromeretics. In *Physical Pharmacy*, 492–521. Philadelphia: Lea and Febiger.

Meury, R. H. 1987. Particle size measurement of pharmaceutical powders using laser light diffraction. In *Particulate and multiphase processes. II. Contamination analysis and control*, ed. T. Ariman and T. N. Veziroglu, 43–54. Berlin: Springer-Verlag.

Nicoli, D. F., and V. B. Elings. 1991. Automatic dilution system. U.S. Patent #4,794,806 (foreign patents pending).

Nicoli, D. F., J. S. Wu, Y. J. Chang, D. C. McKenzie, and K. Hasapidis. 1992. Automatic high resolution particle sizing by single particle optical sensing. *American Laboratory* (July):39–45.

Osol, A., ed. 1980. *Remington's Pharmaceutical Sciences.* Easton, PA: Mack Publishing Co.

Stockham, J. D. 1979. What is particle size: The relationship among statistical diameters. In *Particle size analysis*, ed. J. D. Stockham and E. G. Fochtman, 1–12. Ann Arbor, MI: Ann Arbor Science Publishers.

Stockham, J. D., and E. G. Fochtman. eds. 1979. *Particle size analysis.* Ann Arbor: MI: Ann Arbor Science Publishers.

Swithenbank, J., J. M. Beer, D. S. Taylor, D. Abbot, and G. C. McCreath. 1977. A laser diagnostic technique for the measurement of droplet and particle size distribution. *Prog. Astronaut. Aeronaut.* 53:421.

United States Pharmacopeial Convention, Inc. Report and recommendations of the USP advisory panel on aerosols of the USP general chapter <601> on aerosols. 1991. *Pharmacopeial Forum* (March/April):1703–1712.

Van de Hulst, H. C. 1981. *Light scattering by small particles*. Toronto: General Publishing Co. Ltd.; New York: Dover Publications Inc.

Veals, C. R. 1972. *Fine powders*. New York: John Wiley.

Wadell, H. 1932. Volume, shape, and roundness of rock particles. *J. Geol.* 40:443.

Walton, W. H., and S. T. Beckett. 1977. A microscope eyepiece graticule for evaluation of fibrous dusts. *Amm. Occup. Hyg.* 20:19–23.

Weiner, B. 1979. Particle and spray sizing using laser diffraction. *Soc. Photoopt. Eng.* 170:53.

Weiner, B. B., and D. Fairhurst. 1989. How to choose a particle sizer: A guide. *Brookhaven Instruments Technical Publication No. 327*. Holtsville, NY: Brookhaven Instruments Corp.

Weiner, B. B., and W. W. Tscharnuter. 1987. Uses and abuses of photon correlation spectroscopy in particle sizing. *ACS Symposium Series* No. 332, 49–61. Washington DC: American Chemical Society.

Weiner, B. B., D. Fairhurst, and W. Tscharnuter. 1991. Particle size analysis with a disc centrifuge: Importance of extinction efficiency. *ACS Symposium Series* No. 472, 184–195. Washington, DC: American Chemical Society.

White, H. 1963. *Industrial electrostatic precipitation*. Reading, Mass.: Addison-Wesley.

IX

Collection and Isolation of Particulate Matter

This chapter is intended to provide the pharmaceutical particle analyst with some general insights into the collection and isolation of particulate matter. The analyst can expand upon the concepts introduced depending upon specific requirements. Comprehensive coverage of some of the subjects discussed in this chapter, for example, filtration, would require a separate book and the reader is referred to the reference list if greater depth of information is needed. The pharmaceutical particle analyst is most often a generalist and typically does not need in-depth knowledge of specific techniques of particle collection or isolation. Should the need for detailed information arise, such is readily available from individuals who are specialists, or from the literature. Microfiltration is a complex subject. A wealth of information is available on this topic simply by requesting technical information from filter vendors—Gelman, Pall, Millipore, Sartorius, and others. This information will invariably be provided free of charge, and valuable technical contacts may be made with experts in the applications groups of the various manufacturers. The Millipore Handbook (#AD030,

1992) is a very useful aid in selecting particle isolation and collection techniques. The appropriate section of the text by McCrone and Delly (1973) deals with all aspects of particle collection and the papers by Sokol and Boyd (1968), DeLuca and Bodapatti (1980) and Oles (1978) are useful with regard to collection of particles from pharmaceutical products and environments.

The topics discussed in this chapter are considered in what I believe to be the general order of interest in pharmaceutical particle analysis: microfiltration, physical methods of particle collection, and particle isolation and manipulation. Before getting into specific techniques and methods, I should briefly discuss considerations regarding particulate matter samples in general. First, it is critically important that the sample collected for analysis is representative of the problem to be addressed or of the material to be characterized. If the issue at hand involves particles present in an injectable solution, the analyst should ensure that the units received for analysis contain the particles that constitute the problem. Before beginning any analytical work, the analyst must also ensure that particles to be identified have been adequately described by the person submitting the samples or that the specific problem to be addressed is defined in detail. Ideally, the analyst will be able to personally collect the particulate matter sample for analysis. If the problem is point-generated particulate matter from a filler or component of the process, it is best to have an analyst go to the production area to collect samples. If components of a solution container or device are involved, the parts submitted for analysis should be collected using cleaned forceps and placed in particle-free bags of nylon (not polyethylene) that have been tested for cleanliness. Minimally, telephoned instructions on the method of sampling should be given. In my experience, a sample of particulate matter collected by filtration in another lab and sent in for analysis is liable to be contaminated, and may be suspect on other grounds. The analyst must never forget that a single touch of a finger on a sample can deposit thousands of skin cells. Particle-free gloves are vital if samples must be handed. Despite precautions, any particle laboratory can expect to receive samples collected with various degrees of care and the analyst generally learns to make the best of bad situations.

The experienced particle analyst appreciates the fact that the individuals who submit samples relative to a particle problem can often provide the solution to the problem if the analyst asks the right questions. Location of the particles of interest, circumstances of their occurrence, and their visual appearance often provide the analyst with at least a general idea of the source and identity. An understanding of the process by which an affected solution or device is made is extremely valuable to the analyst in this regard. The color plates in this book show examples of particles commonly collected and isolated from pharmaceutical products.

Filter Structure and Application

The filters used for particle analysis are most frequently one of two types: (1) cast film filters that are spongiform in structure and are made by casting a polymer film containing volatile solvent(s) and pore forming liquids on a smooth surface (Kesting 1971, 1977; Elford 1933), and (2) track etched or nucleation track filters that are produced by etching a thin polycarbonate film that has been exposed to gamma radiation (Fleischer et al. 1964). The latter type are commonly referred to as "Nuclepore" filters based on the name of the original vendor. The generic term *membrane,* which may be used in reference to either of the types of filters by different authors, refers to the thinness of these filters and their generally fragile nature. The book by Brock (1983) is an invaluable basic text and discusses the principles of manufacture of microporous filters of all types, as well as filter function and applications.

The cast film filters often used for particle collection in the lab are open structures with only a small fraction of the membrane volume occupied by the polymer substrate (Figure 1). In a representative filter, of this type, 80% to 85% of the membrane is open space (void volume). This openness provides for a relatively high fluid flow rate. In the days before scanning electron microscopy, it was thought that filters of this type contained cylindrical pores of defined size. Examination of such filters with the scanning electron microscope has revealed that their structure is in fact random, being characterized by a polymer network surrounding spherical or oval voids. Depending on the type of cast film filter considered, the polymer structure surrounding the voids of the filter may be almost complete, or may consist of fibrous strands.

Kesting (1971) described cast film filters as elaborate systems consisting of "open-celled foams. i.e. vacuoles with breached walls. Fastening the cellular network together [are] long hose and chain-like ribs that spread out in three dimensions." The diameters of Kesting's "vacuoles" have no direct relationship to the size of the particles being filtered. The term *interconnected voids* has also been applied in describing the closely adjacent spherical cells of this type of filter. The route followed by a particle in passing through a filter of this type is determined by the flow path in which

Collection and Isolation of Particulate Matter 353

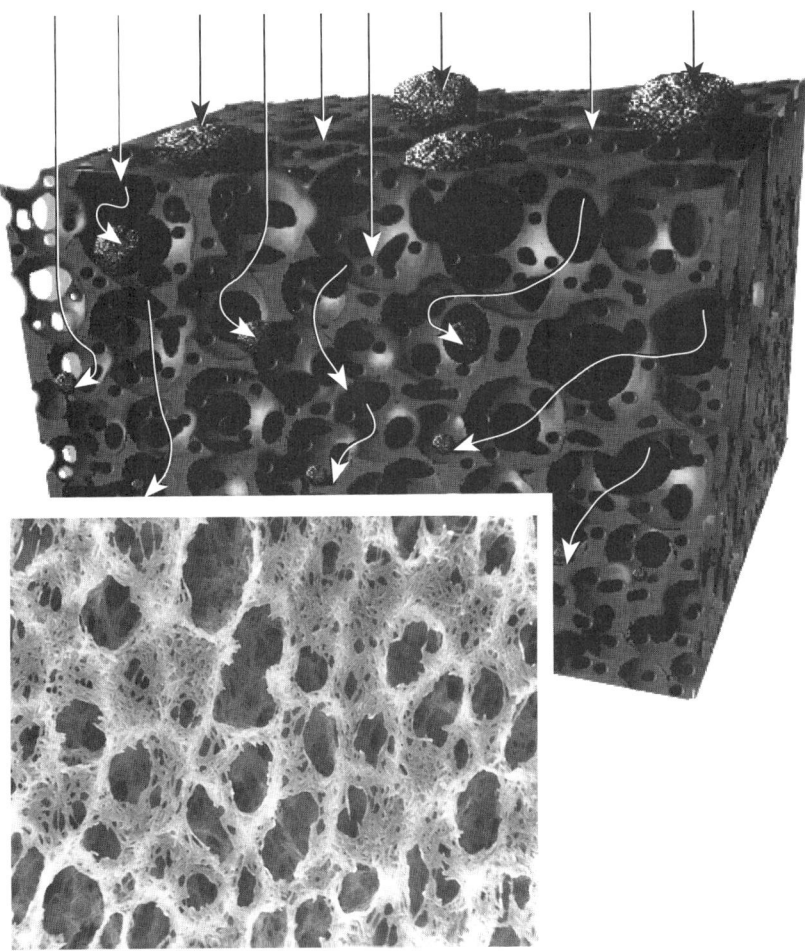

Figure 1. Microporous cast film filter. Inset—Gelman Nylaflo™ filter (photomicrograph courtesy of Gelman Corp.).

---

it is entrained. This flow path is typically complex, changing in direction and velocity numerous times between the upper and lower surfaces of the filter. Filters of this type have also been termed *tortuous path* filters. Although cast film filters are very thin, generally around 150 µm, the filter presents a particle with a relatively thick complex structure. The structure of the surface of these filters may differ from the structure within the depth of the filter. This difference arises from the manner in which membrane filters are made. During solvent evaporation, the side of the filter (in contact with the supporting substrate) will lose solvent at a different rate than filter parts in contact with air, so that pore sizes on the two surfaces differ. The pores or voids within the filter vary in size from one surface to the other. This condition is called anisotrophy; such filters are designated anisotrophic. The side of the filter with smaller pores will be more reflective, and may provide a better visualization of particles.

The open-celled, spongiform structure of cast film filters differs significantly from that of nucleation track (Nuclepore®) membranes, which are made by chemically etching polycarbonate films that have been subjected to localized damage by nuclear radiation (Fleischer et al. 1964). A track-etched membrane filter (Nuclepore®) is shown in Figure 2. The identifying characteristic of this filter is the cylindrical pores of uniform diameter that cause the filter to

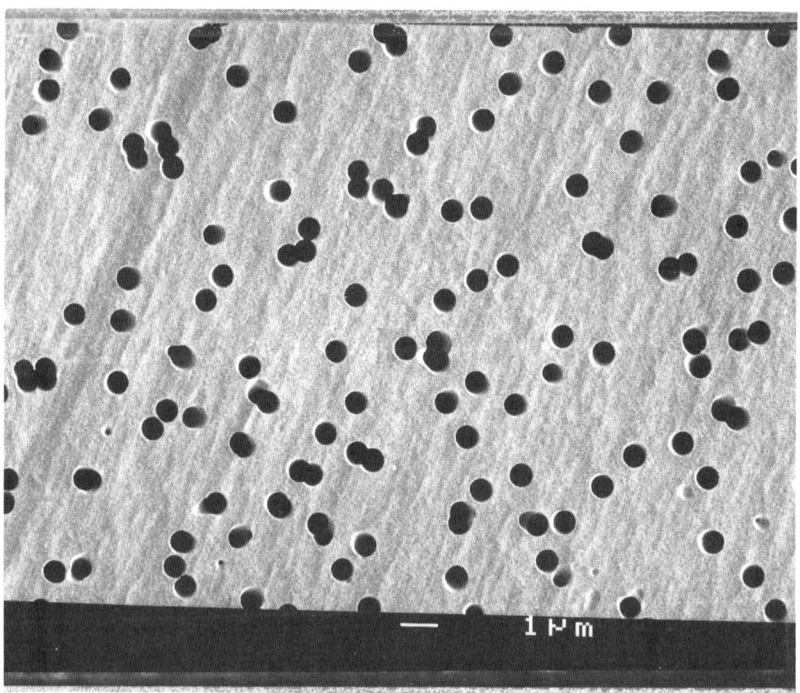

Figure 2. Track-etched membrane filter.

function as a sieve. These filters are suitable for applications in which particles must be trapped on the filter surface. However, as can be seen in the figure, these filters also have less open pore area and consequently lower liquid flow rates than the cast film filters; this characteristic makes them unsuitable for many general filter applications. They also tend to "blind" or become blocked more easily than cast film filters, and their extreme thinness (10 to 15 μm), flexibility, and responsiveness to static electrical charges make handling difficult. Despite their disadvantages, this type of filter is extremely useful for collecting particles for further analysis; the smooth surface allows particles to be easily removed for transfer to the supports used in analytical instruments, such as scanning microscopes or x-ray microprobes.

I must emphasize that this general discussion of microporous filtration media represents an oversimplification of the real situation. Many types of filter media falling into the general category of cast film filters are made by proprietary processes very different from that used to make cellulose acetate, nitrate, or mixed ester filters. Some filters of this type are made by laminating a fragile medium onto a more durable supporting substrate. These details are not essential to the present discussion. The knowledge of most value to the analyst involves the wide range of physical and chemical properties embodied in the different types of filters. Filters for specific applications in a variety of analytical roles may be selected by consulting with vendors or their applications literature.

While the cast film cellulose ester filters and track-etched filters discussed above are useful for the majority of particle isolation procedures undertaken by a pharmaceutical particle analyst, filtration of solvents, acids, or bases may require the use of appropriately resistant filters. If a question arises regarding the selection of a filter with a specific resistance, the ideal first step is for the analyst to consult the vendor catalogs. These catalogs will generally include a tabular presentation of filter types and their resistance to specific solutions. Some of the many other types of microporous filter media are shown in Figures 3–7.

Teflon® (polytetrafluoroethylene or PTFE) filters are made by expanding (stretching) an extruded Teflon® film over a supporting matrix. Polypropylene, polysulfone, and nylon filters are made by a modified cast film process, but have wetting properties and chemical resistance that differ from the conventional cast film cellulose ester or mixed cellulose ester materials. Polypropylene and untreated nylon filters have an avidity for apolar liquids (oils) and may be used to remove such materials from aqueous systems by

356 *Pharmaceutical Particulate Matter*

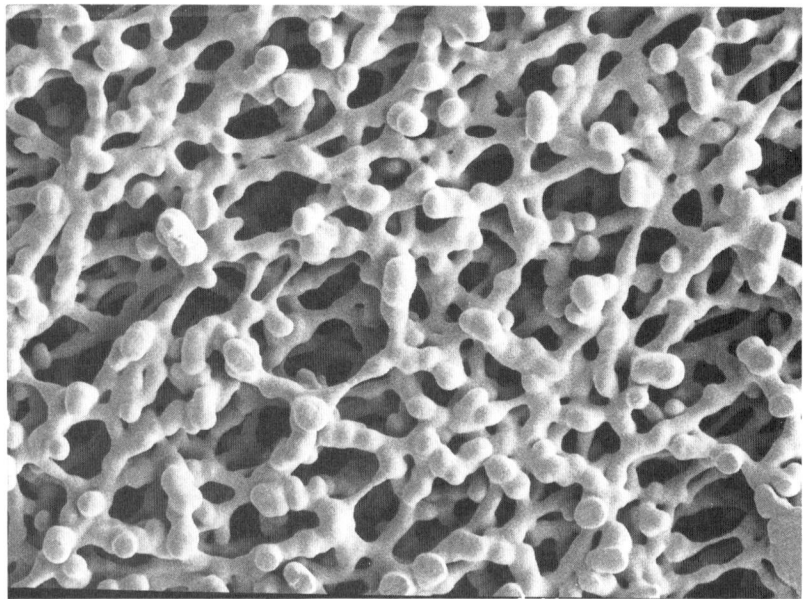

Figure 3. Polysulfone membrane filter.

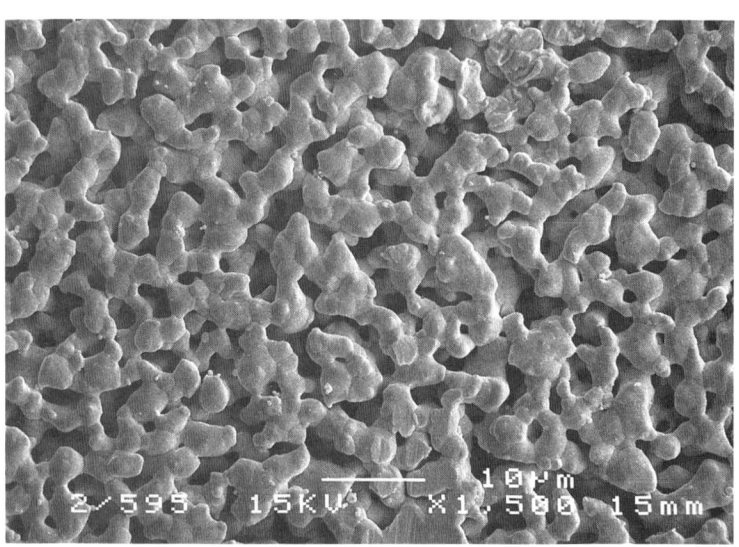

Figure 4. Sintered silver filter.

Collection and Isolation of Particulate Matter 357

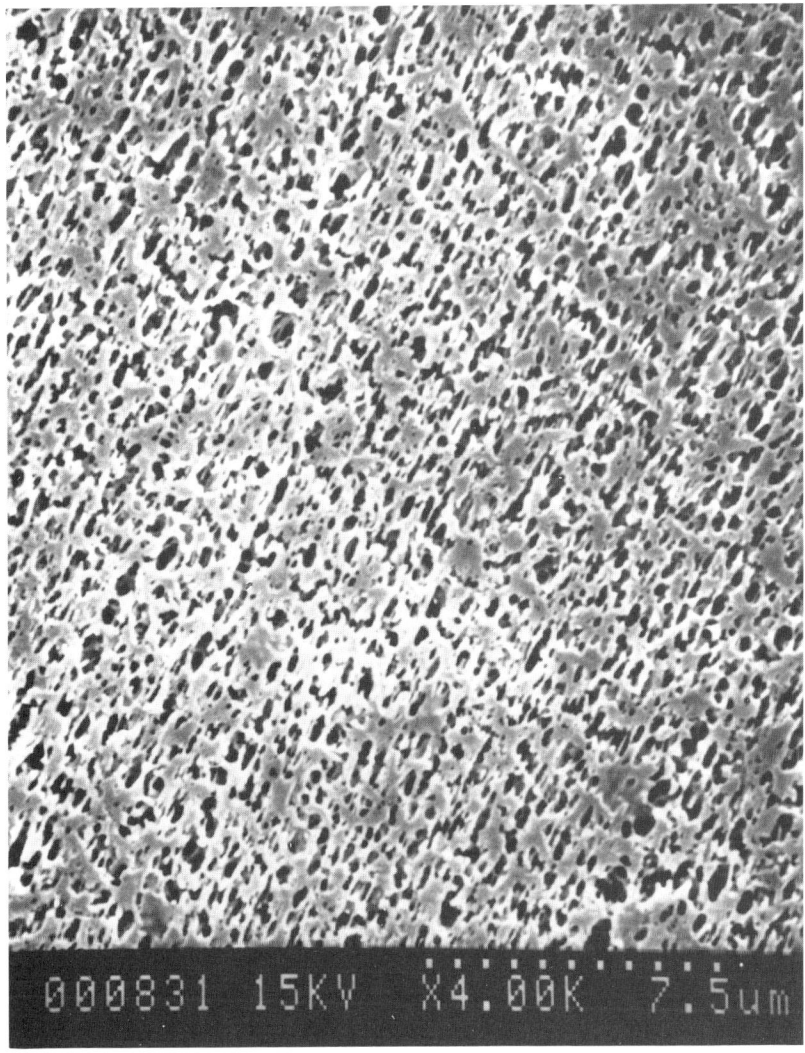

Figure 5. Metricel polypropylene filter (courtesy of Gelman Corp.)

adsorption. Untreated nylon filters have a positive charge and are extremely effective at removing charged materials (including biologicals) from solutions and suspensions. Sintered silver filters are produced by compression of silver particles at high temperature, and the glass Collimated Holes filter (Bares and Lannis 1990)

358 *Pharmaceutical Particulate Matter*

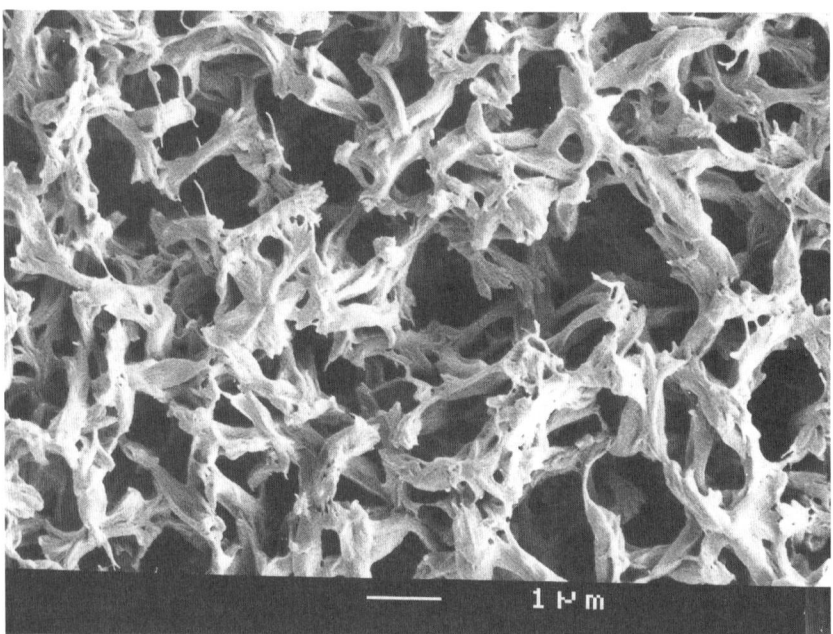

Figure 6.   Nylon membrane filter (Pall Corporation).

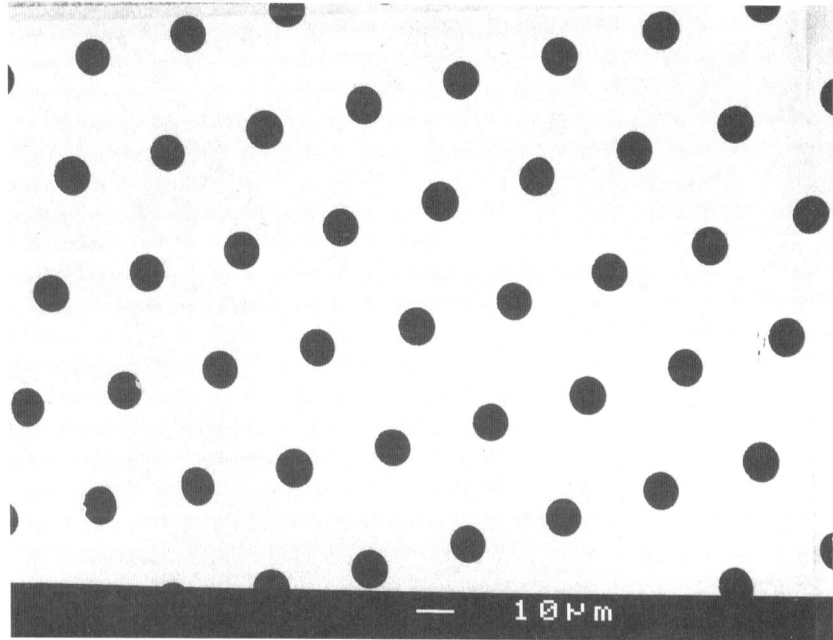

Figure 7.   Collimated holes glass filter.

is made by the proprietary technology (etch-resist) used in manufacture of semiconductor wafers. Each of these filters has properties that may make it useful in special particle isolation endeavors; the analyst is advised to consult the manufacturer's literature for more specific information.

Polysulfone filters are presently offered in both the conventional hydrophobic and inherently hydrophilic types (Supor™, Gelman). The latter material, as well as being far stronger than conventional mixed ester membranes, also offers higher flow rates and does not require a surfactant for wetting. Polymeric microporous filters for analytical purposes are also made from acrylic copolymers, polyvinylidine difluoride, polyvinyl chloride, hydrophilic vinyl-acrylic copolymers, and hydroxyl-modified polyamide.

Retention Ratings, Pore Size, and Porosity

The analyst should have a basic understanding of critical descriptors applied to filter media of different types. These descriptors are retention rating, pore size, and void volume or porosity. The size of particles that the analyst can expect to be retained on a filter with some high degree of efficiency is expressed as the retention rating. Thus, a filter with a retention rating of 0.8 µm would be expected to retain nearly all particles of this size and greater that are contained in a solution to be filtered.

The difference in structure between cast film filters and track-etched (sieve) filters is dramatically illustrated by their retention characteristics (Figure 8). The cut-off or maximum retention is rapidly reached at the retention rating of the track-etched filter; the percent retention of the spongiform cast film filter increases slowly, beginning at a particle size far below the retention rating.

Pore size or pore diameter is directly related to the retention rating and retention characteristics of sieve-type filters such as Nuclepore® or collimated holes glass filter. Obviously, due to the wide variation of pore sizes in cast film filters and the complex structure of this type of media, the pore size measurement is of less value in predicting performance. It should be emphasized that the pore diameters (typically stated in µm) in the manufacturer's literature for cast film analytical filters may be determined in several ways: they may be obtained by direct measurement with an electron microscope based on physical measurements (such as bubble point testing), or determined by challenge with standard particles. This is unlike the case with sterilizing filters, which are tested against organisms to validate their critical function (Lukaszewicz

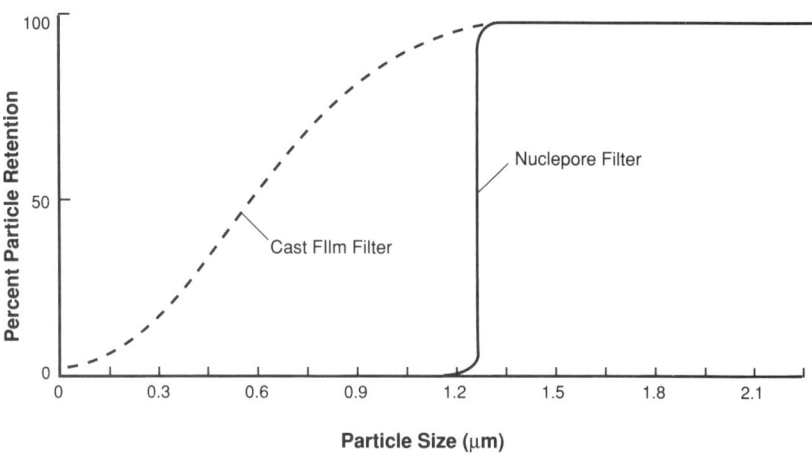

Figure 8. Particle retention curves for filters of different types.

---

and Meltzer 1979). Pore diameters specified are often mean values, and there is a range of sizes on either side of the mean (standard deviation of pore size is typically not specified by the manufacturer).

I will mention bubble point testing briefly, not because it is important in the analytical use of microporous filter media, but because it provides insight into filter structure and function. The cast film filter, despite being made up of a vast array of interconnected voids, generally behaves as though it is composed of a large number of discrete pores. These *pores* are in fact the tortuous path followed by a particle as it passes through the filter or into the depth of the matrix. The bubble point test is most often applied to production filters to ensure filter integrity at the specified retention rating. The test is based on the fact that a liquid held in the pores of a filter requires some pressure to dislodge, with higher pressures required for smaller pore sizes. The pressure required can be calculated as a shown in Figure 9.

A bubble point test is performed by prewetting the filter, increasing the pressure of air upstream of the filter, and watching for air bubbles downstream to indicate the passage of air. The measured pressure at which a steady, continuous stream of bubbles appears is the bubble point pressure. Obviously, the single largest pore in a cast film filter will determine the bubble point. An observed bubble point significantly lower than the bubble point specification for that particular filter may indicate a damaged

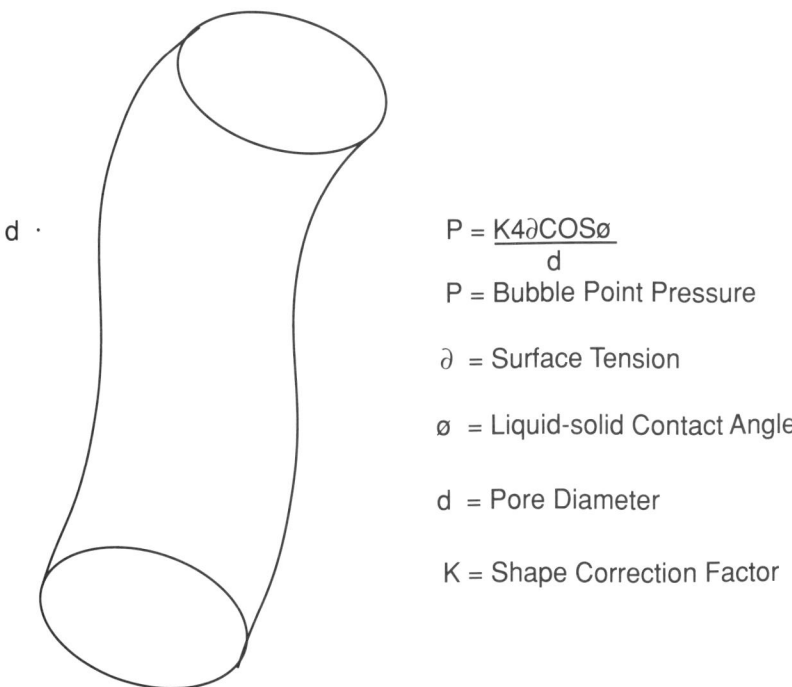

Figure 9. Calculation of bubble point.

(nonintegral) membrane, a system leak, a fluid with a surface tension less than water, or pores larger than spec. Bubble point data for a mixed cellulose ester cast film filter media are shown in Figure 10.

The term *porosity* is often incorrectly applied as a reference to the retention rating of an analytical filter. The retention rating and pore size are distinct from the porosity of a filter. The porosity (or void volume) is that fraction of the filter volume that is open to flow of liquid. Most commercially available cellulose cast film filters have void volumes of 80% or greater. The number of pore openings per unit area of membrane surface is known as the pore density. Pore densities of around 10^8 to 10^9 per cm^2 are generally present in commercially available cast film filters.

Mechanism of Liquid Filtration

Although liquid filtration appears (on initial consideration) to be a simple process, it is actually very complex (Lukaszewicz and

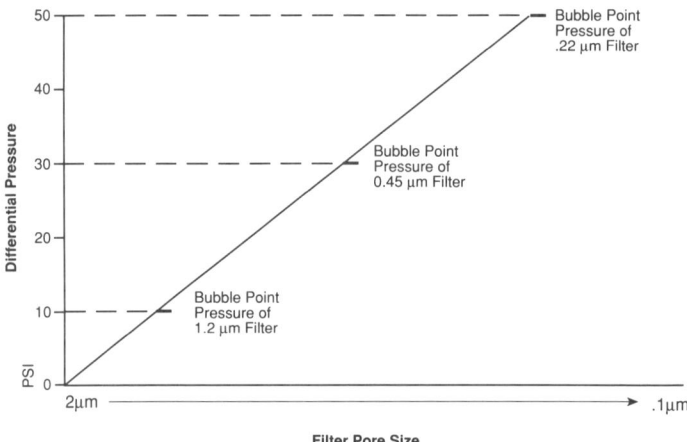

Figure 10. Bubble point data for mixed ester filter.

Meltzer 1979, 1980; Sladek and Leahy 1981). While it is generally not necessary for the particle analyst to understand filter function in detail, general knowledge of how filters work is useful (Michaels 1976; Schmidt 1964). When a liquid containing particles is pulled or pushed through a cast film filter, a complex flow system is set up in which minute streams of liquid move from the solution into and through the pores of the filter and exit the downstream side. Liquid flows more readily through the large pores, so that these pores are preferred in the filtration process (Marshall and Meltzer 1976). Particles suspended in the liquid are carried along in the flowing liquid by inertia. If the particles are small enough to pass through the holes of the filter, they pass out the other side into the filtrate. Particles that are of larger size become impinged upon the surface of the filter, or become physically trapped within the interstices of the filter matrix.

Direct interception of larger size particles occurs, but many particles smaller than the filter pores are also removed (Zierdt 1979). If a particle is smaller than a pore, there is still a high probability that the particle will touch the filter matrix. For such particles that are smaller than a pore, retention will occur if the particle contacts the filter surface and is adhered by electrostatic or van der Waals forces. Sladek and Leahy (1981) measured the depth of penetration of small bacteria (*Pseudomonas diminuta*) into filter media, showing that the bacteria penetrated a considerable depth into the filter before being removed. Penetration was considerably greater in filters with large pores than in filters with small pores, and no significant penetration occurred in filters with a 0.2 μm pore size. Hou et al. (1980) determined the relative significance of mechanical straining (interception) and electrostatic attraction for removing polystyrene beads of various sizes. The results of these two studies illustrate that a membrane filter can function either as a depth filter or as a screen filter, depending upon the particle size in relation to the pore size.

The pH, ionic strength, flow rate, pressure, and temperature of a solution all affect filtration. Most cast film filters possess a significant negative electrostatic charge (up to a hundred volts/cm^2) when they are dry. This charge can be eliminated by use of alpha radiation from a static eliminator or by ionized air. Most of these filters also possess a negative charge when wet if the wetting liquid has a pH value greater than 2–3. Because cells, viruses, and most macromolecules also have negative charges at neutral pH, repulsive forces of an electrostatic nature can develop, which may be stronger than the attraction brought about by static or van der Waals forces. The negative charge on a filter can be reduced or eliminated by raising the ionic strength of the solution to be filtered. This technique can make it possible to remove significant numbers of particles of 1 μm or less in size from water using filters with nominal pores sizes as large as 5 μm to 10 μm.

The electrostatic attraction of a positively charged filter for a negatively charged particle is only important for relatively small particles. The use of filters for sieving (i.e., separating two or more kinds of particles of different sizes) is much more complicated than using filters to retain all particles. Cast film filters do not function as well as sieves because of the wide size range of particles retained. Larger particles retained by a filter may themselves act as filters for the retention of smaller particles that would otherwise pass through. This effect increases in intensity as particles build up on the filter (caking).

As mentioned above, cast film filters may be reasonably uniform in structure throughout their depth, a condition called isotropy, or they may show marked differences in structure from one side to the other, a condition called anisotropy (Kesting et al. 1981; Kesting 1977). Some slight degree of anisotrophy is unavoidable, arising as a result of the manufacturing process (casting onto solid surfaces results in the exposed surface being different in morphology from the surface in contact with the casting support). Cast film filter material sometimes has one side that appears noticeably smoother than the other; the smoother one is the side of the filter that was next to the substrate during the casting process (Elford 1933). An anisotropic filter with a more open structure at the surface than within its depth will permit particles to penetrate into the filter before they are trapped. Flow characteristics are also usually better from the top (more open side) of such filters to the bottom, so that it is desirable to place on anisotropic filter in the filter apparatus with the less reflective side uppermost. In some filters, anisotrophy is intentionally built in to improve solution flow (Marshall and Meltzer 1976). On this type of filter the analyst cannot expect to see particles on the membrane surface unless they are significantly above the retention rating in size.

Based on the above discussion, it should be apparent to the reader that liquid filtration is a totally different process from gas filtration (as discussed in the chapter on environmental particulates). In gas filtration, particles much smaller than the rated pore size are retained with high efficiency (American Public Health Association 1977). Removal of particles occurs by inertial impaction, diffusion, and interception. In liquids, because of the much greater viscosity of the suspending medium, diffusion and inertial impaction are unimportant, and interception is the primary mechanism of retention.

Determination of Retention Ratings

Filter medium is characterized by the diameter of the particle that it can be expected to retained with some high degree of efficiency. Filtration is a statistical phenomenon, and if a suspension of sufficiently high density is used, some particles may appear in the filtrate even if the nominal pore size is smaller than the particle size. This is partly due to the fact that no filter is 100% uniform in structure; some small number of larger holes may be present that have not been detected in quality control procedures. With a high loading of particles, the probability of a particle entering one of these larger holes is increased. Even if 99.999% of the pores in a filter meet specifications, that rare 0.001% event may be sufficient to cause trouble if very dense suspensions are being filtered, or if complete removal of particles is necessary (such as in sterilizing filtration). This consideration of minor importance to the particle analyst. It is conventional in pharmaceutical filtration literature to speak of absolute filters when discussing the use of filters for sterilization purposes. The historical definition of absolute retention has been 100% retention of the challenge organism or particle. True absolute retention at a specific size is very difficult to attain.

Among the conditions that must be specified are the following: test particle used, challenge pressure, concentration, and the detection method used to enumerate particles in the filtrate.

The analyst should be warned that a wide variety of test methods exist and are applied by vendors for determining the retention rating of filters. Nonviable test materials include AC fine test dust, polydisperse glass beads, graded series of monosize latex spheres, and filter media. Intrusion of gases by bubble point or diffusion techniques may also be used for testing. In the case of challenge with particulate matter suspensions, counts obtained upstream and downstream of the material are compared to determine retention ratings. The greatest difficulties encountered with a particulate matter challenge are obtaining an even suspension of the test materials upstream prior to counting, and use of a counting technique with no inherent bias at the size of greatest interest. Light extinction counters are widely applied for this purpose. The use of AC fine test dust is not recommended due to its content of flake-like particles that will be "seen" by a filter as larger than they appear to a particle counter. Bubble point testing is a poor determinant of retention ratings. In a bubble point test, the largest filter pore will be the determinant of the test value; the rating determined in this fashion bears little relation to the performance of a filter in response to a challenge with particulate matter.

Wettability and Refractive Index

Another characteristic of filters that is important in their use for particle collection is their degree of wettability. Filters made of cellulose esters and certain plastics are inherently hydrophobic, and hence are not directly wettable. Such filters may be rendered wettable by the manufacturer's addition of wetting agents that may, in turn, be a source of contamination of a filtered solution. Water can be pushed through a hydrophobic membrane if a sufficiently high pressure is used, but for filters with pores of less than 1 µm in diameter, the pressure required is extremely high and the procedure is generally impractical.

The refractive index of a filter is also important in analytical applications. The whiteness of many membrane filters is due to the high refractive difference between the air in the pores and the polymeric matrix, leading to scattering of the white light that falls on the filter. Refractive indices of 1.51 for cellulose nitrate filters and 1.47 for cellulose acetate filters are representative. If a filter has been dried, it can be made transparent (*cleared*) by filling the void spaces with an oil such as microscope immersion oil. The usefulness of cast film filters for microscopy is often enhanced by adding a colorant that produces a gray (not black, as stated by most vendors), green, or purple filter. Filters with inked grid lines are also widely available and are specified in the USP <788> requirement for large volume parenterals.

Filtration Apparatus

A wide variety of filter holders and filtration funnels are available for use with microporous filters. These differ in size, material of construction, and intended application. The diameter of the filter used is typically determined by the number of particles to be counted and/or the volume of fluid to be filtered. The most common filter diameters available are 13 mm, 25 mm, and 47 mm. The smaller diameters are desirable for filtration of small volumes of liquid, but the analyst should remember that the density of particles on a membrane must be appropriate for the counting procedure to be applied. If only small volumes of sample are available and the particle number in the sample is high, dilution of the sample prior to filtration and use of a larger diameter filter membrane may be indicated. The references by Trasen (1968a, 1968b) give a useful description of filtration techniques.

Filter holders made of metal, glass, or plastic (e.g., polysulfone) are available. The plastic holders are light weight, have adequate mechanical strength, are low in cost, and are easily cleaned. In applications where filters are to be frequently used and cleaned, a plastic filtration apparatus is often chosen. Whether metal, glass, or plastic filter holders are chosen, the equipment employed must be designed for the intended use (low particle shedding characteristics and smooth surfaces) and should be amenable to easy assembly and disassembly. When only aqueous solutions are being filtered, as is most often the case in the pharmaceutical industry, the filtration apparatus can be adequately cleaned by soaking it in a detergent solution, followed by exhaustive rinsing in a stream of distilled water filtered at a retention rating appropriate to the analysis to be performed.

Numerous filter holders for specialized applications are also available. If pressurized gas or process compressed air is to be tested, metal high pressure filter holders that securely lock the filter in a housing and are capable of withstanding the pressures of the system to be evaluated are used. If very small airborne particles (such as fine fibers) are of interest, conductive carbon-filled plastic holders may be obtained that eliminate the adherence of the particles to the material of the holder. Filter holders of all types are available for selection in vendor literature.

Filtration techniques can also be used to isolate particulate matter to be analyzed by chromatography or other means of analysis requiring a liquid sample. This technique is most useful when the particles to be analyzed constitute a dominant mass component of a population, and can be isolated in large numbers on a filter of glass, Teflon®, polycarbonate, or other substrate in which the particles may be dissolved. Once the differential solubility of the particles is determined (such as a solvent that will dissolve the particles of interest but not others present) the filter bearing the particles is extracted by manual procedures or with the aid of ultrasonic or Soxhlet apparatus.

After extraction is completed, the solvent is separated from residual particulate matter by centrifugation and the resulting liquid is evaporated down to the desired volume. In some cases the liquid may be evaporated to as little as 0.5 mL for sampling in microliter aliquots. Extractions from blank filters must be prepared from the same filter lot. Standards should be prepared by dissolving known pure substances in the solvent to be used in the analysis with concentrations to suit the expected range of concentrations in the sample per usual procedures. This procedure may be applied for both GC and HPLC analysis of particle samples. In some cases it may be desirable to fractionate the sample before GC or HPLC is performed. This may be done using liquid chromatography to fractionate the sample for GC analysis, and thin layer chromatography for HPLC analysis.

Collection of Particles for Analysis

The pharmaceutical particle analyst is more often concerned with particle identification than with enumerating particles of different types or different sizes in a population. Sampling for identification may require a less meticulous technique (McCormack et al. 1976). In the simplest case, the entire contents of an affected solution unit can simply be filtered (Michaels 1976; Schmidt 1964). The analyst can often identify particles on the basis of a rapid light microscopic analysis, and if the interest is only in composition of the unknown particles, a small sample may be all that is necessary. The analyst may identify particles *in situ* using instruments, such as an inverted microscope or a hand-held magnifying glass. In the case of an ampoule of drug solution in which visible particles are present, the analyst may simply examine the particles using an inverted microscope. Polarized light may also be used with this instrument, and many commonly occurring extraneous particles in pharmaceuticals (such as paper fibers, cotton, synthetic fibers, glass, metal fragments, rust, skin cells, and rubber) can be identified by this method.

In addition to the techniques for collection of particles discussed in the chapter on microscopy, many other techniques may be improvised for special applications. Bits of filter material may be used to "blot up" liquid droplets for extraction procedures and instrumental analysis. Micropipettes or capillaries can also be used to collect particular liquids by capillary action. A *micro* adaptation of the tape sampling technique may be practical for the isolation of particles for instrumental analysis by x-ray spectroscopy or other electron microscopic techniques. A Formvar® or colloidal solution in a volatile solvent is painted onto a group of particles to be collected. Upon drying, the film is peeled off the substrate with the attached particles and transferred to a carbon or plastic grid for placement in the electron beam instrument. This technique is useful when particles of <10 mm are handled.

Isolation of Particles for Identification

For purposes of identification, some particle samples can be examined directly without further isolation. However, if the particles of interest are imbedded in a matrix or must be removed from a mixture of retentate on a filter, manipulation will be often required. Techniques for isolation and collection of individual particles for analysis involves the use of specialized micro instruments to physically pick up and transfer particles from a filter or other collection substrate to a microslide or sample support for an analytical instrument.

This technique is not new. Louis Pasteur used the microscope to differentiate the optical isomers of tartaric acid. By methodically segregating individual crystals of the two morpho-types, he was able to resolve the optically inactive mixture into the two optically active isomers. This method of isolating individual particles under the microscope using a microneedle, forceps, or another instrument is often essential to identification of particles of interest. Such "particle picking" requires a hood or other HEPA filtered enclosure, a clean work area, a steady hand, a stereomicroscope, and the tools shown in Figure 11. Needle probes and glass fiber brushes are used to pick up single particles. The fine forceps are useful for larger

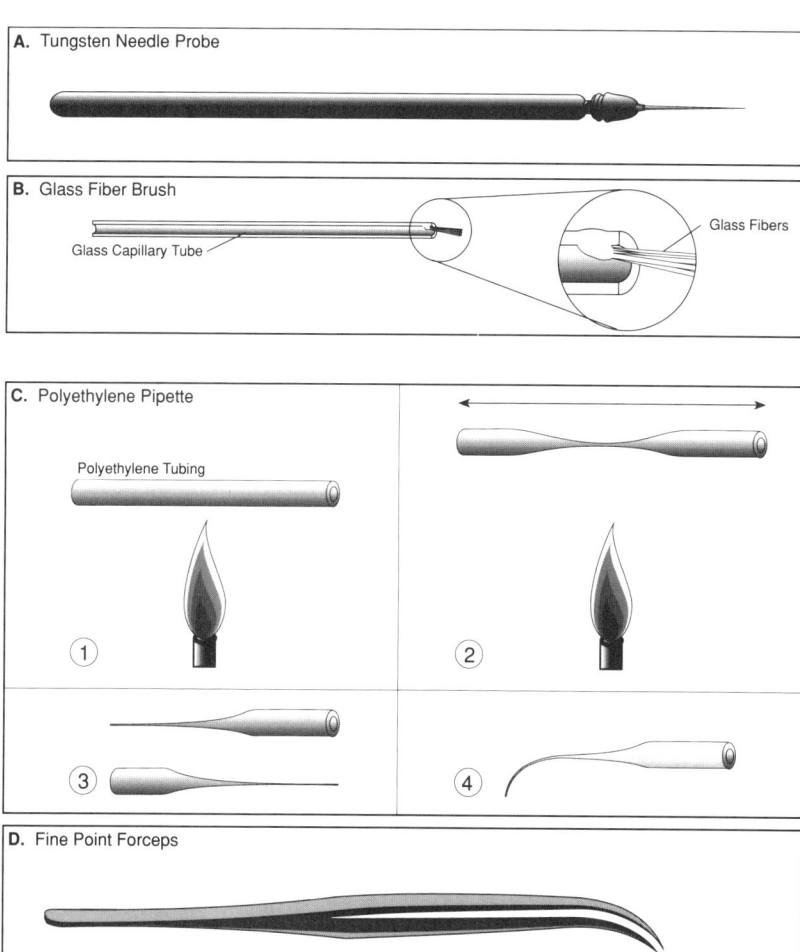

Figure 11.   Tools for particle isolation.

particles. Drawn micropipettes can be used to pick up single particles in a drop of fluid. The techniques for isolating single particles are generally simple, but it is only through careful practice that one acquires the skill necessary for capable particle handling down to sizes of 10 μm and less. The techniques, necessary tools, and the procedures for particle manipulation are discussed in the papers by Teetsov (1977) and DeLuca (1980). Tools specifically designed for particle isolation are available from McCrone Associates, Chicago, IL.

The analyst should always attempt to isolate particles with as little manipulation as possible. Each step in handling risks loss of the particle of interest or the addition of contaminants. One particle should be handled at a time. If the analyst is studying a membrane filter sample by reflected light under a stereomicroscope, specific particles may be removed by touching each with a finely pointed tungsten needle. Adherence of particles to the needle may be enhanced by wetting the tip in a 1% solution of Aroclor® in a solvent such as acetone, and allowing the solvent to evaporate. The coated tip of such a needle with a tip size approximating that of the particle to be isolated is then used to pick up one or several particles under the stereomicroscope. The particles may then be transferred to a small drop of mountant on a clean microscope slide, and after adding a cover slip may be examined with a polarizing microscope. Using a similar technique, particles may be isolated for transfer to a carbon or beryllium mount for examination by scanning electron microscopy or x-ray microprobe, or to a salt plate for analysis by infrared spectroscopy.

The value of the capability for isolation of particles using these physical techniques cannot be overemphasized. The sensitivity limit of microanalytical instruments allow nanogram quantities of material to be analyzed. If a single crystalline particle can be isolated and mounted on the tip of a 10 µm glass fiber, one can obtain an x-ray diffraction pattern. If a clean 10 µm particle can be mounted on a polished beryllium or carbon stub, we can examine it by scanning electron microscopy or analyze it quantitatively with x-ray spectroscopy. Secondary ion mass spectrometry is useful with particles of similar size. Micro FT–IR spectrophotometers can obtain spectra with sharply resolved absorbencies from single particles of 10 µm to 20 µm in size. Experts in x-ray diffraction, electron microscopy, or microprobe analysis are not usually adept at handling single particles of a size that approaches the sensitivity of their instruments. They must depend on particle analysts with this technical skill to acquire samples for these instruments.

There are general procedures and helpful hints regarding particle isolation for the beginner. These include the following:

- Never take your eyes off the particle during a manipulative operation;
- Remove the particle from the needle only by "washing" it off into a microdrop of liquid in which the particle will be trapped;
- Beware of a static electricity; and

- Ensure that the path the needle will take to place the particle on the microscope slide is unobstructed.

Importantly, any particle(s) to be isolated for analysis by instrumental means should be characterized by light microscopy before separation. The mounted particle can then be recognized as the original and not another particle picked up by accident.

Powder Sampling

Bulk powders present special problems in sample preparation. The essential principle to be observed in collecting samples of a bulk powder material is that of ensuring that the sample contains particles of all sizes in the correct concentration proportions. The analyst working with powders must realize the difficulties involved, and understand the ways in which the segregation of different particle sizes in a powder is likely to occur. The sampling procedure must then be designed to minimize the effects of segregation. Sampling of powders is described in some detail in the book by Allen (1990).

In a commonly occurring scenario, the analyst will be asked to collect samples from a drug powder batch that may consist of a number of 50 kg (or larger) drums. This is not a simple task. The powder in the drums has most certainly segregated by size during shipment. A way must be found to sample throughout the volume of powder without introducing contamination. Maintenance of sterility is an overriding consideration when sterile bulk drug powders are to be sampled. For this reason, samples for particle analysis may be collected by the powder manufacturer and shipped separately to the laboratory. This practice is totally acceptable, but assurance must be obtained that the sample supplied is representative both with regard to particle size distribution and levels of extraneous particles.

Scoop sampling (the simplest method) consists of plunging a scoop or other collection tool into the bulk material and withdrawing a sample. This method is likely to result in errors since the whole volume of the sample is accessible to the sampling device, and the sample is typically taken from the surface where it may not be typical of the mass. Large particles that have segregated at the top of a container during shipment will be disproportionately represented in scoop sample. Similarly, sampling at the lower levels of a large container may result in a collection of more fine particles than would be present if the container were thoroughly mixed. Thus, sampling by means of a scoop or spatula is generally unsuitable for collection of a representative sample. A better method is the use of a "thief" to sample from various depths within a large container. A laboratory scale version of this device is shown in Figure 12. Larger models are available for use on drums of powder.

The coning and quartering method of sample dividing (Figure 13) consists of pouring the material into a conical heap and relying on its radial symmetry to give four identical samples when the heap is flattened and quartered with a metal cutter. This method will give reliable results if the heap is symmetrical about a vertical axis, and if the two cutting planes coincide with the axis of the heap. In practice, the heap may not be symmetrical, and symmetry of cutting is difficult to achieve. Vertical size segregation occurs in forming the heap, and any departure from symmetry in the cutting will lead to differences in the size of the four portions into which the heap is cut. The method is very dependent on the skill of the operator. If coning and quartering is possible, the quantity of material available is usually such that it can be separated using a device (such as a chute splitter shown in Figure 14), in which the sample is split into half volumes of decreasing size until the working sample is isolated.

The thief, chute splitter, and cone and quarter methods can be used in applications where small numbers of samples are to be analyzed and the workload is insufficient to justify purchase of a dedicated powder sampling apparatus. If samples of powder material are to be routinely analyzed, specialized motor-driven sample mixing devices (such as a spinning riffler, rotary sample divider, or oscillating sample divider) may be used to obtain uniform and reproducible sampling (Allen 1990).

The standard deviation for numbers of particles counted in specific size ranges varies for the different methods of sampling. Generally, variability decreases with regard to two primary rules of sampling powders: (1) Most reproducible sampling is obtained when the mass of powder to be sampled is in motion; and (2) The best sample for analysis is comprised of many samples of smaller mass taken from the total volume of the bulk material. Measurements based on cone and quarter or scoop sampling approximates 10%. A chute splitter can result in as low as 1–2% variation (SD). The spinning riffler can result in samples for which a 0.1 to 0.3% SD is attainable. Adequate sampling is particularly important when a 50 to 100 kg mass of process material must be reduced stepwise to a gross sample of several kg, a lab sample of 50 to 100 g, and a measurement sample of a milligram mass. Generally, numbers of fines will decrease with the extent to which air is mixed into the

Collection and Isolation of Particulate Matter 373

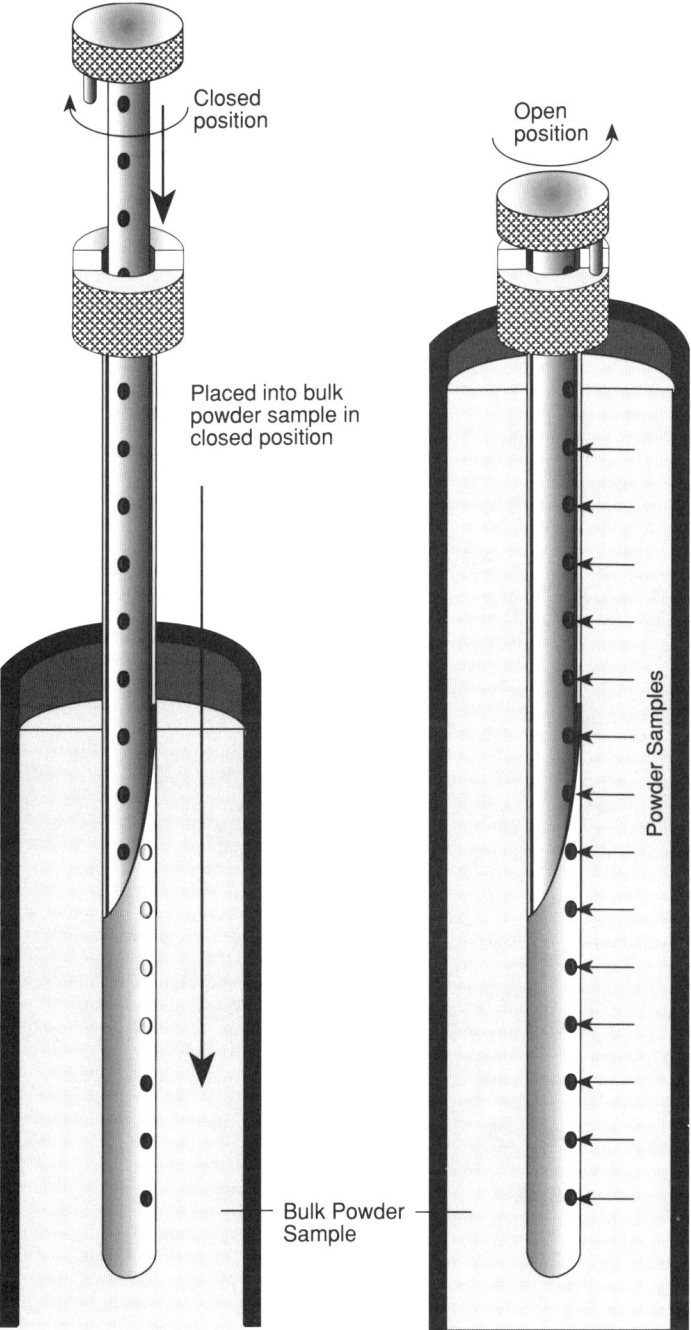

Figure 12. "Thief" for powder sampling.

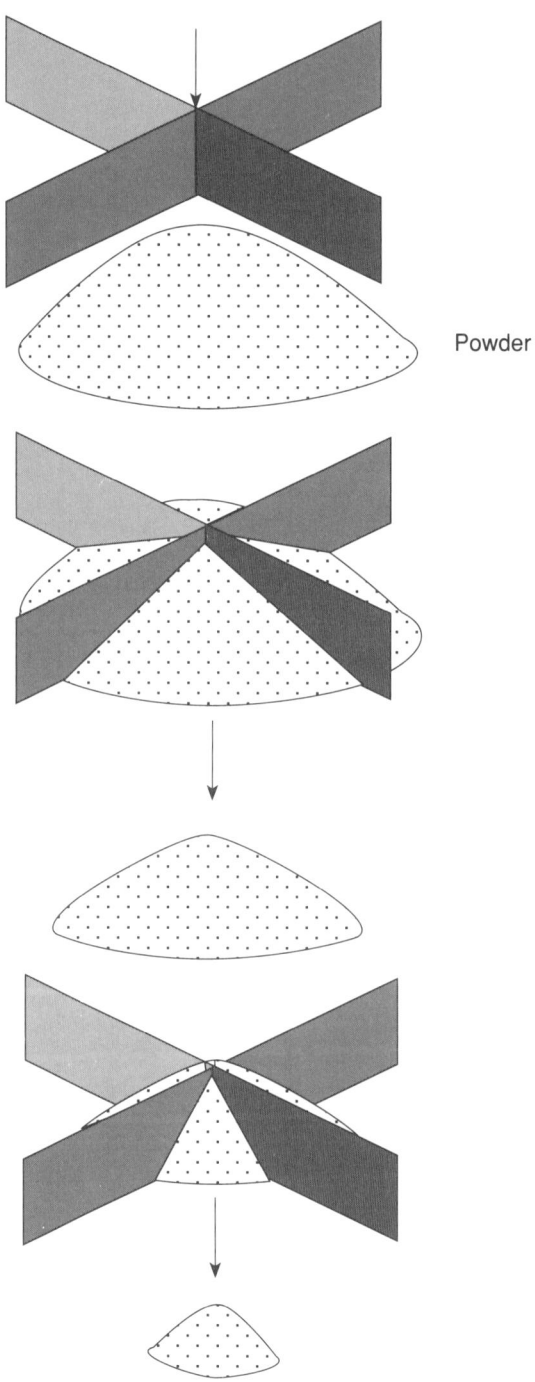

Figure 13. Cone and quarter method of sample collection.

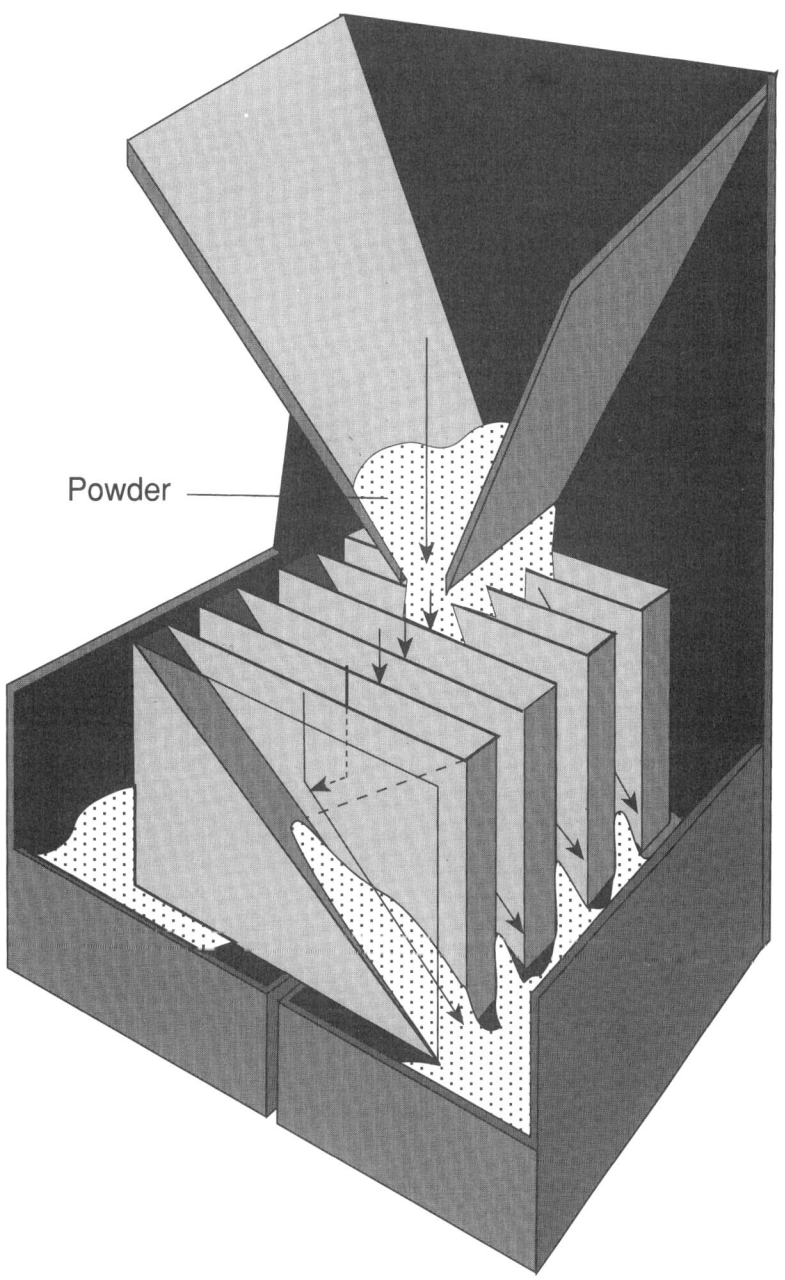

Figure 14. Chute splitter.

sample. Particles segregate when powder is poured into a heap or into a collection vessel.

Once the powder sample is reduced to a workable size, the second difficult problem facing microscopic examination is the preparation of a slide containing a uniformly dispersed, representative sample of the powder. Several methods of accomplishing this are available, but the final result often depends more on the skill and technique of the analyst than the procedure used. If a permanent slide is not required, a useful procedure is simply to place a small sample of the powder on a microscope slide and add a few drops of some dispersing fluid. Some analysts mix the powder in the fluid with a flexible spatula, others roll it with a glass rod. Both procedures may produce fracture of the particles. A preferable alternative is to use a small camel-hair brush. Further dispersing fluid may then be added until the concentration is satisfactory. A drop of the suspension is then placed on another slide with the brush, and a cover slip carefully placed so as to exclude air bubbles. For a semipermanent slide, the cover slip may be sealed with amyl acetate or glue. Silicone oil and glycerol are two other satisfactory dispersing fluids. Some powders may require the addition of a dispersing agent or surfactant to eliminate aggregation.

Another acceptable method for the production of slide mounts is to place a small representative sample of the powder to be analyzed in a 10 mL beaker, add 2 or 3 mL of a solution containing 1–2% collodion in amyl-acetate, stir vigorously, and place a drop of the resulting suspension on the still surface of distilled water in a large beaker. The film produced as this drop spreads and evaporates may then be picked up on a clean microscope slide for examination. A powder material may also be dispersed in a volatile liquid in which it is insoluble, and a drop of the resulting suspension transferred to a slide. When the particulate matter sample is dry, a drop of mounting medium is placed over the particles that may be further dispersed as necessary by sliding a cover slip over the drop of mountant in a circular pattern.

Collection of Particles from Environmental Air

Airborne particles may be counted microscopically and with particle counters. Particles collected onto a filter may be isolated and identified using the technique discussed above with regard to solution-borne particulate matter. Particles may be collected from air in controlled environment areas by the simple use of a vacuum pump attached to an appropriate filtration funnel. A 47-mm stainless steel filter holder is generally a good choice where large volumes of air or air with a high particle burden are to be sampled. The filter holder should be precleaned by the technique discussed earlier, and the filter precounted for background particles. For ease of use or for critical samples, transparent, disposable aerosol contamination monitors are available. These monitors have been precleaned during assembly, and the average surface particle background count is supplied with each lot. The Millipore manual (*Detection and Analysis of Particulate Contamination,* #AD030) referenced at the end of this chapter is available free of charge from Millipore Corporation, (Bedford, MA) and includes particularly useful information on the analysis and enumeration of particles from the air and also catalogs the necessary equipment.

Large quantities of particles removed from the air can be quantitated by gravimetric means. By determining the flow rate of air through the membrane filter and the length of sampling time, the volume of air sampled can be calculated. After counting or weighing the fibers and particles on the membrane filter, the total number counted or weighed is divided by the total sample volume to give counts or weight per unit volume of air. Matched weight monitors, which eliminate the need for preweighing test filters, are available from Millipore for use in gravimetric analysis. Each of these monitors contains two superimposed filters matched in weight to within 0.1 mg.

Vacuum pumps used in aerosol collection should be able to draw enough vacuum to accommodate a range of flow rates from 1 to 150 liters per minute. Flow regulation, pump weight, and operating time are important considerations. Pumps must either be calibrated by a flow meter or be used with a flow-limiting orifice. They should be capable of operating without overheating or changing flow rate over the long periods of time often required in air sampling.

Importantly, flow rate of sampling must be controlled so that the total volume of air sampled can be determined. A simple way to control flow rate is to use flow-limiting orifices such as those available from Millipore. These are inserted into the outlet of either a Millipore 47-mm filter holder, or a Millipore aerosol adapter used with a 37-mm contamination monitor. When a specified level of vacuum is applied, air flows through the filter and orifice at a constant rate. The amount of vacuum required to maintain the correct flow rate for each orifice available is listed in Table I. The applied vacuum must be equal to or greater than the specified level.

Table I. Vacuum Requirement for Function of Flow-Limiting Orifices (Courtesy of Millipore Corp.)

Orifice Flow Rate (L/min)	Minimum Required Vacuum	
	mm Hg	in Hg
1	300	12
2	300	12
3	300	12
4.9	400	16
10	500	20
14	550	22

As mentioned above, filtrative collection of particles may be used either for gravimetric analysis or to collect particles for counting, identification, or other analytical methods. As an interesting example of the latter procedure, the particles of antibiotic powder in the air of an aseptic filling area may be collected on a filter and assayed for antimicrobial activity on the basis of volume of air filtered. Thus, the level of the drug in the air may be related to different airborne count levels, and the numerical variability of drug particles relative to total count variation may be determined. If the process is consistent, the drug component of the total airborne particle count by this means can be shown to represent some constant proportion of the total count so that personnel exposure can be quantitated.

The choice of filters for air monitoring applications is dependent on the purpose for which monitoring is being conducted Pore size and surface texture of a filter, and the analytical method to be applied are important considerations in filter choice. In general, microporous cast film filters will efficiently retain airborne particles with a diameter that is much smaller than the stated pore size of the filter in the same fashion as HEPA filters do. For instance, Millipore Type AA (0.8 µm) mixed ester filter will retain essentially 100% of all particles (>99.99%) drawn onto it. Particles significantly below the retention rating will be collected within the depth of the filter, however, and will be unavailable for analysis. Nuclepore® membranes, as discussed, have a number of advantages for analytical use. Perhaps most notable is the smooth surface on which all particles above the retention rating may be readily detected by SEM. However, the low porosity of these membranes and resulting low flow rates may pose some difficulties for use in air monitoring.

Microscopic Analysis of Airborne Particles

Light microscopy is not currently used to any great extent in analysis of airborne particles. Historically, light microscopic analysis has proven to be of limited use in identifying the small (0.2 µm to 1.0 µm) particles that are often of great interest as airborne contaminants in controlled environment areas. If particles collected on a filter cannot be identified by light microscopy, they must generally be transferred to another substrate for instrumental analysis by SEM–EDXS or other means. While particles of submicron size may be collected on microporous filters by vacuum and the filter subsequently "cleared" to allow microscopic study, this technique is generally too time consuming for routine or frequent use, and the limited resolution of light microscopes constitutes another serious limitation.

The scanning electron microscope is well-suited to investigation aerosol particles. As discussed in Chapter 5, a scanning electron microscope with EDXS capability will provide for rapid identification of particles a fraction of a micron in size, and simultaneously provides morphological information. If particulate matter is to be collected by filtration, the analyst must use care in the selection of a filter due to the necessity of retaining particles on the filter surface. Anisotrophic microporous filters with surface pores larger than their retention rating may retain particles of interest within the depth of the filter matrix rather than on their surface.

There is a variety of commercial equipment available for isolating small particles from the air and collecting them on some substrate suitable for combined SEM–EDXS analysis. This sampling instrumentation includes impingers and impactors, as well as the filter cassettes discussed earlier. The Greenburg-Smith type impinger (Figure 15) and its modifications are probably the most familiar impinger designs. This device has a plate suspended at a fixed distance from a central intake capillary. Impingers can be used to collect particles efficiently down to less than 1 µm in size and are especially useful for sampling fine particle aerosols.

A novel air sampler developed by California Measurements Inc. (Sierra Madre, CA) allows small airborne particles to be collected directly onto stub mounts for examination with a scanning microscope. The design of this device is based on the inertial (cascade) impactors and classifiers used for environmental sampling

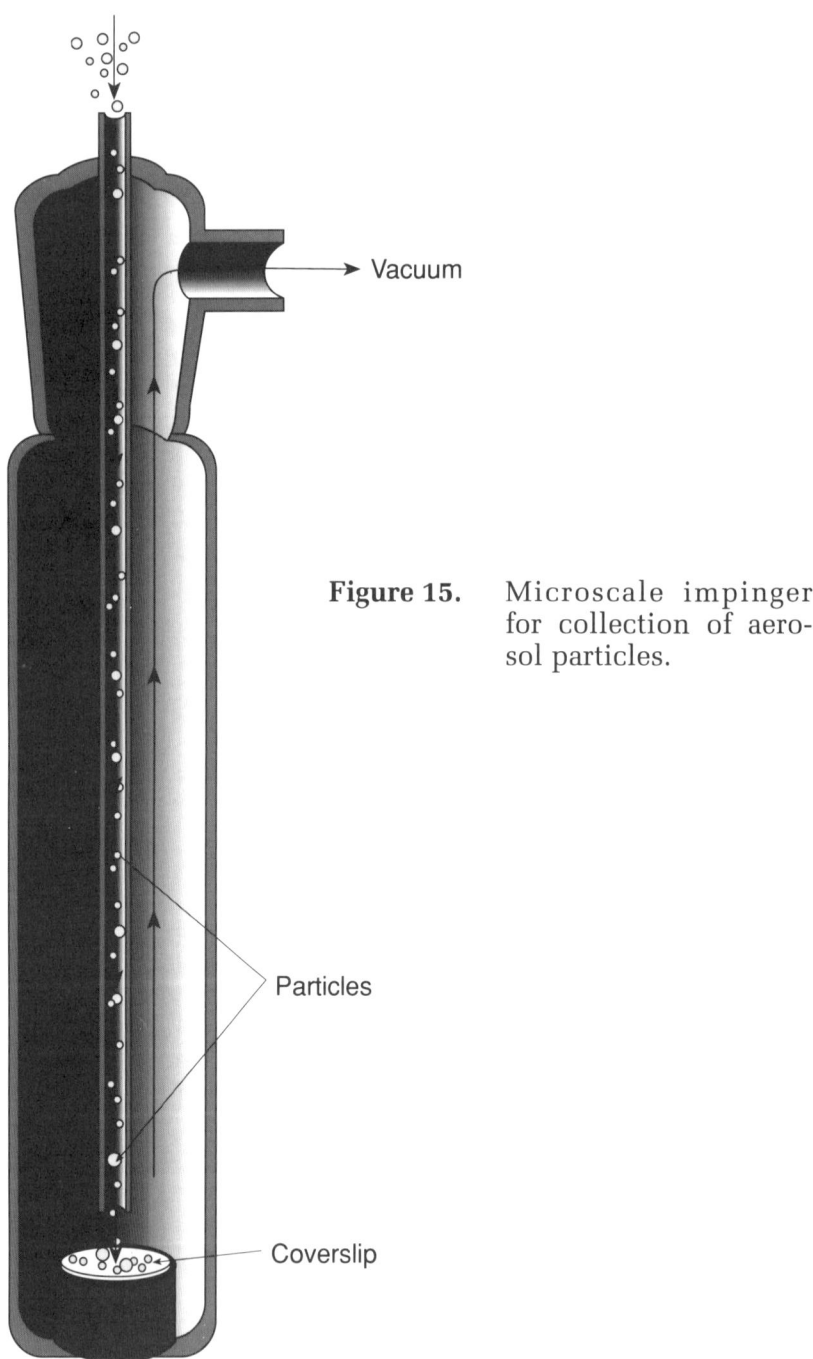

Figure 15. Microscale impinger for collection of aerosol particles.

(Figure 16). The device contains a vertical stack of circular plates with recesses into which the stubs are placed. The plates are placed

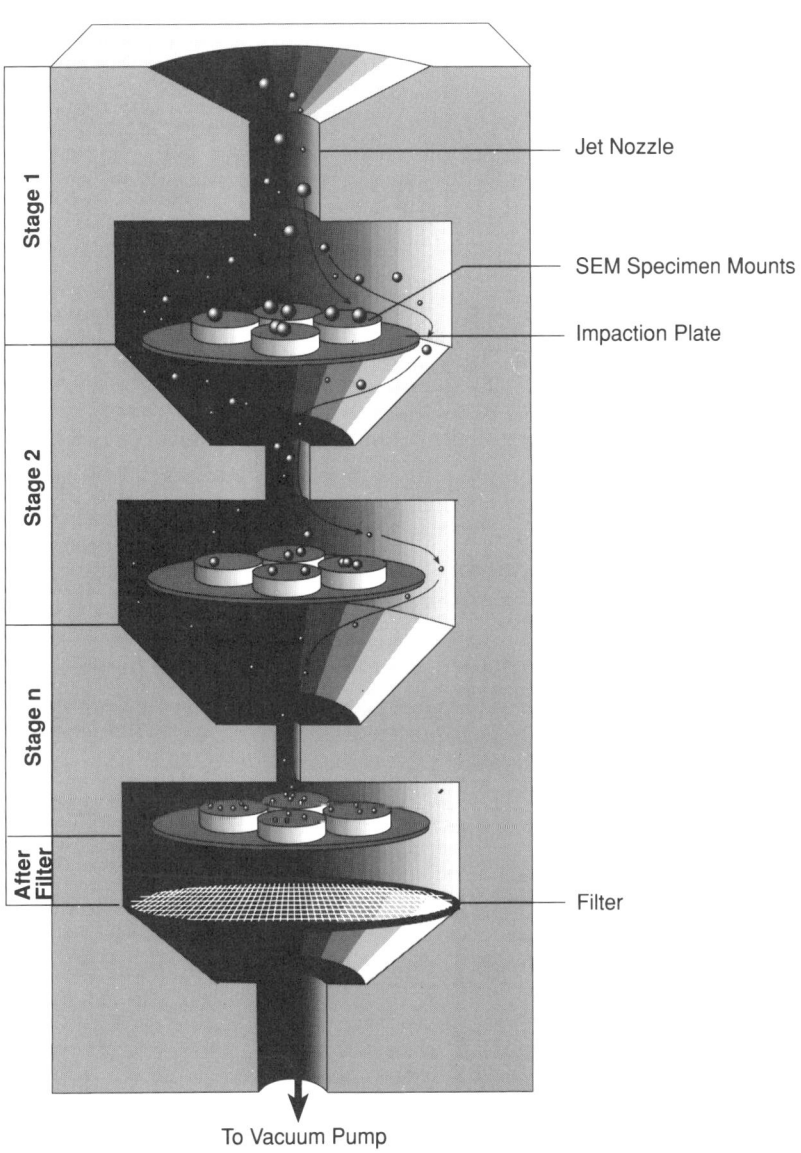

Figure 16. Cascade impactor for collection of fine particles (California Measurement, Inc.).

in a cylindrical enclosure through which air is drawn from top to bottom by a vacuum pump. Based on the geometry of the airflow path over the stubs, smaller or larger particles are collected by inertial impaction. The result, after air is drawn through the device for an appropriate period of time, is a series of scanning microscope stubs bearing size-segregated particles that may be identified and related to a size range in which elevated counts were noted with a particle counter. The use of this device in combination with scanning microscopy (EDXS) provides a specialized but effective approach to identifying small particles present in the air of clean areas such as an aseptic fill complex.

Monitoring of large particles (≥ 10 µm) present in low numbers in controlled environment areas may require special techniques. Surface contamination with large particles can be measured by light microscopic counting and sizing, and for nonaccessible surfaces one can use tape sampling methods. There are also video camera-based techniques and scanning laser light scattering devices for this purpose. In electronics manufacturing, these latter devices may be used for evaluation of the product itself, such as silicon wafers or chips.

One of the most practical methods for monitoring larger particles is based upon microscopic evaluation of "witness plates" that have been exposed to the same environment as the product. Although automated devices for reading witness plates are available, the manual light microscopic evaluation of witness plates is the most useful method for pharmaceutical production environments. The technique provides a simple and effective way of measuring large particle fall-out and particles generated at process points.

The technique is simple in application. Witness plate samplers may be constructed using one of the following materials:

- Black vinyl tape,
- Agar gel,
- Filter paper,
- Polished glass, or
- Aluminum mirrors.

In my experience, the first material works the best. A one-inch square of black double-surfaced vinyl tape is placed in a petri slide container. The surface is washed with 0.2 µm filtered water from a pressure vessel and dried in a HEPA-protected hood. Following the drying of the petri slide with the tape, the section is examined microscopically for cleanliness and exposed for 24 hours or some other appropriate interval in the area to be tested. The number of particles settling on the tape in a given time allows the fall-out rate to be calculated. Multiple plates placed in different process areas can be used to map a controlled environment area for cleanliness.

The Uramec particle fallout photometer (PFO, Figure 17) provides a fast and effective means of reading witness plates. Particle fallout is determined by measuring the amount of light scattered by particles collected on the nonreflective sampling surface dark glass witness plates. Light from an ultrastable halogen lamp is split into two horizontal beams and passed at intersecting angles across the sampling plate. Light scattered by the particles is detected in a photodiode, generating an electronic signal directly proportional to the amount of light scatter. The resulting signal is translated into a PFO value that is displayed on the photometer's digital readout; this value may be correlated with ASTM and other standards for cleanliness.

A built-in microscope permits visual inspection of the particles collected on the sample plate. By mounting a camera on the microscope, photographic documentation of the sample can be obtained and enlarged for closer inspection.

The commercially available aerosol analysis monitors discussed earlier are also very useful for the collection of aerosol particles. These typically consist of a clear polycarbonate cassette with removable cover containing a 25-mm or 37-mm cellulose acetate filter. Ports are provided at the top and bottom of the housing for the application of a vacuum and the entrance of sample air. Upon obtaining elevated counts of airborne particles, these monitors may be placed in the affected clean room or production area and used with a vacuum pump to collect particles for analysis for some specified period of time. As is the case with filters used to collect particles from solution, the filters may be examined directly using a light microscope or sections may be cut from the filter and used as samples for scanning electron microscopy or x-ray spectroscopy.

Most counting techniques used for aerosol monitoring assume a normal distribution of particles on a collection filter. The number of microscope fields to be counted is determined by the number of particles per field and the number of fields at a given magnification. As the number of particles per field decreases, the number of fields counted increases, and vice versa, in order to comply with the statistical needs of the normal distribution. In practice, the number of particles per field is commonly adjusted to between 20 and 30 by sample preparation or by varying the magnification of

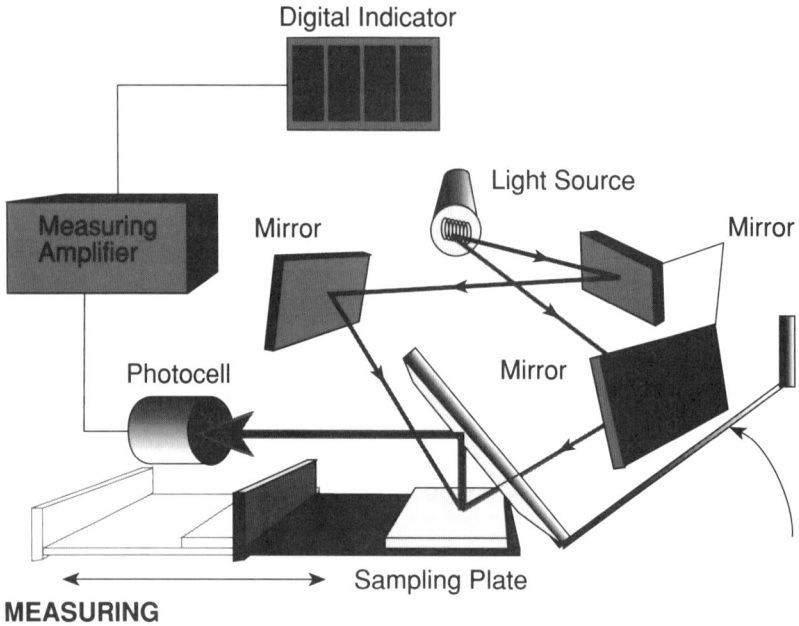

MEASURING

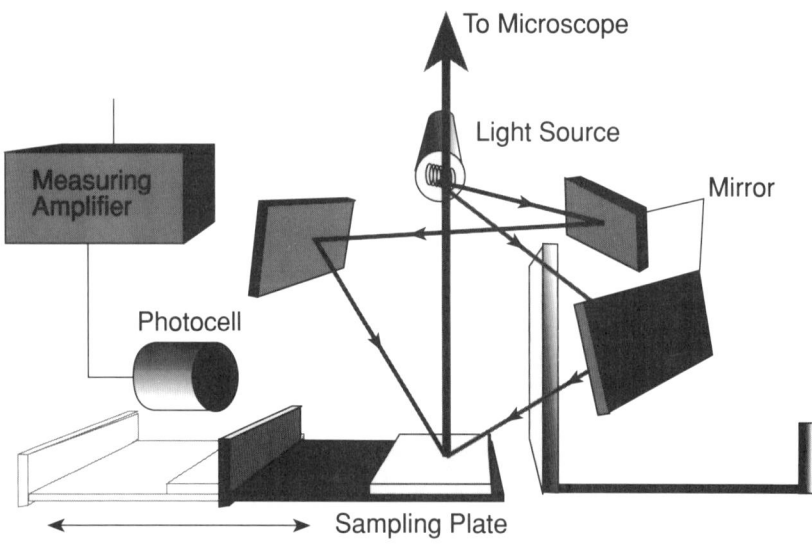

OBSERVATION

Figure 17. Uramec particle fallout meter.

the microscope. Under such conditions, it is sufficient to count 20 to 30 fields in order to achieve confidence levels of 90% to 95%.

Monitoring of Components and Parts

In addition to collecting particles for analysis from solutions, the air, and process points, it may be necessary to collect particles from various physical objects, such as the components of medical devices, closures, or parts of process machinery. The method used here depends primarily on the size of the object to be analyzed and the presence or absence of any surface coatings in which particles might be adhered or entrapped. If the part is large enough to be readily grasped or handled, it may be held in the analyst's gloved hand and rinsed over a filtration funnel with a forceful jet of water from a gun-type solvent dispenser with an integral filter. "Particle free" vinyl gloves are well-suited to this operation, but other types of gloves may be used if care is taken to ensure that after washing in filtered water they add no significant numbers of background particles to the analysis. Larger parts may be rinsed by immersion or by use of a rate jet from a pressure vessel while enclosed in a clean plastic bag of Nylon® or other material that serves to collect the rinse solution for filtration.

If the parts to be tested are small, they may be submerged in a suitably clean wash fluid in an ultraclean glass beaker. Particles may then be removed by sonication or gentle manual agitation and isolated by pouring the wash solution into a filter funnel. It is important to remember that when particles are dislodged, they will settle rapidly, and may be lost at the bottom of the collection vessel unless the solution is poured off fairly rapidly. A second rinse of the collection vessel may also be used to effect a more complete collection of particles. Small objects may be rinsed in groups to collect larger numbers of particles. If particles are adhered to the test articles by oil or grease, aqueous washing may be ineffective in their removal. In this case, detergent solution or a suitable solvent may be used to enhance removal. Freon® is a useful solvent if a silicon oil or grease is involved.

In sampling the surfaces of parts or components, it is practically impossible to quantitatively remove contaminating particles for filtration through a membrane filter. Therefore, it is extremely important to follow the identical rinsing procedure for any given component or system each time the samples are analyzed. The analytical results from such sampling will not yield absolute counts of surface adherent particles, but they will yield meaningful and reproducible data on relative contamination levels.

Sampling of Clean Room Garments

There is an understandably high level of interest in the testing of clean room garments and wiping materials. The pharmaceutical manufacturer most often has an interest either in validating the particle shedding characteristics of garments purchased or verifying the effectiveness of washing when nondisposable woven fabric garments are used. While I have included a brief discussion of testing methodology and particle collection from this source, the pharmaceutical manufacturer should consider requiring the vendor of clean room materials and garments or washing sources to perform particle testing rather than performing these analyses in-house. This opinion is based primarily on the specialized and time-consuming nature of this analysis. A number of appropriate test methodologies are available from ASTM or IES standards.

Generally, fabric materials may be tested either wet or dry. Logically, wiping materials are more frequently tested using a solvent, and garments are most often tested dry. The simplest dry test consists of clamping sections of the material to be tested above the face of a filter in a filtration fixture that allows clean air to be drawn through the fabric and a filter by means of a vacuum pump. Per ASTM Method F51-68, 5 µm filtered air is drawn through five designated 0.01 ft^2 areas of a single thickness of the garment fabric at a rate of 14 liters per minute for 1 minute per area. Loose particulate matter contaminants on or in the garment are impinged on the surface of the filter that is then examined microscopically to determine the number of particles (>5 µm) removed from the garment. For garment monitoring per this standard, it is customary to count and tabulate particles in only two categories:

1. All particles with the major dimension greater than 5 µm, and

2. Fibers (longer than 100 µm with a length-to-width [aspect] ratio exceeding 10 to 1).

Other methods are also available that test the garment or fabric of interest under dynamic conditions. For dry testing, the Helmke drum test is applied by many vendors of clean room gloves, masks, wipers, and garments (Figure 18). Samples to be tested are placed in a rotating drum and are tumbled to release particles. The air in

Collection and Isolation of Particulate Matter 387

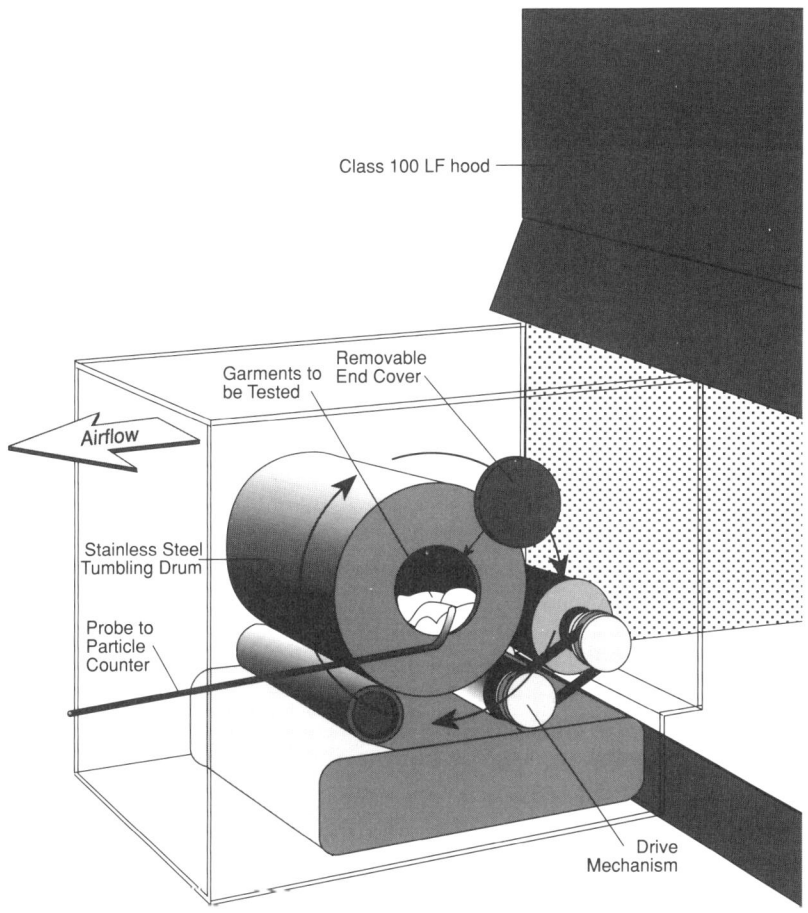

Figure 18. Helmke drum garment test.

the drum is drawn through a sampling probe and the particles ≥0.5 µm released from the samples are counted by a light scattering particle counter. A Helmke drum apparatus or equivalent (as specified in IES RP–CC-003-087-T) is placed in a HEPA-protected hood and the speed of the drum rotation is adjusted to 10 rpm ±0.1 rpm. Alternatively, the air from the drum may be drawn through a filter cassette placed in line between the drum and a vacuum pump and analyzed microscopically.

Yet another method of collection of particles from fabric items in a dry state is based on flexing of the test article. In this procedure the stress is imparted to the wiper by a flexing device, the design of which is based on the Gelbo Flex Tester (as described in IES RP–CC-004-87-T).

The unit consists of a metal and plexiglass enclosure, housing two opposed, cylindrical heads, one stationary and the other attached to a rotating and reciprocating motor-driven arm. When activated, the movable head approaches the stationary one and rotates approximately 180 degrees in the course of its full stroke. A return of the head to its resting position completes one cycle. The rate of flexing is one Hertz.

A sample is mounted in the flexor by wrapping and clamping the ends of the wiper around the heads that are in their extreme open position. Optimally, the width of the section of fabric tested will correspond to the circumference of the flexor heads, yielding a cylinder of the cloth (the edges of which just abut) between the heads. The distance between the heads may be altered by sliding the stationary one on its supporting shaft in the axial direction and locking it in place by means of a set screw. The particles generated by the flexed wiper are collected by an airborne counts sampling probe located beneath the wiper. The counter should sample air at the rate of one cubic foot per minute (cfm) from the chamber in which the wiper is stressed. Thus, if the sample is stressed for one minute (60 cycles), one cubic foot of air will have been drawn from the chamber and the particles it contains counted. The duration of flexing to the sample may be adjusted depending upon the physical characteristics of the wiper, its intended use, and the magnitude of the stress associated with that use.

It has been my experience that dry testing significantly understates the number of particles that might actually be released when a wiper is used in a wet condition. The existence of cohesive forces and static charge, present in all wipers but to different extents, holds particles in place and allows only a portion of them to be removed in the dry state. It has been estimated that approximately one million times more energy would have to be imparted to a dry wiper to remove the same burden of particles as are removed by testing in water. When testing is performed on a wetted sample these forces are dissipated and the release of particles from a wiper more closely approximates what will occur during actual use.

In the simplest application of wet testing, the fabric to be tested is clamped in a filtration funnel apparatus and a specified volume of water is drawn through the cloth by a vacuum and collected in ultracleaned vacuum flask. The solution containing particles from the sample is then filtered for microscopic analysis. Another method makes use of a biaxial shaker of the type commonly employed to mix paint in hardware stores per IES RP–CC-004-87-T. The test fabric is placed in a 4 liter jar with 600 mL of filtered water. The jar and its contents are shaken for 5 minutes; then the particles may be isolated by filtration.

Since the magnitude of the cohesive forces adhering particles to the bulk fabric vary with the composition of the material, and since these forces are eliminated by the characteristics water in a wet test, one would expect that different particle generation of wipers would result in the wet and dry tests. This, in fact, is the case. Typically, fabric with high percentages of synthetic constituents yield relatively low dry particle counts. On wet testing these wipers produce comparatively high counts. On the other hand, those wipers containing cellulosic components gave relatively high particle generation in the dry test and low level of particles in the wet test. This is only an empirical rule of thumb, as the particle generation on any material will be contingent upon other factors as well, including finish of cut edge, handling, and the presence of binders, surfactants, and so forth.

Testing of Clean Room or Surgical Gloves

Gloves used in clean rooms and those used in surgical procedures have received a good deal of interest in the past several years as sources of particulate matter. Gloves are readily tested for particle shedding characteristics by the test described in IES RP–CC-005-87-T. The test described in the recommended practice is based on rinsing particulate matter from a tested glove into 700 mL of filtered deionized water; particles removed are enhanced by mechanical agitation using a paint shaker or other means. Particles in size ranges of 0.5 µm to 150 µm are enumerated by instrumental counting or by microscopy and compared to eight limit sets that relate to particles/cm^2 of glove surface.

The reader interested in testing gloves is directed to the standard. The single further observation I will make relates to the enumeration of particles washed from gloves using instrumental counting. No counter is available with the required dynamic range for this testing based on a single type of sensing. Particles must be counted in categories of 0.5 µm to 5.0 µm up to 50 µm–150 µm. Thus, the use of different sensors will be required to cover the entire range, or Hiac/Royco's hybrid light scattering-light extinction sensor (Microcount 05; dynamic range of 0.5–350 µm) may be used. In either case, the calibration of the light scattering sensor used for the 0.5 µm to 5.0 µm size range will be especially critical for the reasons discussed in the earlier chapter on instrumental counting. The analyst must keep in mind that: (1) slight differences in calibration will result in significant variation in counts in this range due to the extremely high numbers of small particles present, and (2) a difference in refractive index between submicron particles from gloves and latex calibration particles used may result in a level of bias that renders particle size number data invalid or of decreased usefulness.

Summary

A wide variety of particle isolation and collection methods is available to the pharmaceutical particle analyst. The most commonly used analytical path involves the isolation of particles from solution by filtration onto a microporous filter followed by isolation of the particle(s) of interest using a fine-pointed transfer probe. Once the particle is isolated, it may be analyzed by polarized light microscopy, x-ray spectrometry, or other instrumental means. Specialized methods are also available for the collection of particles from surfaces, containers, process points, garments, and the atmosphere.

References

Allen, T. 1990. *Particle size measurement,* 4th Ed. New York: Chapman and Hall.

American Public Health Association. 1977. *Methods of air sampling and analysis,* 2nd Ed. Washington, D.C., p. 984.

ASTM Standard F51-68. 1989. *Standard test method for sizing and counting particulate contaminants in and on clean room garments.* Philadelphia: American Society for Testing and Materials.

Bares, D., and M. Lannis. 1990. The potential of sieve filters for particulate determination. In *Proc. Int. Conf. on Particle Detection, Metrology and Control,* p. 467–501. Arlington, VA.

Brock, T. D. 1983. Membrane filtration: A user's guide and reference manual. *Sci. Tech. Inc.* Madison, WI, p. 381.

DeLuca, P. P., and S. Bodapatti. 1980. Guidelines for the identification of particles in parenterals. *FDA Guidelines* No. 3 (July).

Detection and analysis of particulate contamination (Literature #AD030). 1991. Bedford, MA: Millipore Corp.

Elford, W. J. 1933. The principles governing the preparation of membranes having graded porosities. *Transactions of the Faraday Soc.* 33:1094–1106.

Fleischer, R. L., P. B. Price, and E. M. Symes. 1964. Novel filter for biological materials. *Science* 143:249–250.

Hou, K., C. P. Gerba, S. M. Goya, and K. S. Zerda. 1980. Capture of latex beads, bacteria, endotoxin, and viruses by charge-modified filters. *App. and Environ. Microb.* 40:892–896.

IES Recommended Practice RP–CC-003-87-T. *Garments required in clean rooms and controlled environmental areas.* Mt. Prospect, IL: Institute of Environmental Sciences.

IES Recommended Practice RP–CC-004-87-T. *Wipers used in clean rooms and controlled environments.* Mt. Prospect, IL: Institute of Environmental Sciences.

IES Recommended Practice RP–CC-005-87-T. *Recommended practice of clean room gloves and finger cots.* Mt. Prospect, IL: Institute of Environmental Sciences.

Kesting, R. E. 1971. *Synthetic polymeric membranes.* New York: McGraw-Hill.

Kesting, R. E. 1977. Asymmetric cellulose acetate membranes. In *Reverse osmosis and synthetic membranes*, ed. S. Sourirajan, 89–111. Ottawa, Canada: National Research Council of Canada Publication Number 15627.

Kesting, R. E., A. Murray, A., K. Jackson, and J. Newman. 1981. Highly anisotropic microfiltration membranes. *Pharm. Tech.* 4:53–60.

Lukaszewicz, R. C., and T. H. Meltzer. 1979. Concerning filter validation. *J. of the Paren. Drug Assoc.* 33:188–194.

Lukaszewicz, R. C., and T. H. Meltzer. 1980. On the structural compatibilities of membrane filters. *J. of Parent. Drug Assoc.* 34:463–472.

Marshall, J. C., and T. H. Meltzer. 1976. Certain porosity aspects of membrane filters: Their pore distribution and anisotrophy. *Bull. of Paren. Drug Assoc.* 30: 214–225.

McCormack, J., J. E. C. Harris, and H. J. Sullivan. 1976. Single particle characterization by optical microscopy and associated techniques. *Proc. Analyst. Div. Chem. Soc.* 13:344–348.

McCrone, W. C., and J. G. Delly. 1973. The light microscopy atlas. *The particle atlas,* Vol. 2, 2nd Ed. Ann Arbor, MI: Ann Arbor Science Publishers.

Michaels, A. S. 1976. Synthetic polymeric membranes: practical applications: past, present and future. *Pure and App. Chem.* 46:193–204.

Oles, P. J. 1978. Particle analysis and identification in the pharmaceutical industry. *Microscopy* 26:41–48.

Schmidt, W. H. 1964. Control and analysis of particulate matter by membrane filtration. *Bull. of Paren. Drug Assoc.* 18 (6):25–31.

Sladek, K. J., and T. J. Leahy. 1981. Retention of bacteria by membrane filters. Annual Meeting of the Society of Food and Dairy Microbiologists, 4–9 October, in Montreal, Canada.

Sokol, M., and J. Boyd. 1968. Sampling techniques in analysis for particulate matter. *Bull. of Paren. Drug Assoc.* 22:9–12.

Teetsov, A. S. 1977. Techniques of small particle manipulation. *Microscope* 25:103–113.

Trasen, B. 1968a. Detection and reduction of particulate matter in pharmaceuticals. *Chem. Eng. Progress* 64 (2):64–68.

Trasen, B. 1968b. Membrane filtration technique in analysis for particulate matter. *Bull. of Paren. Drug Assoc.* 22:1–8.

Zierdt, C. H. 1979. Adherence of bacteria, yeast, blood cells, and latex spheres to large-porosity membrane filters. *Applied and Environ. Microb.* 38:1166–1172.

X

Process Control of Particulate Matter

In the preceeding chapters, two basic principles regarding the occurrence of particulate matter in pharmaceutical products have been presented. First, there is no indication that the levels of particles present in large volume injections (LVI), small volume injections (SVI), or administration sets currently produced under GMP in the United States or abroad represent any significant issue to the patient. The conduct of millions upon millions of courses of intravenous therapy with no adverse effects due to particulate matter have empirically shown that currently marketed materials are safe and efficacious. Second, pharmacopeial particulate matter limits do not control particle numbers in finished product. While these limits may in some cases prevent substandard product from entering the marketplace and from being administered to patients, particles in marketed product can, in fact, only be controlled by the conscientious application of GMP by the manufacturer. This chapter represents an extension of my previous discussions of particulate matter control and elimination by manufacturers of medical products.

There has historically been a significant level of interest in particulate matter for the purpose of process evaluation (Hayashi 1980a, 1980b). Manufacturers of both injectable products and medical devices monitor particle burden of product to ensure that processes are running within the validated target limits. The key concern in this regard is that an increase in the level of particles in product may be an indication that the process by which the product is manufactured is not well-controlled. Levels of both visible and subvisible particles have been considered as useful measures of the degree of process control. In an early study, Brownley (1967) reported on the use of process control charts to evaluate rejection rates in visual inspection. In addition to data for the total number of rejects, he discussed the use of charts for specific types of visible particulate matter (such as fibers and glass), and stated his belief that the parenteral manufacturer could benefit from this type of information in assessing the cumulative capability of process operations to produce a high quality product. As an index of quality, others have suggested that the data on the level of subvisible particles would be more helpful than the results of visual inspection due to the high level of variability inherent in visual inspection assays and the low numbers of visible particles present in product (Davis et al. 1970).

In the U.S., management of the regulatory agency has repeatedly emphasized that enforcement activity is directed primarily at the process rather than the finished product. This reflects the agency's acceptance of the principle of process control of particulate matter. High variability regarding finished product particle burden or high levels in respect to the limits serve to direct investigators back to process points that are not adequately controlled. Ample grounds for enforcement activities directed at an uncontrolled (non–GMP) process are already available without further limits or requirements. These may be found in

- The Federal Food, Drug, and Cosmetic Act (as amended), United States Code, Title 21;
- The Code of Federal Regulations, Title 21, Part 221, Current Good Manufacturing Practice for Finished Pharmaceuticals; and
- USP <1077> Good Manufacturing Practice for Finished Pharmaceuticals.

Process Design

Process design incorporates not only the consideration of process machinery, environmental cleanliness, and filtration, but that of container and closure cleanliness as well. Currently available process technology for both SVI and LVI production incorporates the potential for significant reductions of the nonviable particle burden in product. The harsh reality of the capital outlay required for modernization typically results in applied technology lagging behind the latest developments in manufacturing processes. The delayed implementation of process advances does not affect product quality, but may significantly impact production efficiency. The manufacturer is able to incorporate new technology most cost effectively only in the design of new facilities. As a result, given the current world economy, the application of new technology may move relatively slowly.

The current manufacture of pharmaceutical products incorporates an extremely wide range of processes. In addition to the general categories of terminally sterilized and aseptically filled products, one must consider dry powder drugs, emulsions, protein and electrolyte solutions, and total parenteral nutrition formulations. The preparation of pharmaceutical grades of water is also of extreme importance. Sterilization may be performed by steam, filtration, or other means; there are also a bewildering variety of container types available. Design of a manufacturing process for elimination of particulate matter involves consideration of basic principles that are common to many types of products and containers. Invariably, the ultimate result achieved with regard to particle control and elimination will relate to the thoroughness of planning before production is begun.

Process design for elimination of particles will ideally commence when a manufacturing facility is on the drawing board, so that elimination of particulate sources and exclusion of particulate matter from the product can be built into the manufacturing line. As we all know, the ideal is often not the case in the real world. Too often one is faced with the problem of reducing particulate matter levels inherent in an "old" process that started running a decade or more ago, when higher levels of process-related particulate matter were acceptable. Often progress in process design based on particulate matter control must be made step-wise as new lines or facilities that will use an existing process are built or as process lines are upgraded.

The design of processes to eliminate particulate matter is emphasized in Japan, Europe, and the United States. Although the approach to process design for particle elimination is somewhat different in Japan than in western nations, there is no evidence that the product quality achieved in this regard differs. The Japanese approach to particulate matter elimination through process design is interesting (Hayashi 1980a, 1980b; Ishikawa 1976). Many Japanese pharmaceutical manufacturing plants (and processes) are newer than their U.S. or European counterparts. The majority of the LVI solutions sold in Japan are marketed in blow molded (blow-fill-seal) polyethylene bottles. The processes for blow molding and filling of these units are designed to totally exclude environmental particles. The polyethylene container also incorporates stoppers that are made from rubber with extremely low levels of additives. Furthermore, the vendors of stoppers are required to furnish stoppers that are extremely clean, and in many cases, ready for use. Process-generated particles are low in number due to the specific design of the process machinery and the use of laminar airflow enclosures of the type typically used in Western countries for aseptic filling operations.

As well as controlling environmental particles, the Japanese design for filling and product handing machines incorporates minimal potential for particle generation. Filling machines are run under manufacturing conditions before delivery to the purchaser and particulate matter generation is monitored. The filling machinery used for LVIs invariably incorporates a high level of container protection from particulate matter, and represents a high level of development of existing technology. As a result of these design steps and a uniform 100% automated manual visual inspection, Japanese product contains very low levels of visible particles (Mochida et al. 1984; Tsuji and Lewis 1978).

Many particle-reduction measures are effective only when they are installed in a total system, the cost justification of which must be undertaken by a comprehensive approach. In Japan, manufacturers identify an investment vehicle—extra capacity, a new product manufacturing consolidation, quality (it is never high enough), obsolescence, and so forth. Instead of attempting to address this need in isolation, the firm undertakes an aggressive overall assessment to see if the investment in the latest manufacturing and processing technology is justified. Not infrequently, a manufacturing system is put in place and validated with as much as 50% additional capacity, built in from the start. System usage tends to increase quickly, particularly for flexible systems, and thus system capacity is not the limiting factor in the rate of return in investment. This approach is feasible in Japan where the companies involved are privately owned. Their management is not subject to the short-term scrutiny of economic analysts, and has more latitude to pursue long-term goals.

European and American corporations historically have used direct and indirect labor savings as the primary economic justification for investment in new equipment and manufacturing systems. In this consideration product quality, yields, overhead, sterile space requirements, long-term operating cost, manufacturing consolidation, and potential for growth are all significant economic concerns.

Process control of particulate matter is closely tied into the facility in which the process is conducted. The predominant planning principle applied in the design of new facilities in the west has been the "integrated" approach. With this approach, the prevention of particulate matter in parenterals requires a review of the total manufacturing system. Accordingly, it is necessary to consider all process elements for their potential impact on particulate matter. This includes the design of buildings and the control of environmental conditions, the performance of equipment, process specifications, the selection of packaging components, raw material specifications, utilities systems, work practices and procedures, and the execution of quality management activities; all of these are critical to the elimination of particles from product.

Many production facilities currently in operation are not adequate to meet future market standards. The decision is often made, after a technology assessment and an extensive survey of current practice, to build a new "state-of-the-art" manufacturing plant rather than to expand and upgrade existing facilities. This decision represents a commitment by the manufacturer to incorporate the highest possible quality standards, and reflects a belief shared with the Japanese that quality results from excellence in design and planning. If vendors sell in the world marketplace, they will be required to comply with known and anticipated quality standards and the GMPs of the different markets served. The simplest approach is designing products that meet the standards of the most critical marketplace. In the view of most manufacturers, quality and productivity (and hence cost) are complimentary objectives, and optimum achievement in either of the two areas is heavily dependent upon the performance in the other.

Although there are some philosophical differences in these two approaches, the end result with regard to the particle burden of finished product is closely similar. Large volume injection product manufactured in domestic (U.S.) and European plants of the major manufacturers can be expected to show a very low particle burden at the ≥ 10 µm and ≥ 25 µm sizes, a level equivalent to that of its Japanese counterparts.

Process Control

The design of the production process for injectable products with respect to elimination of particulate matter involves a process design consideration that provides for elimination of all particulate sources (Brownley 1967). Sources of particulate matter in the process include not only the environment and objects that contact the product, but the product itself; the following comprises a partial list of potential particle sources:

- The environment;
- Process piping and vessels;
- Container materials (glass, plastic);
- Closure;
- Assembly procedures;
- Contaminants from drug raw material;
- Drug degradants;
- Buffers; and
- Excipients, diluents.

The concept of making product under GMP conditions has three pivotal features: (1) developing a manufacturing process from which sources of particulate matter are eliminated or rigorously eliminated, (2) careful validation of that process to perform as designed, and (3) monitoring of the process and its key parameters at levels of testing sufficient to detect deviations from the design quality levels. Implicit critical components in the elimination of particles from the GMP-controlled process are:

- Raw material and component quality;
- Personnel as part of the quality process;
- Supplier (vendor) alliances for quality; and
- Regulatory personnel educated with regard to process control and GMP.

The term *process* assumes that a process or total manufacturing operation or procedure has been defined for a specific product. Therefore, the *process* consists of not only machines but of containers, devices, drug formulations, developmental work, raw materials, mix conditions, and so forth. Each requirement listed for a given process must have a specified measurement. The (extremely) important quality principles to be observed in the basic steps of process design were discussed in the preceding section; design of the product itself is also extremely important. Saving time in getting a new product to market at the cost of thorough process design is a false economy. Any time-to-market saving will be more than offset if product particulate matter issues surface in the marketplace, with attendant loss of customer confidence due to recalls and the loss of revenue from scrapped product. This unfortunate situation can occur if GMP was lacking in either design or execution of the product.

Statistical Process Control

Each process applied in the production of an injectable product can be characterized in terms of key process parameters that vary over specific ranges from batch to batch. These variables are constantly monitored to ensure process control. The application of statistical principles to the analysis of monitoring data is the basis of statistical process control (SPC). SPC supports manufacturing of products that are defect-free and completely conform to requirements. The strategy of SPC is useful in the monitoring and control of particulate matter. Wheeler and Chambers (1992) provides an excellent presentation of the process and is highly recommended in this regard.

The SPC methodology applied today was begun by Dr. Walter Shewhart at Bell Labs in the 1920s. Shewhart believed variability was either within limits set by chance, or outside those limits. If it was outside, he believed that the source of variability could be identified. This was based on his studies of the laws of variation in nature. In these studies Shewhart used statistics to describe how variation affected sample outcomes. When he applied the same principles to manufacturing data, he found that such data did not always behave the same way that natural data did. Out of this inconsistency he formulated a distinction between chance and assignable variation.

In a manufacturing process making a series of parts, each has measurable dimensions or other descriptors. If these parts are periodically selected and measured, the measurements vary because the materials, machines, operators, and methods interact to produce variation. Such random variation is relatively consistent over time because it is the result of many contributing factors. Shewhart called these factors random or chance causes, and thought of the resulting variation as "controlled variation."

In addition to chance causes, other specific factors may occasionally have a large impact on product measurement. These factors might be machines out of adjustment, raw materials that are different, differences in machinery, differences between workers, or differences in the environment due to physical location or management structure. Shewhart argued that such factors were identifiable, and that the impact of such "assignable" causes would be sufficient to cause a significant and definable pattern of variation.

As philosophical guides for manufacturing, the engineering concept of variation and Shewhart's concept of variation have little in common. They have different objectives and different results. The engineering concept of variation has the object of meeting specifications. This naturally results in products that vary as much as possible, because anything within "specs" is considered "good enough." In contrast, the object of Shewhart's concept is process consistency, and this naturally results in products that are as consistent as possible. Therefore, it makes no sense to try to reconcile these two concepts of variation. Management must adhere to one or the other as a guiding principle: mere conformance to specifications or a continuous process of improvement.

Dr. W. Edwards Deming worked with Shewhart at Western Electric. He realized the power of Shewhart's variability control techniques and began to talk of the need for American industries to make greater use of statistical analysis in their manufacturing processes. In 1947, Deming went to Japan at the request of the government to help prepare for a census. While there, he met with statisticians and business managers. Japan's economy was in shambles. Faced with the necessity of completely rebuilding their industry, Japanese leaders were seeking the help of every expert available to them. They asked Deming how their reputation as makers of inferior products could be changed, and how they might make an impact on world markets. Deming told them that they could become an important economic force in the world by using statistical methods in their manufacturing. This advice was taken seriously. Whereas Shewhart had used the terms *assignable cause* and *random cause* to refer to the two sources of variability, Deming applied the terms *special cause* and *common cause* to describe the same two sets of variability sources.

The Japanese were again exposed to the concepts of statistical process control in 1949 through the efforts of Dr. Ichiro Ishikawa, the Director of the Union of Japanese Scientists and Engineers (JUSE). Realizing that more education was needed before the program could be implemented. Ishikawa invited Deming back to

Japan to give seminars under the sponsorship of JUSE. In collaboration with Ishikawa, Deming met with top Japanese industrialists to insure their support in making the use of statistical methods a success. Because of Deming's reputation, and the respect the industrialists had for Ishikawa, their support was assured.

Deming's concepts are presented in *Quality, Productivity, and Competitive Position* (1982). The ASQC handbook (1983), the Ford handbook (1984), and the books by Duncan (1974), Grant and Levenworth (1980), Wheeler and Chambers (1986), and Taylor (1991) discuss both principles and application of SPC. This includes manual assembly processes, semi-automatic processes, continuous production processes, and production lines that are fully automated. Similarly, it offers a means of controlling both total product quality as well as individual parameters such as particulate matter. The specific principles related to particle control are closely related to quality assurance of chemical test data (Taylor 1987) and to industrial principles (Charbonneau and Webster 1978).

With regard to managing variation, it is unimportant whether we choose to use the Shewhart or Deming terminology; what is important is that sources of variation be identified and eliminated. Process variation is what causes defects and prevents us from consistently achieving high quality products. To evaluate whether a process is stable or unstable, we have to determine what "causes of variation" it contains.

- **Random causes of variation** are always present in a process. They are imparted by the process design and behave like a constant system of chance events. A stable process contains only common causes of variation.

- **Assignable causes of variation** are not attributable to process design and do not behave as chance events. An unstable process contains assignable causes of variation.

The most important tenet of this approach to process control is that it requires the manufacturer to move away from a focus on lot quality and product acceptance decisions (Juran and Gryna 1979, 1980; Juran et al. 1979). Instead, the focus is on process quality and process acceptance. The attribute and variable acceptance sampling plans currently applied by many manufacturers, whether based on an acceptable quality level (AQL) or on some other such index, are aimed at product acceptance. Product acceptance is generally an after-the-fact strategy and too frequently involves the sorting and scrapping of defective product. Defect elimination cannot be achieved by a product acceptance approach, but it is achieved only by process acceptance and process control. Process acceptance is based upon an evaluation of process output to validate that the process is stable and capable, and that it continues to operate in that manner over time. Only a consistent process validated for quality of output is accepted for use. An added benefit of this approach is that the actions required to keep a process stable will also result in continuing process improvement.

All processes for the production of pharmaceutical products result in product that vary in characteristics with regard to particle burden. The variation in particle burden results from a complexity of factors present in the process (machines, materials, peoples, and environment). In Shewhart's terminology the causes of the variation can be divided into two categories:

1. Variation due to assignable causes, and
2. Variation due to inherent (random) causes.

Assignable causes with regard to particulate matter are exemplified by particle sources that produce particulate matter of a single type in product. An example of an assignable cause is the generation of glass particles in SVI product by a filling needle. Another example is an occurrence of drug-related insolubles in dry vials due to degradation or stopper-solution interactions. In the latter case, the cause involved relates to formulation rather than production conditions.

Variation due to random causes is the sum of the inherent variation in the process parameters after assignable causes have been eliminated. Individually, the variation each of these random causes are of decreased consequence in comparison to assignable causes, and taken together, they produce a random scatter in the data. Individual random causes are typically more difficult to identify than assignable causes, and basic changes may be required in the process to eliminate them; to identify the random causes, special engineering studies and detailed particle identification must often be undertaken. These sources often cannot simply be "controlled" out because of the limitations or costs of the technology involved. A random cause of extraneous particles in product might be the chance occurrence of particles in the environment at process points; other random factors include human or instrumental variation in count data collected, in natural set-up and adjustment differences across several similar machines, or in slight variations in raw material over time. Importantly, some random causes

Process Stability and Capability

The result of SPC is a stable process. This concept applies to particulate matter burden as well as other parameters (Figure 1). A stable process is consistent. Output from the process is the same from hour to hour, week to week, and month to month. The average does not shift significantly upward or downward, and the process range does not increase or decrease. A stable process is predictable. Costs are predictable. Production is predictable.

The differences among measurements of product characteristics such a length, width, strength, or particle burden, indicate the presence of variation. If statistical distributions of these measurements remain the same over time, we say the process is stable and will consistently produce products with characteristics that fall within the distribution. The same is true of particulate matter. On the other hand, if the distributions change over time, we say the process is unstable (Figure 2); assignable causes are typically responsible. If a process is unstable, knowledge of today's process

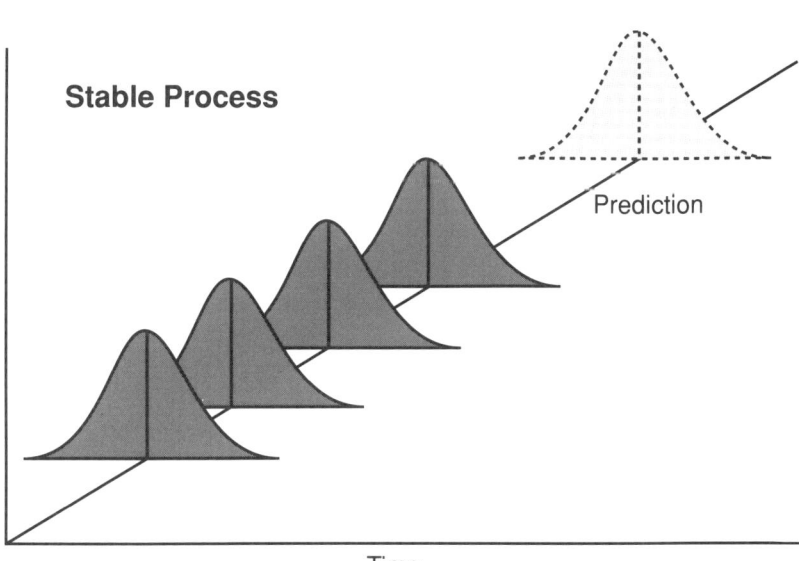

Figure 1. The stable process.

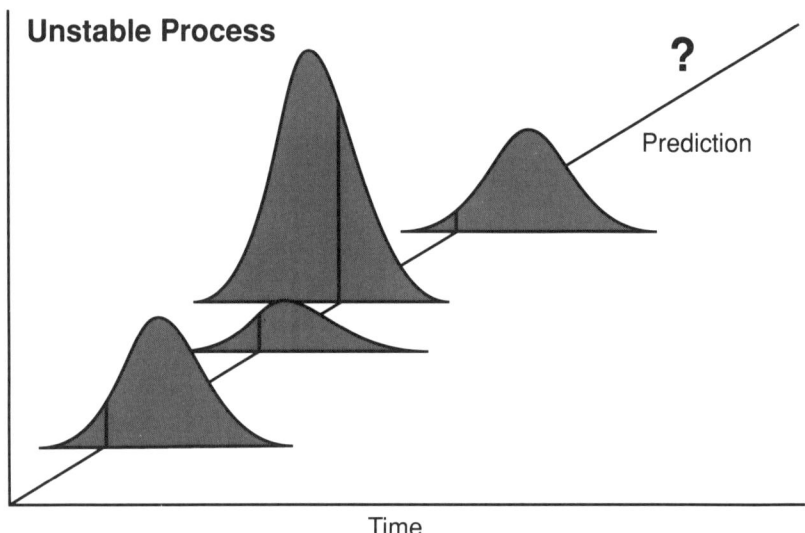

Figure 2. Unstable process.

---

gives you no ability to predict future costs and production capacity.

Finally, if the statistical distributions of measurements of product characteristics fall within the limits of product requirements, we say the process is capable. Of necessity, a process must be stable before it can be capable. A capable process consistently produces products that meet requirements. Every unit made is virtually defect-free (Figure 3). Even with an extremely capable process, there always remains some decreased probability of generating a defect. The wide "skirt" of the distribution for a process that is stable, but not capable, is due to random causation of variation.

Thus, the theory of SPC application involves:

1. Use of SPC to attain a stable process through the control and the elimination of assignable causes of variation; followed by

2. Development of a capable process, such as a process that consistently generates product within a designated control limits set.

As mentioned earlier, there is a very important philosophical perspective to observe in the use of the terms *assignable* and

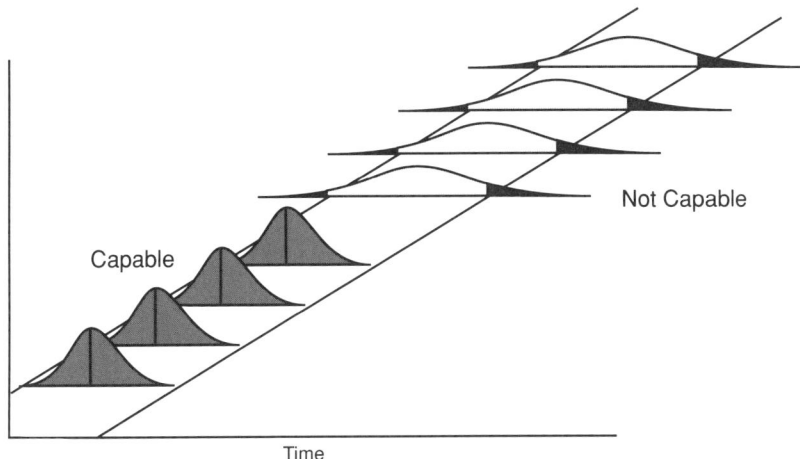

Figure 3. Capable and noncapable processes.

random with regard to sources of process variability. Typically, assignable causes are those that are most readily detected when a process (newly implemented or already in place) is reviewed for the purpose of achieving greater stability. Random causes often turn out to be uninvestigated due to their lower contribution to the overall capability. Stated another way: For any process, in regard to particulate matter generation, there will exist a number of sources of particulate matter that may be ranked based on their percentage contribution to the total variation. If in a total of 10 sources of particulate matter, 2 contribute 65% of the total process variability, the manufacturer may be satisfied to eliminate those 2 sources and define the remaining 8 as random in nature. This approach has historically proven effective in many instances, with significant increases in process stability being achieved with the removal of a small number of particulate matter sources that contribute relatively large numbers of particles to the finished product.

There is an inherent difficulty with this approach. Following the removal of the 2 major sources of variability from the process, the 8 remaining retain their original ranking order of importance; but now they contribute proportionately more of the total particle burden detected in the product and hence are more important as individual variables. These remaining sources will be more difficult to investigate and sort out. The manufacturer, understandably, may decide not to proceed further in the study due to the diminishing marginal utility of further improvements, and the fact that the process is already capable within established limits. If, however, further investigation is pursued using well-designed experiments, the result will be identification of more "assignable" causes and a further decrease in total variability of the process. This in turn will result in a more capable process, lower mean particle burden, and decreased costs.

This concept is important enough to justify an example. Suppose that a manufacturer has implemented a new dry powder filling line to process a recently approved dry powder dosage form. The initial particle analysis study performed indicated a mean particle burden of 50 particles/mL ≥10 µm in the reconstituted product. Following initial particle identification studies, the major contribution is found to be insolubles present in the dry powder drug, and finely divided fragments of plastic bushing material from the high speed fillers employed. The elimination of these two (obvious) sources of variability results in a decrease of the mean particle burden to 20 particles/mL ≥10 µm in size. This is a dramatic improvement within internal limits, but control charting indicates that the range of counts obtained in testing 20 units from each batch is still undesirably broad. This suggests the continued existence of a significant variable or a large number of random sources that contribute low levels of particulate matter. Both situations are deemed unacceptable and further investigation is undertaken.

Particle identification suggests the particles remaining in the product are from a number of sources. A detailed overview of the process by a problem elimination term determines that the particulate matter level in containers stoppered and capped without drug is less than 5 particles/mL at the ≥10 µm size. Previous tests on the drug material itself in the initial particulate matter elimination studies have shown this material to now be extremely clean, contributing on an average less than 5 particles/mL after reconstitution. Evaluation of the hopper filling operation suggests the plastic bags in which the bulk drug is contained is a primary suspect as the most significant remaining particulate matter source. This is borne out by inspection trips to the facility where the drug is manufactured, and visits to the vendor of the bags. In the production process for the drug, the layout of the packing station is such that bags are held open and exposed to both environmental and point-generated particles while waiting to be filled. At the facility where the bags are made by a blown film extrusion process, unfiltered air is used to inflate the film, resulting in large number of particles adhering to their inner surface.

This situation is corrected by (1) switching to bags made of a different type of plastic (nylon) that is known to have an extremely low particle burden, and (2) protecting the bags during filling. Two important points regarding sampling and identification of particles should also be made. Particles related to the container in which bulk drug powders is shipped may not be detected when a thief or similar device is used to sample from the mid-volume of a mass. Also, mixed particle populations of contaminant particles do not necessarily represent multiple sources.

Control Charting

The concept of charting data related to process variability is well known and is applicable to particle count data as well as other critical aspects of the process (ASTM E-11). The control chart for particle count data in its simplest application is a linear plot of process or product particle counts against batch or other logical subgroups. Environmental particle counts per time interval (hourly, daily) may also be plotted in order to establish reference limits and allowable variation (control limits) in counts in a specific process. This procedure is a simplistic and powerful tool for process control.

Control charts show both short-term variation due to assignable causes and the longer-term variation (trends) associated with the evolution of a process. Charts are useful for both process monitoring and improvement.

A key principle to be observed in control charting is the definition of appropriate sample subgroups. For production of injectable products and particle count data, a very useful exercise is to group particle count data by rational subgroups and plot the subgroup data consecutively in order of production, or versus time. Based on this type of study, a control chart is developed and control limits can be placed on the chart. Following initial process definition studies, time-ordered subgroups are plotted during subsequent steps of process monitoring at a much reduced frequency.

Subgroups of samples should be established so that the output represented by the data within the subgroup is produced under as homogeneous conditions as possible. The subgroups should be set up so that if an assignable cause should occur, it has a high likelihood of appearing as a difference between subgroups. Filling machine operation is one critical determinant of product particle burden. If a process uses four filling machines, it is reasonable to take separate sample groups from the output of each machine. Within a subgroup, data will be from the same machine. Between subgroups, data is gathered from each machine, and represents a different subgroup. An assignable cause for high particle counts in the output from one machine would be indicated by shifts in that machine's subgroup's average or an increase in particle counts.

A sample of how particle count data (or other variable measurements) may be analyzed as variables is provided by the following procedure:

1. Define appropriate sample subgroups (batch, shift, output of one filler or line, etc.).
2. Determine the subgroup size, n.
3. Collect the data. It should be consecutive production with a minimum subgroup n of 50 units.
4. For each subgroup, calculate the average ($\overline{X}$) and standard deviation (s).

$$\overline{X} = \frac{X_1 + X_2 + X_3 + \ldots X_n}{n}$$

Where: $\overline{X}$ = Mean of Individual Measurements
n = Total Number of Measurements, and

$$s = \sqrt{\frac{\sum_{i=1}^{n}(X_i - \overline{X})^2}{n - 1}}$$

5. Plot the subgroup averages and standard deviations on separate charts.

6. Calculate the grand average ($\overline{\overline{X}}$) and average standard deviation ($\overline{s}$) for the sets of the data:

$$\overline{\overline{X}} = (\overline{X}_1 + \overline{X}_2 + \ldots \overline{X}_k) \div k$$

$$(\overline{s}) = (s_1 + s_2 + \ldots s_k) \div k$$

where k = number of subgroups

7. Plot the grand average ($\overline{\overline{X}}$) as the center or control line on the chart of averages.

8. Calculate the upper and lower control limits based on the sample standard deviation with control limits set at

3 standard deviations above and below the mean according to

$$\overline{\overline{X}} \pm \frac{3(\overline{s})}{\sqrt{n}}$$

Draw the limits (UCL, LCL) on the $\overline{X}$–s chart (Figure 4).

9. Analyze the chart for statistical control. For the process to be in control there must not be any points outside of the control limit or any patterns with the control limits.

10. Calculate the capability potential index (*Cp*) of the process. In the case of the upper and lower specification limits:

$$Cp = \frac{USL - LSL}{6\,(\overline{s})}$$

where *USL* = upper specification limit and *LSL* = the lower specification limit. In the case of an upper specification limit and process target:

$$Cp = \frac{USL - \text{target}}{3\,(\overline{s})}$$

In the case of a lower specification limit and process target:

$$Cp = \frac{\text{target} - LSL}{3\,(\overline{s})}$$

In the case of a upper specification limit without a process target:

$$Cp = \frac{USL - \overline{\overline{X}}}{3\,(\overline{s})}$$

In the case of a lower specification limit without a process target:

$$Cp = \frac{\overline{\overline{X}} - LSL}{3\,(\overline{s})}$$

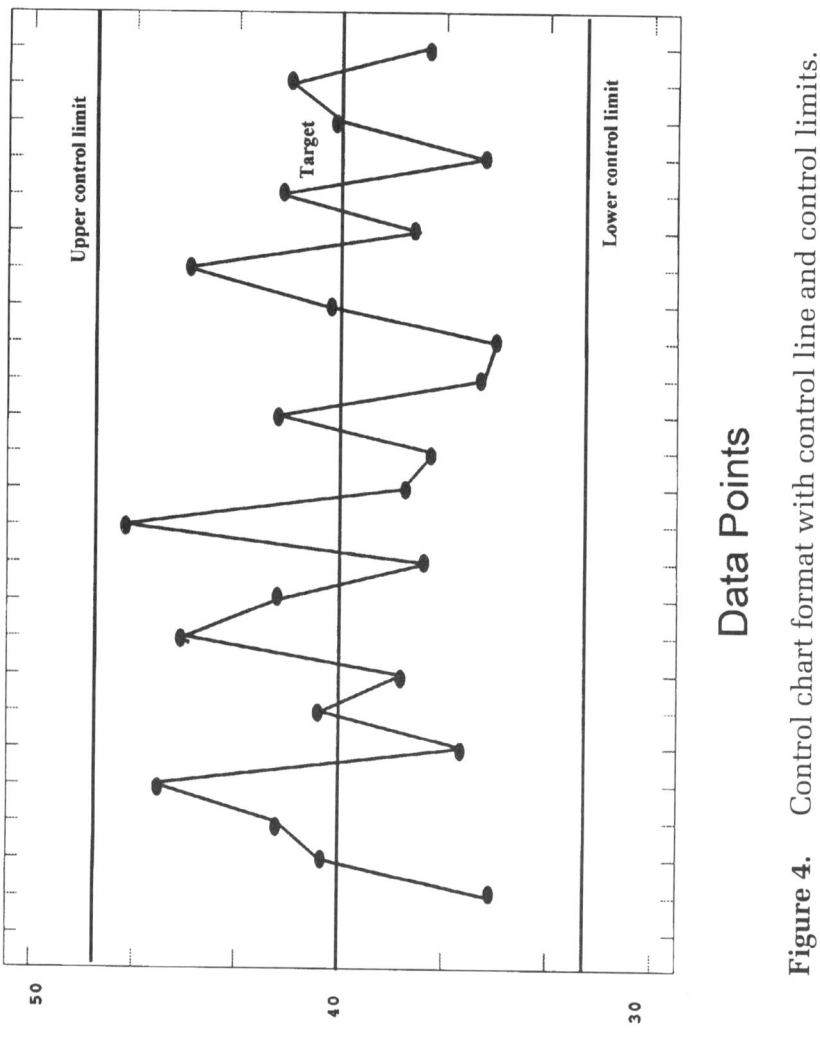

Figure 4. Control chart format with control line and control limits.

11. If $Cp \geq 1.5$, the process is capable. Otherwise, take steps to reduce the inherent variation. Data from the potential study should also be used to assess if there are problems in centering the process as evidenced by the position of the calculated mean and the presence of nonconforming items in the sample. Centering problems must be solved before starting the performance study.

An example of SPC and control charting may be applied to particle count data from injectable product is provided in Table I and the control chart of Figure 5. The data represents a portion of a process validation study in which sample units were collected from 10 filling heads and tested by light extinction counting. While the N of 10 units is smaller than would normally be chosen for this purpose, this data is illustrative of the principle involved.

Table I. Data (≥10 µm Particle Counts per mL) from Process Validation

(samples [subgroups] taken across batch)

Filling Head Number

Unit #	1	2	3	4	5	6	7	8	9	10
1	11	9	2	18	18	11	2	12	28	29
2	8	14	7	21	4	10	6	13	25	31
3	7	12	12	19	16	9	5	15	14	27
4	6	11	17	20	7	8	5	11	26	26
5	12	7	16	22	12	7	4	9	18	37
6	9	14	13	22	8	11	7	10	21	31
7	11	16	12	17	8	10	3	8	24	42
8	7	12	3	16	25	9	1	12	28	28
9	7	10	5	17	29	9	2	13	26	29
10	11	9	7	19	8	8	8	12	21	34
($\bar{X}$) Mean	8.90	11.40	9.40	19.10	13.50	9.20	4.30	11.50	23.10	31.40
SD (s)	2.18	2.76	5.32	2.13	8.33	1.32	2.31	2.07	4.56	4.97
Range	6	9	15	6	25	4	7	7	14	16

Several interesting observations may be made on inspection of the data in Table I and the charts. The mean counts for heads 1, 2, 6, and 8 do not appear to be significantly different to a particle analyst familiar with count data from light extinction particle counters. Means range from 8.9 to 11.5 counts per mL and SD ranges from 1.32 to 2.76. Thus, these groups would appear on initial inspection to provide an indication of what is achievable for the process. Other filling heads show different counts and variability. Head number 7 has a mean of only 4.3 counts per mL, but the large relative standard deviation (RSD) suggests that the units generated may not differ significantly in mean counts from those of heads 1, 2, 6, and 8. Head 3 has a mean count close to those of the latter, 9.4, but a much higher SD. Heads 4, 9, and 10 give units with a particle burden that is most certainly higher than that of the fillers, particularly in consideration of the lower RSD. In this case,

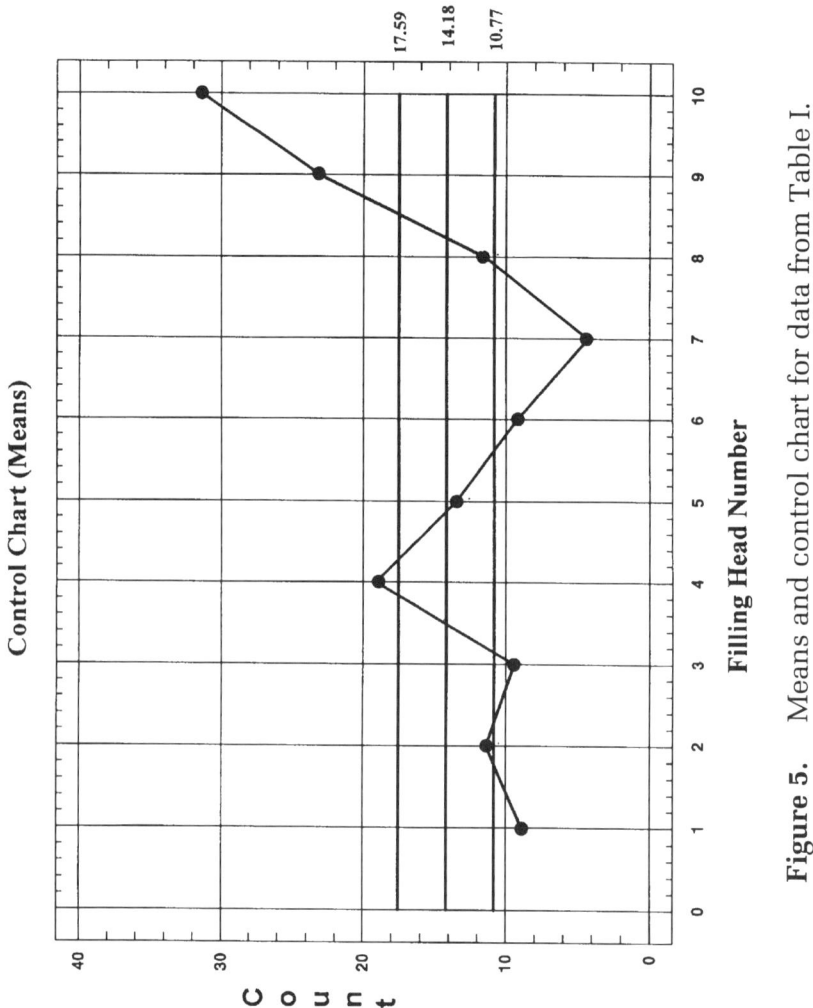

Figure 5. Means and control chart for data from Table I.

investigation of the higher particle counts from these fillers is warranted in order to bring the count levels in line with the mean of heads 1, 2, 6, and 8. In this investigation, it must be ensured that a process variable unrelated to the filling operation (e.g., bottle washer, sterilizing tunnel) is not responsible for these higher counts.

This consideration of the particle burden produced by ten individual filling heads on a single production line also allows us to make some interesting observations on the capability of the process. First, if individual filling heads had not been considered separately as a first approximation, we might have drawn misleading conclusions regarding the between-unit particle burden variability of product from the line as well as the average particle burden of product from the line. The mean count for all ten fillers is 14.18 particles per mL ≥10 µm in size. This illustrates how errors in judgment may be made by compressing one level of variables within a higher level variable. On discovering the variability between filling heads during process validation, a necessary step would be to determine the cause of variability between fillers and then correct the factors resulting in the higher counts from fillers 4, 9, and 10. Elimination of this variability will have a number of benefits. Both process variability and product quality in regard to particle burden will be improved. Additionally, once variability between units from the different fillers is reduced to a level below significance, the output of the line rather than that from individual filling heads may be sampled, and SPC will be much simplified.

Control charting of the line output can be conducted according to several approaches. Typically an $\overline{X}$–s or means control chart will be used. Control limits may also be established based on range ($\overline{X}$–r chart) or standard deviation (s chart). For an X–r chart an appropriate number of units are sampled, and the particle count ranges are plotted on the control chart that has a central horizontal $\overline{\overline{X}}$ line based on data collected during process validation and control limits placed at ± the average range value times a constant. The s chart has only an upper control limit. These calculations are explained in the references by Wheeler and Chambers (1986) and Taylor (1991). The sample size selected will be based on the process variability and the level of the mean counts with regard to alert or compendial limits placed on the process or based solely on a consideration of the between-unit variability observed with samples tested during process validation.

Additional useful information may be obtained by construction of $\overline{X}$–r and s control charts from the filling head data (Figures 6 and 7). The mean standard deviation is 3.59. The UCL for the s chart is 6.23. Filling head number 5, which is very close to the mean value, is obviously more variable than the other filling heads by both the SD and range plots. This data indicates that excessive variability of filling head 5 is worthy of investigation as well as the high average values from filling heads 4.9 and 10.

Additional examples of control charted particle count data from controlled (stable) and uncontrolled (unstable) processes on a batch basis is shown in Figures 8 and 9. This data has been collected on a

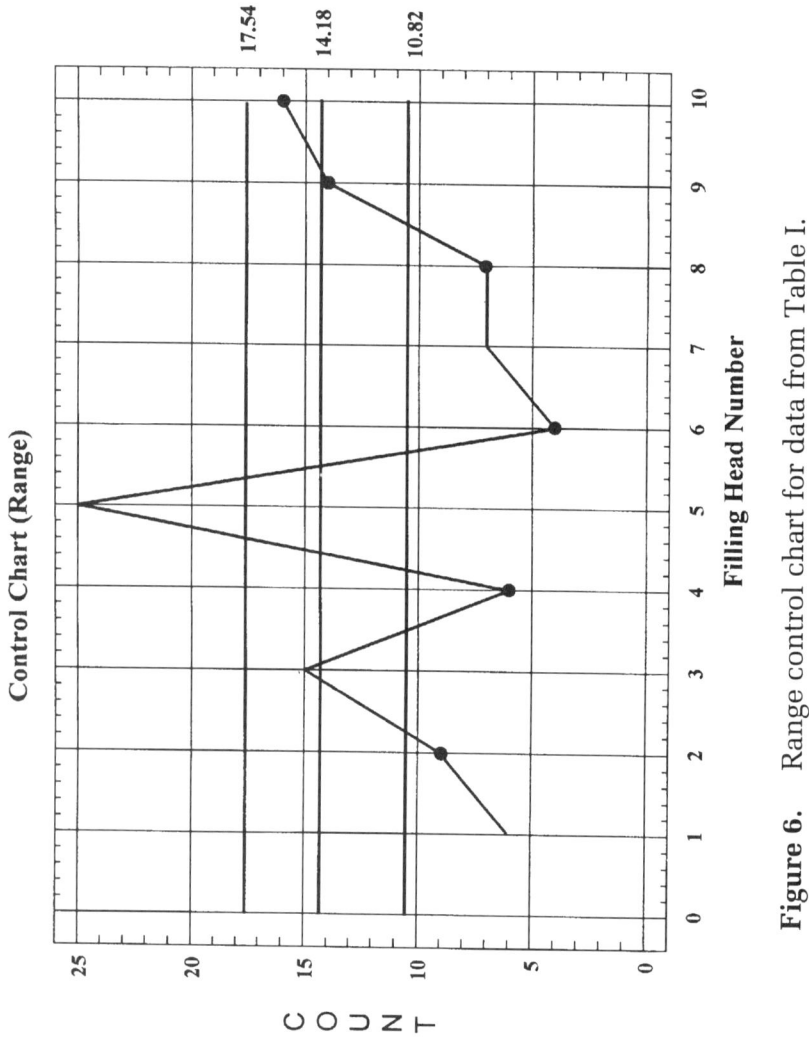

Figure 6. Range control chart for data from Table I.

batch basis, with 24 batches tested using a N of 10 samples for batch. Batch sampling of this sort will be effective only after specific process point variables, such as those related to the individual filling heads, are eliminated.

Invariably, process validation studies that are used to define process capability will involve far larger numbers of samples than will the trending or monitoring activities related to process control.

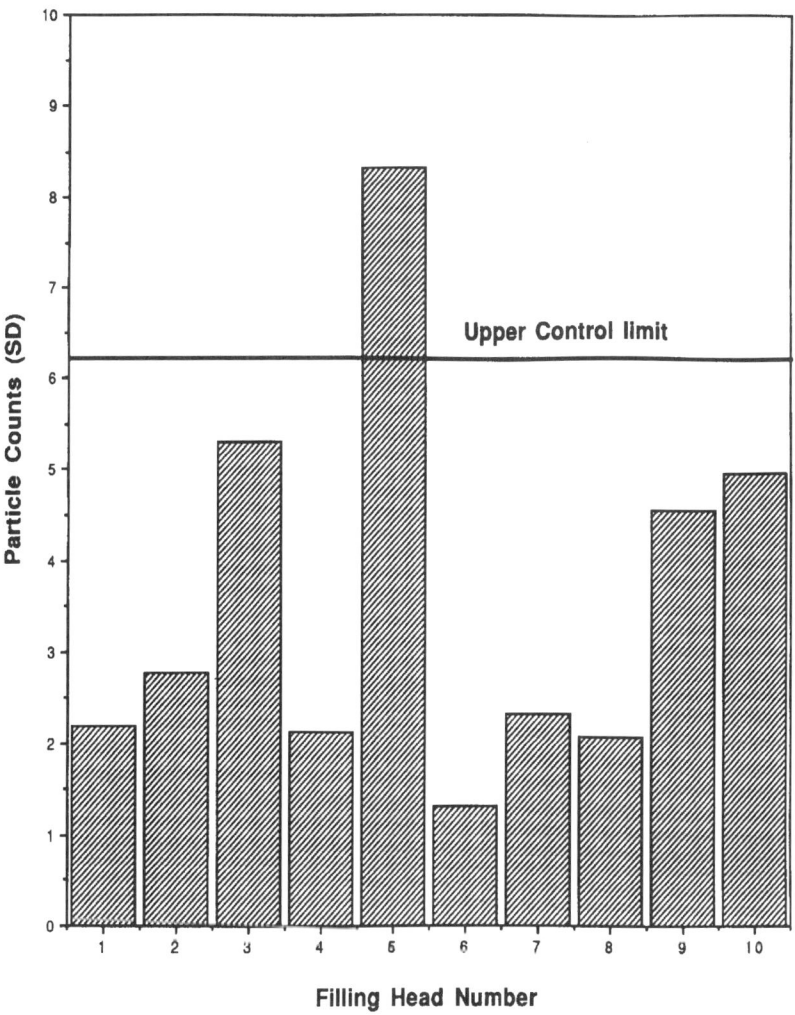

Figure 7. SD control chart for data from Table I.

As an example, for a process that has been appropriately validated and runs with a low level of variability regarding particle burden, 10 units may be a sufficient sample for batch of 30 to 50 K units. The validation itself may entail as many as 500 samples for validation of the process to run a batch of this size. The statistical analysis required to define sample sizes necessary to detect changes of critical magnitude in particle burden (and other parameters) are

416 *Pharmaceutical Particulate Matter*

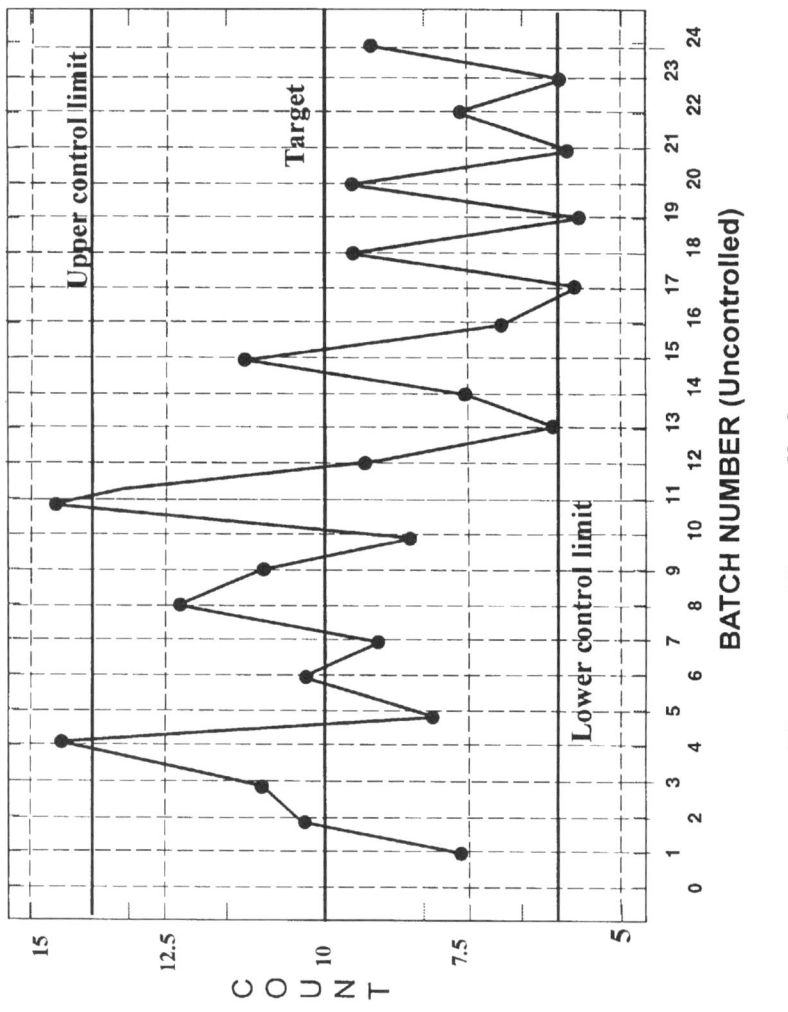

Figure 8. Uncontrolled process.

straightforward and widely used by quality assurance statisticians; the best course in this endeavor and others is to obtain guidance from these professionals in the initial establishing of sampling plans. A critical nonstatistical consideration here is that the number of units even in a validation study must bear a realistic numerical relationship to the size of a batch that will be filled in production. As an example, a run of 1000 units is unlikely to suffice as a realistic validation for 100 K unit batches in the

Process Control of Particulate Matter 417

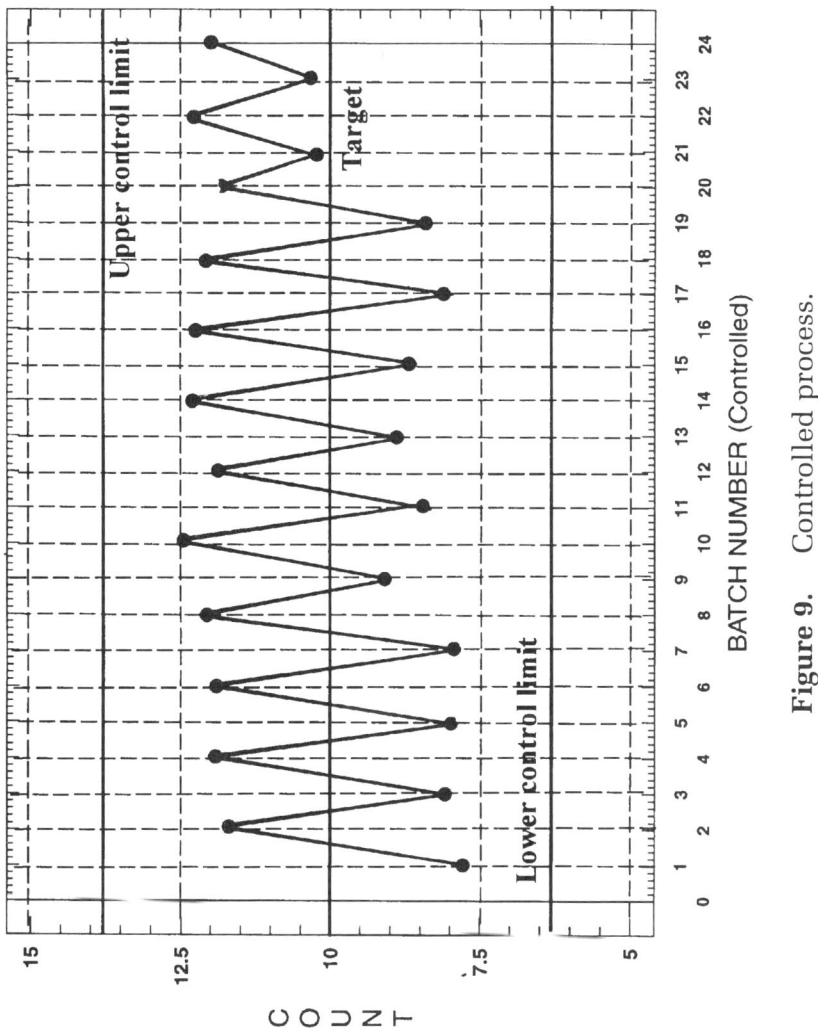

Figure 9. Controlled process.

perception of a regulatory investigator. This aspect of validation is currently receiving a high level of scrutiny by the regulatory agencies.

Parameters descriptive of process variability as well as sample means should be control charted. It is just as important, if not more so, to ensure the process variability is under control as it is to keep the mean on target! The minimum effort should include an $\overline{X}$-s chart. Range of sample observation, or relative standard deviation (RSD) may also be used for this purpose. The SD is typically the best choice for this purpose. The generation of the different types of charts is detailed (with examples) in the text by Taylor (1991). The range of sample observations is readily calculated, but the description is sensitive to sample size, with large sample groups from a given population showing a larger range. The SD is relatively insensitive to sample size. The RSD, also referred to as the coefficient of variation or CV, is a less suitable measure of variability, since it is a percentage relationship between the mean and SD and does not reflect the numerical variability of a process. The layout of the control chart is identical to that of the X control chart. The CV may be less useful with regard to particulate matter because the SD tends to be proportional to the mean, making the CV constant. In SPC, however, we are testing for instability. If the process is stable, $\overline{X}$, SD, and Range (given a constant N) do not change, making their respective charts applicable. The sampling distribution of CV is not nearly so well-behaved, leading to its infrequent use in studies of particulate matter burden.

The application of control charts to particle count data is quite similar to that found with other process variables. One of the peculiarities of particle count data is that zero count values are commonly encountered with regard to large particle sizes. The easiest way to deal with this is simply to base statistical considerations on particle sizes at which counts are sufficient for conventional statistical treatment. The 10 µm count for most domestically (U.S.) produced LVI is typically satisfactory for this purpose, but large numbers of single digit data points are encountered if 1 mL test volumes are considered. The use of large sample aliquots so that higher numbers of counts are collected will serve the same purpose. The use of counts from a smaller size threshold for control charting is based on the assumption that counts at the different sizes are linked in some predictable fashion. This assumption is generally, but not invariably, true.

If zero count values must be dealt with, the particulate matter level parameter becomes an attribute rather than a variable. In this case, we can make a good-bad or a pass-fail judgment based on whether or not particles occur. This is the situation faced in visual inspection procedures whereby the presence of a particle is recorded as a "fail" and absence of particles is a "pass." In the chapter on visual inspection, the probabilistic handling of the type of data was discussed. This is generally not applicable to subvisible counts due to the destructive nature of the test and the lack of opportunity for repeated reinspection. Importantly, attributes do not allow trending on predictions to be performed with data. These manipulations are key benefits of the control charting process (the basic value of the SPC process is assessing whether a process has changed).

The fact that particle counts within a given size category represent a non–Gaussian distribution has little or no effect on the SPC process. Mean counts are invariably used for control charting, and the means of Poisson or log-normal distributions follow a Gaussian distribution. The nonnormal distribution of particle counts may result in some problems if ranges of data points are plotted, since Poisson or log-normal distributions have wider ranges than Gaussian populations with a similar mean due to the long "tail" on the right side of the distribution. Any issues related to the nonnormal distributions of the log of the count values or the log +1 is plotted in lieu of the data points themselves.

A control chart is one of the most sensitive of all in-process monitoring tools. It is useful in uncovering previously unobserved variations due to assignable causes other than the one being investigated. The concept is well presented in the ASTM Handbook (1976). The primary benefit of the control charting procedure in process validation is process definition. In this role, the control chart defines the attainable level of particle burden to be expected from the process and the variability of the particle burden. When the product for which the control chart has been developed goes into production, the manufacturer will continue to chart the product particle burden using batch release (monitoring) data. This ensures that the process remains in control and continues to operate in the fashion that was validated during product development. Monitoring, by definition, involves much lower levels of testing than is required for validation (Taylor 1991). Consistent process control will set the stage for increased process capability as discussed in the Ford Motor Company's book regarding process control and capability (1984).

In addition to charting particle count data from release testing, the manufacturer should have in place an action plan that provides for the elimination of the cause of any elevation of particle burden that may occur. Specific actions that may be taken are described in more detail in the chapter on process- and product-related particles. Generally the action plan will involve:

- Process description with identification of points that impact particle levels;
- Identification of critical environmental monitoring parameters that relate to particle burden;

- "Plan of attack" to isolate process factors responsible for elevation of particulate matter;
- Analytical processes to identify and source particles;
- Sampling plans to evaluate the effects of particulate matter reduction measures; and
- Criteria for problem elimination.

There are two critical observations that should be made regarding the specifics of SPC with particle count data. In addition to the two compendial size ranges of interest per the USP (≥10 µm; ≥25 µm) a number of sizes may be of interest in process validation. For the BP, the ≥2 µm and ≥5 µm sizes would be a consideration. Similarly, larger particles (25 µm to 50 µm) might be tracked if these were shown to have some relationship to the occurrence of visible particles. As has been discussed in preceding chapters, the distribution of extraneous particles in a unit of product may be complex, and the variability of counts in one size range may be totally different from that in another.

Batch Sampling

Yet another extremely critical aspect of the process control of particulate matter is the testing (monitoring) that will be applied to ensure that product manufactured in a batch basis conforms to requirements. In this regard, the introduction to the <788> particulate matter requirement in USP XXII states that a manufacturer must elaborate a statistically valid sampling plan from which inferences may be drawn regarding units of a batch that are not tested. Thus, the burden of determining specifics regarding sample size and test method is placed on the manufacturer. A fact not to be overlooked here is that with a validated and controlled process in place, the assurance of batch suitability can be obtained by testing a relatively small number of units (Blanchard et al. 1978; Tsuji and Lewis 1987).

Significantly, the USP particle assays for parenteral solutions are limits tests, and are intended to indicate only whether or not the product tested meets or exceeds the compendial limits. The USP tests are not intended to provide a critical estimate of the numbers of particles per mL in a parenteral solution unit; for example, whether units in a batch contain a mean of 40 or 50 particles ≥10 µm per mL. Hundreds of units from a typical batch of injectable product would have to be tested using a critically designed assay if this were the goal. Importantly, data obtained will always be method dependent (Mochida et al. 1984).

What the FDA and other regulatory groups expect from the application of such tests in release or stability study testing is a result that gives a high degree of confidence that the mean count of the batch from which tested units are taken does not exceed USP limits (Munson 1990). The USP <788> tests as applied by most manufacturers generally provide this high degree of confidence. This confidence in results of testing is due both to sampling plans that involve testing of appropriate numbers of samples and to the low levels of particulate matter present in most products in comparison to compendial limits that have been achieved by the manufacturer's drive to increase product quality. The misconception on the part of some manufacturers and regulatory investigators that larger numbers of particulate matter samples are better is based on a failure to understand the statistical principles of the test and the result that the USP tests are intended to provide. Larger numbers of samples may provide a more powerful estimate of the true mean particulate matter count at ≥10 µm and ≥25 µm, but do not provide any practical advantage with regard to estimating whether a batch is within limits.

The requirement for a 10-unit pool sample in the USP <788> requirement for SVI is particularly unfortunate. This section of the methodology was written with a superficial understanding of sampling theory applicable to parenterals. The 10-unit sample was selected primarily on the basis of the small volume of some SVI units (e.g., 1-mL ampoules, 5-mL powder vials) and the necessity for pooling to obtain an adequate sample for a 10-mL test volume. Some consideration was also given to the elimination of variability between units of dry powder dosages. The pooling method thus provides no measure of between-unit variability and is thus useless for predicting batch suitability or ensuring that above limits units are not released. As larger units are pooled, the two 5-mL sample aliquots prescribed in the test give an increasingly unsuitable estimate of the count of the pooled volume. As an example, the pooling of ten 100-mL units results in a solution pool of 1 L that must be counted using a 10-mL sample.

I have included the following discussion of sampling theory as an aid in selection of statistically valid sampling plans as directed by the Pharmacopeia. I would respectfully remind the reader, however, that regulatory investigators may be singularly narrow-minded with regard to adherence to the pharmacopeial requirements. Thus, selection of a sample size other than 10 units for SVI product subject to USP limit may be criticized in an inspectional observation, to which a response will have to be generated. At the manufacturer's discretion, optimized sample schemes may be described in informational communications to the agency, thus preventing difficulties during later inspections.

The pooling of sample units is a particularly problematical issue, since pooling masks individual sample variability and precludes any observation of between-unit variability that is essential to prediction of whether or not an individual unit of the tested batch will exceed limits. In the case of developing a valid sampling plan that allows extrapolation of data to untested units, a valid sample plan is critical. Importantly, the reader is directed to the General Notice Section of USP XXII (p. 5). The manufacturer who exercises GMP control of particulate matter need not perform particulate matter testing per the USP <788> to ensure that requirements are met. Such assurance may be obtained from either "process validation" or from "in-process controls." Statistically sound, critically designed sampling plans constitute in-process controls of the most critical effectiveness.

I should also observe, in this regard, that widely accepted sampling schemes are available that have known probabilities of detecting defects when defects occur at a certain level in a population. Examples are the sampling plans provided in Military Standard 105-E. One issue with application of this standard regards their definition of a "defect." These standards are directed at sampling for attributes, that is, defective and nondefective samples. While it is possible to apply the sampling plans as specified in the standards by defining a subvisible particle count in excess of a specific number as a defect, more appropriate sampling plans may be developed on the basis of the historical mean counts at a certain size for a specific type of product, the distribution of these counts, and probabilistic considerations. This latter approach results in sampling plans well-suited to the product being tested. When a sampling plan of this nature is to be developed, it is essential that a statistician well versed in quality testing and the nature of the test used to collect the data be involved.

Consider the case of a manufacturer who produces SVI units (<100 mL) of saline and dextrose product in glass bottles. The appropriate USP limit for such units is 10,000 particles per container ≥ 10 µm, and 1000 particles per container ≥ 25 µm. This equates, for a 100-mL container, to 100 particles/mL and 10 particles/mL at the ≥ 10 µm and ≥ 25 µm sizes respectively. The manufacturer knows that the product typically evidences particle counts far below these limits (typically less than 10 particles/mL ≥10 µm, and less than 1 particle/mL ≥25 µm). Further, the manufacturer is convinced that the process by which these units are made is stable and well controlled. In this situation, considerable latitude is available to the manufacturer in defining a batch release assay other than the 10-unit sample pool specified by the USP for SVI product.

In this example, it may be advantageous in terms of time requirements for testing, the amount of product expended in testing, and strength of data obtained for the manufacturer to decrease the number of units tested and to test individual units instead of pooled units. In the initial statistical consideration by the manufacturer in our example, it becomes obvious that the testing of individual units provides a better estimate of the particle burden of individual units and the variability of particle burden between units than does a pooled sample. This may be explained as follows: if X represents the particle count per 5 mL of sampled volume, there will be some overall rate of particle detection (λ). Thus, we know that our count distribution may be modeled as a Poisson distribution with rate λ. If we pool ten 50-mL units and then test two 5-mL sample aliquots, we are in effect creating two independent Poisson random variables X_1 and X_2. Hence, the average determination has a true variance of $\lambda/2$. If we take three independent samples from each of five units, we are in essence generating fifteen variables $X_{1,1}$; $X_{1,2}$; $X_{1,3}$; $X_{2,1}$; ..., $X_{5,3}$ that are independent and distributed as Poisson random variables. The average determination of these fifteen samples has a true variance of $\lambda/15$. Hence, the 5-unit sample plan provides a more precise estimate of the particle count than a 10-unit pool.

Thus, the first step taken in the development of a statistically valid sampling plan by the manufacturer is to test individual units instead of a solution pool. Initially, 10 individual units are measured by a light extinction procedure and the mean particle count per mL of fluid for both 10 µm and 25 µm particles is determined. If the average count exceeds the USP limit (100 and 10 counts per mL respectively for a 100-mL unit), then the lot is rejected as having too high a level of particulate matter. The next step in a statistical analysis of particle count data for this or any other type of product is to generate a plot of particle numbers/mL at the compendial ≥10 µm and ≥25 µm sizes versus frequency of occurrence. Figure 10 illustrates the distribution of 10 µm light extinction count data from product made by the manufacturer in our example. This data distribution is generally typical of terminally filtered SVI product; the count data invariably fit an asymmetric

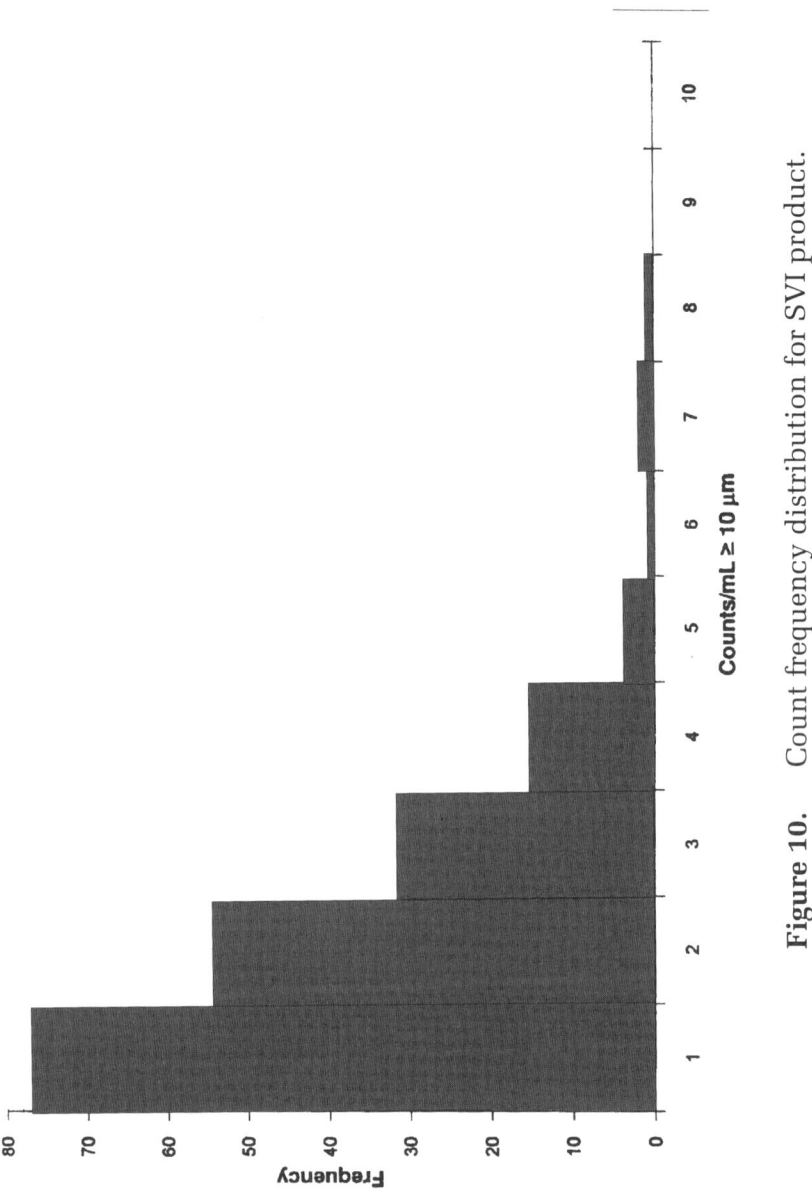

Figure 10. Count frequency distribution for SVI product.

curve that is skewed to the right with lower counts occurring with a much higher frequency. A plot of this type allows the distribution of count data to be determined and probability of failure to be predicted. For the data in Figure 10, the highest count observed was eight particles/mL ≥10 μm; the USP limit at this size range for a 50-mL unit is 200 particles/mL.

Once the distribution of count data (Poisson, log normal, negative binomial, etc.) is known and the mean, variance and SD of counts are determined, probability of exceeding limits based on samples of different sizes may be calculated. At this point, the probability of a result that exceeds limits when the true mean count is at some given level below the USP limit (false rejection) and the probability of a result that is below the limits when the true mean is above the limit (false acceptance) may be determined. The concept of a warning or alert limit is critical to this or any other sampling scheme in which a number of samples much lower than the total number of units in a batch will be tested. For example, based on the distribution of a historical data set, an appropriate alert limit may be established such that if the mean count of a sample group exceeds the alert limit, $P \geq 0.01$ that the true mean count exceeds the product limit. The smaller the sample size used, the lower will be the alert limit at which probability of failure of product limits is greater than 0.01.

The internal alert limits usually used in practice by manufacturers, however, are invariably much less than the USP limits. The manufacturer in our example might select an alert limit of 35 particles per mL (10 μm) or 3 particles per mL (25 μm). Since these alert limits are so much lower than the actual compendial limit, it has been suggested that sampling done with a smaller number of units would not adversely affect the performance of the test. Here we will consider two sample sizes, 10 units and 5 units, and compare their respective error rates in determining particulate matter level.

Assume that the number of counts per mL in a single unit is distributed as a Poisson random variable with some average number of counts per mL. Thus, for a single sample the average count $X = Po(\tau)$, the average count may then be characterized as a Poisson variable with mean $n\tau$ where n is the number of units sampled. That is,

$$\text{Prob}(X = k/n) = \text{Prob}(\Sigma X_i = k) = e^{-m} (n\tau)^k / (k!)$$
$$\text{for } k = 0, 1, 2 \ldots.$$

The average count will thus have a true mean of τ and a variance of τ/n. If we halve the number of samples, we will increase the variability and the likelihood that a lot with an average particle count that exceeds limits is accepted. The major concern here is accepting a lot as good when, in actuality, the mean particulate matter burden in that lot exceeds specifications. It is obvious that the chance of this increases as the sample size decreases. The remaining question is whether or not that increase is important enough to justify the larger sample size.

Table II presents the percentage of lots that would be accepted under the decreased sampling scheme given some true average particle count. For each value of τ three sample sizes are reported: 1 unit, 5 units, and 10 units. As can be seen when τ is close to the limit (34 to 40 for 10 µm and 3 to 4.5 for 25 µm), the difference between the sampling plans is evident. For example, if the true mean particle count were 40 for 10 µm particles, then a 10-unit sampling plan would be preferred. Such a plan would result in false acceptances of a lot no more than 1 out of 170 tests. A 5-unit test would incorrectly accept these lots 1 out of 25 times.

Table II. Probability of Accepting[a] a Lot Under Various Schemes

(True mean is real number of particles (per mL) for a given lot.)

Sample Size	True Mean (10 µm)	Acceptance[b] Probability (%)*	True Mean (25 µm)	Acceptance Probability (%)[b]
1	5	100.00	0.5	99.825
5	5	100.00	0.5	100.00
10	5	100.00	0.5	100.00
1	10	100.00	1.0	98.101
5	10	100.00	1.0	99.993
10	10	100.00	1.0	100.000
1	15	100.00	1.5	93.436
5	15	100.00	1.5	99.539
10	15	100.00	1.5	99.980
1	20	100.00	2.0	79.403
5	20	100.00	2.0	82.106
10	20	100.00	2.0	97.423
1	20	100.00	2.5	75.758
5	20	100.00	2.5	80.603
10	20	100.00	2.5	86.331
1	29	88.409	3.0	65.723
5	29	99.314	3.0	80.603
10	29	99.972	3.0	54.835
1	31	79.364	—	—
5	31	94.795	—	—
10	31	98.815	—	—

Sample Size	True Mean (10 μm)	Acceptance[b] Probability (%)*	True Mean (25 μm)	Acceptance Probability (%)[b]
1	34	61.174	—	—
5	34	66.724	—	—
10	34	71.754	—	—
1	35	54.479	3.5	53.663
5	35	52.009	3.5	32.754
10	35	51.421	3.5	22.694
1	36	47.783	—	—
5	36	37.284	—	—
10	36	31.062	—	—
1	40	24.241	4.0	43.347
5	40	3.940	4.0	15.651
10	40	0.586	4.0	6.169
1	44	9.675	—	—
5	44	0.097	—	—
10	44	0.001	—	—
1	46	5.617	4.5	34.230
5	46	0.009	4.5	6.341
10	46	0.000	4.5	1.160
1	50	1.621	5.0	26.503
5	50	0.000	5.0	2.229
10	50	0.000	5.0	0.159
1	54	0.388	5.5	20.170
5	54	0.000	5.5	0.694
10	54	0.000	5.5	0.017
1	100	0.000	10.0	1.034
5	100	0.000	10.0	0.000
10	100	0.000	10.0	0.000
1	200	0.000	20.0	0.000
5	200	0.000	20.0	0.000
10	200	0.000	20.0	0.000

[a] Alert limit of not more than (NMT) 35 particles/mL 10 μm and NMT 3 particles/mL 25 μm
[b] Calculated based on a Poisson distribution of count data
* 100.00% is used to express probability of acceptance instead of 100% because 100% (1) implies that the probability is exactly 100% and (2) that the probability is ≥99.995%. The latter is the true statement. Thus, 100.00% implies ≥99.9995%.

The apparent superiority of the 10-unit test is only true for a narrow range of τ values near the limit. If the true mean number of particles is much greater than the limits set, it does not really matter which test is used as the change of incorrectly accepting a lot falls to zero quite rapidly. This is more true of the 10 μm particles than the 25 µm particles. For either size of particle, note that the USP limits are far above the true means listed in Table II. Any lot that had mean particulate matter levels near the USP limits would surely fail the test whether 5 or 10 were sampled. The added power of a 10-unit test is only useful for those lots whose mean falls in the questionable range near the 35 and 3 count limits. Smaller sample size lots that are just over the alert limits would be more likely to be accepted, but it is very unlikely that any of these "bad" lots would have particle counts near the USP limits.

Given this result, the manufacturer decides to perform a test on 5 individual units using an alert limit of 35 particles/mL ≥10 µm and 3 particles/mL ≥25 µm.

Summary

The development and maintenance of a high quality pharmaceutical product depends upon the use of a comprehensive approach to particulate matter control. This approach must be based on an accurate assessment of product quality and careful control of both the manufacturing environment and formulation. Visible inspection and subvisible counting techniques have progressed to the point where an objective assessment of particulate matter quality is possible. Advances in analytical techniques have made particle identification more feasible and an understanding of particle formation an attainable goal. With regard to particulate matter control in pharmaceutical products and manufacturing environments, it may be assumed that the remainder of the 1990s will bring steady progress toward an order of magnitude of 10-fold or greater in the level of cleanliness. This process will be driven, as always, not only by quality considerations, but by factorable cost considerations as well. Happily, the next decade promises a willingness on the part of the regulatory body in the United States to accept innovation and streamlining of validation of change.

Finally, it is essential that the reader keep in mind several basic precepts with regard to the control and elimination of particulate matter in pharmaceuticals. First, at the low levels of particulate matter found in current products manufactured in the United States, there is no issue with regard to patient effects of particulate matter. Some low particle burden in parenteral products is unavoidable. If products as manufactured were totally free of particles, administration of the solutions (i.e., entering containers, use of needles, tubing, and medical devices) would still result in a particle burden in solutions infused. Most importantly, no amount of monitoring of particles in solutions or environments, nor capability for particle identification can substitute for GMP control of manufacturing that denies particles access to product in the first place. GMP rather than monitoring or regulatory and compendial requirements controls particles. It is the manufacturer's commitment to product quality that has resulted in the current high quality levels, cost effectiveness, and efficacy of parenteral solutions.

References

ASTM Committee E-11 on Statistical Methods. 1976. ASTM Manual on *Presentation of data and control chart analysis (STP-15D),* 4th Revision. Philadelphia: American Society for Testing and Materials.

Blanchard, J., J. A. Schwartz, D. M. Byrne, and D. B. Marx. 1978. Comparison of two methods for obtaining size distribution characteristics of particulate matter in large-volume parenterals. *J. Pharm. Sci.* 67:340.

Brownley, C. A. 1967. Statistical analysis of parenteral product rejects. *Bull. Paren. Drug Assoc.* 21:77.

Charbonneau, H. C., and G. Webster. 1978. *Industrial quality control.* Englewood Cliffs, NJ: Prentice Hall.

Davis, N. M., S. Turco, and E. Snively. 1970. A study of particulate matter in I.V. infusion fluids. *Am. J. Hosp. Pharm.* 27:822.

Deming, W. E. 1982. *Quality, productivity, and competitive position.* Cambridge, MA: Massachusetts Institute of Technology, Center for Advanced Engineering Study.

Duncan, Acheson J. 1974. *Quality control and industrial statistics*, 4th Ed. Philadelphia: Richard D. Irwin, Inc.

Ford Motor Company, Inc. 1984. *Continuing process control and process capability improvement.* Dearborne, MI: Ford Motor Company, Statistical Methods Office.

Glossary and tables for statistical quality control. 1983. Milwaukee, WI: American Society for Quality Control, Statistical Division.

Grant, E. L., and R. S. Levenworth. 1980. *Statistical quality control,* 5th Ed. New York: McGraw-Hill, Inc.

Hayashi, T. 1980a. Studies on the particulate matter in parenteral solutions. Part 1. Occurrence and size distribution of particulate matter in parenteral solutions. *Yakuzaigaku* 40:62.

Hayashi, T. 1980b. Studies on the particulate matter in small volume injections. Part 3. Evaluation criteria on quality of particulate matter in small-volume injections. *Yakuzaigaku* 40:133–140.

Human and veterinary drugs: Current good manufacturing, packing, or holding (Code of Federal Regulations 21). 1978. *Federal Register* 43FR190:45014–45089.

Ishikawa, I. 1976. *Guide to quality control.* Asian Productivity Association. Available from Unipub, P.O. Box 433, Murray Hill Station, New York, NY 10016.

Juran, J. M., and F. M. Gryna, Jr. 1979. *Juran's quality control handbook,* 4th Ed. New York: McGraw-Hill, Inc.

Juran, J. M., and F. M. Gryna, Jr. 1980. *Quality planning and analysis*, 2nd Ed. New York: McGraw-Hill, Inc.

Juran, J. M., F. M. Gryna, Jr., and R. S. Bingham, Jr., 1979. *Quality control handbook,* 3rd Ed. New York: McGraw-Hill, Inc.

Military Standard 105-E 1989. Sampling procedures and tables for inspection by attributes. *Department of Defense document Mil-Std-105-E.* Washington, D.C.: The Government Printing Office.

Mochida, K., H. Isaka, and S. Tsuji. 1984. Insoluble particulate matter test for small-volume injections. *Iyakuhin Kenkyu* 15:305–318.

Munson, T. E. 1990. FDA perspectives on particulate matter testing in small volume injections. In *Proc. PDA Int. Conf. on Particle Detection, Metrology, and Control,* 827–837. Arlington, VA.

Taylor, J. K. 1987. *Quality assurance of chemical measurements.* Lewis Publishers, p. 328.

Taylor, W. A. 1991. *Optimization & variation reduction in quality.* New York: McGraw-Hill, Inc.

Tsuji, K., and A. R. Lewis. 1987. Evaluation of acceptance criteria for particulate limits for small-volume parenteral products. *J. Pharm. Sci.* 67:50–65.

Wheeler, D. J., and D. S. Chambers. 1992. *Understanding statistical process control.* Knoxville, TN: Statistical Process Controls, Inc.

XI

Medical Devices

The discussion in the preceding chapters has been directed almost entirely toward injectable materials. This is reasonable, since the majority of published information on the subject of particulate matter in medical products pertains to large and small volume injections. The fact that less has been published regarding particles in medical devices is reflective of the health care professional's generally decreased level of concern over the infused particle burden arising from this component of intravenous (I.V.) therapy.

In the current world marketplace, there are a large number of medical devices intended to serve a wide range of needs. Devices of various types incorporate into their construction polymeric tubings, electronic components, molded parts, elastomeric injection sites and closures, filters, metal fittings, sponges, cotton or polymeric plugs, check valves, capillary fibers, catheters, and needles. Some products classified as medical devices are purely structural replacements (e.g., metal or ceramic hip joints). Others incorporate complex grafting structures, hydrogels, selective filters, electronic controllers, and bioreagents. Particulate matter is most certainly not an equal concern for all device types.

The variety of medical products categorized as "devices" is so wide as to cause difficulties in any general discussion, or with regard to any uniform application of regulatory requirements. To simplify matters, this chapter is concerned primarily with devices that have a solution path that comes in contact with injectable solutions, blood, or dialysate (i.e., materials administered to a patient via a route other than a normal body opening). I will refer to this general device category as parenteral-type devices or solution contact devices. With regard to particulate matter, this broad grouping may be usefully subdivided into several subcategories. The most obvious category includes solution transfer sets used in a pharmacy, solution and blood administration sets, syringes, and other drug delivery devices. A second category includes oxygenators, autologous transfusion devices, blood warmers, and like devices applied in surgical procedures. The third group consists of chronic use devices such as central venous catheters, transfer sets used with continuous ambulatory peritoneal dialysis (CAPD) therapy, and hemodialyzers.

Just as there is no evidence to indicate that the low levels of particles present in injectable products manufactured under CGMP are a hazard to patients, there is also no indication that any significant patient health issues are related to the particulate matter from parenteral-type devices. While a very limited number of studies have suggested that occasionally specific devices may have high particle burdens (Knopp et al. 1982; Page et al. 1970; Dimmick et al. 1976), recent comprehensive studies of Gour (1987) and Di Paolo et al. (1990) show that a wide range of parenteral-type devices have low solution contact path particle burdens.

In the Gour study, the majority of a wide range of tested devices met the acceptability criteria imposed by the investigator of a maximum of 25 particles ≥10 µm, and 5 particles ≥25 µm per mL of eluent. Di Paolo et al. (1990) commented that intravenous administration sets are potential sources of substantially lower particulate matter contamination than the infused solutions themselves, and that an in-line filter in a set functions effectively not only in removing particles from devices, but from the infusate solutions as well.

Since the aim of the latter study was to test relatively large numbers of various types of administration sets, an electronic particle counter was chosen. This enabled the authors to examine a large number of sets in a relatively short time. It should be pointed out that this type of equipment is not generally well-suited for qualitative examination of devices for particulate matter, or for reliable counting of larger (≥25 µm) particles. Indeed, this consideration has prompted the German Standards Institute (Deutsches Institut fur Normung; DIN), to recommend the use of a light microscope to analyze particles in intravenous administration sets.

During the past decade, considerable interest has been expressed by regulatory and compendial groups in the U.S., Canada, the U.K., and Europe regarding the need for particulate matter requirements for medical devices. Most recently, the USP has proposed a requirement for disposable single-use syringes. A number of widely accepted requirements for devices (e.g., those of AAMI and ISO) are already in place, and it seems unlikely that additional requirements are needed. The majority of the few documented occurrences of high levels of particulate matter in specific devices are based on large (visible-sized) particles. The most appropriate test method would thus appear to be a microscopic assay performed on the total eluent volume of a flush solution passed through a device. The principles outlined in the preceding chapters regarding the monitoring and control of environmental and process-related particles also apply directly or indirectly to medical device manufacture. Similarly, the sections regarding particulate matter analysis and enumeration by various means are applicable to particles isolated from devices.

Parenteral-Type Devices

Presently, the primary concern of both regulatory agencies and manufacturers are devices that have a contact path for blood or solutions that will be infused directly into the venous circulation of a patient. This category includes administration sets, blood sets, dialyzers, I.V. catheters, needles, syringes, and other indirectly related products (such as devices for CAPD). Examples of devices of this type are as follows:

- Sets (administration, recipient, blood)
- Sets (dialyzer, oxygenator—inlet, and outlet)
- Hollow fiber dialyzers
- Bubble oxygenators
- Membrane oxygenators
- Pump cassettes
- Cell elimination filters
- Cardiotomy reservoirs
- Heat exchangers
- Empty plastic containers for I.V. solutions
- I.V. catheters
- Needles
- Central catheters

- Extracorporeal tubing
- Vascular grafts
- Extension sets
- Pharmacy compounding sets
- Solution transfer sets
- Autotransfusion devices
- Balloon catheters

Sources and Control of Particulate Matter in Devices

Many of the particles associated with medical devices originate at process assembly points; typically a much a smaller number comes from the environment. Each component part assembled into devices typically contributes some variable level of unique particles. Interestingly, because of the distinct sources of particles found in devices, mixed particle populations composed of subvisible 1 μm to 50 μm particles (representing the inherent burden of components), and small numbers of larger particles of visible size (predominantly process-related) may occur. Currently manufactured parenteral-type devices span a range of complexity from single administration sets and extension sets to blood oxygenators, extracorporeal circuits, blood warmers, and autotransfusion devices. Large numbers of individual component parts may be included in devices of the latter types. Even simple devices may incorporate parts made from several different types of polymeric material (Table I).

Table I. Polymeric Components of Medical Devices

Rigid Plastic	Flexible (Tubing)	Elastomers
Styrene	PVC	Synthetic natural rubber
Impact styrene	Polyethylene	Butyl rubber
Acrylic	Polypropylene	Halobutyl rubber
Clear ABS	Nylon	EPDM
Rigid PVC	Polyurethane	Neoprene
Polycarbonate	Silicone	Silicone
Polysulfone	Teflon®	Styrene-butadiene
Polyester	Natural rubber	Nitrile
Nylon	Synthetic natural rubber	Thermoplastic elastomers (TPE)
Polypropylene	Hytrel	
Polymethylpentene		
Cellulosics		
Rigid urethane		
Ektar®		

Specific polymeric materials are selected for an application based on their characteristics relative to the following criteria: (1) resilience; (2) flexibility; (3) printability; (4) transparency; (5) tensile strength; (6) working pressure; (7) resistance to heat, physical forces, and chemicals; and (8) bonding properties. Cost and resistance to the gamma radiation, ethylene oxide, or chemical agents that are applied for the purpose of sterilization are also concerns. For some applications, the particle-generating properties of materials may also be a critical concern.

A number of sources of particulate matter in devices may be suggested based on the nature of the components and the assembly processes applied. Medical grade tubing (silicone, vinyl, polyurethane, polyisoprene or other) may have an inherent particle burden based on its composition or the process by which it is formed. Additionally, whenever tubing is cut by any means, particles are generated. Injection-molded rigid plastic parts, such as spikes and connectors, may have an associated particle burden originating from fillers or reinforcing agents that may segregate at surfaces, or from minor ingredients that can "bloom" out. The method of collection of injection molded parts is also critical. As an example, rigid plastic parts with sharp edges that are allowed to drop from the mold into a receiving pan lined with a polyethylene bag can be expected to generate particles from the soft polyethylene. Plastic parts may be washed prior to assembly or may be produced by a "clean" molding process; the latter is invariably a better approach due to particles being eliminated rather than attempts being made to remove them using washing procedures of variable effectiveness.

Elastomeric device components (such as injection sites, diaphragms, and valves) are subject to the same general considerations as stoppers with regard to particle generation. These include blooming or migration of low molecular weight components and surface adherent particles such as fibers. Filters may be particularly problematic sources of particles; fibrous filters used for blood transfusion invariably shed fibers, and the fragile nature of microporous membrane material makes it liable to generate particles when it is cut or pressed into a housing. Sintered plastic filter media is prone to shed particles of incompletely sintered material, and cutting hollow fiber filters can generate fragments of the microporous medium. Large plastic parts tend to develop static charges in handling or molding and can attract and persistently adhere fibrous particles such as paper or cotton. These large particles may create a conspicuous visible defect if they adhere to external surfaces of a device. Metal needles and cannulae sometimes bear abrasive particles on their surfaces from sharpening, or contain particles within the lumen due to the forming process. The silicone lubricants (grease or oil) applied to the piston seal of disposable plastic syringes may form agglomerates with particulate matter present in the device, and silicone oil microdroplets may be counted if light extinction counters are applied in enumerating particles in the effluent from a syringe.

Control of particulate matter in assembly processes is critical for devices. The protection of components at each assembly station is important, since a supply of parts is typically held in close proximity to the point at which they will be used. The protection of parts during handling and storage in particle-free bags becomes increasingly critical as more assembly steps are involved, since the potential for the access of process-related particles to the device is increased with the number of assembly steps. The negative aspects of human contact with devices during manufacture may be more important than is the case with parenteral solutions, due to the difficulty of protecting the device solution contact path during assembly, and to the higher number of manual operations generally required. The reader has been previously advised concerning the particle-generating properties of feeder bowls, which are widely used in device manufacture. Automatic or robotic assembly of devices is, in general, superior to manual assembly; but machines will also generate particles from their moving parts and from the device components that they handle.

Those working with control and elimination of particulates from devices and components are familiar with flash or molded parts as a source of particulates. Flash from molding processes may be firmly attached to a noncritical area of an affected plastic part and thus constitute a cosmetic defect rather than a functional or particulate matter issue. If it is released during assembly or use of a device, however, flash has serious negative implications regarding the process. The same may be said of "angel hair"—the long thin filaments of polymer that are produced by drawing of melted plastic during heat-sealing or piercing. Both types of particles are relatively easy to source, identify, and control.

Some process machinery, such as tubing cutters or vibratory feeder bowls, is an obvious potential source of particulate matter. Other machinery used in manufacturing will also prove capable of generating particulate matter that may gain access to the solution path. Examples include tubing expanders, leak testers, printers, and slitters. Sonic welding or cutting, and radio frequency (microwave) sealing may serve to either generate, detach, or disperse particles. Packaging machinery often generates fragments of plastic (Tyvek®) or coated paper due to the cutting and drawing processes involved;

although sets are most often closed at this point in manufacture, negative customer perceptions may result from this type of particulate matter.

Troubleshooting a process to isolate the source of particulate matter or to define individual contributions to the total particle burden is sometimes necessary. There are generally three steps involved in this type of assessment. The first (essential) step is simply observing each process point in operation. The general level of cleanliness of work surfaces is important, as is that of specific areas that contact exposed portions of the device. The presence of paper fibers is usually an indication of a problem, as are unprotected device components that are exposed to contamination from an operator or by personnel traffic while awaiting assembly. The second step is verifying observations by the use of witness plates that are left in place for some interval in the critical areas, then evaluated microscopically. Collection of particles may also be effected by the use of filter cassettes attached to a vacuum pump as discussed in a previous chapter. In this application the cover of the cassette should be removed so that maximal surface area of the filter is exposed.

The last step is to survey static electrical potential. This step is crucial in assessing the vulnerability of the components to airborne particles at a given process point. A static potential of thousands of volts is sometimes generated on the surface of large plastic parts during handling or molding. The function of this charge in attracting particles from any great distance is questionable, but static potential will attract particles over short distances and can result in persistent adherence of particulates to critical surfaces. Any process step involving plastic sheeting or exposed flat plastic surfaces is suspect; static can be generated by the movement of belts, turntables, and rollers or by other movement of plastic surfaces against one another. Static may be dissipated by ionized air sources used in combination with vacuum nozzles that collect particles loosened by the ionized air. Ionizing grids on the face of high efficiency particulate air (HEPA) filters are effective in reducing static charges over short distances (less than 1 meter). Different means of static dissipation may be evaluated with the assistance of vendors of this type of equipment, who are sufficiently knowledgeable. Control of humidity is critical in this regard.

Process Design

In earlier chapters, the principles of particulate matter control in the manufacture of parenteral products were discussed. Since principles regarding devices differ substantially from injectable products in some specific areas, a brief discussion is appropriate. With the wide range of medical devices manufactured, there are a large number of assembly processes and variations of those processes. This situation holds in our present limited consideration of devices having a solution path that contacts infusion solutions or blood. As was the case with parenteral solutions, minimal particle burden in the final product can be achieved far more cost-effectively through process design than by particle removal operations (such as component washing), rigorous inspection procedures, or an after-the-fact "cleanup" of problem process points.

The simplistic approach to the goal of particle elimination involves the acquisition of clean components and subassemblies from vendors, and their clean fabrication into devices. These two steps are equally important. The obtaining of clean components will not happen by chance, but requires the vendor's understanding of the customer's requirements and a commitment to this endeavor. Economic factors will obviously be a concern, and it is extremely important that the parties involved accept the fact that cleaner components will result from judicious process design and control, and that a higher level of cleanliness need not be synonymous with higher costs. When particle issues arise with a given device, in the field or during manufacture, there is often an unfortunate tendency to focus troubleshooting efforts and resources only on the immediate problem. This approach frequently provides only temporary elimination of the particle source responsible and may result in another problem at a later date at a different process point or with a different vendor. This retrospective approach is not cost effective, and results in higher per-unit costs for the finished product.

In the case of many devices, the design of the process for particulate matter elimination is simpler than back-tracking to identify, source, and eliminate particles once detected. Consider the design of a process to assemble a simple administration set consisting of two 1-meter lengths of tubing, a "Y" injection site (with integral drip chamber), a spike, a needle, and an over-the-needle catheter. There are, thus, seven components that will be assembled, and each must be considered separately and carefully in the course of process design.

Most frequently, the manufacturer of the device purchases bulk tubing that will be cut to length on site. Cutting of tubing is notorious for the generation of elongate, crescentic fibrous particles that mysteriously appear in drip chambers or within in-line filter housings. The cutting mechanism is as critical as the sharpness and durability of the blade used. A regimen for blade changes and careful selection of the cutting machine and blade type (steel or ceramic) is called for; with some materials, laser cutting may have advantages. The bulk tubing used (both with regard to composition and extrusion process) should be chosen for a low inherent particle burden. With some tubings, extrusion aids (slip agents) may constitute a significant component of the released particulates. Therefore, the execution of the extrusion process to include a consideration of die temperatures, cool rate, and control of buildup of char or low molecular weight components of the polymer on the die is very important. Bulk tubing rolls cannot be assumed to be immune to particulate matter contamination during storage, handling, and shipping simply because the tubing lumen is closed to the environment. Any adherent material on the tubing surface has the potential for building up at a critical process point and being carried into the lumen of the device, or being transferred to critical areas of the device on the hands of the assemblers (touch contamination).

The remaining components of the set must be received with vendor assurance of cleanliness based on process control and monitoring during production. The catheter needle tubing should be made by a process that minimizes lumen roughness and particulate matter, and sharpened by a process that ensures removal of any residual abrasives and/or metal fragments. Assembly of the needle into its hub must be conducted under conditions that provide minimal access of particles to the hub or needle shaft. Injection molding of the spike should be done under clean molding conditions that provide for collection of the part and its attachment to a clean-molded drip chamber with maximal control of particulates. The rubber chosen for the septum of the "Y" site should give minimal particle generation when penetrated by a needle, and should be free of any additives (modifiers or processing aids) at a level sufficient to produce "bloom" during sterilization or storage. The access of particles to this and other elastomeric parts must be carefully controlled, due to the tendency of these materials to adhere particles with which they come in contract. If the vendor of our "Y" site uses a vibratory feeder bowl to pass the septa singly into the assembly station, this area should receive careful scrutiny as a potential contributor of particles. Feeder bowls invariably require cleaning at periodic intervals to prevent them from becoming reservoirs for particulate matter. A particular concern here may be achieving a balance between sufficient surface lubrication of the septa to ensure feeding through machinery, and an excess of a material (such as silicone or slip agent) that will generate particles.

With regard to assembly of the device, specific safeguards related to restricting generation and transport of particles and their contact with the product will be observed. In the absence of automated assembly, personnel should be required to wear smock or jacket overgarments, and depending on the potential for touch contact with product, particle-free gloves. Components awaiting assembly must be protected from particles in the air, both those generated by the process, and those generated by or adherent to the surfaces of the containers in which the components are held. Depending on the particle levels generated at the assembly point, ionized air blowdown of the point, and vacuum removal of process-generated particles may be employed. Work surfaces at assembly points should be carefully watched for any buildup of particulate matter.

Even with effective local measures for cleaning and particle removal, HEPA protection of process points is desirable. Although HEPA airflow is not sufficient to remove particles from a work surface or component, it minimizes the float time of particles such as fibers and establishes a flow of clean air onto and around the process point. Modular HEPA enclosures with side curtains provide an economical way to achieve this protection. Periodic cleaning (with lint-free cloths and a suitable solvent) of work surfaces, assembly mandrels, punches, and other equipment is also effective in reducing work station particle levels.

Monitoring of particle levels on components (by the vendor) and in finished device product (by the device manufacturer) play an important role in ensuring that a process continues to operate as designed. Monitoring of particulates should not be confused with 100% inspection, whereby some nondestructive analysis is applied to all units manufactured. Monitoring signifies a low level of testing that is applied to ensure that a minimal particle burden is maintained, as assured by a consistent, controlled, and validated GMP process. Given the existence of a consistent, controlled process that has been validated to result in low levels of particles, testing of low numbers of samples suffices to assure that the process is running within limits. Total testing of any device product is ineffectual as a particulate matter control measure; process control is the only approach capable of achieving particle elimination.

Patient Concerns

With parenteral-type devices, our primary concern is particulate matter that can be washed from the solution contact path and thus infused into a patient along with the particulate matter burdens derived from large or small volume injections, admixtures, and so forth. Importantly, the particulate matter burden to which a patient receiving parenteral therapy is exposed is a function of the total process of solution administration, including the techniques of admixture, addition of drug, and vein access. Thus, limiting the patient particle loading cannot be reliably achieved by limiting particulate matter related to individual components of the system, such as parenteral solutions or administration sets. We cannot consider the particle burden delivered to the patient as dependent upon any single physical component of the system that delivers a parenteral solution.

The only completely effective approach to minimizing exposure of patients to particles involves the use of in-line disposable filters of IV infusion systems. Terminal filters are effective in reducing patient exposure to all types of particulates resulting from the infusion process, not merely the components present in parenteral devices, solutions or infusion sets. Filters have proven useful in some cases in reducing the incidence of phlebitis related to infusate particle burden (Falchuk et al. 1985; Barnett et al. 1983). However, these few cases of patient benefit do not justify the wide-scale use of in-line filters. Current intravenous therapy practice, based on more recent research and in-house studies conducted in large hospitals, dictates the use of terminal filters only in the case of some few specific drugs and for TPN admixtures. A number of economical, disposable in-line filters presently on the market are suitable for this application as needed, and a wide range of sets that incorporate such filters are available. In recent years the efficiency of these filters has increased, while technical advances and competitive pressure has driven their cost down.

A word regarding the relative cost effectiveness of in-line filters is also in order. The cost of additional compendial or regulatory particulate matter requirements placed on solution or device manufacturers must eventually be passed on to the health care consumer. In the case of most manufacturers, this increased cost will not result in any predictable patient benefits, whereas the use of filters is a measure of proven effectiveness in limiting patient particulate matter exposure. No matter how restrictive, particulate matter limits on solutions or devices are not capable of controlling the total particulate matter burden administered to patients. In contrast to the uncertain measure of particulate matter control provided by particle limits on solutions and devices, the use of in-line filters when indicated is an economical, effective method of improving the quality of patient care.

Analysis of Particulate Matter in Devices

Parenteral-type devices may be analyzed by a number of different methods. Since the main concern is particulate matter washed from the device solution contact path in use, a reasonable analytical circumstance is one in which a volume of flush solution (equal to that of the use volume of the device) is passed through the device under "as used" conditions. For a simple administration set, this might involve water (or 0.9% sodium chloride) passed through the set at a head pressure of approximately 1 meter, at a flow rate of 120–150 mL/hour. To facilitate the analysis, a higher flow rate that may be more effective in removing particles is typically used. Several methods have been suggested by compendial groups, standards organizations, and manufacturers associations. Two of these are summarized below.

British Standards Institution Method (1986)

I. Sample

   Test 5 sets of the product.

II. Apparatus

   The following apparatus and materials are required:

   1. Straight-sided borosilicate beakers of 200 mL graduated capacity

   2. A top-loading balance, measuring in divisions of 0.1 g or less

   3. A sodium chloride intravenous infusion BP containing 9 g of sodium chloride per liter

   4. An instrument capable of counting the number of particles suspended in a known volume of electrolyte solution having equivalent sphere diameters equal to or greater than 2 μm and equal to or greater than 5 μm

III. Method

   A. Run approximately 100 mL of sodium chloride infusion into the beaker in small aliquots, rinsing and discarding the infusion.

   B. Collect 150 mL of the infusion in the beaker and determine particle counts at 2.0 μm and 5.0 μm. **Note:** The test should not proceed until consistent conditions have been obtained, and periodic checks should be made to ensure that these criteria are maintained.

C. Empty the beaker and drain in the inverted position or use a fresh, clean beaker.

D. Handling the set as little as possible, remove the connector protector and squeeze the filter chamber before inserting the connector into the infusion supply. Invert the set before releasing the filter chamber so that air can escape down the set and is not trapped. It is essential that the flow control be opened to release air, and closed before reinverting so as not to lose fluid. The filter chamber should be full of sodium chloride infusion and the drip chamber half full. If more infusion is needed in the set, remove the connector, gently squeeze the filter chamber to remove air, replace the connector, and release the filter chamber.

E. Arrange the set so that the connector is 1.0 m to 1.1 m above bench height, and the beaker on the balance is 700 mm to 900 mm from the infusion source and drip stand.

F. Collect 200 g of infusion in the beaker at a drip rate of 9 g/min to 11 g/min, taking care to collect the first few drops issuing from the set.

G. Immediately determine particle counts at 2.0 µm and 5.0 µm on five replicate samples from the solution to the beaker using a Coulter counter or light extinction counter.

HIMA–PMA Method (1980)

I. Test Preparation

A. Test Environment

All procedures should be performed in a laminar flow hood equipped with HEPA filters that are certified to meet Class 100 conditions. The laminar hood should operate 24 hours a day for reliable results.

B. Apparatus Preparation

1. All solvents (water and isopropyl alcohol) used to clean the apparatus must be filtered through a

membrane filter (with a maximum pore size of 2.0 μm) into the precleaned, pressure-dispensing vessels. The solvent dispensers are fitted with membrane filters as specified.

   a. Water—25 mm, 1.0 μm, white, plain
   b. Isopropyl Alcohol—25 mm, 1.0 μm or 2.0 μm, white, plain

C. Filter Holder Assembly

   Clean the filtration apparatus and accessory items before use, as follows:

   1. Wash filtration apparatus with a warm solution of liquid detergent (dilute as per package instructions).
   2. Rinse in 0.45 mm filtered water.
   3. Before each use, ultraclean the filtration apparatus utilizing pressure vessels and a "gun" with a 0.45 μm filter.
   4. Rinse with filtered isopropyl alcohol.
   5. Follow with a final rinse of 0.45 μm filtered water.

D. Membrane Filter Assembly

   1. Clean the inside top and bottom of the petri slide with filtered purified water. Set aside to dry in the laminar flow hood with the top of the petri slide ajar.
   2. Rinse the blades of the unserrated forceps with a forceful stream of filtered purified water.
   3. Using the cleaned forceps, remove a 0.8 μm black-gridded filter from the package. Holding the filter in a vertical position and starting at the top of the nongridded side), sweep a stream of filtered water back and forth across the surface, working slowly from top to bottom, so that the particles will be rinsed downward off the filter. Repeat the process on the gridded side.
   4. Place the cleaned membrane filter (grid side up) on the support screen of the base. Place the ultracleaned funnel on the base and secure with the spring clamp.

5. Repeat the above steps for each membrane filter and assembly.

E. Reservoir Assembly (Figure 1)
1. Attach an ultraclean piece (approximately 2" in length) of clear plastic tubing to the flat end of an ultraclean, long or short point connector.
2. Place a 1.20-µm (or smaller retention rating) filter into the 47-mm in-line filter holder and assemble the filter holder as required.
3. Insert the inlet of the in-line filter holder into the plastic tubing that is attached to the long or short point connector.
4. Attach an ultraclean piece (from 2–6" in length) of clear plastic tubing into the outlet of the in-line filter holder.
5. Using a hemostat, clamp the plastic tubing that is attached to the long or short point connector (Note: a roller clamp will also serve this purpose).
6. Insert the exposed end of the long or short point connector into the stopper of a 1000 mL IV bottle of Sterile Water for injection, USP.

II. Method
A. Blank Analysis
1. A blank analysis should be performed on the apparatus rinse water at the beginning of the test period, and after each solvent-dispensing filter change. A blank analysis should be performed on the eluate water from the I.V. bottle setup at the beginning and end of every test day.
2. After assembling the test apparatus and filtration equipment, discharge and discard 100 mL of apparatus rinse water from the filter jet solvent dispenser.
3. Fill the filter holder with 50 mL of rinse water and vacuum through an 0.8-mm porosity gridded membrane filter. Remove the membrane filter from the filter holder, place in an ultraclean petri slide, and set aside to dry in the laminar flow hood with the cover slightly ajar.

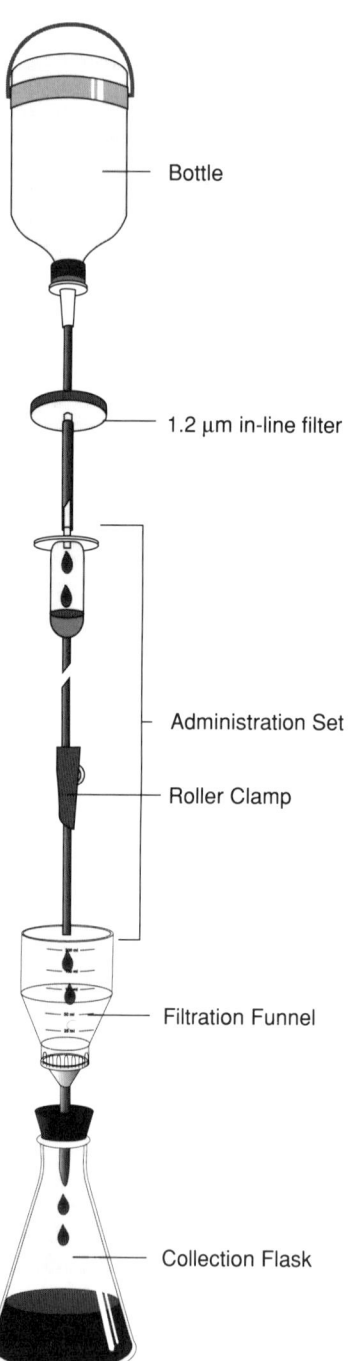

Figure 1. Test procedure for device particulate matter assay.

4. Examine the membrane filter microscopically at 100× magnification for particulate matter. The particulate matter should not exceed 5 particles ≥10 µm, or 2 particles ≥25 µm, and no fibers.

B. Test Procedure

1. After assembling the test apparatus and filtration equipment, attach the test sample to the plastic tubing that is attached to the outlet of the in-line filter assembly.
2. Flush the lumen of the test sample with 50 mL of eluate water, and collect the solution directly into the filtration funnel that houses a 0.8-µm black-gridded membrane filter.
3. Turn on the vacuum and filter the solution until approximately 10 mL of eluate remain in the funnel.
4. Flush an additional 50 mL of water through the test sample and vacuum filter as above.
5. Repeat this procedure until 1000 mL of filtered water has been flushed through the test sample.
6. After all 1000 mL of eluate have been filtered, rinse the funnel walls with 25 mL of apparatus rinse water, using care not to direct the stream of water onto the filter surface.
7. After turbulence has dissipated, vacuum filter the rinse water.
8. Turn off the vacuum and remove the filter carefully with ultraclean unserrated forceps, and place onto a petri slide using a piece of double sided tape.
9. Allow the filter membrane to dry in the laminar flow hood with the cover slightly ajar.
10. Upon drying, count the particulate matter contained on the membrane filters as follows:
    a. Position the incident light illuminator at an angle of 10°–20° to ensure maximum definition of particles for counting and sizing.

b. Using 100× magnification, count the particles lying within the entire effective filtration area in the following size ranges: 10–<25 μm and ≥25 μm. Additionally, count and size the fibers in a separate "fiber" category.

Tests have also been developed by the Association for the Advancement of Medical Instrumentation (AAMI) for blood filters and autotransfusion devices. These are generally similar to the method above that has been proposed for administration sets and are summarized briefly below. It is essential that anyone wishing to perform analyses per these standards purchase copies from AAMI, so that specifics of the analysis may be followed.

Autologous Transfusion Devices (AAMI, ATG-1991)

In summary, the test is specified as follows:

All operations are performed in a laminar flow hood equipped with high-efficiency particulate air (HEPA) filters. The test apparatus includes all components of the device as supplied by the manufacturer, which are filled to their maximum volume during the test according to specified use procedures. The flush liquid is introduced into the system by gravity or pumping apparatus, as required, until the device is filled.

Particles in the total volume of effluent from the device are collected onto a 0.8-μm retention rating filter membrane in a vacuum filtration apparatus, both of which have been previously cleaned. A blank membrane with a volume of test fluid equivalent to that used in the device is counted in conjunction with the analytical membrane. A vacuum may be used to assist in filtration through the test membrane. After the analysis, the test membrane is removed from the filtration apparatus, placed in a petri dish container with the cover slightly ajar, and dried in the laminar flow hood. The particles collected on the membrane surface are counted microscopically. The particle/fiber counts for all particles larger than 10 mm in diameter, for those larger than 25 mm in diameter, and for all fibers is calculated as:

$$\text{Particle/Fiber Count} = \frac{\text{Count Test} - \text{Count Control}}{\text{Total Test Fluid Volume}}$$

The apparatus tested is allowed to provide no more than the following particulate burden: 50 particles per mL for particles larger than 10 µm; 5 particles per mL for particles larger than 25 µm; and 6.5 per mL for fibers. It is worthy of note in this procedure that the flush volume used is determined by the volume of the device, rather than being arbitrarily specified, and the limit chosen for ≥10 µm and ≥25 µm particles is the USP LVP limit.

Blood Filters (AAMI BF 7-1989)

This test is also performed in a laminar flow enclosure equipped with high-efficiency particulate air (HEPA) filters. The flush liquid is Water for Injection, USP, filtered through a 0.8-µm retention rating filter prior to its introduction into the device. A blank analysis is performed in conjunction with the test, using the same filtration apparatus and filter type used for the flush water from the device. Thhe blank count must not exceed 10% of the limits counts as specified. A total volume of 2500 mL of the flush water is passed through the filter at a rate of 500 mL/minute. The analysis membrane is counted microscopically, and the difference between the test and blank counts is calculated for particles larger than 10 µm in diameter, larger than 25 µm in diameter, and for all fibers.

The shed particle burden for the tested filter cannot exceed the following levels:

1. 0.90 particle per milliliter of solvent flush larger than 10 mm;
2. 0.35 particle per milliliter of solvent flush larger than 25 µm; and
3. 0.65 fiber per milliliter of solvent flush.

Choice of Particle Counting Methods

The methods summarized above have in common the use of a filtered flush solution supply for the test, and quantitation of particles in the collected flush solution. The test method applied in enumerating particles from the solution path of a device is a critical consideration. It must be emphasized that the light-extinction counting method is generally unsuitable for testing devices. This assessment is largely based on the fact that particulate matter populations from devices are heterogeneous and poorly characterized, and may contain large particles that are either not counted or are down-sized by the counter. The microscopic assay is the method of choice since it allows particulate matter to be both enumerated and characterized.

The microscopic method would appear to be particularly appropriate in view of the fact that the small number of customer complaints received on devices involve large particles. The case concerning particles in the disposable syringes cited in the Canadian HPB Medical Devices Alert No. 55 (1983) and loose particles in the blood lines of the extracorporeal sets cited in Medical Devices Alert No. 58 (1983) are good examples. The cleanliness of the syringes and blood lines reported was *visually* unacceptable. Only a microscopic test will reproducibly detect and size large particles. Automatic particle counters are efficient and generally free from observer bias, but they are subject to errors of their own. Microscopic examination yields information both on the configuration of the particles and their origin. Keep in mind that the yield of particles in the rinsing process will depend to some extent on the type of rinsing fluid—pure water, detergent, or electrolyte—and on the rinsing action, and on the volume of solution used. One point of view is that the rinsing medium and action should be as stringent as possible in order to recover the greatest number of particles. Another view is that the medium and rinsing action should simulate those to which the device will be exposed during use. The numbers of particles rinsed from a tested device can be expected to decrease significantly with increasing flush volume. With simple solution administration sets and most other devices, the first 100 mL of flush solution typically removes 90% or more of the total particle burden. The analyst must be aware of this factor when designing flush assays for specific devices so that the particles per mL in the device are not calculated based on unrealistically low flush volume. The obvious effect of this error will be an overestimate of the shed particle burden.

GMP Control of Device Particulates

The GMP requirements for visually acceptable product have proven sufficient to control the cleanliness of medical devices. Both the U.K. and U.S. regulatory agencies presently provide general guidelines for the control of particulate matter in device manufacture. In the U.K. these are based on the Guide to Good Manufacturing Practices for Sterile Devices and Surgical Products (1981). FDA guidelines are issued in accordance with Title 21 of the Code of Federal

Regulations Chapter 1, and describe procedures of general acceptability to FDA regulations for a subject matter within its statutory authority. Guidelines are not legal requirements. A person who follows an agency guideline may be assured that the procedures or standards will be acceptable to the FDA. Procedures and standards other than those in the guidelines may be used as long as the proper validation studies have been performed that demonstrate the finished product meets appropriate standards.

Good Manufacturing Practice, for devices as well as for injectable products, represents the sum total of those activities necessary to ensure that products meet established requirements for quality, safety, and performance. The principles and key elements of GMP control of device manufacture are outlined below:

I. Principles of GMP for Device Manufacture

   A. An integrated system of manufacture and quality assurance
   B. Separate management responsibilities for production and quality assurance
   C. Suitable premises, equipment, and materials
   D. Trained personnel
   E. Documented procedures for manufacture and quality assurance
   F. Appropriate batch and product records
   G. Adequate transport and storage
   H. A recall system
   I. A system for auditing the operation of Good Manufacturing Practice

II. Environment

   A. Control and/or classification of manufacturing areas
   B. Positive pressure environment (air flow and velocity)
   C. Temperature/humidity control
   D. Filtered air (HEPA, other)
   E. Construction—walls, lights, ceiling, floors, equipment
   F. Particle count monitoring

- G. Microbial environment monitoring
- H. Cleaning and sanitation
- I. Validation
- J. Corrective action program
- K. Static charge (ionization)

III. Process
- A. Compressed air (oil-free, etc.)
- B. Water quality
- C. Control of extraneous materials such as cardboard
- D. Transfer practices
- E. Equipment design for particulate matter generation and removal
- F. Sampling/testing
- G. Validation

IV. Component Control
- A. Wash versus nonwash
- B. Package protection of raw materials
- C. Use of dryers, and so forth, for particle control after wash
- D. Storage requirements
- E. Sampling control
- F. Sampling/testing

V. Personnel Control
- A. Uniforms (captive versus noncaptive)
- B. Polyester smocks versus cotton uniforms
- C. Hair covers
- D. Masks (where necessary)
- E. Gloves
- F. Shoe covers

G. Flow of personnel

H. Training related to particulate matter sources

I. Health requirements for visual inspectors and other product contact personnel

Current Regulatory Issues

It is interesting to review the results of recent FDA inspections of device manufacturing facilities. They provide some indication of the concerns of the FDA thinking regarding device particulate matter issues. First of all, there seems to be a general acceptance on the part of investigators that subvisible particulate matter is not a concern in devices. This viewpoint has been borne out by a majority of the studies conducted, including most notably those of Di Paolo et al. (1990) and Gour (1987). There is, however, considerable regulatory interest in the occurrence of visible particles both within the solution contact path of devices and in the packing of administration sets and other items.

It is likely that the agency's general perception regarding particulate matter in devices is not dramatically different from that of most device manufacturers. Broadly speaking, the role of the investigator who visits a device manufacturing plant is to ensure that devices are made, processed, stored, and handled according to approved procedures, and that GMP is followed by the manufacturer. While particulate matter (particularly of visible size) may be used as a "first pass" indicator of difficulties, its most significant impact point for the investigator is that if process control is lacking, GMP may have been violated. The occurrence of particulate matter may provide the investigator with clues that lead to specific process difficulties.

Specific examples of this approach are provided by the occurrence of material entirely foreign to the process within the package of a device or in the device itself. The occurrence of human hair or fibers from street clothing (e.g., wool) implicates gowning practices. The presence of insect parts or plant material suggests that air classification between clean and less clean production areas have not been maintained, or that particulate matter from areas outside the plant has not been denied access. The presence of animal hair may point to inappropriate laundering of smocks or protective garments. Fragments of packaging material may indicate inadequate housekeeping at critical process points. These materials all provide indications of potential process difficulties that may be the basis of inspectional observations.

There have been a number of indications that the perception of agency management in regard to particulate matter also bears key similarities to that of device manufacturers. The agency doubtless realizes that there is no "magic number" with regard to levels of particles in or on devices or within packaging. The occurrence of particulate matter must be judged on a case-by-case basis with:

- Use of the device;
- Location of particles;
- Nature of process;
- Amount of particulate matter;
- Type of particulate matter; and
- GMP implications.

All of the above need to be considered. There is also a realization that the importance of particulate matter differs dramatically dependent upon the use of a device (i.e., an implantable device, blood contact device, or a device that enters a sterile field is likely to be judged far more critically than a simple disposable solution administration set). The agency policy in this regard is sufficiently flexible so that enforcement action may be taken at a low level of particulate matter for one type of device, while another type of device with a higher level of inherent particulates (such as an autologous transfusion device) may be deemed acceptable with significantly higher levels of particles.

Some recent inspection results reflect a high level of scrutiny of visible particulate matter, with the emphasis placed on the presence of particles in packaging and an external surface of device equal to or greater than that placed on particles in the devices themselves. Not only are devices such as administration sets being closely scrutinized, but also devices such as heat exchangers, cooling jackets for surgical laser systems, procedure trays, nebulizers, and the like. The basic rationale involved in this enhanced concern over visible particles seems to be the investigators' perception that the presence of visible particles in device packaging is reflective of undesirably high levels of process-related particles, that in turn indicates non–GMP manufacturing conditions.

Two decades ago there was an active interest in the effects of high numbers of monotypic particles (e.g., starch, talc) in surgical wounds in the causation of granulomas (see the review by Ellis

1990). The sources of these materials have largely been controlled or eliminated through the use of low-powder or powder-free gloves; the majority of the particulate matter to which a surgical patient is exposed consists of material inherent in the procedure performed.

Independent of device-related particles, there are numerous opportunities for particles to enter the operative field and, therefore, the incision. Some number of these undoubtedly enter the patient's circulation. Although many of these particles are large, they do not cause complications (Adwers 1992); and yet they represent major "doses" of large particulate matter or foreign bodies that are enclosed in the surgical wound. To name just a few:

- The patient's own body hair. Whether or not the surgeon believes in shaving the skin prior to the operation, shaved or shed body hair is commonly observed in the operative field during abdominal surgery. It seems to have no appreciable effect on wound healing or the incidence of post-op wound infections.

- Fibers from sterile drapes, gowns, hats, and masks (disposable cloth). Particles in this category are commonly observed, especially with any friction contact between two or more pieces.

- Particles and fibers from gauze sponges, lap packs, and dressings.

- "Char" from laser or electro-cautery coagulation and cutting devices. This is so common that a sandpaper pad is provided for the surgeon to clean the carbonized material off the cautery tip during the operation.

- Absorbable hemostatic materials and debris from oxidized cellulose and collagen-based products used to aid in control of bleeding from cut or abraded tissues.

- Particles shed from plastic devices. This type of particle is due to frictional contact between plastic and metal tools or sheaths.

- Sutures (absorbable or permanent).

- Surgical staples and clips.

- Bone chips. This type occurs in large numbers during orthopedic procedures.

- Fragments of gallstones and or renal stones.

Certainly this list is not all-inclusive, or meant to imply that the presence of a significant amount of foreign matter cannot potentially complicate the wound-healing process. However, in general surgery, particulate matter is commonly seen in the operative field and is simply of no consequence. It is treated by the body as foreign material despite how it arrived there. Most of this material, if not actively absorbed by the reticuloendothelial system, is encapsulated in a fibrous envelope and thus effectively partitioned from the body economy.

Considering these observations, it is difficult to believe that small numbers of sterile particles, that may on rare occasions be found in or on a device intended for surgical use, would cause any problems. This seems all the more obvious when one compares the small numbers of particulates from this source to the previously described list of much larger foreign materials that are not associated with patient injury.

Attendant to perceived problems with visible particulate matter, investigators have been demonstrating a new level of initiative in inspecting device manufacturing facilities. Conditions of manufacture, judged acceptable on previous inspections, have during later inspections been judged unacceptable. Investigators have, on numerous occasions, used magnifying glasses in inspections. There has been some suggestion by investigators that the presence of any visible particles (either within a device or its package) constitutes grounds for rejection of the product; that is, an unwritten requirement for zero visible particles is being enforced. The terms *adulterated* or *contaminated* have been applied to product bearing visible particles. The term filth has also been used to indicate presence of visible particles. This author is confused by the use of the term filth in reference to process inherent particulate matter related to medical devices produced under CGMP. In general, filth connotes foul or dirty matter, refuse, a dirty or corrupt condition, or putrid matter. *Webster's New Collegiate Dictionary* defines *filth* as "foul or putrid matter" with *putrid* being defined as "rotten." The definition of *particulate matter,* however, is "of or relating to minute separate particles," with *particle* defined as "a minute quantity or fragment; a relatively small, or the smallest discrete portion or amount of something." Thus, the use of the word filth as a generalized descriptive term for particulate matter is a misuse of the term. In a 1943 case of the United States versus Swift and Company, the courts found that "Congress intended that the word *filthy* as used in the Act should be construed to have its usual and ordinary meaning and should not be confined to any scientific or medical definition."

FDA personnel have referenced 21 CFR Section 351(a)(1) to support the use of the word *filth* to characterize particulate matter. Section 3512, which references "filthy, putrid, or decomposed substance(s)" relates to unsanitary conditions, and is generally understood to mean substances that are biological or chemical in nature; it is unlikely that Congress intended that substances, such as fragments of device components, or packaging materials should be termed *filth*. Thus, it is difficult to understand why the FDA would associate visible particulates found in and on the disposable medical devices with filth. Most particulate matter found in and on the surface of medical devices is matter derived from the product or from a production process. To define clean particles of plastic, paper, Tyvek®, or other packaging materials as *foul and dirty matter, refuse, or putrid matter* would seem to be far outside the bounds of the definition.

Whether or not the Safe Medical Devices Act of 1990 provides grounds for the increased severity of device-related regulatory inspections is open to speculation. There is no doubt, however, that there are some technical problems relating to the approach being used by the agency. The detection of visible particles in devices and their packaging materials is subject to an even higher number of critical variables than is the case with injectable products. It is, in every sense of the word, impossible to create a uniform requirement for visual inspection of devices due to the wide variation in physical construction, size, and application. It is quite conceivable that a complex device with a high solution path particle burden might easily pass a visual inspection due to the opacity of its components, while a simple device that could be more critically inspected because of its transparency would be deemed "unsuitable" based on the detection of a single visible particle. Any official requirement, expressed or implied, for the total absence of visible particles would be impossible to uniformly enforce. Such a requirement would be more unrealistic for devices than for injectables, where the circumstances of inspection are much more straightforward. While the application of GMP in device manufacture results in extremely low levels of visible particles, the manufacture of devices with no visible particles is beyond the scope of GMP and beyond the capabilities of contemporary manufacturing processes. Thus, the strict enforcement of such a requirement would result in the disruption of the flow of device products into the marketplace.

The issue of particles in packaging materials, such as blister packs or pliable film coatings, represents a severe problem for industry. The presence of a single visible particle exterior to the solution path of a device represents no risk to a patient. The difficulty of total elimination of particles from packaging materials is so great as to represent an impossibility for any production method that will be economically practical. Thus, the cost versus benefits issue is raised once again. Importantly, the applications of GMP to packaging of devices is far less specific than with the actual manufacture of devices themselves. A high level of technical refinement is often used in the creation of a package that is a durable sterile barrier for a device, and applied by automated machinery. Total particle elimination from high speed packaging operations represents an extremely difficult task. High speed packaging machinery is extremely cost-effective, but is almost impossible to protect against static electricity and the consequent attraction and adherence of small numbers of visibly-sized particles. Particle control in this regard is critically dependent on the control of point-generated particles in cutting, drawing, and sealing operations, and in the control of static electricity through humidity, ionized air, and other measures.

The present philosophy of the FDA with regard to particulate matter in devices may be summarized as follows. In general, the agency does not believe that an imminent hazard health exists with respect to particulates, and does not have information or complaints that would suggest an industry-wide problem. Nonetheless, the issue of particulates in now of a higher priority than in the past and will be approached more systematically. The FDA intends to increase its level of understanding and sophistication regarding particulates as part of an overall effort to minimize the level of "filth" in medical devices. Compliance activities will be handled on a case-by-case basis, depending on whether the FDA believes that a company has established and adhered to effective procedures and processes to control particulate matter contamination. The FDA has clearly stated that the emphasis would be on the process rather than on final product. The FDA will not be specifying numerical limits or *action levels*. However, the agency will have some *threshold* in mind that will relate to the industry's capability to control particulate matter levels. If the FDA believes that industry capability has improved, the threshold levels may consequently be decreased.

A summary observation regarding device regulatory issues related to particulate matter is that given the current regulatory climate, any manufacturer of medical devices should have a monitoring plan for visible particulate matter in place. This plan should include sampling methods, test methods, and accept-reject criteria based on appropriate attribute testing standards (e.g., Mil Std 105-E). The concept of CGMP is extremely important and is a matter that manufacturers' organizations must take seriously. An investigator who sees a high level of monitoring of critical and environmental control at Plant A on Monday will be favorably impressed; this favorable impression will rapidly give way to dissatisfaction during a visit to Plant B on Tuesday, if the second manufacturer does not have similar controls in place. Thus, consistency between processes and inspection measures and industry standards regarding particulate matter control will be critical with regard to the outcome of inspections.

Device-Related 483s

Indeed, in the absence of USP requirements for particulate matter in devices, FDA auditors have found ample grounds for enforcement activities based simply on whether or not device production adheres to GMP. Some issues that have arisen are the following:

- Failure to monitor particulate matter levels of finished product;
- Failure to establish alert and action limits for particle counts resulting from monitoring;
- Failure to maintain environmental controls on particulate matter;*
- Absence of a documented system for dealing with customer complaints;
- Inadequate housekeeping procedures;
- Failure to monitor and trend airborne particulates;
- Presence of cardboard in production areas;
- Lack of directional air movement;
- Lack of specific dress codes and hygiene procedures; and
- Failure to implement GMP procedures for both supervisory and workforce GMP training. (This training should cover the GMP regulations themselves, product knowledge, and quality awareness issues.)

---

* Section 820.46, Environmental Control, of the GMP regulation, is considered by the FDA to be a "discretionary" requirement; that is, the degree of environmental control to be maintained must be consistent with the intended use of the device and details of how to achieve this control is left to the manufacturer to decide." ("Discretionary GMP requirements" are those that may or may not apply to the manufacturer of a specific device.)

Device Specific Particulate Matter Issues

In any consideration of the exposure of patients to particles originating in medical devices, it is necessary to discriminate carefully between types of devices being considered. Complex devices with an extensive solution or blood path contact surface have the potential for generation of larger numbers of particles than administration sets or disposable syringes (Bain and Abethell 1988). Indeed, the majority of reports dealing with generation of particles by devices pertain to complex single-use devices such as oxygenators (Allardyce et al. 1966; Ashmore 1968; Page et al. 1970) and extracorporeal circuits (Clark et al. 1976; Hoenich et al. 1990; Knopp et al. 1982; Pastoriza-Pinol et al. 1979). Pumped sets have on occasion been implicated in generating particles due to mechanical damage (spallation) of the set's inner surface by the pump (Barron et al. 1986; Boretos 1971; Leong et al. 1982).

In the case of the complex types of devices listed above, it is likely that any particle problems might be alleviated by careful device design and material selection. It would seem that the inclusion of appropriate filters between the patient and the device is essential (Loop 1976; Dimmick et al. 1976), based on the nature of the procedures in which oxygenators and extracorporeal circuits are used; particularly the tendency of blood exposed to polymeric surfaces to generate thrombus (microemboli). Such filters have proven effective both in autotransfusion and in transfusion procedures (Goldiner et al. 1972).

Chronic use devices, such as dialyzers, also have been scrutinized for particle shedding characteristics and particulate matter issues (Caiazza 1988; Hoenich et al. 1990; HPB Alert #58, 1983), due to the long-term exposure of the patients involved. Here the simple expedient of flushing the device before use per the manufacturer's instruction eliminates concerns (Inagaki 1987). It is interesting to note that despite the widespread use of hemodialysis therapy, documented instances of adverse effects on patients from particles are lacking. Syringes, another widely used disposable device, have been evaluated with regard to both the shedding of particles and microdroplets of silicone oil (Chatelau and Berger 1985; Illum 1980). Here again, even in cases of long-term use (e.g., insulin administration), evidence of harmful effects on patients is lacking. The mode of application of a device and the use procedure appears in some instances to be a more critical issue than the particle burden of the device (Illum et al. 1978a, 1978b).

Consideration Regarding Particulate Matter Requirements

During the past decade, there have been a number of discussions between industry and the various regulatory authorities regarding whether or not particulate matter requirements for devices are necessary or desirable. In general, a comparison of the particulate matter levels in medical devices to the particulate matter levels acceptable (per the USP monograph) for LVI or SVI indicates that devices do not significantly contribute to the particulate matter levels to which the patient is exposed. Additionally, it would seem that products produced under controlled conditions meet customer expectations, as evidenced by the total absence of customer complaints regarding subvisual particulates and the very low number of complaints received related to large (visible) particles. This low number of complaints is impressive based on the fact that millions of devices are used annually.

Difficulties associated with the development of particulate matter measurement required for devices include: differences in: (1) the physical properties of devices, (2) use procedures, and (3) the potential hazards involved. This further complicates establishment of a standard, and it becomes evident that a single standard or requirement for devices could not possibly address the wide range of product types available. A Dacron® vascular graft, and a winged catheter needle would not be expected to exhibit similar particulate matter levels—especially since the Dacron® vascular graft has some potential to release particles throughout its life span. Other medical devices (syringes and blood oxygenators) have materials (such as silicone or surfactants) purposely applied to aid in the product's function (Ernerot 1965). Eliminating these additives to control particulate matter could adversely effect the function of the product. Failure to allow for particles generated as a result of the additives within an allowable limits range would result in an unwarranted rejection of the product.

The main points that underscore the general lack of need for requirements are:

- The absence of any clinical evidence indicating that particulate matter requirements on medical devices would benefit patients;
- The impracticality of requirements for devices due to the many different types of devices and the lack of any uniformly applicable test method;

- The fact that only GMP will control device particulate matter burden (requirements may represent cost without benefits); and
- Present availability of GMP plans for device manufacture (e.g., the 1981 DHSS guide) that have proven capable of controlling device particulate matter burden.

An evaluation of the cost-benefits ratio should also be made to ascertain if the costs expended to comply with a standard are equal to the expected benefit. In a worst-case scenario, small companies might be unable to continue operating due to inordinate cost increases. Increased manufacturing costs as a result of implementation of an additional standard of unsubstantiated benefit would inevitably result in increased cost to the consumer. This would appear to be particularly undesirable at this time, when the medical community around the world is attempting to control costs. Process controls and effective implementation of current applicable GMPs continue to be the medical device industry's methods of choice for control and reduction of particulate matter levels.

The basis for an eminently reasonable solution to the issue of particles in devices for both the manufacturer and the regulatory agency may be found in the enforcement of the GMP requirements currently in place. While low numbers of visible particles in devices or within packages may be expected for devices manufactured under GMP conditions, the occurrence of large numbers invariably indicate that some defect in application of GMP exists. Thus, enforcement (and control) of the particulate matter must be based on scrutiny of the process, rather than attempting to quantitate defects by inspection.

Importantly, particle limits for devices also cannot be based on an arbitrary relationship to present USP particle limits for injectable products, but must be based on a rational technical approach involving method validation and testing. Any particle standards developed must be practical and achievable by the manufacturers. Suitable device particle standards cannot be developed without an approach that incorporates the following elements:

- Sorting medical devices into appropriate categories. One particle limit is not suitable for the large variety of intravenous medical devices.
- Developing and validating the test methodology for each device category.
- Performing round-robin product surveys for each category.

This sound scientific approach is neither quick or easy; nor is it arbitrary. It would result in information on which particle standards could be based. But first, it should be demonstrated that an actual clinical need exists, before determining that a standard needs to be developed. If a need is identified for a specific product, controls should logically be established for that product. Any proposals for limits must be tempered with the knowledge that there is no significant evidence regarding any clinical effect of particles from devices.

A sample approach does exist for the control of the particle burden received by the patient. Today a wide range of filters are available that prime easily, bind very little drug product, and maintain acceptable flow rates throughout use. As discussed earlier, application of these filters in the small number of cases where their use is indicated will provide a means of totally eliminating any patient issues. Filtration is a far better alternative approach to particle control than particle standards with regard to intravenous therapy. In-line filtration can reduce the amount of particles received by a patient to a level lower than that contributed by the cleanest component. This requirement alternative is more cost effective and results in substantially less patient particle exposure than particle standards for intravenous medical devices and injections. It has the added advantage of reducing the contamination introduced by the practitioner during the use of the device. It is true that a filter will increase the cost of each administration slightly. However, the larger marketplace demand would likely cause higher volume manufacture, resulting in less expensive filters.

Safe Medical Devices Act of 1990

The Safe Medical Devices Act of 1990 (PL 101-629) became law on November 28, 1990. This legislation culminated years of efforts by Congressman Henry Waxman (D–CA), chairman of the Subcommittee on Health and the Environment of the Committee on Energy and Commerce of the U.S. House of Representatives. Congressman Waxman and Congressman John Dingell (D–MI), chairman of the Energy and Commerce Committee, had worked for three years toward what they considered improvements in FDA's regulation of medical devices. As was expected, this revision of the Medical Device Amendments of 1976 increased the regulatory pressures on one of a diminishing group of industries that are still competitive in the international marketplace. Although the new law has some beneficial aspects, there are some provisions of the law that, in the words of Secretary of Health and Human Services, Louis Sullivan, "appear to impose heavy burdens on FDA and industry without matching improvements to public health" (i.e., cost without any foreseeable benefit).

It is not possible to predict what effect the new law will have with regard to the occurrence of particulate matter in devices, and the generation of requirements. Although the user problems that stimulated the Act arose chiefly from functional issues related to a small number of devices, particulate matter in devices will probably receive closer scrutiny as a result of its passage. Undoubtedly, some number of user reports will involve occurrence of particulate matter in devices even though the particulate matter is not concerned with serious injury or illness. There is no definition provided of what constitutes a "reasonable probability" or a "serious adverse health consequence." The latter could conceivably be extended to include the occurrence of particulate matter. Special FDA controls could presumably include the implementation of particulate matter monitoring procedures in the manufacturing of devices, or possibly the implementation of limits without USP involvement; post-market surveillance of reportable items might conceivably involve occurrence of observation for particulate matter.

The law also requires device users to report incidents involving death, serious injury, or serious illness related to devices. Serious illness and serious injury are defined as: (1) being life threatening; (2) resulting in permanent impairment of a body function or permanent damage to a body structure; or (3) necessitating immediate medical or surgical intervention to prevent permanent impairment of a body function or damage to a body structure. In order to provide the FDA flexibility in dealing with devices, the new law allows application of controls other than performance standards. Special controls may include post-market surveillance; patient registry; and development and dissemination of guidelines, recommendations, and other actions the FDA deems necessary to provide such assurance.

In the past the FDA has not had a mandatory recall authority. They have relied upon threats of seizure, injunction, or criminal prosecution to cause companies to recall a product. While the FDA has published recall guidelines in 21 CFR, Part 7, these are voluntary. The recall authority provided by the 1990 legislation is one of the most significant provisions in the new law. This section actually allows the regulatory agency to order immediate cessation of distribution of a device and recall with no due process. This order is allowed where there is deemed to be a "reasonable probability" of serious adverse health consequences. No definition of what constitutes a "reasonable probability" or a "serious adverse health consequence" is provided.

Another provision that would necessitate significant effort is the establishment of a system to track patients with implants or other devices whose failure would be likely to have serious adverse health consequences. While on the surface this requirement seems rational, and indeed may be highly desirable for some products, it could be subject to misuse through over-application in the current overzealous enforcement environment. The agency may now require a manufacturer to conduct post-market surveillance of any device introduced or delivered into interstate commerce after January 1, 1991. The post-market surveillance provision is limited to the following devices: (1) permanent implants, the failure of which may cause serious adverse health consequences or death; (2) those intended for use in supporting or sustaining human life; (3) or those that potentially present a serious risk to human health. Post-market surveillance is intended to provide an "early warning system" that allows for the early identification of potential problems with medical devices within a reasonable time of their first marketing.

The next several years will be critical as FDA develops policies and regulations to implement the new law. Hopefully, with cooperation between the agency and industry, conscientious compliance by industry will evolve, and the health care end-user will be benefitted by the new law (without restriction of the industry whose overzealous regulation would only serve to disadvantage the patient). If the new law is to be prevented from becoming a serious detriment to the medical device industry, the FDA must be prepared to handle additional responsibilities demanded of them without delays in product approvals or overly stringent enforcement practices. These potential negatives are highly undesirable, but are a possible outcome given the agency's shortage of resources.

Summary

Particles in parenteral-type medical devices originate from a wide variety of sources; critical components of their control include:

- Process design;
- Material selection;
- Component vendor certification;
- Process monitoring; and
- Adherence to GMP.

The particle burden of parenteral-type device sets is low in comparison to the potential particle contribution from other I.V. therapy components (such as small volume injections). The only reasonable control of particles in devices is effected by GMP and process monitoring-not additional regulatory requirements. Requirements should be developed only in cases where a need can be clearly established based on clinical evidence.

Since GMP (rather than level of testing or limits) determines the particle burden of devices, the only effective control of particulate matter in devices will result from conscientious implementation of GMP by all device manufacturers. For manufacturers that presently have well-defined GMP programs of proven effectiveness, it seems likely that compendial limits (and additional testing) will only result in higher production costs that will reflect no benefits in the form of reduced particulate matter burden.

References

Adwers, J. R. 1992. Personal communication.

Allardyce, D. B., S. H. Yoshida, and P. G. Ashmore. 1966. The importance of microembolism in the pathogenesis of organ dysfunction caused by prolonged use of pump oxygenator. *J. Thorac. Cardiovasc. Surg.* 52:706–715.

American national standard for autologous transfusion devices. ATG-1991. 1991. Arlington, VA: Association for the Advancement of Medical Instrumentation.

American national standard for blood transfusion microfilters. BF7-1989. 1989. Arlington, VA: Association for the Advancement of Medical Instrumentation.

Ashmore, P. G., V. Svitek, and P. Ambrose. 1968. The incidence and effects of particulate aggregation and microembolism in pump oxygenator systems. *J. Thorac. Cardiovasc. Surg.* 55:691–697.

Bain, R., and J. A. Abethell. 1988. Particle contribution from infusion devices. *Brit. J. Pharm. Pract.* 10:40–42, 46, 48.

Barnett, M. I., N. A. Armstrong, D. C. James, and B. K. Evans. 1983. Particle contamination from administration sets. *Brit. J. Parent. Ther.* 4 (16):8–17.

Barron, D., S. Harbottle, N. A. Hoenich, A. R. Morley, D. Appleton, and J. F. McCabe 1986. Particle spallation induced by pumps in hemodialysis tubing sets. *Artif. Organs* 10 (3):226–235.

Boretos, J. W., and F. R. Wagner. 1971. Particle fragmentation generated in pump sets. *J. Biomed. Mat. Res.* 5:411–412.

B. S. 2463 (Draft), Transfusion equipment for medical use, Part 2, Specification for giving sets. 1986. London: British Standards Institution, page 20.

Caiazza, S., A. Giangrande, P. Cantu, A. Castiglioni, L. Paoletti, and G. Donelli. 1988. Particle migration from haemodialysis circuits: Electron microscopy and microprobe analysis. *Biomater. Artif. Cells Artif. Organs* 16 (4):721–729.

Chatelau, E. A., and M. Berger. 1985. Pollution of insulin with silicone oil: A hazard of disposable syringes. *Lancet* 1:1459.

Clark, R. E., D. R. Deitz, and J. G. Miller. 1976. Continuous detection of microemboli during cardiopulmonary bypass in animals and man. *Circulation* 54: III74–III78, 78–83.

Dialyzer blood lines containing loose particulates. 1983. *Medical Devices Alert No. 58* (April 19). Canada: Health Protection Branch.

Dimmick, J. E., K. E. Bove, J. McAdams, and G. Benzing. 1976. Fiber embolization, a hazard of cardiac surgery and catheterization. *New Engl. J. Med.* 292:685–687.

Di Paolo, E. R., B. Hirsch, and A. Pannatier. 1990. Quantitative determination of particulate contamination in intravenous administration sets. *Pharm. Weekbl.* 12 (5):190–195.

Ellis, H. 1990. Hazards of surgical glove dusting powders. *Surgery, Gynecology and Obstetrics* 171:521–527.

Ernerot, L., and E. Sandall. 1965. The shedding of particles from syringes. *Act. Pharm. Sueccica.* 2:411–420.

Falchuk, K. H., L. Peterson, and B. J. McNeil. 1985. Microparticulate-induced phlebitis: Its Prevention by in-line filtration. *N. Engl. J. Med.* 312 (2):78–82.

Goldiner, P. L., W. S. Howland, and C. Ray. 1972. Filter for prevention of microembolism during massive transfusions. *Curr. Research, Anesthesia and Analgesia* 51 (5):717–725.

Gour, L. 1987. Particulate matter in parenteral type medical devices. *Pharmacopeial Forum* (May/June): 2506–2522.

Guide to good manufacturing practices for sterile medical devices and surgical products. 1981. London: Department of Health and Social Security, Her Majesty's Stationery Office, page 72.

HIMA/PMA task force final report on particulate in intravenous equipment. 1980. Washington, D.C.: Health Industry Manufacturers Association, page 82.

Hoenich, N. A., J. Thompson, J. McCade, and D. Appleton. 1990. Particle release from haemodialysers. *Int. J. Artif. Organs* 13 (12):803–808.

Hoenich, N. A., J. Thompson, E. Varini, J. McCade, and D. Appleton. 1990. Particle spallation and plasticizer (DEHP) release from extracorporeal circuit tubing materials. *Int. J. Artif. Organs* 13 (1):55–62.

Human and veterinary drugs: Current good manufacturing, packaging or holding (Code of Federal Regulations 21). 1978. *Federal Register* 43FR190:45014–45089.

Illum, L. 1980. Characterization of particulate contamination released by application of parenteral solutions. III. Particulate matter from syringes. *Arch. Pharm. Chem. Sci. Ed.* 8:109–119.

Illum, L., V. G. Jensen, and N. Moller. 1978a. Characterization of particulate contamination released by application of parenteral solutions. I. Particulate matter from administration sets. *Arch. Pharm. Chem. Sci. Ed.* 6:93–108.

Illum, L., V. G. Jensen, and N. Moller. 1978b. Characterization of particulate contamination released by application of parenteral solutions. II. Particulate matter from cannulea. *Arch. Pharm. Chem. Sci. Ed.* 6:169–178.

Inagaki, H., T. Hamazaki, H. Kuroda, and S. Yano. 1987. Foreign particles contaminating dialysers and methods of removing them by rinsing. *Nephron.* 46 (4):343–346.

Intravenous therapy guideline. 1985. Ottawa, Ontario: Health Services Directorate, Health Service and Promotion Branch, page 74.

Knopp, E. A., F. G. Baumann, D. Pratt, R. Faden, F. P. Catinella, I. M. Nathan, P.X. Adams, J. N., Cunningham, Jr., and F. C. Spencer. 1982. Release of particulate matter from extracorporeal tubing: Ineffectiveness of standard arterial line filters during bypass. *J. Cardiovas. Surg.* 23 (6):470–476.

Leong, As-Y., A. P. S. Disney, and D. W. Gove. 1982. Spallation and migration of silicone from blood-pump tubing in patients on hemodialysis. *N. Engl. J. Med.* 306:135–140.

Loop, F. D., J. Szabo, R. D. Robinson, and K. Urbanek. 1976. Events related to microembolism during extracorporeal perfusion in man: Effectiveness of in-line filtration recorded by ultrasound. *Ann. Thorac. Surg.* 21:412–420.

Page, U. S., J. C. Bigelow, C. R. Carter, and R. L. Swank. 1970. Emboli (debris) produced by bubble oxygenators: Removal by filtration. *Ann. Thorac. Surg.* 9:18–22.

Pastoriza-Pinol, J. V., J. MacMillan, and B. F. Smith. 1979. Analysis of microembolic particles originating in the extracorporeal circuit before bypass. *J. Extracorp. Technol.* 11:221–228.

Safe Medical Devices Act of 1990. 1990. Washington, D.C.: U.S. Printing Office.

Transfusion equipment for medical use. 1985. *International Standard ISD/DIS/1135.* Paris: International Organization for Standardization, p. 176.

Visible solids in disposable syringes. 1983. *Medical Devices Alert No. 55* (March 17). Canada: Health Protection Branch.

XII

Patient Issues Related to Particulate Matter

This subject frequently arises when particulate matter in injectable products is discussed. There is no evidence to suggest that any risk to patients is presented by the extremely low levels of particles in the parenteral products currently marketed in the U.S. or other countries that conform to requirements of the major compendia and CGMP. Nonetheless, the consideration of patient risk remains a foremost concern to manufacturers of injectable products and medical devices as well as to compendial groups and regulatory agencies. While this subject is somewhat peripheral to the efforts of the particle analyst, it is of sufficient interest to merit brief discussion in this book.

In beginning this discussion, it is critical that we separate the consideration of physiological effects of particulate matter from other issues related to injectable products. The latter category includes sterility, adverse reactions related to specific drugs or individual patients, and miscellaneous product quality issues. It is also critical to an objective consideration of possible effects of particles on patients that we separate historical issues raised by early authors (e.g., Garvan and Gunner 1963, 1964) from the present situation. Similarly, the ill effects observed (when drug abusers have infused crushed tablet material, or when patients have been mistakenly infused with suspensions of insoluble drug material intended for intramuscular injection) do not equate to patient risk in an appropriately conducted course of intravenous therapy (Griffen et al. 1951; Johnston and Waisman 1965; Burton et al. 1965; Butz 1969).

The available data that assists us in drawing conclusions regarding effects of particulate matter on patients is found in four areas: (1) transport of particles in the circulatory system; (2) the few reported instances of human harm resulting from infusion or injection of particles; (3) animal experiments; and (4) human studies involving two unrelated subjects, that is, liposomal dosages and the incidence of infusion thrombophlebitis. In this chapter, I have briefly considered physiological factors related to particulate matter and the findings of studies in each of these categories.

Circulatory Transport

The manner in which the human body deals with foreign particles is a key consideration in this discussion of particle effects on patients. The mammalian blood circulation system consists of two interconnected circulatory systems, one (arterial) at a higher pressure than the other (venous). The heart pumps blood through both simultaneously. A particle introduced into a peripheral vein in the arm will travel along the venous system toward the right side of the heart. Since veins increase in size as they approach the heart, it is unlikely that any particle would lodge in a vein prior to the pulmonary circulation at this point. After passing through the heart the particle enters into the pulmonary artery, and then the extensive capillary bed of the lung. Particles passing through the capillaries of the lung would be expected to enter the pulmonary venous circulation, return to the heart, then be distributed to other organs of the body. Depending upon the size of an insoluble particle, it will eventually lodge in a capillary at some tissue site, or be ingested by circulating phagocytic cells or by tissue phagocytes such as the Kupfer cells of the liver or alveolar microphages.

Arteries constantly branch and divide as they supply oxygenated blood to the tissues and organs. The smallest arterial blood vessels are found in the capillary beds, in which the diameter of the vessels approximates the diameter of the red blood cells. The capillary walls are distensible and the flexible erythrocytes can distort to pass through constrictions significantly smaller than their normal discoid diameter of 7 μm. In theory, occlusion of a capillary by some foreign particle larger than about 10 μm in diameter might conceivably cause the vessel downstream of the blockage to collapse, and a particle larger than about 50 μm could potentially cause multiple capillaries to close down. This blockage of capillaries could result in denial of oxygenated blood to a tissue or part of a tissue. However, it must be noted that the damage resulting from vessel occlusion will depend to a large degree on the amount of collateral circulation that is available to that tissue. Blocked single capillaries are unlikely to cause any biological effect, since there are nearly always available alternative circulatory pathways feeding the same tissue site. It is interesting to note in this regard, that radiopaque particles of 1500 μm and larger in size are routinely applied in preoperative embolization of arteriovenous vascular malformations of the brain without ill effects for the patient (Russell and Levy 1987).

Animal studies summarized in a following section of this chapter suggest that the lung constitutes an increasingly effective barrier to particulate matter, as particles of larger size than 10 μm are considered. Thus, inert particles with diameters larger than 10 μm and many smaller particles may be entrapped in the capillary beds of the lung, and to a lesser extent in the spleen and liver. In the lung, there is an active mechanism for passing the trapped particles through the capillary walls so that they are excreted into the sputum and mucus and continuously swept upwards and out of the lung. Further, the alveolar macrophages are highly active phagocytes, and particles would be expected to be removed by these cells, that can actively pass from the pulmonary circulation into the air space. The lung also has an extensive collateral circulation, and an unrealistically high particulate matter load would be required to close down a sufficient area of the lung to cause any physiological damage. Infusion of a single unit of stored blood results in the deposition of particulate material in the lung that is far in excess of the particle burden resulting from multiple courses of intravenous therapy; even so, adverse effects due to single units of blood or a small number of units have not been reported.

In light of this consideration, it would seem that particles of 50 μm and larger (particularly if administered in large numbers) could reasonably be expected to lodge in alveolar capillaries, with a consequent decrease in pulmonary function. This would occur with large capillaries being blocked and the function of multiple capillaries being restricted by single, large particles. This situation would not be expected to result with administration of a parenteral solution containing small numbers of particles at much smaller sizes. The effects of sub 10-µm particles passing through the lungs and lodging in capillary beds in other organs, or being phagocytosed by tissue phagocytes are not clear.

Human Injury by Particles

Concerns for safety of patients receiving IV therapy were first addressed in the works of Garvan and Gunner (1963, 1964). Since these initial reports, numerous papers have been published on this topic and a significant number of review articles (Backhouse and McCollum 1986; Davis and Turco 1971; Gross and Carter 1966; Gross 1967; McCollum 1985; Turco and Davis 1973; Doris et al. 1977; Garvan and Gunner 1971; and Brewer 1966), have been written concerning the clinical significance of particulate matter. Although there has been a great deal of controversy about this subject, it must be concluded that injection of very high numbers of foreign particles into the venous circulation is harmful. The primary evidence for this can be found in the literature on drug abuse. Injections of crushed tablets, capsules, and other solid dosage products have often resulted in serious consequences (Butz 1969; Burton et al. 1965; Johnston and Waisman 1965). For example, one drug user died after an intravenous injection of Darvon® capsules (Hopkins 1972), presenting evidence of severe pulmonary dysfunction. In another report, Douglas (1971) and co-workers found that three of seven addicts who injected drugs had abnormal roentgenographic indicators, pathologic foreign body emboli, and granulomas; the remaining had abnormal pulmonary function. Emboli have also been observed in the eyes of drug abusers (Atlee 1972).

There is some evidence to associate cellulosic particles (fibers) with physiological response (Adams et al. 1965). Here again, the only danger would seem to be with extremely high levels of fibers. Fibers are effectively nonexistent as contaminants in currently produced injectables. During the routine histological examination of human necropsies, VanGlahn and Hall (1949) found cellulosic particles associated with six cases of cardiac embolism over a 20-year period, with the only common factor being intravenous therapy over the 10 days prior to death. Experimentally, these authors demonstrated that foreign-body granulomatae were formed in animals after the injection of large numbers of cellulose fibers. This has been confirmed by other workers (Wartman 1951).

The classical investigations associated with cellulosic contamination were those of Garvan and Gunner (1963, 1964), who concluded that capillary granulomatae were unlikely to produce an immediate clinical effect in the patient. The major risk was considered by these investigators to be due to postoperative pulmonary infarctions. Critical evaluation of this study shows that the authors were concerned with grossly contaminated solutions (representative of another era of injectable product manufacture) and often did not provide details of the microscopic identification procedures used.

Animal Studies

The results of numerous animal experiments have also been reported. The references of Brewer (1966); Geisler et al. (1973); Hozumi et al. (1983); Kanke et al. (1973); and Schroeder et al. (1978a, 1978b) will provide the reader with review material. In these and other animal studies performed to date, massive doses of particulate matter have typically been injected into species including dogs, rabbits, rats, mice, and hamsters. Infused particles have included glass beads, cotton fibers, paper fibers, polystyrene latex spheres, paper fragments, and other insoluble substances. In addition to differences in the type and shape of the particulate matter, the particle sizes infused ranged from a few microns to several hundred microns. Although these studies suggest in general that excessive levels of particulate matter in intravenous solutions could potentially cause adverse effects, they do not relate in any way to the current clinical situation involving human patients and current injectable products. One of the earliest studies of this type, King et al. (1933), injected an overwhelming dose of 250 mL of a 0.8 mg/mL suspension (0.2 g) of powdered silica intravenously into a dog, which died 6 hours later. This bizarre experiment gave rise to a variety of clinical complications including:

- Phlebotomy;
- Spleen enlargement;
- Hemorrhage in the kidney;
- General thrombi and agglutination of platelets;
- Pulmonary emboli producing death in some cases by mechanical obstruction of the flow of blood through the lungs; and
- Foreign body granulomatae.

Adverse effects from the injection of particles are not easily demonstrated. Brewer and Dunning (1947) performed work with rabbits involving a three-year period of administration of powdered glass. Their results indicated that microemboli, thrombi, and granulomas may be produced by this means. In some of the higher-dose groups, the liver and spleen showed some enlargement with respect to controls, but all organs appeared histologically normal. The lungs of some animals were found to contain as much as 2% wet weight of glass after a year's continuous administration of the powdered glass suspensions. These animals showed no ill effects. Subsequently, Gnadinger (1957) used rabbits in a similar study and he also found no evidence of foreign body reactions, granulomate formation, or pyrogen response.

Gross, in a paper published in 1967, reported results observed when twenty young adult and healthy beagle dogs were injected intravenously with small quantities of ground-up filter paper, of such size as would pass through an 18 gauge needle (75 microns or less in diameter), and similar preparations of an unspecified plastic material used to coat rubber stoppers in commercially available bottles of intravenous injectables. The animals that received 2.5 mg or more of particulate matter of either type presented numerous pulmonary granulomas that were demonstrable as early as 5 days after a single injection of 10 mL of saline containing these impurities. It should be observed that these experiments also represent totally unrealistic conditions in regard to current patient exposure to particles. The quantity of paper fibers used was extremely high—2.5 mg of ground paper represents millions of paper filters. Further, the unidentified stopper coating material used likely represented a reactive substance, possibly a polyamide material. Importantly, objective assessment of these and earlier reports in which harmful effects were noted involved a rapid administration of the test particles, so that aggregation effects would logically be suspected to be involved. Indeed, the critical effect of rate of administration appears to have been almost uniformly overlooked as a critical parameter in the majority of animal experiments formed.

A study conducted by the Parenteral Manufacturers Association (Geisler 1973) involved the intravenous injection of inert polystyrene spheres into rats within a short period of time. Necropsies were then performed at various intervals from 1 hour to 28 days following injection. The results were summarized as follows:

- Thirteen of 18 rats injected with 8×10^6 particles per kg at a particle size of 40 μm died within five minutes.

- Rats showed normal blood studies, organ weights, and pathologic criteria after being injected with either

8×10^5 particles size 0.4 µm to 10 µm, or 4×105 particles per kg of particle size 40 µm.

- Particles in the 4 µm size range were found in the lung, liver, and spleen.
- Particles in the 10 µm size range were found primarily in the lung, although some particles were also found in five other organs.
- Particles in the 40 µm size range were found in the lungs and myocardial tissue.

This study, as was the case with previous research, involved the injection of large numbers of 40 µm particles into the animals that showed ill effects. Considering the overwhelming dose, far above that resulting in any course of human I.V. therapy, the ill effects were not remarkable.

Schroeder et al. (1978a, 1978b) intravenously administered polystyrene microspheres to dogs at different levels, and monitored a variety of clinical signs including arterial blood pressure, arterial blood pH, blood gases (O_2 and CO_2), leucocyte count, heart rate, and ECG. No significant changes were observed during the sphere administration and for three hours afterwards, and the only untoward effect noted was a slight increase in leucocyte count after an extremely high dose of 2.4×10^9 spheres. After four weeks the animals were sacrificed. No evidence of organ damage due to the particles could be demonstrated, indicating that the inert spheres of 3–25 µm infused had no effects physiologically. It is interesting to consider the lack of any observed effect of the relatively massive experimental doses of particles administered in short periods of time in this and other studies, in light of the low total numbers of particles contained in currently produced parenteral solutions. Whereas Schroeder et al. administered levels of 10^9 particles with no effect, the maximum number of particles received from a 1-L large volume intravenous solution conforming to USP requirements would be 50,000 greater than 10 µm. In prolonged administration of parenteral solutions that would reasonably be expected to result in a "worst-case" exposure of a patient to particulate matter, thousands of units would be required to approximate the level of exposure achieved in animal experiments.

Liposome Research

Investigations of the use of liposomes or microspheres as potential drug delivery systems have contributed to our knowledge of the fate of infused particles, and are reviewed in the book by Davis et al. (1984). Other publications that provide information of interest on this subject include those of Bommer and Bradfield (1984). They concluded that blood clearance of particles (in the range of 10 µm in size and less) is by phagocytosis, irrespective of the chemical nature of the particle-blood interface. Phagocytic macrophages of the reticuloendothelial system (RES) are located in the liver and spleen as well as the lung. Using ^{41}Ce-labeled polystyrene microspheres, Kanke et al. (1980) studied the fate of beads of 3, 8, 15, and 25 µm diameter particles infused intravenously into beagle dogs. These authors found a prolonged retention of particles larger than 8 µm in the lung, implying this to be a critical size regarding the passage of particles through the pulmonary vascular bed. Smaller particles were collected in the liver and spleen by phagocytosis. Particles larger than 12 µm were not extensively phagocitized, suggesting that there may be an upper size limit to the phagocytosis of inert particles.

Phagocytosis requires energy and oxygen was found to be consumed in proportion to the number of particles ingested by the cells and their size (Schroeder et al. 1978a). After examining effects produced by different sizes of spheres, the authors concluded that particles smaller than 0.25 µm produced no significant increase in leucocyte respiration. It was found that particles smaller than about 0.4 µm could not be detected in any of the tissues examined histologically. Interestingly, particles larger than 10 µm also produced no measurable effect on leukocyte respiration.

Particles smaller than 100 nm (0.1 µm) are capable of leaving the systemic circulation by passing through gaps or fenestrations between the endothelial cells in the walls of the blood vessels. These openings are of varying size, depending on the organ considered. The larger gaps are in the liver, spleen, and bone marrow. These openings allow the natural lipid emulsions (or chylomicra) to escape from the bloodstream into the liver hepatocytes. Capillary fenestrations are smaller in the pancreas, intestines, and kidneys; and particles of only 50–60 nm are allowed to pass through. Studies of clearance kinetics and the distribution of particles throughout the body have been carried out on polystyrene-divinylbenzene copolymer beads produced with a range of particle diameters. Schoenberg et al. (1961) injected doses of up to 1.6×10^{12} particles per kg body weight of beads with diameters from 0.5 µm to 1.17 µm. Clearance efficiency was unaffected by either the particle diameter or the dose; 90% of the particles being cleared within 90 minutes of administration, and the remainder taking up to 18 days to be cleared. It was suggested that this secondary slower clearance stage was due to the development of an equilibrium between the phagocytosis, and reentry into the circulation from the cells of the RES in the liver and spleen.

Infusion of Blood-Related Materials

In the past decade, there has been considerable interest in the effect of microaggregates and proteinaceous debris in stored blood or platelet concentrate on patients receiving large scale transfusions during surgery. A similar interest is associated with the autologous transfusion process associated most notably with open heart surgery (Bisio et al. 1982).

When whole blood is stored, protein materials (including fibrin) coagulate to form amorphous insoluble material and red cells, platelets, leukocytes, and fibrin strands form microaggregates ranging from 20 μm to 500 μm in size. Numbers of microaggregates and levels of acellular debris increase with duration of storage. Upon infusion of stored blood, these particulate materials are introduced into the vasculature of the patient receiving the transfusion. Connell and Swank (1973) observed significant levels of arterial-venous blood shunting in the lungs of recipients transfused with stored blood in excess of approximately 30% of their total blood volume. Evidence of capillary occlusion in the lungs of recipients of transfusions of unfiltered blood, which may contain thousands of 20 μm microaggregates per mL and hundreds of larger microaggregates, is not surprising. In the 1980s it became common practice to filter transfused stored blood through Dacron® wool depth filters, with an 80 μm or 40 μm retention rating. This procedure eliminated the adverse effects previously observed, although patients probably continue to receive numbers of microaggregates below the retention rating of the filters used. This infused particle burden is certainly several orders of magnitude greater than that resulting from an average course of intravenous therapy, by conservative estimate. Further, the infused microaggregates are biologically active due to the enzymes and other reactive chemicals released by the cells of microaggregates upon lysis.

The storage of platelet concentrate similarly results in the formation of microaggregate material (Galbasov et al. 1989). The infusion of unfiltered platelet concentrate may result in the formation of ultrastructural changes, similar to those observed in situations known to lead to pulmonary dysfunction, such as following massive transfusion, hypovolemia, sepsis and hypoxia. Application of

40 µm Dacron® filters has proven to be efficacious in elimination of adverse reactions in the lung from this source.

A further interesting demonstration of the human body's ability to deal with particulates is provided by the intraoperative autologous transfusion procedure applied in thoracic surgery and other operations. In this procedure, blood released into the surgical cavity by surgery is aspirated into a collection reservoir, filtered through a 20 µm to 80 µm filter, and returned to the patient's circulation. This blood most certainly carries with it significant numbers of particles in the ≥10 µm range, including those originating from the surgical sources described in the preceding chapter.

Phlebitis and Particles

Peripheral vein phlebitis or thrombophlebitis, a localized erythrematous reaction at the site of infusion (redness at site and along the vein, elevated skin temperature, tenderness) has been observed as a complication of I.V. therapy (Brown 1970; Collin et al. 1973). In 1971, Davis et al. carried out a study of intravenous fluids, and concluded that plastic containers gave rise to fewer particles in solution than those in glass. These authors observed that the addition of devices and drug additives increased the number of particles, and suggested that final (in-line) filtration before infusion appeared to be effective in reducing the incidence of peripheral vein phlebitis. This final observation was confirmed by Ryan et al. in 1973, and was shown to have clinical significance whereby the use of a 0.45 µm final filter reduced the incidence of phlebitis in patients receiving intravenous fluids over several days. Turco and Davis (1973) also demonstrated a decrease in particle burden of infusion fluids by using in-line 0.22 µm filters.

Over the past two decades, investigations related to the influence of final in-line filtration with 0.2 µm filters on the incidence of infusion phlebitis, suggest some relationship of infused particles and phlebitis. A number of the studies performed (e.g., Falchuk et al. 1985) have suggested that the number of particles in the intravenous medications were directly related to an earlier onset of phlebitis in patients receiving these drugs via the intravenous route. Other authors have questioned the economic viability of in-line filters, and asked whether the uncertain danger from particles justifies the increased cost. More recent research (Rypins et al. 1990; Maddox et al. 1983; and Gotz et al. 1985) into the causes of infusion phlebitis has lead to the conclusion that in-line filtration is definitely not broadly effective in reducing the incidence of the reaction. Knowledge that has evolved out of studies of phlebitis and particulate matter conspicuously includes the fact that phlebitis is a much more complex reaction than originally supposed. The definition of phlebitis, the nature of the drug infused, vascular access procedure, vein used for infusion, osmolarity of infused solution, type of catheter, patient sensitivity, and microbiological issues have all been determined to be critical factors that may singly or in combination outweigh the effect of particulate matter. The role of in-line filters in the adsorption of pyrogens that might be responsible to some extent for phlebitis has not been thoroughly investigated.

Conclusions Regarding Patient Risk

Based on the basic investigations conducted up to the present time, and in available literature, conclusions regarding the danger to patients from particles are the following:

- Even with the vastly increased use of LVPs in recent years, there is no documented evidence of patient harm resulting from the administration of intravenous therapy, on either a chronic or short-term basis.

- There is evidence, some of it conflicting and confusing, that particulate matter in parenterals may potentially give rise to clinical problems.

- There is strong evidence that the quality levels of parenterals have improved greatly within the past 25 years (the post–Garvan and Gunner era).

- The use of in-line filters appears to be justified only when certain medications and admixtures are being administered.

Summary

Reports of clinical ill-effects related to massive inadvertent administration of particles must be separated objectively from our consideration of issues that might arise due to the low numbers of small particles currently present in injectables, administration sets, or other medical products produced under CGMP. The results of studies, in which levels of particulate matter many orders of magnitude higher than those to which patients are exposed were administered to animals before any effects were noted, can hardly be regarded as convincing evidence of patient hazard. Jonas (1966) concluded that:

> Particulate matter in large volume parenteral solutions should be viewed as potentially hazardous to the patient. The degree of danger will depend upon the quantity, physical characteristics, and biological properties of the particles as well as by the chance location of the particle in the vascular system of the patient.

Based on the extremely low level of particles present in currently produced injectable products, it would seem that the "potential hazard" must be considered nonexistent. With these current low levels, the consideration of patient effect becomes simply one of exposure of the patient's vascular system to extremely low quantities of nonreactive material at a low rate of infusion. The quantities of inert particles present in domestically produced LVP product equates to approximately 1.2×10^{-8} g/mL or .012 mg/L of administered solution. For a 70 kg individual, this equates to a dosage level of 0.17 ppb on a body weight basis. This level of exposure is so far below the levels at which harmful particle-related effects have been observed with experimental animals, human drug abuse, or unintentional injection of suspended material, the two situations are totally unrelated with respect to ill effects on patients. Importantly, in a number of animal studies that have been cited indicating the harmful effects of particles, the effect rate of administration of test particles was unrealistic with regard to any course of intravenous solution administration. Not only the extremely high levels of particles administered might also be suspected of resulting in particle agglomeration.

The possibility that clinical ramifications would occur related to the use of parenterals containing levels of particles that are typical of current product appears beyond the realm of possibility. As Turco and Davis suggested in their review article (1973), the possible effects of low levels of particles on patients cannot be determined in the absence of controlled studies on humans. No studies have been, or are likely to be reported. Control human tissue samples are difficult to obtain because of disease, environmental pollutants, and the difficulty of determining how many intravenous solution units a subject has received. Thus, excluding the studies involving drug abusers, there is no evidence of harm to humans due to injected particulate matter.

Similarly, there would seem to be no issues associated with chronic administration of intravenous therapy. Given that only a few thousand particles 10 µm in size are likely to be infused per liter of intravenous solution, and the fact that doses of 10^9 particles of various types have resulted in no demonstrable effects in experimental animals of much smaller than human body mass, there appears to be little grounds for concern. The same principles of GMP that control particles at low levels in pharmaceutical products ensure that the particle burden of infused materials is not an issue to the patient.

References

Adams, D. F., B. D. Tord, and J. Kosek. 1965. Cotton fibre embolism during angiography. *Radiology* 84:678–683.

Atlee, W. E. 1972. Talc and cornstarch emboli in eyes of drug abusers. *J. Amer. Med. Assoc.* 219:49–51.

Backhouse, C. M., and C. McCollum. 1986. Particles in PT: cause for concern? *Brit. J. Par Ther.* 7 (12):136–143.

Bisio, J. M., R. S. Connell, and M. W. Harrison. 1983. The formation and effect of stored platelet concentrate microemboli on pulmonary ultrastructure. *Sur. Gyn. and Obstet.* 154:342–347.

Bommer, J. W. B., and J. Bradfield. 1984. The reticulo-endothelial system and blood clearance. In *Microspheres and drug therapy: Pharmaceutical, immunological and medical aspects*, 25–38. ed. S. S. Davis, L. llum, J. G. McVie, and E. Tomlinson. Amsterdam: Elsevier.

Brewer, J. H. 1966. Particulate matter: Toxicology. *Bulletin Parent. Drug Assoc.* 20:35–52.

Brewer, J. H., and J. H. F. Dunning. 1947. An in vitro and in vivo study of glass particles in ampoules. *J. Amer. Pharm. Assoc.* (Sci. Ed.) 36:289–293.

Brown, G. 1970. Infusion Thrombophlebitis. *Brit. Clin. Pract.* 24:197–200.

Burton, J. F., E. S. Zwadzki, H. R. Wetherell, and T. W. Moy. 1965. Mainliners and blue velvet. *J. Forensic Sci.* 10:466–472.

Butz, W. C. 1969. Pulmonary arteriole foreign body granulomata associated with angiomatoids resulting from the intravenous injection of oral medication, e.g., propoxyphene hydrochloride (Darvon®). *J. Forensic Sci.* 14:317–326.

Collin, J., D. E. F. Tweedle, C. W. Venables, F. L. Constable, and I. D. A. Johnston. 1973. Effect of a millipore filter on complications of intravenous infusions: A prospective clinical trial. *Brit. Med. J.* 2:456–458.

Connell, R. S., and R. L. Swank. 1973. Pulmonary microembolism after blood transfusion; an electron microscopic study. *Ann. Surg.* 177:40–47.

Davis, N. M., and S. Turco. 1971. A study of particulate matter in I.V. infusion fluids—phase 2. *Am. J. Hosp. Pharm.* 28:620–623.

Davis, S. S., L. Illum, J. M. McVie, and E. Tomlison, eds. 1984. *Microspheres and drug therapy: Pharmaceutical, immunological and medical aspects.* Amsterdam: Elseiver.

Doris, G. G., B. A. Bivins, R. P. Rapp, D. L. Weiss, P. P. DeLuca, and M. B. Ravin. 1977. Inflammatory potential of foreign particulates in parenteral drugs. *Anesthesia and Analgesia Current Researches* 56:422–428.

Douglas, F. G. 1971. Foreign particle embolism in drug addicts. *Ann. Int. Med.* 75:865–872.

Falchuk, K. H., L. Peterson, and B. J. McNeil. 1985. Microparticulate-induced phlebitis: Prevention by in-line filtration. *N. Engl. J. Med.* (Jan 10) 312:78–82.

Galbasov, Z. A., E. G. Popov, I. Y. Gavrilov, and E. Y. Pozin. 1989. Platelet aggregation: The use of optical density fluctuations to study microaggregate formation in platelet suspensions. *Thrombosis Res.* 54:215–223.

Garvan, J. M., and B. W. Gunnor. 1963. Intravenous fluids: A solution containing such particles must not be used. *Med. J. Australia* 2:140–145.

Garvan, J. M., and B. W. Gunner. 1964. The harmful effects of particles in intravenous fluids. *Med. J. Australia* 2:1–6.

Garvan, J. M., and B. W. Gunner. 1971. Particulate contamination of intravenous fluids. *Brit. J. Clin. Pract..* 25:119–121.

Geisler, R. M., P. J. Garvin, B. Klamer, R. U. Robinson, C. R. Thompson, W. R. Gibson, F. C. Wheeler, and R. G. Carlson. 1973. The biological effects of polystyrene latex particles administered intravenously to rats—A collaborative study. *Bull. Parent. Drug. Assoc.* 27 (3):101–117.

Gnadinger, E. 1957. A new procedure for the control in injection solutions. Ph.D. diss., University of Strasbourg.

Gotz, V. P., K. H. Rand, and B. S. Kramer. 1985. Effect of filtering amphotericin B infusions on the incidence and severity of phlebitis and selected adverse reactions. *Drug Intell. Clin. Pharm.* 19 (June):436–439.

Griffen, G. D., H. E. Essex, and F. C. Mann. 1951. Experimental evidence concerning death from small pulmonary emboli. *Int. Abs. Surg.* 92:313–314.

Gross, M. A. 1967. The danger of particulate matter in solutions for intravenous use. *Drug Intelligence* 1:12–13.

Gross, M. A., and C. J. Carter. 1966. The pathogenic hazard of particulate matter in solutions for intravenous use. In *Proc. Symposium on Safety of Large Volume Parenteral Solutions,* 31–35. Washington, D.C.

Hopkins, G. B. 1972. Pulmonary angiothrombotic granulomatosis in drug offenders. *J. Amer. Med. Assoc.* 211:909–911.

Hozumi, K., K. Kitamura, T. Kitade, and S. Iwagami. 1983. Localization of glass particles in animal organs derived from cutting of glass ampoules before intravenous injections. *Microchemical Journal* 28:215–226.

Jonas, A. M. 1966. Potentially hazardous effects of introducing particulate matter into the vascular system of man and animals. In *Proc. Symposium on Safety of Large Volume Parenteral Solutions,* p. 23–30. Washington, D.C.

Johnston, W. H., and J. Waisman. 1965. Pulmonary cornstarch granulomas in a drug user. *Arch. Pathol.* 92:196.

Kanke, M., G. H. Simmons, D. L. Weiss, B. A. Bivens, and P. P. DeLuca. 1973. Clearance of ^{41}Ce labelled microspheres from blood and distribution in specific organs following intravenous and intraarterial administration in beagle dogs. *J. Pharm. Sci.* 67 (4):508–513.

King, E. J., and H. Stantial. 1933. The biochemistry of silicic acid. I. Determination of Silica. *Biochem. J.* 27:990–1014.

Maddox, R. R., J. F. John, L. L. Brown, and C. E. Smith. 1983. Effect of in-line filtration on post infusion phlebitis. *Clin. Pharm.* 2 (Jan–Feb):58–61.

McCollum, C. 1985. The nature and clinical effects of particulates in intravenous medications. In *Proc. Europ. Conf. on Visible and Subvisible Particles in Parenteral Products,* 43–48. European Org. Q.C.

Russell, E. J., and J. M. Levy. 1987. Direct catheter redirection of a symptomatic errant intracranial silastic sphere embolus. *Radiology* 165:631–633.

Ryan, P. B., R. P. Rapp, P. P. DeLuca, W. O. Griffen, J. D. Clark, and D. Cloys. 1973. In-line final filtration—A method of minimizing contamination in intravenous therapy. *Bull. Parent Drug. Assoc.* 27:1–14.

Rypins, E. B., B. H. Johnson, B. Reder, I. J. Sarfeh, and K. Shimoda. 1990. Three-phase study of phlebitis in patients receiving peripheral intravenous hyperalimentation. *Am. J. Surg.* 159 (2):222–225.

Schoenberg, M. D., P. A. Gilman, V. R. Mumaw, and R. D. Moore. 1961. The phagocytosis of uniform polystyrene latex particles (PLP) by the reticuloendothelial system (RES) in the rabbit. *Brit. J. Experim. Pathol.* 42:486–495.

Schroeder, H. G., B. A. Bivins, G. P. Sherman, and P. P. DeLuca. 1978a. Physiological effects of subvisible microspheres administered intravenously to beagle dogs. *J. Pharm. Sci.* 67 (4):501–507.

Schroeder, H. G., G. H. Simmons, and P. P. DeLuca. 1978b. Distribution of radiolabeled subvisible microspheres after intravenous administration to beagle dogs. *J. Pharm. Sci.* 67 (4):508–513.

Turco, S., and N. M. Davis. 1973. Clinical significance of particulate matter a review of the literature. *Hospital Pharmacy* 8:137–140.

VanGlahn, W. C., and J. W. Hall. 1949. The reaction produced in the pulmonary arteries by emboli of cotton fibers. *Am. J. Pathol.* 25:575–580.

Wartman, W. B., R. B. Jennings, and B. Hudson. 1951. Experimental arterial disease. I. Reaction of the pulmonary artery to emboli of filter paper fibers. *Circulation* 4:746–766.

Appendix I

Photomicrography of Particulate Matter

Damian Neuberger, Ph.D.
Research Scientist
Baxter Healthcare Corp.

There are numerous microanalytical techniques available to the particle analyst for the identification of particulate matter. These include the following seven techniques:

1. Scanning and transmission electron microscopies,
2. Optical microscopies, including polarized light microscopy,
3. Fourier transform infrared microspectroscopy (micro FT–IR),
4. Energy and wavelength dispersive x-ray spectroscopies,
5. X-ray diffraction,
6. Ion probe analyzers, and
7. Electron spectroscopy for chemical analysis (ESCA) and the related process Auger spectroscopy.

Of these techniques, polarized light microscopy (PLM) is generally the most accurate and rapid method for the identification of particulate matter isolated from parenteral solutions. If it is of sufficient size, any particle can be characterized by this method and compared with known reference particles. Once learned, isolated particles can often be very quickly identified on sight by the experienced microscopist. This process is essentially the same one that allows us to identify on sight everyday items we encounter at home or work.

In some cases, other analytical instruments may be able to provide a characterization of the chemical composition, but not the specific identity of the particle or its source. For example, micro FT–IR may be able to identify a particle as cellulose, but the application of PLM could reveal that the particle is an aggregate of cotton fibers. Similarly, the many forms of silicon dioxide (SiO_2) can be chemically characterized by EDXS, but the specific form is most easily identified by PLM. To illustrate the importance of the other analytical tools, the suspected presence of talc aggregated with rubber on a latex glove may be quickly confirmed by the characteristic magnesium and silicon peaks in its EDXS spectra.

Rapid and accurate identification of unknown particles depends largely on the analyst's ability to remember the morphological features and microscopic characteristics of many different particles. Photomicrographs of reference particles serve to train and assist the microscopist in the identification of isolated particles. To demonstrate the role of photomicrography in the identification of particulate matter, this section (see four-color plates near the middle of this book) presents illustrations of some common particles encountered in parenteral products. A discussion of some of the basic techniques and instrumentation used to prepare photomicrographs is also presented.

Sample Preparation

The isolated particulate matter to be photographed is mounted between a clean glass microslide and coverslip in an appropriate mounting medium. Aroclor 5442, one of the Meltmount series mounting media[1], Pro Texx™ (Lerner Labs), or water may be selected depending on the refractive index (n_D) of the particle and other requirements of the final image. For example, to show Becke lines for all the particles in a population with different refractive

---

[1]McCrone Accessories & Components, 850 Pasquinelli Drive, Westmont, IL 60559; (708) 887-7100.

indices, a mounting liquid with a n_D higher or lower than that of all the particles must be selected. The microslide can be cleaned by a number of techniques, but one of the easiest is to press a piece of transparent adhesive tape to the mounting surface of the slide and immediately remove it. This lifts off all the particulate matter on the slide as well as fingerprints and other oily residues. Another excellent technique is to thoroughly rub the slide with a paste of Bon Ami® scouring powder. Rinse the slide for 1–2 minutes under running warm tap water followed by a rinse in distilled water. The slide can be leaned against an inverted beaker or placed in a clean slide staining rack to dry. The particle is placed on the cleaned slide in a drop of mounting media and a coverslip is carefully lowered to avoid entrapping air bubbles.

Instrumentation

It is beyond the scope of this section to describe the proper use of the polarizing light microscope. The microscopist may review the procedures for alignment and use of the polarized light microscope in several excellent reference texts[2,3,4]. Prior to particulate matter analysis and photomicrography, the microscope must be carefully aligned and Köhler illumination established.

In all types of photography, lighting is the most critical aspect to quality results. Köhler illumination, introduced by August Köhler in 1893, provides the brightest, most even illumination from a heterogeneous (coiled tungsten filament) light source. This system requires a small centerable lamp filament, an adjustable condenser lens to focus the filament, an adjustable field diaphragm in front of the lamp condenser, and a removable ground glass. In practice, the lamp filament is focused on the substage (condenser) diaphragm and in the back focal plane of the objective lens while the field diaphragm, which acts as a self-luminous source of bright even illumination, is focused at the plane of the specimen (Figure 1).

Since most polarized light microscopes manufactured today have an attached lamphouse, the set-up procedure for Köhler illumination will be described for this type of system.

---

[2]W. C. McCrone and J. G. Delly, *The Particle Atlas*, 2nd ed., *An Encyclopedia of Techniques for Small Particle Identification*. Vol. I, *Principles and Techniques*. (Ann Arbor, MI: Ann Arbor Science Publishers, Inc., 1973).

[3]J. G. Delly, *Photography Through the Microscope*. Publication P-2, 9th ed. (Rochester, NY: Eastman Kodak Co., 1988).

[4]W. C. McCrone, L. B. McCrone, and J. G. Delly, *Polarized Light Microscopy* (Ann Arbor, MI: Ann Arbor Science Publishers, Inc., 1978).

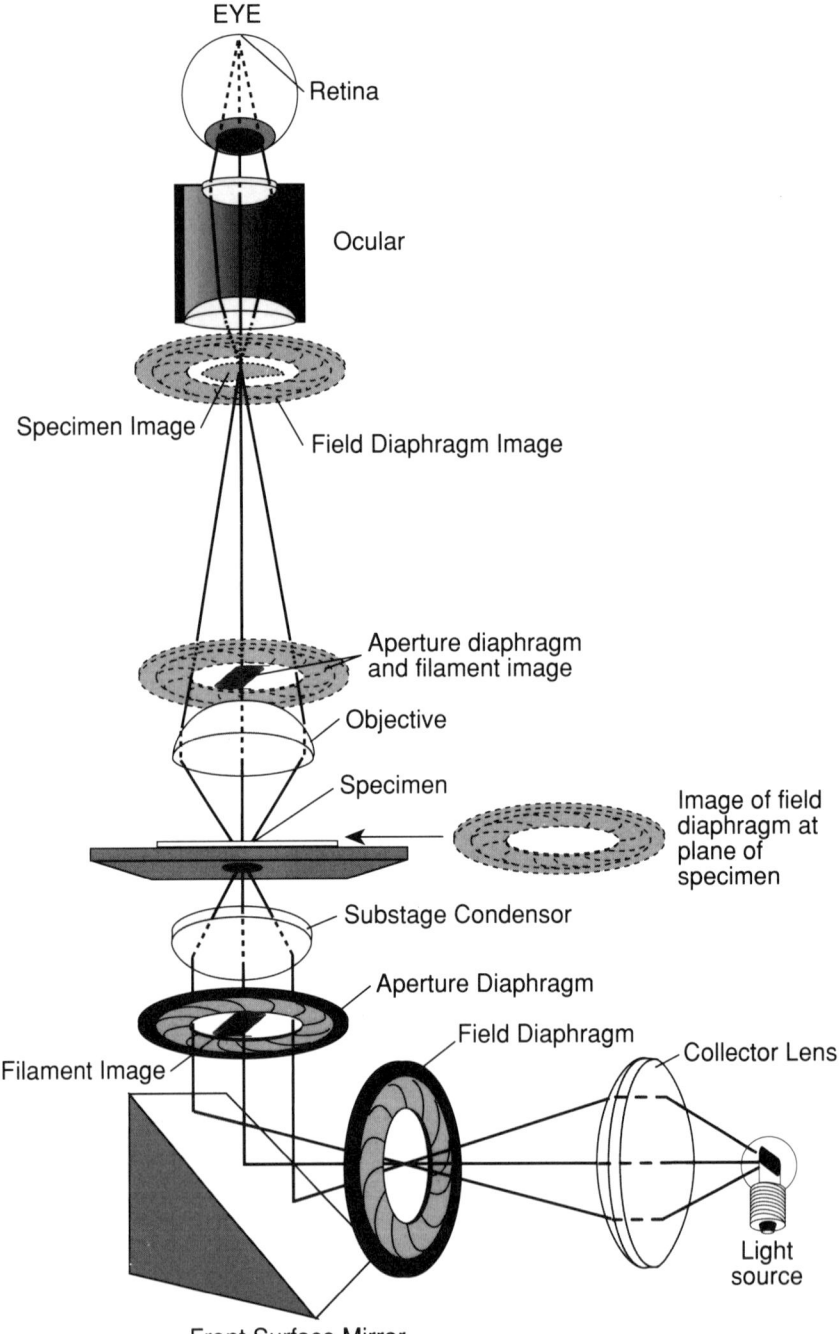

Figure 1. Köhler Illumination.

1. Remove all filters and diffusers from the illuminating path.

2. Set the filament voltage to approximately 80% and fully open the field and substage diaphragms.

3. Place a piece of thin paper, such as lens tissue, translucent plastic, frosted glass, etc., over the opening where the light exits from the base of the microscope below the condenser assembly. Center the lamp to provide an evenly illuminated opening.

4. Place a test specimen that contains good contrast on the microscope stage, select the 10× objective and set into position any corresponding auxiliary condenser lenses used for this objective.

5. Adjust the binocular tubes for interpupillary distance and diopter correction (eyepiece focus) as described in Chapter IV. Obtain a focused image.

6. When using a polarized light microscope with a rotating stage and centerable lens mount nosepiece, center the rotation of the image by adjusting the alignment screws on the stage and objective lens mounts. Generally, the lowest magnification objective lens is in a fixed mount and the shorter focal length lenses are in centerable mounts. The rotation of the stage is first centered with the fixed position lens in place and the remaining lenses are then individually centered so that image rotation is on axis.

7. Close the substage (condenser) diaphragm.

8. Open the field diaphragm and move the lamp housing back and forth along the optical axis or adjust the lamp condenser lens until the filament image is in sharp focus on the substage (condenser) diaphragm. This can be usually viewed from below either directly or by using a small mirror.

9. Open the substage diaphragm to illuminate the specimen. Adjust the brightness by adding neutral density filters or changing the transformer voltage. Focus the specimen.

10. Close the field diaphragm and center it using the condenser alignment screws. Raise and lower the condenser to focus the field diaphragm image (the edge of the aperture).

11. Open the field diaphragm to just fill the field of view and move the specimen until a clear area is located.

12. Insert the Bertrand lens (an auxiliary lens located below the eyepieces) or remove an eyepiece and insert a focusing telescope (used to center phase contrast annular rings). If neither optic is available, remove an eyepiece and view the back focal plane of the objective lens directly.

13. Establish a sharply focused image of the filament in the back focal plane of the objective lens by focusing the lamphouse condenser lens or moving the filament along the optical axis. Center the filament using the lamphouse adjustments to fill the back focal plane of the objective lens. Return the microscope to normal orthoscopic viewing conditions.

14. Finally, adjust the substage diaphragm to achieve the final image. This is one of the most important aspects of critical microscopy as it establishes the numerical aperture of the objective lens and thus determines the depth-of-field, contrast, and resolution—the quality of the final image. The condenser aperture must be adjusted for each lens and specimen to achieve the optimum compromise between contrast and resolution. Remove one eyepiece and observe the back focal plane of the objective lens as the condenser aperture is slowly closed from full open. Observe the diameter of the condenser aperture and compare it to the specimen image. As the aperture is closed, the specimen will, at some point, begin to show increasing contrast; note the position of the edge of the aperture diaphragm in the back focal plane of the objective lens. As the diaphragm is further closed, the image will develop increased contrast and depth-of-field, but will lose resolution and, with increasingly smaller aperture diameter, show diffraction zones around small image details.

15. The aperture position where changes in image contrast can just be readily discerned is often close to the optimal setting; however, the photomicrographer must find the best compromise, being careful not to excessively close the diaphragm.

Most photomicrographic systems today incorporate the use of an automatic leaf shutter module to control exposure. To this module, one or more camera backs may be attached, either 35 mm, $2^1/_4$ square roll film, $3^1/_4$ by $4^1/_4$ film, or 4×5 film backs. The Nikon

FXA photomicroscope (Figure 2) incorporates the camera mechanism, the microprocessor camera control, and facilities for one video camera and three film camera backs (a 4 × 5 and two 35 mm are shown). This system exemplifies the state-of-the-art photomicroscope, available from most manufacturers, that provides a microprocessor controlled camera system to monitor film speed, film type, lamp voltage, imprint data on each exposure, and so forth. In addition these photomicroscopes may also provide for autofocus of objectives, motorized nosepieces and condensers, and automatic adjustment of condenser diaphragm. If automatic exposure control is not available, then a suitable exposure meter[5] must be used to determine shutter speed. Some photomicrographic systems (e.g., Olympus PM-10ADS) also incorporate a color temperature meter so that color temperature may be more critically set by adjusting lamp voltage. The use of a quality leaf shutter is critical for the elimination of vibration. Although microscopists have used single lens reflex (SLR) camera bodies, a SLR may introduce vibration through the motion of the mirror and the shutter. In contrast, a high quality leaf shutter is generally less prone to introducing vibration into the system. In any case, always perform an actual test of any system to determine the level of vibration. Allow the microscope/camera system to stabilize before taking an exposure and use cable releases, self-timers, or remote electronic controls to actuate the shutter.

Film

The selection of film depends on the final use of the photomicrographs. There are several film components that must be considered in its selection: black & white (B&W) or color film, film format, speed, color rendition, color balance, resolving power, contrast, and granularity. Although B&W and color films can be used, the latter are necessary to record interference colors. Polaroid® color print and slide films may be used when immediate results are necessary; however, instant color negatives for enlargements and reprints are not yet available. Color reversal (slide) films and negative films produced by several manufacturers may also be used to provide higher resolution, lower granularity images suitable for high magnification projection and enlargements. Film format will be determined by the choice of camera back. Film speed must be considered when photographing moving specimen samples or if the

---

[5]McCrone Accessories & Components, 850 Pasquinelli Drive, Westmont, IL 60559; (708) 887-7100.

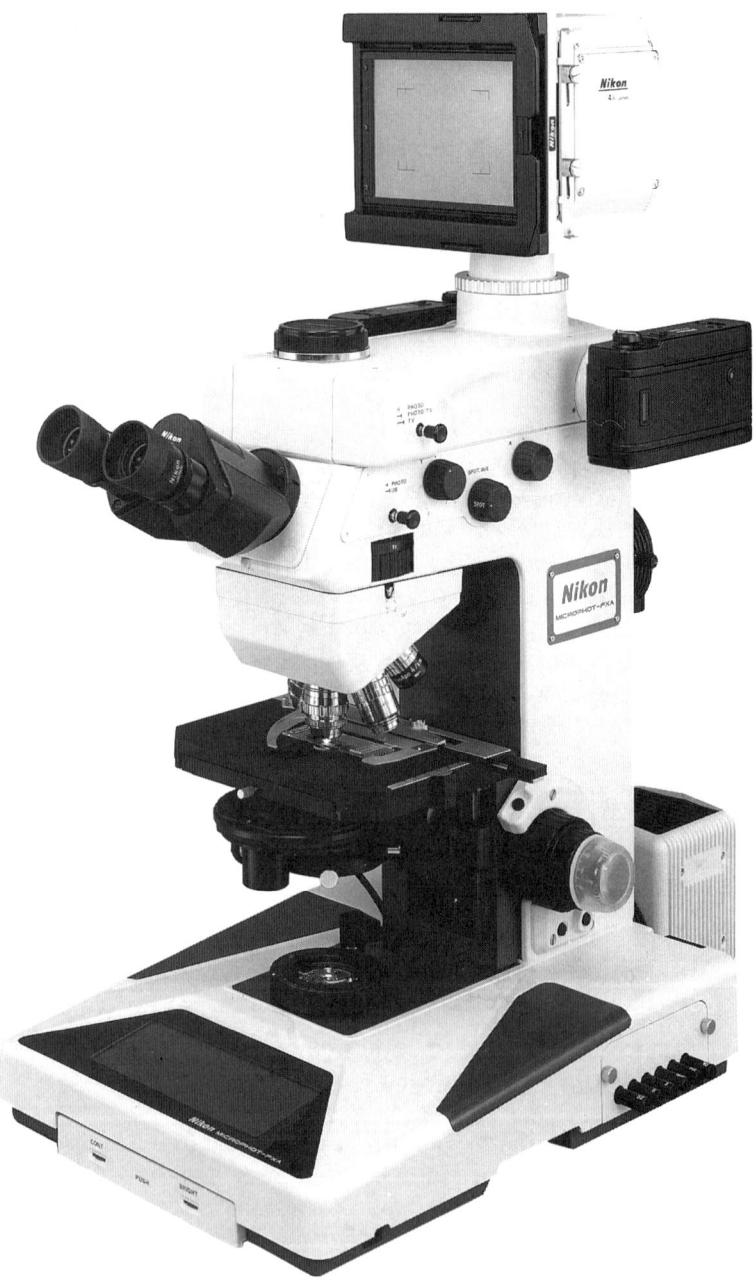

Figure 2. Nikon Microphot-FXA with built-in photo system. Photo courtesy of Nikon, Inc., Melville, N.Y.

illumination is very low, such as in the case of PLM or fluorescent microscopy. Speed should also be considered if problems are encountered with reciprocity failure (the shift in color balance and exposure time with long or short exposures). Color rendition is reflected in the way a film reproduces the specimen colors depending on the film's spectral sensitivity; daylight color reversal films offer a greater selection. For optimum results with color films, a professional grade of film should be purchased in volume for each lot and refrigerated until used (be sure to allow at least two hours for the film to reach ambient temperature before use). This will allow for the user to initially determine the filtration necessary to obtain the proper color balance of the film; this filter pack can then be used for the rest of the batch.

A photomicroscope illuminator is generally a tungsten light source (3200°K) for which Type B film is balanced. However, the selection of film depends on many factors; the final choice may preclude the use of tungsten balanced film (the specimen colors to be recorded may require a film with a particular spectral sensitivity that is not available in tungsten color balance).

Resolving power is the ability of a film emulsion to record closely spaced features as separate entities. This aspect of a film's capabilities is usually expressed as the number of line pairs per millimeter that are distinguishable in the photograph. The resolution determined for a given film is strongly linked to the image contrast that is related to the subject, film characteristics, processing, and so forth. Granularity is a characteristic that relates to the size of the emulsion grains formed following development and to the irregular distribution in the emulsion. The level of graininess will depend on processing variables that will, in turn, also effect speed and contrast of the film. Each of these factors must be considered and the choice of film based on the final use of the photomicrographs.

Light Balancing Filters

These filters adjust color temperature of the illuminator by absorption and concomitant shift of the spectrum. The No. 81 series (81, 81A, 81B, and 81C that lower the color temperature by 100, 200, 300, and 400°K increments respectively) are used when the light source color temperature is higher than the film. For example, if the illuminator is 3400°K and the film is 3200°K, an 81A filter would be used. If the illuminator color temperature is lower than the film, then a No. 82 series filter would similarly be used. A test series must be made to determine the necessary correction for the voltage selected, usually close to the value recommended by the instrument manufacturer. Any changes in the intensity of the illumination must then be made using neutral density filters because any change in voltage will change the color balance.

Color Compensating Filters

Shifts in the final color rendition can occur as the result of several factors—type of film and film batch, color temperature, lenses, heat absorbing filters, diffusion filters, UV emissions, stains, mounting media, and microslides. Color compensating (CC) filters are used to correct for these slight to sometimes significant color shifts. A series of color compensating filters are available in different densities (05, 10, 20, 30, and 40) of magenta, cyan, yellow, red, green, and blue. A test series must be made for each new batch of film and instrument system to determine the proper CC filtration to yield the desired results. The initial test series should consist of the color balance filter previously determined and a 10CC filter of one of the six CC colors. The measured exposures should be bracketed by ±1 stop in 1/3 stop increments for each of the six CC filter colors and the results should be viewed on a graphic arts–type light box balanced for 5500°K. The filtration requirements can be further delimited using a Kodak Color Print Viewing Kit that has six cardboard holders, each with a CC5, CC10, and CC20 filter of one of the six CC colors. The exposures on the test roll are viewed with various combinations of CC filters (color and density) to determine, more closely, the exact filtration required to provide, for example, a neutral gray background. It is also helpful to have a series of neutral density filters to compare two test frames that differ not only in color compensation but also in density. A second or third series of test exposures may have to be made to determine the final filtration requirements. This process may have to be repeated when the color balance is critical for a particular specimen. Finally, the test film must be processed consistently according to the manufacturers requirements. If the film is being processed by an outside laboratory, obtain the services of one that stringently controls their color processing line.

An excellent source and thorough discussion of practical information to the photomicrographer is the Eastman Kodak Publication P-2, *Photomicrography Through the Microscope.*[6]

---

[6] J. G. Delly, *Photography Through the Microscope.* Publication P-2, 9th ed. (Rochester, NY: Eastman Kodak Co., 1988).

Polarized Light Techniques

There are a variety of polarization techniques, four of which will be described, used to prepare polarized light photomicrographs of anisotropic and isotropic particulate matter. One of the principle problems encountered in polarized light photomicrography is that the conditions for optimum illumination of isotropic particles and anisotropic particles are not the same, that is, isotropic particles are best imaged with bright-field illumination, whereas anisotropic particles present the most information between crossed polarizer and analyzer (crossed polars). A further complication to polarized light photomicrography occurs with a heterogeneous population of particles exhibiting low to high birefringence. This results in a high light intensity ratio (high contrast) that may be beyond the capabilities of the recording film. One solution for these problems is to slightly uncross the polars.

Partially Uncrossed Polarizer and Analyzer (Polars)

In order to image both isotropic and anisotropic particles, the polarizer and analyzer can be slightly uncrossed by about 10–14° from the crossed position. This technique lightens the background from black to a shade of gray that permits isotropic particles to be seen. Although the interference colors of anisotropic particles will be almost the same as when the polars are crossed, they will, nonetheless, be reduced in intensity by the presence of the polarized light that is not stopped by the analyzer. Since each of the illustrations in this section represents a single type of particulate matter, it was not necessary to image both isotropic and anisotropic particles at the same time. This technique was selected to illustrate anisotropic particles oriented so as to show extinction; this is not possible with the techniques described below. Partially uncrossed polars also can be used to show the relationship of birefringent particulate matter to adjacent structures. For example, the presence of talc or starch in histology sections would require partially uncrossed polars to show the surrounding isotropic tissue. However, this can result in light intensity ratios of 15:1 and be difficult to record on films that are generally limited to ratios of 3:1 or 4:1. Under these circumstances, the darker areas of the image will be underexposed and may exhibit a green color shift as a result of reciprocity failure.

Parallel Polars

When the polarizer and analyzer are placed parallel to each other, a bright-field background is obtained and both anisotropic and isotropic particles are visible. Anisotropic particles will show complementary interference colors to those seen between crossed polars; however, weak birefringence will be difficult to see against the bright-field background. Another disadvantage to this technique is that anisotropic particles oriented so as to be at extinction cannot be readily distinguished from isotropic particles.

Crossed Polars with Quarter-Wave Compensator

The addition of a quarter-wave plate compensator is another approach to imaging both anisotropic and isotropic particles and fibers. However, this method also cannot distinguish between anisotropic particles at extinction and isotropic particles.

Circularly Polarized Light (Crossed Quarter-Wave Compensators)

This technique places the sample between crossed quarter-wave plate compensators that are themselves between crossed polars; the quarter-wave compensators are oriented at 45° to the vibration direction of the polars. The light emerging from the polarizer/lower quarter-wave compensator is circularly polarized. This type of illumination is also obtained from commercially available circular polarizer filters used on autofocus cameras. Circularly polarized light produces interference colors at all rotation positions. Since extinction does not occur, isotropic particles and anisotropic particles at extinction may be differentiated. Still, this method has the disadvantage of being unable to image isotropic particles. To provide a small amount of bright-field illumination to lighten the background, the polars may be slightly uncrossed (as previously described) or a small hole of a size appropriate for the objective aperture may be cut in the polarizer.

Illustrations

An Olympus Vanox microscope with a PM-10ADS camera system and polarized light optics was used to take the photomicrographs of particulate matter. **(Refer to the four-color plates near the middle of the book and the descriptions below.)** Kodak Ektachrome Professional Daylight EPR 135 daylight film with the addition of an 81A + 20B + 5M filter pack was used due to the unique color shift when the polars were partially uncrossed. Additional instrument settings included polars uncrossed by 14° (except Exhibit L, epithelial cells, which was between crossed polars) and a 10V transformer setting for the 100W quartz halogen illuminator. The amorphous material (Exhibit A), microporous filter fragments (Exhibit E), and rust particles (Exhibit K) on membrane filters were photographed using episcopic dark-field illumination (a 100W quartz halogen illuminator at 8V) and Kodak Ektachrome Professional Tungsten EPY 135 film without additional filter pack. As previously noted, the Vanox camera system is fitted with a color temperature meter so that the illuminator voltage can be optimally set to match the color balance of the film selected.

Exhibit A. Amorphous material. This tan, yellow, or light brown–colored amorphous material may be filtered from dextrose solutions and SVI reconstituted dry powder drugs. This material may appear as faintly visible discolorations on the filter membrane or as a more substantial membranous, amorphous material as shown in this micrograph. This material is formed as a result of a complex reaction of reducing sugars with amino acids to form numerous compounds, among which are furfural derivatives and N-glycosides. Magnification ×140.

Exhibit B. Cotton. These fibers are transparent and colorless and are flattened into regularly to irregularly twisted ribbons with a central lumen or canal. The cross-section profile ranges from narrowly elliptical to circular, the latter exhibiting a smaller cell lumen. Cotton fibers are not wood-type fibers, but cotton seed trichomes (hairs), approximately 12 to 60 µm long (depending of the variety of cotton) and 10–35 µm wide. The cell wall of cotton fibers consist of a primary cell wall and a thick secondary wall of almost pure cellulose. The surface of the fiber wall occasionally has transverse markings, but the cell wall does not have pits. A characteristic feature of cotton fibers is the lack of extinction between crossed polars. The refractive indices are 1.578 (parallel) and 1.532 (perpendicular). Magnification ×179.

Exhibit C. Polyester (Dacron®). These transparent, colorless, cylindrical fibers have a smooth surface except where delustering pigment particles are exposed on the surface or have become detached (resulting in an irregular surface texture). The cross section of this fiber is donut-shaped. The refractive indices are 1.700 (parallel) and 1.550 (perpendicular); birefringence is very high for a fiber, 0.150; elongation is (+); extinction is complete. The interference colors for these fibers are high, fifth-order light green and rose. The fibers shown here are 45–48 µm in diameter. Magnification ×179.

Exhibit D. Diatoms (from diatomaceous earth). Diatoms are mostly unicellular organisms (some colonial forms occur) of freshwater and marine habitats. There are an estimated 5600 extant (living) and 35,000 extinct species of diatoms. The cell walls of diatoms are unique double shells (frustules) composed of polymerized, opaline silica ($SiO_2 \cdot nH_2O$); the two halves (valves) fit together, one on top of the other, similar to a petri dish. Scanning electron microscopy has shown the shells to be delicately marked with large numbers of minute, intricately shaped depressions, pores, or passageways that connect the living protoplasm within the shell to the outside environment. These markings, which serve to classify species, have been used by microscopists to test the quality of objective lenses. The valves are colorless, transparent, and usually isotropic; they may be circular, oval, cresentic, linear, triangular, or square. The silica shells of diatoms have accumulated over millions of years to form diatomaceous earth, a fine, powdery, substance used as an abrasive, filtering, or insulating material. Magnification ×355.

Exhibit E. Filter fragments. These white, opaque, irregular particles range in size from 5 µm to 120 µm and were shed from a microporous membrane filter. The particles exhibit a microporous morphology, characteristic of the type of manufacture, when examined under higher magnification optical microscopy or scanning electron microscopy. Magnification ×69.

Exhibit F. Glass fibers. These fibers are smooth, colorless, transparent, isotropic cylinders. The cross-section profile is round and 15–30 µm in diameter. The refractive index is usually about 1.55, but can vary widely depending on the composition of the glass (approximately 1.52 for borosilicate glass and higher for soft glasses). The broken ends of glass fibers usually show a sharp transverse or diagonal fracture, but may be chipped consistent with their brittle nature. Magnification ×69.

Exhibit G. Hair (Human, Caucasian, blond). These fibers consist of a outer cuticle composed of layers of tightly overlapping scales surrounding a layer of tightly packed cells called the cortex. The central core or medulla is made up of loosely packed cells and will appear dark opaque if filled with air. The medulla may be continuous (especially in larger hairs), discontinuous, or absent. The cuticular scales in human hair do not protrude much from the shaft. The cross-section profile varies in shape from circular to oval and hair types vary depending on area of the body, age, sex, and race. Hairs may be transparent to almost opaque; refractive indices are about 1.554 (parallel) and 1.542 (perpendicular); birefringence is 0.012 and sign of elongation is (+). Extinction is usually complete and parallel but, depending on the shaft morphology, may not be uniformly complete. Human hair ranges in size from 50 to 150 µm in diameter. Magnification ×91.

Exhibit H. Polyamide (Nylon). These are smooth, transparent cylindrical filament yarn fibers with a trilobal cross-section profile. The refractive indices are 1.574–1.576 (parallel) and 1.523 (perpendicular); birefringence is 0.051–0.053; elongation is (+); extinction is parallel and complete. The interference colors for these fibers are second order yellow through third order yellow-green. The fibers shown here are 51–65 µm in diameter. Nylon fibers are manufactured in a variety of cross-section shapes, including round and tetralobal. Although the polyamide fibers are colorless, they may be dyed various colors in final use. Magnification ×91.

Exhibit I. Acrylic (Orlon®, delustered). These fibers are smooth, colorless, transparent cylinders with a flattened dog-bone cross-section profile. Other fibers may be trilobal or mushroom-shaped in profile. This fiber sample contains delustering pigments. Refractive indices are 1.510–1.520 (parallel) and 1.517–1.523 (perpendicular), birefringence ranges from 0.002–0.005. Orlon is one of the few fibers with a negative (-) sign of elongation; extinction is parallel and complete. Interference colors are low, first order gray. These fibers are approximately 30 µm in diameter, but can range from 18 to 54 µm. Magnification ×179.

Exhibit J. Rayon. These colorless, transparent, striated-appearing cylinders exhibit a multilobed cross section that can be determined by optical sectioning. Fibers range in size from 9 to 38 µm. Refractive indices for these fibers are 1.535–1.555 (parallel) and 1.514–1.535 (perpendicular); sign of elongation is (+) and birefringence ranges from 0.028 to 0.037. The interference colors for these 20 µm fibers are first order yellow to indigo. Magnification ×138.

Exhibit K. Iron oxide. These particles, commonly identified as rust particles, were filtered onto a Millipore® membrane and photographed with dark-field episcopic illumination. The particles (mostly yellow, orange, and various shades of bright red to brown red) are opaque aggregates of rounded to equant grains; a few metal gray to black iron particles are also present. These particles are soluble in HCl and their identification can be confirmed by the presence of Fe and O peaks in spectra obtained by energy dispersive X-ray spectroscopy. Magnification ×140.

Exhibit L. Epithelial cells (skin fragment). The surface of human skin consists of cornified flattened cells that flake off as scales or individual cells; dandruff scales are an example of sheets of epithelial cells. The scales are folded, curled, flat, polygonal to irregular in shape, transparent, and colorless to light tan. Interference color is a very weak gray with about a 100 nanometer (nm) retardation. Epithelial cells exhibit characteristic bands or striations of moderately birefringent collagen bundles within the cells. Extinction can be seen for portions of the collagen bundles in this skin fragment. Skin fragments often contain adherent particulate matter, such as hair and textile fiber fragments, talc, starch, and other particulate matter components of cosmetics, powders, and ointments. Magnification ×138.

Exhibit M. Corn starch. These particles are transparent, colorless, mostly subspherical to polyhedral grains ranging in size from 5 to 20 µm. The refractive index is approximately 1.53. Starch is composed of long, unbranched, helically coiled polysaccharide chains, which may be the basis for the grain formation. The result of this type of development is that a dark cross pattern is seen between crossed polars. Starch grains may show a concentric layering of starch around a centric to eccentric dark central point (hilum). The morphologic variation of starch is so extensive that its origin may be identified as to species of plant and plant part. A starch identification may be confirmed by the iodine-potassium iodide (I_2KI) test in which starch stains a blue to deep purple color. Magnification ×275.

Exhibit N. Talc, USP, $Mg_3(Si_2O_5)_2(OH)_2$. These birefringent particles are colorless, transparent to translucent plate-like particles, and translucent aggregates of fibrous blades (on edge, the thin, flat, plate-like particles look like long, narrow needles). The fibrous aggregates have incomplete undulose extinction. Refractive indices of talc particles (monoclinic steatite) are reported[7] to be 1.539 (a), 1.589 (b), and 1.589 (g); birefringence is 0.050; the sign of elongation is (-). Particles in this sample ranged from 2.5 to 105 µm. Magnification ×138.

Exhibits O and P. Wood fibers. Softwoods (conifers) and hardwoods (dicots) have basic structural differences. The terms *hardwood* and *softwood* do not express the degree of density of these woods; balsa, a tropical dicot, is one of the softest woods, and slash pine is harder than some of the hardwoods. Chemical fibers are those that are prepared by dissolution of the intercellular binding material (middle lamella) by chemical treatment (maceration),

---

[7] W. C. McCrone and J. G. Delly, *The Particle Atlas*, 2nd ed., *An Encyclopedia of Techniques for Small Particle Identification.* Vol. II, *The Light Microscopy Atlas.* (Ann Arbor, MI: Ann Arbor Science Publishers, Inc., 1973).

resulting in relatively intact cells. The fiber-like cells described for each wood represent examples in a range of morphological variation that can make identification difficult for some types of isolated fibers. The refractive indices of fibers range from 1.53–1.58; all of these elongated fibers have a (+) sign of elongation.

Exhibit O. Hardwood chemical fibers. Dicot woods exhibit a greater variety of types of thick-walled fiber-like cells than do coniferous woods. These include vessel elements, tracheids, and fibers. Vessel and tracheary elements have thick secondary walls, lack the living protoplasts at maturity, and have pits in their walls that exhibit a black cross-shaped (✦) pattern between crossed polars. Interference colors are often first order gray. In addition, vessels generally have perforations in the end walls of the cells, but they may also be found on the lateral walls. Since perforations are holes in the cell wall, they do not exhibit polarization patterns as do the pits. Vessels are broad and flattened as a result of product processing whereas tracheids are narrow and flat, with more highly tapered end walls. Fibers are long, narrow, tapered cells with a polygonal cross-section profile and exhibit low, second order interference colors. Most isolated dicot fiber-like cells have originated from paper or paper products. Magnification ×91.

Exhibit P. Softwood chemical fibers. The principle feature of coniferous woods is the absence of vessels (described for hardwoods). Three types of thick-walled cells are characteristic of softwoods: (1) long, tapered, flattened, colorless, transparent tracheids with large, circular bordered pits (not perforations); especially on the tapered end walls that exhibit a black cross-shaped (✦) pattern between crossed polars, interference colors are often first order gray; (2) long, tapered, colorless, transparent thick-walled fibers that exhibit higher order interference colors (second-order series) with good extinction; and (3) shorter, more rectangular-shaped ray tracheids with sloped end walls and bordered pits; interference colors are also first-order gray. Extinction in softwood fibers is parallel and nearly complete. Most isolated conifer fiber-like cells have originated from paper or paper products. Magnification ×69.

Appendix II

Vendor and Equipment Information

This vendor listing is not intended to be comprehensive, but rather is to serve as a starting point in a search for lab equipment useful in the analysis of particulate matter, supplies for the "clean" laboratory, clean room garb, and other essential materials and instruments. More detailed lists of where to purchase specific items can be found in such pharmaceutical or clean room trade publications as *Clean Rooms, Pharmaceutical Technology, Medical Device and Diagnostic Industry,* and in journals such as *The Journal of Parenteral Science and Technology.*

Particle Counters (Airborne and Solution)

Climet Instruments Company
1320 W. Colton Ave.
Redlands, CA 92374
(725) 793-2788

Coulter Electronics
601 W. 20th Street
Hialeah, FL 33010
(800) 327-6531

Hiac/Royco World Headquarters
11801 Tech Road
Silver Spring, MD 20904
(800) 638-2790 or
(301) 680-7000

Malvern Instruments Inc.
10 Southville Rd.
Southborough, MA 01772
(508) 480-0200

Met One
481 California Ave.
Grants Pass, OR 97526
(503) 479-1248

Particle Measuring Systems, Inc.
1855 S. 57th Court
Boulder, CO 80301
(910) 940-5891

Rion Co., Ltd.
20-41, Higashimotomachi
   3-chome
Kokubunji, Tokyo 185, Japan
0423-22-1133

TSI Inc.
Industrial Test Instruments
   Group
P. O. Box 64394
St. Paul, MN 55164
(800) 876-9874 or
(612) 490-2888

Light Extinction Counter Sensors

Russell Laboratories
3314 Rubio Crest Drive
Altadena, CA 91001
(818) 797-6163

Counter Calibration Software

Berdovitch & Associates
307 S. Milwaukee Ave.
Wheeling, IL 60090
(708) 459-3320

Calibration Materials

Bangs Laboratories, Inc.
979 Keystone Way
Carmel, IN 46032
(317) 844-7176

Coulter Electronics, Inc.
601 W. 20th Street
Hialeah, FL 33010
(800) 327-6531

Duke Scientific Corp.
1135-D San Antonio Rd.
Palo Alto, CA 94303
(415) 962-1100

GMC, AC Rochester Division
P. O. Box 1001
Flint, MI 48556
(313) 236-5000

Interfacial Dynamics Corp.
4814 NE 107th Ave., Suite B
Portland, OR 97220
(800) 323-4810 or (503) 256-0076

Japan Synthetic Rubber Co.,
   Ltd.
Specialty Materials Dept.
2-11-24
Tsukjii, Chuo-ku, Tokyo
03-5565-661 0

National Institute of Standards
   and Technology
Office of Standard Reference
   Materials
Chemistry Bldg., Room B311
Gaithersburg, MD 20899
(301) 975-2000

Powder Technologies Inc.
 (PTI)
1119 Riverwood Drive
P. O. Box 1464
Burnsville, MN 55337
(612) 894-8737

Polymer Laboratories, Inc.
Technical Center
Amherst Fields Research Park
160 Old Farm Road
Amherst, MA 01002
(413) 253-9554

Polyscience Inc.
Paul Valley Industrial Park
400 Valley Road
Warrington, PA 18976
(800) 523-2575 or
(215) 343-6484

Whitehouse Scientific
The Whitehouse
Whitechurch Road
Waverton, Chester
C H 3 7 P B (UK)
44-0-244-332-626

Visual Inspection Systems

P. W. Allen & Company
25, Swan Lane, EVESHAM,
Worcs, WRII 4PE, UK

Brevetti C.E.A., s.p.a.
Via BTG. Monte Baldo 24
36100, Vicenza, Italy
0444-562241-562560

Eisai U.S.A. Inc.
Glenpointe Centre East
300 Frank W. Burr Blvd.
Teaneck, NJ 07666-6741
(201) 692-0999

Production Equipment
17 Legion Place, P. O. Box 236
Rochelle Park, NJ 07662
(201) 845-4475

Seidenader Equipment Inc.
35 Airport Park
Morristown, NJ 07960
(201) 267-8730

Strunk/Robert Bosch Corp.
121 Corporate Blvd.
South Plainfield, NJ 07080
(201) 753-3700

Takeda, United Chemical
Machinery Supply Co.
1520 Route 37 West, Suite 2
P. 0. Box 4142
Toms River, NJ 08756-4142
(908) 349-3131

Image Analysis

Artek Systems Corporation
(Vendor for Omnicon System)
170 Finn Court
Farmingdale, NY 11735
(516) 293-4420

Cambridge Instruments, Inc.
P. O. Box 123
Buffalo, NY 14240-0123
(716) 891-3000

Noran Inc.
2551 West Beltline Highway
Middleton, WI 53562
(608) 831-6511

Olympus Corporation
Precision Instrument Division
4 Nevada Drive
Lake Success, NY 11042-1179
(516) 488-3880

Quantex Corporation
252 North Wolfe Rd.
Sunnyvale, CA 94086
(408) 733-6730

Electrical Zone Sensing Counters

Coulter Electronics, Inc.
P. O. Box 2145
601 W. 20th St.
Hialeah, FL 33010
(800) 327-6531

Particle Data, Inc.
P.O. Box 265
Elmhurst, IL 60126
(708) 832-5653

Laser Diffraction Particle Analyzers

Christison (Fritsch) Scientific
  Equipment Limited
Albany Road
East Gateshead Industrial
  Estate
Gateshead NE8 3AT
(091) 477-4261

Coulter Electronics
601 W. 20th St.
MC 195-10
Hialeah, FL 33010
(800) 327-6531

Horiba Instruments, Inc.
1021 Duryea Ave.
Irvine, CA 92714
(714) 250-4811

Leeds & Northrup
Sumneytown Pike
North Wales, PA 19454
(215) 699-2000

Malvern Instruments Inc.
10 Southville Rd.
Southboro, MA 01772
(508) 480-0200

Sympatec GmbH
D-3392 Clausthal-Zellerfeld
Burgstatter Strabe 6
05323-717-0

Lamma Instrumentation

Leybold Heraeus
5700 Mellon Rd.
Export, PA 15632
(412) 327-5700

R. J. Lee Group
350 Hockberg Rd.
Monroeville, PA 15146
(412) 325-1776

Light Microscopes

Bio-Rad
19 Blackstone Street
Cambridge, MA 02139
(617) 864-5820

Nikon Inc. Instrument Group
623 Stewart Avenue
Garden City, NY 11530
(516) 222-0200

Olympus Corporation
4 Nevada Drive
Lake Success, NY 11042-1179
(516) 488-3880

Reichert Scientific
  Instruments
Microscopical Optical Consulting, Inc.
P. O. Box 586

Valley Cottage, NY 10989
(914) 268-6450

Wild Leitz
Wild Heerbrugg Ltd.
9435 Heerbrugg (Switzerland)
071-703131

Carl Zeiss, Inc.
One Zeiss Drive
Thornwood, NY 10594
(914) 747-1800

X-Ray Spectrometers

EDAX International, Inc.
A North American Philips
   Company
150 West Center Court
Schaumburg, IL 60195
(708) 705-9878

EG&G Ortec
100 Midland Rd.
Oak Ridge, TN 37830
(615) 482-4411

Kevex Corporation
1101 Chess Drive
Foster City, CA 94404
(415) 573-5866

Link Systems (USA) Inc.
P. O. Box 50810
3290 W. Bayshore Rd.
Palo Alto, CA 94303
(415) 856-2726

Mattson Instruments, Inc.
1001 Fourier Drive
Madison, WI 53717
(608) 831-5515

Nicolet Instrument Corporation
Analytical Division

1834 Walden Office Square
Suite 100
Schaumburg, IL 60173
(800) 634-6929 or
(708) 397-5200

Noran Instruments, Inc.
2551 W. Beltline Highway
Middleton, WI 53562-2697
(608) 831-6511

Peak Instruments, Inc.
P. O. Box 1256
Princeton, NJ 08542
(609) 924-7946

Perkin-Elmer Corp.
761 Main Ave.
Norwalk, CT 06859-0012
(203) 762-1000

Princeton Gamma-Tech, Inc.
1200 State Rd.
Princeton, NJ 08540
(609) 924-7310

Electron Microscopes

AMRAY
160 Middlesex Turnpike
Bedford, MA 01730
(617) 275-1400

Hitachi Scientific Instruments
460 E. Middlefield Rd.
Mountain View, CA 94043
(415) 961-0461

JEOL (U.S.A.) Inc.
11 Dearborn Rd.
Peabody, MA 01960
(508) 535-5900

U.S.A. Cambridge Instruments,
   Inc.

40 Robert Pitt Drive
Monsey, NY 10952
(914) 356-3331

Photon Correlation Spectrophotometers

Brookhaven Instruments Corporation
750 Blue Point Road
Holtsville, NY 11742
(516) 758-3200

Malvern Instruments Inc.
10 Southville Rd.
Southborough, MA 01772
(508) 480-0200

Otsuka Electronics Co., Ltd.
3-26-3, Shodai-Tajika
Osaka, 573 Japan
0720-55-8550

Santa Barbara Technology
   (Nicomp)
135 Nogal Dr.
Santa Barbara, CA 93110
(805) 968-1497

Laser Light Scattering Liquid Counters

Spectrex Particle Counters
3594 Haven Ave.
Redwood City, CA 94063
(415) 365-6567

Micro (Submicron) Particle Samplers

California Measurements, Inc.
150 East Montecito Ave.
Sierra Madre, CA 91024
(815) 355-3361

Microfiltration Supplies

Buckbee-Mears St. Paul
A Unit of BMC Industries, Inc.
245 E. 6th Street
St. Paul, MN 55101
(612) 228-6400

Collimated Holes, Inc.
460 Division Street
Campbell, CA 95008
(408) 374-5080

Gelman Sciences
600 S. Wagner Road
Ann Arbor, MI 48106
(800) 521-1520 or
(313) 665-0651

Millipore Corp.
80 Ashby Rd.
P. O. Box 9125
Bedford, MA 01730-9125
(800) 225-1380 or
(617) 275-9200

Pall Filtration
2200 Northern Blvd.
East Hills, NY 11540
(800) 645-6532 or
(516) 484-5400

Sartorius Corp.
140 Wilbur Place
Bohemia, Long Island, NY
   11716
(516) 563-5122

Clean Room Supplies

Baxter Healthcare Corporation
Industrial Division
27200 North Tourney Rd.

Valencia, CA 91355
(805) 253-7463

Berkshire Corporation
River Street
Great Barrington, MA 01230
(800) 242-7000 or
(413) 528-2602

Clean Room Products, Inc.
1800 Ocean Avenue
Ronkonkoma, NY 11779
(516) 588-7000

Clestra Cleanroom Technology
4003 Eastbourne Drive
Syracuse, NY 13206
(315) 437-2152

E.I. Du Pont De Nemours &
  Company
Fibers
Laurel Run Building
P. O. Box 80, 705
Wilmington, DE 19880-0705
(302) 774-1000

Teijin Shoji America, Inc.
  (Garb)
42 W. 39th St., 6th Floor
New York, NY 10018
(212) 840-6900

Texwipe
650 E. Crescent Ave.
P. O. Box 575
Upper Saddle River, NJ 07458
(201) 327-9100

Particle Analysis Equipment (General)

McCrone Associates
850 Pasquinelli Dr.

Westmont, IL 60559
(708) 887-7100

Powder Analysis Equipment

Gilson Company, Inc.
(Agent for Futsch GMBH)
P. O. Box 677
Worthington, OH 43085-0677
(800) 444-1508

Hosokawa Micron Division
10 Chatham Rd.
Summit, N.J. 07901
(201) 273-6360

Malvern Instruments, Inc.
200 Turnpike Rd.
Southborough, MA 01772
(508) 480-0200

Micromeritics Instrument Corp.
1 Micromeritics Dr.
Norcross, GA 30093
(404) 662-3633

Quantachrome
5 Aerial Way
Syosset, NY 11791
(516) 935-2240

Rotex Inc.
1394 Knowlton St.
Cincinnati, OH 45223
(513) 541-1236

Seishin Enterprise Co., LTD.
Nippon Brunswick Bldg. 5-27-7
  Sendagaya
Shibuya-ku, Tokyo, Japan T155
03(350)5771

Shimadzu Scientific Instruments, Inc.,
7102 Riverwood Dr.
Columbia, MD 21046
(410) 381-1227

W.S. Tyler, Inc.
P.O. Box 8900
3200 Bessemer City Rd.
Gastonia, NC 28053
(704) 629-2214

Secondary Ion Mass Spectrometers

CAMECA INC. USA
2001 West Main Street
Stamford, CT 06902
(203) 348-5252

Laboratory Robots

Bohdan Automation, Inc.
1500 McCormick Boulevard
Mundelein, IL 60060
(708) 680-3939

Zymark Corp.
68 Elm Street
Hopkinton, MA 01748
(508) 435-9500

Additional Sources of Supplemental Information and Standards

American Institute of Aeronautics and Astronautics (AIAA)
370 L'Enfant Promenade, S. W.
Washington, DC 20024
(202) 646-7400

American National Standards Institute (ANSI)
11 West 42nd Street, 13th Floor
New York, NY 10036
(212) 642-4900

American Society of Heating, Refrigerating, and Air-Conditioning Engineers (ASHRAE)
1791 Tullie Circle, NE
Atlanta, GA 30329
(404) 636-8400

American Society of Mechanical Engineers (ASME)
345 E. 47th Street
New York, NY 10017
(212) 705-7722

American Society for Testing and Materials (ASTM)
1916 Race Street
Philadelphia, PA 19103
(215) 299-5400

Association pour la Prevention et l'Etudie de la Contamination (ASPEC)
Secretariate d'ASPEC
1, Cite Paradis, rue Paradis
75010 Paris
France
011-33-1-424-70375

British Standards Institution (BSI)
Maylands Avenue
Hemel Hempstead,
Hartfordshire HP2 4SQ
England
011-44-2-230442

Commission of the European
   Communities (CEC)
Office for Official Publications
   of the European Communities
2 rue Mercier
L 2985, Luxemborg
011-352-43011

Defence Research Establish-
   ment Suffield (DRES)
National Defence
Ralston, Alberta
Canada
(403) 544-4000

Deutsche Institut for Normung
   (DIN)
Deutsche Elektrotechnische
   Kommission In DIN Und
   Vde
Stresemannallee-15
D-600
Frankfurt am Main 70
Germany
011-49-69-63080

Food and Drug Administration
   (FDA)
Division of Drug Quality
Compliance
Center for Drugs and Biologics
5600 Fishers Lane
Rockville, MD 20857
(301) 443-1544

Institute of Electrical and
   Electronics Engineers (IEEE)
445 Hoes Lane
P.O. Box 1331
Piscataway, NJ 08855-1331
(908) 981-0060

Institute of Environmental
   Sciences (IES)
940 East Northwest Highway
Mt. Prospect, IL 60056
(708) 255-1561

International Organization for
   Standards (ISO)
CP-56
Rue de Varembe
CH-1211
Geneve 20
Suisse
011-41-22-749-0111

International Society of Pharmaceutical Engineers (ISPE)
3816 West Linebaugh Avenue
Suite 412
Tampa, FL 33624
(813) 960-2105

Japan Air Cleaning Association
   (JACA)
Tomoe-Ya Building No. 2-14
1-Chome, Uchi-Kanda
Chiyodaku, Tokyo, 101
Japan
011-81-33-996165

Japanese Industrial Standards
   (JIS)
4-1-24
Akasaka
Minato-Ku, Tokyo, 107
Japan
011-81-3-3583-8005

National Institute of Standards
   and Technology (NIST)
U.S. Department of Commerce
Gaithersburg, MD 20899
(301) 921-2805

National Technical Information Service (NTIS)
U.S. Department of Commerce
5285 Port Royal Road
Springfield, VA 22161
(703) 487-4600

R³-NORDIC
Dr. Bengt C. Ljungqvist, Pres.
Building Services Eng.,
KTH (Roepe Inst. of Tech.)
S-100 44
Stockholm, Sweden
011-46-8-790-8586

Schweitzerische Gesellschaft fur Reinraumtechnik
Seestrasse 5
Postfach
CH-8700 Kusnacht
Switzerland
011-41-1-911-0055

Society of Automotive Engineers (SAE)
400 Commonwealth Drive
Warrendale, PA 15096
(412) 776-4841

Standards Association of Australia (SAA)
Standards House
80 Arthur Street
North Sydney, New South Wales
Australia
011-61-2-963-4111

Verein Deutscher (VDI)
VDI-Gesellschaft Technische Gebaude Ausrustung
Graf-Recke Strasse 84
D-400 Dusseldorf
Germany
011-49-211-62140

Software for Data Reduction

CA–Cricket® Graph™
Computer Associates International, Inc.
1240 McKay Drive
San Jose, CA 95131
(408) 432-1727

EXECUSTAT®
Stratregy Plus Inc.
5 Independence Way
Princeton, NJ 08540
(800) 452-1832

LOTUS
Lotus Development Corporation
55 Cambridge Parkway
Cambridge, MA 02142
(617) 253-9150

Microsoft® EXCEL
Microsoft Corporation
One Microsoft Way
Redmond, WA 98052-6399
(206) 635-7070

STAGRAPHICS®
STSC, Inc.
2115 East Jefferson Street
Rockville, MD 20852
(800) 232-STAT

Appendix III

Trademarks

Analyslide®	Filter examination and storage container Gelman Sciences, Ann Arbor, MI 48106
Aroclor®	Mounting media Monsanto Co., St. Louis, MO 63167
Bev-A-Line®	Hytrel®-lined flexible PVC tubing Thermoplastic Processes, Inc., Stirling, NJ 07980
Bon Ami®	Polishing cleanser Faultless Starch/Bon Ami Co., Kansas City, MO 64101
CA-Cricket® **Graph**™	Graph Computer Associates International, Inc., San Jose, CA 95131
Coulter®	Coulter Electronics, Inc., Hialeah, FL 33010
Coulter Counter®	Electronic particle counter Coulter Electronics, Inc. Hialeah, FL 33010
Dacron®	Polyester fiber DuPont Chemicals, Wilmington, DE 19898

Darvon®	Darvon-N, propoxyphene napsylate USP, Eli Lilly, Indianapolis, IN 46285
Easy-Lab®	Lab automation software Zymark Corp., Hopkinton, MA 01748
EXECUSTAT®	Data analysis system Strategy Plus, Inc., Princeton, NJ 08540
Elzone®	Particle measurement system Particle Data, Inc., Elmhurst, IL 60126
Extar®	Polyester-based polymer Eastman Kodak Co., Kingsport, TN 37662
Flanders®	Filter Flanders Filters Inc., Washington, NC 27889
Formvar®	Polyvinyl formal plastic Monsanto Co., St. Louis, MO 63167
Freon®	Precision cleaning agent E. I. DuPont De Nemours & Co., Wilmington, DE 19898
Gelman®	Gelman Sciences, Ann Arbor, MI 48106
Gore-Tex®	Expanded PTFE W. L. Gore and Associates, Inc., Newark, DE
HIAC/Royco®	Division of Pacific Scientific Company, Silver Spring, MD 20904
Hytrel®	Polyester elastomer DuPont Chemicals, Wilmington, DE 19898
Lotus®	Software Lotus Development Corp., Cambridge, MA 02142
Meltmount®	Mounting media Cargille Laboratories, Cedar Grove, NJ 07009
Metricell®	Microporous polypropylene media Gelman Sciences, Ann Arbor, MI 48106

Micromeretics®	Micromeretics Corp., Norcross, GA 30093
Microsoft® Excel	Worksheet analysis, exchanging data, customizing, automating Microsoft Corporation, Redmond, WA 98052-6399
Microsoft® Word	Word processing program Microsoft Corporation, Redmond, WA 98052-6399
Millipore®	Millipore Corp., Bedford, MA 01730
Nuclepore®	Track-etched membranes Costar Corp., Cambridge, MA 02140
Orlon®	Acrylic fiber DuPont Chemicals, Wilmington, DE 19898
Pall®	Pall Corporation, Long Island, NY 11542
Permount®	Microscope slide mounting medium Fisher Scientific, Pittsburgh, PA 15219
Plexiglas®	Acrylic sheet Rohm and Has Co., Atlanta, GA 30338
Polaroid®	Instant film Polaroid Corporation, Cambridge, MA 02139
Scotch®	Transparent tape 3M Commercial Office Supply Div., St. Paul, MN 55144
Spectrex®	Spectrex Corp., Redwood City, CA 94063
STAGRAPHICS®	Statistical graphics system STSC, Inc., Rockville, MD 20852
Supor®	Inherently hydrophilic polysulfone membrane Gelman Corporation, Ann Arbor, MI 48106
Teflon®	Fluorocarbon resin DuPont Chemicals, Wilmington, DE 19898

Triton® X-100	Detergent Rohn and Haas Co., Philadelphia, PA 19105
TSI®	TSI Incorporated, St. Paul, MN 55164
Tween® 20	Detergent ICI America, Inc., Wilmington, DE 19897
Tygon®	Plastic tubing Nortar Performance PLastics, Wayen, NJ 07470
Tyvek®	Speenbonded polyolefin DuPont Tyvek, Wilmington, DE 19880
Ultipor®	Nylon microporous filter medium Pall Corp, Glen Cove, Long Island, NY 11542
Zymate®	Robotic system Zymark Corp., Hopkinton, MA 01748

Name Index

A

Abendroth, P., 243
Abethell, J. A., 460
Abramson, L. R., 6, 323
Adams, F., 172
Adams, D. F., 473
Adwers, J. R., 455
Akers, M. J., 3, 10, 237
Aldrich, D. S., 144, 237, 240, 249, 253
Alexander, D. M., 257
Allardyce, D. B., 460
Allen, T., 267, 300, 308, 330, 334, 341, 372
Amaker, P., 52
Anderson, M. E., 160
Anger, V., 121
Aoyama, T., 248
Archambault, G. F., 22
Archimedes, 267, 278
Ashline, K. A., 245
Ashlund, B., 22
Ashmore, P. G., 460
Atlee, W. E., 473

B

Backhouse, C. M., 237, 473
Bain, R., 460
Bangs, L. D., 78
Barber, T. A., 5, 57, 70, 78, 100, 316
Bares, D., 357
Barnett, M. I., 10, 53, 441
Barron, D., 460
Beckett, R. K., 135, 136
Beddow, J. K., 274, 278, 312
Bemer, D., 204
Benjamin, F., 1
Berger, M., 460
Bisio, J. M., 478
Blackwell, H. R., 30
Blanchard, J., 53, 70, 72, 77, 420
Blesner, J., 207
Bloss, F. D., 177
Boardman, R. P., 279
Bodapatti, S., 121, 132, 160, 249, 351
Bollinger, R. O., 160
Bommer, J. W. B., 477
Borchert, S. J., 1, 10, 32, 33, 44, 144, 237, 244, 249
Borden, P., 229
Boretos, J. W., 460
Bottlinger, M., 201
Boucher, C. L., 33
Bovey, E., 126, 135
Boyd, J., 351
Boymund, P., 52
Bradfield, J., 477
Bragg, L., 179, 180
Brewer, J. H., 31, 243, 257, 473, 474

Brock, T. D., 252, 352
Brown, G., 479
Brownley, C. A., 44, 394, 398
Buerger, M. J., 181
Buettner, H., 204
Burton, J. F., 471, 473
Buseck, P. R., 163
Butz, W. C., 471, 473
Bzik, T. J., 214

C

Caiazza, S., 460
Caldow, R., 207
Capellan, J. M., 172
Carstensen, J. T., 268
Carter, C. J., 473
Carver, L. D., 54, 60
Castaing, R., 173
Chambers, D. S., 401, 413
Chamot, E. M., 121
Charbonneau, H. C., 401
Chatelau, E. A., 460
Choate, S. J., 274
Chrai, S., 70
Clark, R. E., 460
Coates, V. J., 304
Coll, H., 330
Collin, J., 479
Connell, R. S., 478
Conzemius, R. J., 172
Cooper, D. W., 200, 207, 219
Cotter, R. J., 165, 171
Cournoyer, R., 166
Crowl, V. T., 334
Curry, C. J., 166

D

Dahlinder, L., 243
Damme, P. A., 248
Danielson, J. W., 248
Davies, C. N., 223
Davies, P. J., 257
Davies, R., 271
Davis, N. M., 240, 394, 477, 479, 481

Davis, S. S., 473
De Broglie, 148
DeLuca, P. P., 1, 5, 50, 57, 102, 121, 131, 135, 138, 160, 243, 245, 300, 323, 351, 369
DeMalka, S. R., 4
Delly, J. G., 102, 135, 137, 351, 489, 496, 502
Deming, W. E., 400, 401
DiGrado, C. J., 53
Digaetano, T. N., 44
Dimmick, J. E., 432, 460
Dingell, J., 463
Di Paolo, E. R., 432, 453
Dixon, A. M., 231
Dodds, A. W., 22
Dodge, L. E., 306
Dolcher, D., 240, 258
Doris, G. G., 473
Douglas, F. G., 473
Draftz, R. G., 101, 135, 138, 160
Drewel, M., 304
Duke, S. D., 78
Duncan, A. J., 401
Dunning, J. H. F., 31, 243, 257, 474

E

Edmundson, I. C., 269, 298
Elford, W. J., 352, 364
Elias, H. G., 306, 311
Elings, V. B., 324
Ellis, H., 454
Endicott, C. J., 10
Erike, A., 173
Ernerot, L., 70, 237, 243, 246, 255, 257

F

Fairhurst, D., 298, 309
Falchuk, K. H., 441, 479
Farlow, N. H., 159
Fayed, M. E., 268
Fiegl, F., 121
Fink, D. G., 279
Fitch, H. D., 216

Fleischer, R. L., 352, 354
Fochtman, E. G., 268
Fong, W., 123

G
Galbasov, C. A., 478
Gallant, R. C., 73
Garvan, J. M., 470, 473
Gavrilovic, J., 173, 175
Geisler, R. M., 474, 475
Gennaro, A. R., 268, 341
Gnadinger, E., 475
Godding, E. W., 26
Godfray, M. F., 121
Goldiner, P. L., 460
Goldsmith, S. H., 70
Gotz, V. P., 479
Gour, L., 432, 453
Graf, J., 160
Grant, E. L., 401
Green, H., 243
Gregg, S. J., 330
Greiner, J., 200
Griffen, G. D., 471
Gross, M. A., 473, 475
Grotzinger, S. J., 207
Groves, M. J., 4–6, 10, 77
Grundelman, G. P., 70
Gryna, F. M., 401
Gunner, B. W., 470, 473

H
Hall, J. W., 473
Hallock, W. K., 257
Hamilton, R. J., 136
Harfield, J. G., 53
Harthcock, M. A., 165
Hasegawa, K., 243, 244
Hatch, T., 274
Hausdorff, H. H., 304
Hayashi, T., 34, 257, 393, 396
Heinrich, K. F., 162
Henley, M. W., 77
Herdan, G., 268
Heywood, H. A., 136, 274, 275
Hillencamp, F., 172

Hinds, W. C., 219
Hiraoka, K., 258
Hirleman, E. D., 306, 309, 311
Ho, N. F. H., 1
Hoenich, N. A., 460
Holmes, B., 160
Hopkins, G. B., 473
Hopkins, G. H., 50
Horioka, M., 248
Horvath, H., 204
Hou, K., 363
Hovenac, E. A., 204
Hozumi, K., 474
Humecki, H. J., 165

I
Illum, L., 460
Inagaki, H., 460
Ishikawa, I., 396, 400, 401

J
James, R. W., 181
Jensen, L. H., 177
Johnson, K. T., 10
Johnston, W. H., 471, 473
Jonas, A. M., 481
Juran, J. M., 401

K
Kalm, M., 1
Kanke, M., 474, 477
Каspor, G., 201
Kaufmann, R., 172
Kaye, B. H., 279, 300, 330
Keady, P. B., 211
Kerker, M., 304
Kesting, R. E., 352, 363
King, E. J., 474
Kinsman, S., 52
Kirnbauer, E., 101, 134
Klein, H. J., 34
Knapp, J. Z., 6, 22, 28, 30–32, 34, 300, 323
Knollenberg, R. G., 73, 204, 207, 298
Knopp, E. A., 432, 460

Köhler, A., 489
Korbl, J., 243
Kowalsky, R. J., 243
Kramer, W., 22
Kruger, R. F., 172
Kushner, H. K., 22, 30–32, 34

L

Lacy, M. E., 165
Lanier, J. M., 126
Lannis, M., 357
Laplace, 335
Layendecker, E. B., 78
Leahy, T. J., 362
Lechene, S. P., 158
Leong, As-Y., 460
Levenworth, R. S., 401
Levy, J. M., 472
Lewis, A. R., 396, 420
Lieberman, A., 89, 201, 208, 222, 298
Liebl, H., 173
Lines, R. W., 51, 52
Liu, B. Y. H., 204, 208, 228
Lloyd, P. J., 267
Long, P. L., 165
Loop, F. D., 460
Luerkins, 278
Lukaszewicz, R. C., 359, 361
Luscher, R., 242

M

Maddox, R. R., 479
Marshall, J. C., 362, 364
Martin, J. S., 102
Martin, A., 267, 281
Martyn, G. W., 34
Mason, C. W., 121
Mastenbroek, 26
McCollum, C. N., 237, 473
McCormack, J., 120, 367
McCrone, W. C., 101, 102, 120, 121, 125, 146, 351, 489, 502
McFadden, P., 309
McHugh, J. R., 173
Mellstrom, G., 243, 246
Meloy, T., 274, 278, 312

Meltzer, T. H., 251, 360, 362, 364
Meserschmidt, R. G., 165
Meury, R. H., 306
Michaels, A. S., 362, 367
Mochida, K., 396, 421
Montague, W., 204, 208
Montanari, L. F., 50, 54
Muggli, R. Z., 165
Muhlen, E., 5
Mulford, D. F., 136
Munson, T., 3
Munson, T. E., 212, 213, 421

N

Nicoli, D. F., 324
Nishida, S., 241
Nishimura, R., 241

O

Oles, P. J., 121, 160, 351
Osol, A., 268
Otter, L., 268

P

Page, U. S., 432, 460
Pasteur, L., 368
Pastoriza-Pinol, J. V., 460
Peterson, M. C., 241
Pflag, S. C., 10
Porter, M. C., 135
Portnoff, J. B., 77
Post, J. E., 163

R

Rebagay, T., 57, 102, 135, 245
Reuter, E. W., 34
Roseman, T. J., 249
Rubow, K. L., 225
Russell, E. J., 472
Ryan, P. B., 479
Rypins, E. B., 479

S

Sandell, E., 22, 29
Saylor, H. M., 31
Scheuler, B., 172
Schmidt, W. H., 362, 367

Schoen, D. R., 255
Schoenberg, M. D., 477
Schroeder, H. G., 50, 57, 102, 474, 476, 477
Sharp, J., 237
Shewhart, 399–401
Sing, K. S., 330
Sladek, K. J., 362
Smart, J. D., 257
Sokol, M., 351
Sommer, H. T., 59, 204, 207, 208
Sorenson, R., 3, 212–213
Speed, W., 243
Stewart, I. M., 102
Stockham, J. D., 268, 269, 283, 288
Stokes, G., 328, 330
Stout, G. H., 177
Sullivan, L., 464
Surkyn, P., 172
Swank, R. L., 478
Swithenbank, J., 309
Szymanski, W. W., 201, 208

T

Taylor, S. A., 10
Taylor, W. A., 401, 413, 418, 419
Tchao, T., 241
Teetsov, A. S., 123, 369
Trasen, B., 121, 135, 137, 366
Tscharnuter, W. W., 309
Tsuji, K., 396, 420
Turco, S., 240, 473, 479, 481

U

Ugelstad, J., 81
Uhlir, A., 45
Umhauer, H., 201

V

Valvani, S. C., 245
Van de Hulst, H. C., 304
VanGlahn, W. C., 473
Veals, C. R., 267
Veltman, A. M., 257

W

Wadell, H., 274
Wagner, P. E., 201
Waisman, J., 471, 473
Walton, W. H., 136
Warner, R. R., 158
Wartman, W. B., 473
Watson, H. H., 136
Waxman, H., 463
Webster, G., 401
Weiner, B. B., 298, 309, 311, 329
Wen, H. Y., 201
Wheeler, D. J., 401, 413
White, H., 288
White, R. D., 245, 248,
Whitlow, R. J., 242
Wilkison, M. C., 81
Williams, A., 10
Williams, J., 57
Wilson, R. G., 173
Winchell, A. N., 120
Winchell, H., 120
Winding, O., 160
Wischnitzer, S., 146
Wood, W. M., 53

Y

Yakowitz, M. L., 242
Yalkowsky, S. H., 245
Young, R. W., 50
Young, 335

Z

Zierdt, C. H., 362
Zweers, J. R., 228

Subject Index

10-unit pool sample, 421
5-hydroxymethyl furfural, 245

A

AC fine test dust, 84
Accept Zone, 31
Acceptable quality level (AQL), 401
Acceptance criteria, 214
Accuracy, 302
Achromatic lenses, 103
Achromats, 103
Adherent material, 439
Administration sets, 432
Adsorbate, 331, 333
Adsorbent, 330, 331, 333
Adsorption, 330–334
Adsorption isotherm, 331
Adverse reactions, 470
Aerodynamic particle sizing, 342, 343
Aerosol analysis monitors, 383
Aerosol particles, 188, 200, 379, 380
Aerosol photometer, 200
Aerosol population analysis, 338
Agglomerates, 279
Agglomeration, 239, 280, 328
Aggregates, 279
Aggregation, 239
Air bubbles, 53, 73

Airborne contaminants, 187
Airborne particles, 188
Airborne particulate cleanliness classes, 218
Airy disc, 110
Alert limits, 425
Allen liquid viewer, 27, 28
Alternative count standards, 85, 86
Alveolar capillaries, 472
Alveolar macrophages, 472
Amorphous particles, 69
Ampoules, 16, 32, 33, 38, 243, 256–258
Analysis of particulate matter in devices, 442–448
Analyzer, 118
Animal studies, 472, 474–476
Anisokinetic sampling, 219
Anisotropic crystal, 118, 120
Aperture diaphragm, 112
Apertures, 52
Apochromats, 103, 105
Arithmetic mean, 284
Aroclor®, 124, 370
Aseptic fill areas, 219, 231
Aseptic practices, 231
Aseptic processing, 213
Assignable causes of variation, 400–402
Astigmatism, 148

Subject Index   525

Attribute, 418
Autocorrelation function, 311
Autodilution, 324
Autologous transfusion devices, 432, 448
Automated (Machine) Inspection, 34–44
Automated inspection, 16
Automated light extinction counting, 87
Average diameters, 294, 295, 297, 298

B

BiS and BiS$_2$, 246
Barium sulfate, 248, 249
Batch sampling, 420, 421
Becke line, 121, 122
Between-Instrument variability, 72, 95
Between-analyst variability, 95
Birefringence, 118
Black and white background light box 25
Blood filters, 449
Blood-related materials, 478
Blow-fill-seal, 258
Blown film extrusion process, 406
Borosilicate glass, 243
Bragg's law, 159, 180
Breadth, 275, 276
Bremsstrahlung, 158
British standard method, 313
Bunny suit design, 232

C

CGMP, 456, 458
Calibration, 50
Calibration curve, 63–66
Capillaries, 471–473
Capillary orifice, 225
Cartridge filters, 251–253
Cascade impactor, 379, 381
Cassegranian microscope, 165
Cassegranian optics, 169
Cast film filters, 352–355

Cellulosic particles, 473
Centrifugal pumps, 250
Chromatic aberration, 103, 106, 148
Chute splitter, 372, 375
Circular area diameter, 135
Circulatory transport, 471
Closures, 240–242
Cognitive shape descriptors, 272
Coincidence counting, 72
Cold aerosol, 199, 200
Collection of particles, 376–379
Collimated Holes filter, 357, 358
Combustion particles, 189
Commercial standards, 82
Common cause, 400
Comparison calibration, 208
Comparison standards, 101
Compendial Requirements, 44, 45
Components of medical devices, 434
Compound magnifying system, 102–107
Compound microscope, 104, 105
Compressed air, 223
Condensation nucleus counter, 200
Condenser lenses, 111, 112, 150
Coning and quartering, 372, 374
Constructive interference, 117
Containers, 240, 242, 243
Contamination control, 188
Continuous/multiplexed air sampling, 209
Control charting, 407–420
Controlled environment areas, 189
Cost-benefits ratio, 462
Coulter counter, 51–54
Coulter principle, 17–18, 50–53
Critical inspection volumes, 42
Critical micelle concentration, 244, 245
Crystallization, 182, 239, 243, 247
Crystallized particulates, 244
Crystallized powders, 246
Cubic crystals, 118
Curvature of field, 105, 107
Cutting of tubing, 438, 439

D

DOP challenge, 200
Dacron®, 12
Dark-field condenser, 114
Dark-field microscopy, 112, 114
Dead-legs, 250
Degassing, 336
Degradation, 239
Destructive interference, 117
Detection, 204
Detection limits of manual inspection, 31, 32
Detection efficiency and sensitivity, 34
Device-related 483s, 459
Dialyzers, 433, 460
Diaphragm or time-pressure fillers, 250
Diffraction, 110
Diffusion, 194
Digitized image, 316
Dilution procedures, 86
Diode array, 204
Disc centrifuges, 328, 329
Dispersion staining, 122
Disposable syringes, 13–15, 433, 460
Distribution of extraneous particle counts, 294
Documentation, 254
Doppler anemometry, 311, 312
Drug abuse literature, 473
Dynamic range, 302

E

Eisai, 35–38
Elastomeric device components, 434, 435
Electrical zone sensing, 50
Electromagnetic lenses, 149–151
Electron microscopy, 145–160
Electronic particle counters, 50, 432
Electrostatic attraction, 363
Elemental composition analysis, 162
Elongation ratio, 275
Emulsion polymerization, 78, 79, 81
Emulsions, 17, 268
Energy-dispersive spectrometer, 159
Ensemble measurements, 302
Enumeration of particles, 7, 134
Environmental air, 376
Environmental particle monitoring, 201
Environmental particulate matter, 7
Episcopic, 112, 113
Equivalent spherical diameters, 269–271
Error sources, 70–73
Erythrematous reaction, 479
Extinction, 118–220
Extracorporeal circuits, 460
Extraneous particles, 239, 240
Extrinsic particles, 6
Eyepiece, ocular, 103
Eyepoint, 103

F

False acceptance, 425
False rejection, 425
Fast atom bombardment, 169
Federal Standard 209-D, 190, 212–217, 219
Federal Standard 209-E, 215–217, 219, 226, 228
Feret's diameter, 127, 128
Field diaphragm, 131
Field test, 199
Filling heads, 411–415
Filling machines, 253, 396
Filling needles, 253
Filter holders, 366, 367
Filter structure, 352
Filter efficiency, 197
Filters, 192–200, 250–253, 352–367, 441
Filters—anisotrophic, 354
Filtration, 131–135, 250–253

Filtration apparatus, 366
Flake-like particles, 69
Flash, 436
Flatfield objectives, 107
Flow rate, 55
Formation of particles, 239
Formvar®, 161
Fractal analysis, 279
Fraunhofer diffraction, 306

G

Gas adsorption, 330
Gaussian distribution, 284, 286
General classification of particles, 269
Good Manufacturing Practice (GMP), 1–4, 188, 393, 398
Graticule, 126
Gravimetric analysis, 377
Gray zone, 31
Grid, 161

H

HEPA filter particle retention, 197, 198
HEPA filters, 187, 192–194, 196–198
Hiac/Royco CHM-type sensor, 60
Hiac/Royco HR-type sensor, 60, 61
Hot stage microscopy, 125
Hydrophobic, 365

I

Image analysis, 312, 316–318
Image formation, 104
Immiscible fluids, 72
Impaction, 194
In-line filters, 441
Infrared microspectrophotometry, 165–167
Infrared microscopes, 166
Infused particle burden, 431
Inhalers, 338
Inspection devices, 26, 27
Inspection machines, 34–43
Inspection procedure, 24, 25

Instrumental drift, 86
Intensity fluctuation spectroscopy (IFS), 309
Interception, 194, 362
Interference, 116–118
Intermittent (manual) sampling, 209
Interpupillary distance, 129
Intrinsic particulate matter, 6
Iron hydroxide, 248
Isokinetic sampling, 216, 219
Isolation of particles, 123, 368–371

J

Jet sieving, 322

L

Laminar airflow, 194, 195
LAMMA, 169–172
Large particle monitoring, 229
Large volume injection (LVI), 4, 5, 239
Laser cavity, 59
Laser diode sensors, 59
Laser velocimeter, 343
Laser versus white light aerosol counters, 203–208
Lattice planes, 178
Leaks, 198, 199
Length, 275
Lens aberrations, 103
Light extinction counting, 5, 54–75, 323–328
Light scattering effects, 56, 72
Liposomes, 476–478
Liquilaz sensor, 74
Log-log, distribution of particles, 5
Log probit plot, 288, 292
Lyophilized materials, 247
Lyophilized powders, 246

M

Magnetic lens, 152
Magnification, 102
Mandatory recall authority, 464

Martin's diameter, 128, 129
Mass spectrometry, 169
Maximum horizontal intercept, 128
Measurement of particle size, 127–129
Measures of central tendency, 283
Mechanical vibrations, 59
Mechanisms of filtration, 194
Median ($d_{1/2}$), 284
Medical devices, 12
Medical grade tubing, 435
Mercaptobenzothiazole, 241
Mercury porosimeter, 334, 335
Micro FT–IR, 165, 166, 168
Microaggregates, 478
Microfiltration, 350
Micromesh sieves, 320
Microscope calibration, 126
Microscopic assay, 433, 450
Microscopic particle counting, 129–134
Microscopically determined diameters, 271
Microspheres, 83
Mode (d_o), 284
Modular HEPA enclosures, 440
Monitoring of components, 385
Monochromatic light, 59
Monodisperse polystyrene latex dispersions, 83
Multiplexed air sampling, 209, 210
Multiplexed sensors, 209, 210

N

Nephelometry, 304, 305
Nicol prism, 116
Non–Gaussian distributions, 284
Nonenvironmental particle sources, 238
Nonlinear response curve, 67
Nucleation track filters, 352
Nuclepore® membranes, 352, 354
Numerical aperture, 110

O

Objective lenses, 107
Oculars (eyepieces), 111
Optical particle counters (OPC), 187, 201–207, 213, 219, 221, 222, 226, 228
Oxygenators, 432, 460

P

Packaging materials, 240–243
Parenteral-type devices, 432–434
Particle control measures in aseptic fill areas, 208
Particle fallout photometer, 383, 384
Particle picking, 368
Particle shape, 70, 271–281
Particle size standards, 77–87
Particle-reduction measures, 396
Particle-size distributions, 281–298
Particulate matter control, 6–8
Particulate matter limits, 2
Particulate matter requirements for devices, 461–463
Pattern recognition, 278
Percent detection of particles, 37
Permount, 124
Personnel monitoring, 231, 232
Phagocytic cells, 471
Phagocytosis, 477
Philosophy of the FDA, 458
Phlebitis, 479, 480
Photodetector, 62, 75
Photodiode, 36, 54
Photomultiplier tube (PMT), 153
Photomultiplier tube detector, 309
Photon correlation spectroscopy, 17, 309, 310
Physiological effects, 470
Piston-type fillers, 250
Plano objectives, 107
Platelet concentrate, 478
Poisson distribution, 286
Polarization of light, 116, 118
Polarization of reflected light, 115
Polarized light microscopy, 115, 125
Polarizer, 118, 119
Polarizing light microscope, 119, 121

Poly- (diethyleneglycol) isophthalate, 253
Polycarbonate, 367
Polydisperse material, 86
Polydisperse sphere suspensions, 87
Polymerization, 79, 80
Polypropylene filters, 355, 357
Polystyrene latex sphere, 79, 80
Polystyrene microspheres, 476, 477
Polystyrene spheres, 475
Polysulfone filters, 355, 356, 359
Pore size, 344, 338, 359–365
Porosimetry, 330–338
Porosity, 335, 359, 361
Powder sampling, 371–376
Powdered silica, 474
Precipitation, 239, 243
Precision, 302
Problem process points, 438
Process control, 12, 398–403, 407–428
Process design, 7, 239, 394–397, 437–440
Process point-generated particles, 249–253
Product-container interactions, 248
Projected area diameter, 128
Pulmonary circulation, 471
Pulmonary function, 472

Q

Quadrupole mass spectrometer, 173, 174
Quasi-elastic light scattering (QELS), 309

R

Radiation, 158
Random causes of variation, 400–402
Range control chart, 414
Ratio of container surface area to solution, 242
Reflected illumination, 112

Refraction/reflection, 66
Refractive index, 56, 107, 114, 115, 121, 122, 365
Regulatory issues, 453–459
Reject zone, 31
Rejection probability, 30
Remote particle monitoring, 208–212
Reproducibility, 33, 302
Resolution, 56, 68, 71, 148, 302
Resolving power, 110
Responsive curve of OPC, 204
Retention ratings, 359–361, 364
Reynolds numbers, 226, 227
Rinsing of glassware, 133
Robot system, 88
Robotic assembly of devices, 436

S

SD control chart, 415
Safe Medical Devices Act of 1990, 463–465
Sampling effects, 71, 72
Sampling for large particles, 259, 260
Sampling of clean room garments, 386–389
Sampling probe velocity, 219–223
Scanning electron microscopy (SEM), 144, 146, 152–160
Scattering, 66, 304
Scoop sampling, 371
Screening, 194
Secondary ion mass spectrometry (SIMS), 172–177
Sedimentation, 239, 328
Sedimentation and impaction, 226
Semiachromats, 103
Semiapochromatic lenses, 105
Semiautomatic machines, 28
Sensing zone, 59
Sensitive zone, 76
Sensitivity, 67
Sensor, 54
Septa, 439
Shape factor, 276
Sieve fractions, 319

Sieving, 292, 300, 303, 318–323
Signal generation, 155–158
Silicone oils, 2, 241
Sintered plastic filter media, 435
Size-number distribution, 290, 292
Skin cells—shedding, 189
Small volume injections (SVI), 3, 5, 14, 16, 57, 58, 239, 244, 245
Sodium phosphate, 243
Solenoids, 149, 150
Solution and formulation components, 243–246
Solution transfer sets, 432
Sonic flow restriction, 225
Sonic sifter, 321
Source lifetime, 59
Special cause, 400
Spectrex (prototron) system, 75–77
Spherical aberration, 103, 106, 148
Stable process, 403, 404
Stage micrometer, 126
Standard latex particles, 81
Standards, 4, 8–10, 12
Static electrical potential, 437
Static volumetric method, 331
Statistical handling of data, 214
Statistical process control (SPC), 399–404
Sticky tape, 124
Stokes number, 223
Stoppers, 240–243
Storage and handling of standard particles, 81, 82
Straining, 194
Surfactants, 82
Suspension polymerization, 79
Swollen emulsion process, 80, 81
Syringes, 12–15, 432, 433

T

TPN admixtures, 441
Teflon® filters, 355
Testing of gloves, 389, 390
Testing of HEPA filters, 197–201, 365

Thickness—particle, 275
Thief, 372, 373
Thietan-2-one, 246
Thin film support, 116, 161
Thin film interference, 117
Thresholds, 52, 54, 55
Thrombophlebitis, 479
Time-of-flight spectrometer, 170, 171
Tortuous path filters, 353
Total parenteral nutrition (TPN), 17
Transmission electron microscopy (TEM), 144, 146–149, 152
Troubleshooting a process, 437
Tube material selection, 229
Tubing transport of particulate samples, 226
Tubular extrusions, 242

U

USP <788> microscopic particulate matter test, 129–132
USP light extinction test, 57, 58
USP particle count reference standard (PCRS), 84, 85
USP requirements—history, 8, 9
Unstable process, 401, 404

V

Validation of the robotic assay, 89, 92, 93
Vector components, 118
Verification, 212
Vibratory feeder bowl, 436, 439
Video imaging, 38
View volume, 59, 62
Virtual image, 103
Visible particulate matter, 257, 454
Visual inspection, 15–17, 22–34

W

Wavelength, 110, 111, 149, 157, 159
Wet sieving, 321, 322

Wettability, 365
White light extinction sensors, 59, 60, 204
Wire probe, 169
Witness, plates, 259
Working distance of objectives, 109

X
X-ray spectra, 163, 164
X-ray diffraction camera, 180
X-ray diffraction crystallography, 177–183
X-ray spectroscopy, 160–165

Y
YAG laser, 171